This volume consists of a number of authoritative reviews on the effects of thermal energy on all types of living organisms and biological molecules. The rapid developments taking place in all areas of biology are placing an ever greater premium on the availability of review articles, especially when, as in the case of this work, the approach cuts across established divisions within biological science. The papers presented are by accepted authorities in the field, and together comprise a comprehensive work of considerable value to all researchers in biological, physiological, and related fields.

THERMOBIOLOGY

THERMOBIOLOGY

Edited by

ANTHONY H. ROSE

Department of Microbiology
University of Newcastle upon Tyne, England

1967

ACADEMIC PRESS · LONDON and NEW YORK

ACADEMIC PRESS INC. (LONDON) LTD.

BERKELEY SQUARE HOUSE

BERKELEY SQUARE

LONDON, W.1.

U.S. Edition published by

ACADEMIC PRESS INC.

111 FIFTH AVENUE

NEW YORK, NEW YORK 10003

Made and printed in Great Britain by
William Clowes and Sons, Limited, London and Beccles

Contributors

BARNETT, S. A., *University of Glasgow, Scotland.*

BELDING, H. S., *University of Pittsburgh, Pittsburgh, Pennsylvania, U.S.A.*

BRANDTS, J. F., *University of Massachusetts, Amherst, Massachusetts, U.S.A.*

BROOM, B., *Middlesex Hospital Medical School, London, W.1., England.*

BUNT, J. S., *Institute of Marine Science, University of Miami, Florida, U.S.A.*

CHAPMAN, D., *Unilever Research Laboratory, The Frythe, Welwyn, Herts, England.*

CLARKE, K. U., *University of Nottingham, Nottingham, England.*

DUMBELL, K. R., *The Wright-Fleming Institute of Microbiology, St. Mary's Hospital Medical School, London, W.2. England.*

FARRELL, J., *University of Newcastle upon Tyne, England.*

FRY, F. E. J., *University of Toronto, Toronto, Canada.*

LANGRIDGE, J., *Commonwealth Scientific and Industrial Research Organization, Canberra, A.C.T., Australia.*

LING, G. N., *Pennsylvania Hospital, Philadelphia, Pennsylvania, U.S.A.*

MACFADYEN, A., *University College of Swansea, Wales.*

MCWHINNIE, M. A., *De Paul University, Chicago, Illinois, U.S.A.*

MCWILLIAM, J. R., *Commonwealth Scientific and Industrial Research Organization, Canberra, A.C.T., Australia.*

MOUNT, L. E., *Institute of Animal Physiology, Babraham, Cambridge, England.*

ROSE, A. H., *University of Newcastle upon Tyne, England.*

SZYBALSKI, W. T., *University of Wisconsin, Madison, Wisconsin, U.S.A.*

Preface

Few biologists would deny that temperature is one of the most important environmental factors that affect the activities of living organisms. Studies on the effects of temperature on the activities of individual organisms have been carried out for many years, but the past decade has seen a marked upsurge of interest in the subject. There were many reasons for this renaissance. The availability of suitably controlled and monitored apparatus was undoubtedly an important factor. At the same time, there has been a growing interest in the ecology of organisms both in terrestrial environments and in the oceans; nor have biologists been slow to anticipate the possibilities for the existence of life on other planets. Studies on the effects of temperature on individual plants, animals and micro-organisms, and on the behaviour and distribution of these organisms in complex ecosystems, form an integral part of ecology. Unfortunately, because of the time-honoured fragmentation of biological science into botany, zoology and microbiology, many of the data on the effects of temperature on, for example, plants, are unknown to biologists who are principally interested in other types of organism. It was with the hope that biologists might wish to become acquainted with work on the effects of temperature on organisms other than those with which they are primarily concerned, and with the responses of biological macromolecules to temperature, that I undertook to edit this book.

In order that the book should be of most value to biologists, it was essential that it be written not by one or two authors but by a team of contributors each a specialist in his or her own field. I should like to thank all contributors for their willing co-operation in this venture. I am also greatly indebted to Miss Judith Farrell for valuable discussions during the planning of this book and for timely editorial assistance, and to the staff of Academic Press Inc. (London) for their never-failing co-operation. Finally, I wish to thank my wife, Jane, my sons Aidan and Simon, and my daughter, Sarah, for help in preparing the index.

ANTHONY H. ROSE

Newcastle upon Tyne
December 1966

Contents

1*

*All temperatures quoted in this book
are in degrees Centigrade*

Chapter I

Introduction

A. H. ROSE

*Department of Microbiology, University of
Newcastle upon Tyne, England*

Thermal energy or heat is obviously one of the most important environmental factors that affect the activities of living organisms. All organisms are continually subjected to some degree of heat, and it is the magnitude of this degree that is important to the organism. Man's awareness of the general effects of heat on living organisms almost certainly came quite early in his development, probably during his first attempts to cook food. Further knowledge accumulated quite empirically, much of it being recorded in cookery books. Definitive information on the effects of heat on living organisms came only after the construction and development of suitable instruments for making accurate measurements of temperature. Galileo invented his thermoscope around A.D. 1600. But it was not until 1848 that William Thomson (later Lord Kelvin) placed the concept of temperature and the theory of temperature measurement on a sound thermodynamic basis, and laid the foundations for experiments on the effect of temperature on living organisms. In the years that followed, a vast amount of information was reported on temperature effects on living organisms.

Life as we know it developed in an aqueous environment, and the need for liquid water restricts the temperature range in which organisms can grow and be metabolically active to the range $-2°$ to $100°$, a range sometimes referred to as the "biokinetic zone". But biologists quickly realized that the temperature limits for growth and activity of individual plants and animals were much narrower, and much of the earlier work in thermobiology was concerned with recording the temperature ranges for growth and activity of individual organisms. Among the earliest observations made was that some animals, including man, can maintain body temperature at a fairly constant value, despite reasonably wide variations in the environmental temperature. These animals are known as *homeotherms*. Plants, micro-organisms and lower orders of animals, on the other hand, do not have this capacity, and the temperature of their tissues is determined largely by the environmental temperature. These organisms are described as *poikilotherms*. Some poikilotherms can develop over a wide range of temperatures, and are referred to as *eurythermal* to distinguish them from *stenothermal* organisms, growth of which is restricted to a much narrower range of temperatures.

Biologists have derived quantitative expressions to describe the effects of temperature on living organisms. The earliest, and probably the most obvious way, was in the form of the *temperature coefficient* or Q_{10} value, which is the ratio of the rate of a metabolic process (e.g. growth or an enzyme reaction) at one temperature to the rate at a temperature 10° lower, i.e.

$$Q_{10} = \frac{k_{t+10}}{k_t}$$

In this equation, k is the velocity constant and t the temperature. Q_{10} values were first calculated for chemical reactions, and only later were they applied to biological processes. A generalized, and far more sophisticated, way of describing the effect of temperature on biological processes came when the Arrhenius equation, which like the temperature coefficient had been formulated originally to describe the effects of temperature on the rates of chemical reactions, was applied to biological processes. Some examples of Arrhenius plots are given in Chapters 3 and 6.

During the past decade, there have been important developments in two main areas of thermobiology. The tremendous advances that have been made in our understanding of the properties, behaviour and synthesis of biological macromolecules have led to a great amount of work being done on the effects of temperature on cell components, including proteins, nucleic acids, lipids and, very importantly, water. Molecular thermobiology is still very much in its infancy, but there can be little doubt that it is destined to make an important contribution to other areas of thermobiology. Another branch of biological research in which thermobiology is making important contributions is ecology. The problems here are complex. The biologist needs to integrate data on the effects of temperature on individual organisms, much of it obtained in the artificial environment of the laboratory, if he is to understand the effect of temperature on the complex cycles and food chains that operate in natural environments.

Information on the effects of temperature on living organisms is very widely scattered throughout the literature. Fortunately, many of the areas have been reviewed from time to time, and these articles have provided useful summaries of individual areas of thermobiology. Also, a number of texts have been published, bringing together data from some or all of the major areas of thermobiological research. These texts (Bělehrádek, 1935; Johnson, Eyring and Polissar, 1954; Precht, Christopherson and Hensel, 1955; Johnson, 1957) should be perused for reviews of the earlier literature on thermobiology. But research in several areas of the subject has made very rapid strides in the past decade, and the present book was conceived in an attempt to bring together reviews on all aspects of thermobiology, particularly the rapidly developing subjects of molecular thermobiology and the ecological importance of the thermal energy.

Each contributor to the present volume was given complete freedom in the treatment of his or her subject matter. Inevitably, the accounts presented reflect, in some part, the interests of the authors. Bearing in mind the very voluminous literature on thermobiology, and the need to restrict the size of the volume, there must be omissions. Moreover, some specialists will almost certainly feel that their particular subject has received a somewhat cavalier treatment. Nevertheless, I hope that bringing together in this way, accounts of the effects of temperature on all types of living organisms, and on their component molecules, will initiate processes of cross-fertilization in which, for example, the biologist can acquaint himself with some of the more recent work on the effects of temperature on proteins and lipids, while the molecular thermobiologist will be able to read of the truly vast number of problems which he, or his successors, will want to explain in molecular terms.

References

Bělehrádek, J. (1935). "Temperature and Living Matter", 277 pp. Gebrüder-Borntraeger, Berlin.
Johnson, F. H. Ed. (1957). "Influence of Temperature on Biological Systems", 275 pp. American Physiological Society Inc., New York.
Johnson, F. H., Eyring, H. and Polissar, M. J. (1954). "The Kinetic Basis of Molecular Biology", 874 pp. John Wiley and Sons, New York.
Precht, H., Christopherson, J. and Hensel, H. (1955). "Temperatur und Leben", 514 pp. Springer-Verlag, Berlin.

Chapter 2

Effects of Temperature on the State of Water in the Living Cell

Gilbert N. Ling

Department of Molecular Biology in the Department of Neurology, Division of Medicine, Pennsylvania Hospital, Philadelphia, Pennsylvania, U.S.A.

I. Introduction

The subject of the effect of temperature on the state of water in the living cell poses a difficult problem for the review-writer whose usual task consists of drawing together into a coherent account the ideas and experimental findings of the majority of workers in an area. This is not possible with the present subject. There is not even a consensus of opinion on the structure of pure water itself (see Frank, 1965); as regards the state of water in living cells, the situation is even more obscure.

The majority of cell physiologists have followed the direction of the classical membrane theory introduced by Pfeffer some 80 years ago. The implicit assumption of this theory was that proteins and other bio-macromolecules exercise negligible influence on the properties of the water within the cell. Until relatively recently, this assumption was apparently supported by the bulk of experimental observation on the subject (see, however, the reports by Fischer and Suer, 1938; Ernst, 1928; Nasonov, 1962; Troschin, 1958; and Gortner, 1937, 1938). But, within the last decade or so, the situation has changed radically. Rapid advancement of modern techniques has made possible a variety of studies of protein–water interaction using a wide range of experimental methods. These include small-angle X-ray scattering (Beeman, 1961), sedimentation and electrophoresis (Jacobson, 1953, 1955), dielectric measurements (Ritland et al., 1950), density measurements (Hearst and Vinograd, 1961), and nuclear magnetic resonance studies (Berendson, 1962). The results of these studies unanimously support the notion that proteins and other biomacromolecules orient water molecules to a considerable extent (see also Forslind, 1952; Szent–Györgyi, 1957; Klotz et al., 1958; Klotz 1960). Most of these studies have been carried out on proteins in solution in vitro. Since the typical living cell contains a high percentage of protein (around 20% of the wet weight), these results imply that cell water must possess a much higher degree of organization than pure liquid water.

The problem of the state of water in the living cell reflects the rapid and profound transition now under way in our concept of the living cell. This concept has emerged from an early phase in which cell behaviour and properties have been interpreted in terms of descriptive biological parameters, such as membrane permeability and metabolic pumps, into a phase in which they are interpreted in terms of the more fundamental parameters of modern physics. Through the evolution of modern physics, man has succeeded within the last 40 years in commanding a high degree of understanding of the inanimate world; our comprehension of the biological world must eventually merge with and complement this understanding.

In the following account, I shall first briefly describe the effects of temperature changes on the structure of pure water and aqueous solutions to provide a basis for a discussion of the effects of temperature changes on the water in the living cell. Since large-scale investigation of this problem has barely begun, much remains for the future; at this stage few of our conclusions can be considered final.

II. Effects of Temperature on the Structure of Water and Aqueous Solutions

A. TEMPERATURE EFFECTS ON CO-OPERATIVE ORDER–DISORDER TRANSITIONS

A proper increase in temperature causes liquid water to turn into steam; with a proper decrease in temperature, water freezes into ice. Such *phase transitions* occur within narrow ranges of temperature which are referred to as the melting or the boiling point. These abrupt transitions occur because a shift of temperature is accompanied by a shift in the relative magnitude of the molar Gibbs free energy for the alternative state. For example, the value of the molar Gibbs free energy is favourable for water to assume the ice structure below the melting point, but unfavourable above the melting point; the water–steam phase transition is similarly determined by the value of the molar Gibbs free energy. Such ordinary phase transitions are sometimes referred to as transitions of the first order because the change of Gibbs free energy with temperature during the transition is continuous, but the change of entropy, the negative first-order derivative of the Gibbs free energy with respect to temperature, is discontinuous.

Another type of transition also occurs within a narrow range of temperature, but on the basis of a different mechanism. This type is referred to as *co-operative* transition. Ordinary phase transition discussed above is considered to be independent of the proportion of molecules in either of the two alternative states. Co-operative transition, on the other hand, arises from precisely such a dependence. Ordinary phase transitions usually involve changes of density; co-operative changes usually do not.

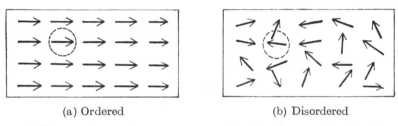

(a) Ordered   (b) Disordered

FIG. 1. A diagram illustrating co-operative order–disorder transition in a magnet. An individual atom (circled) assumes the ordered (a) or disordered (b) orientation, depending on the orientation of the other atoms in the system.

The mechanism of co-operative transition can perhaps best be understood by using the example of ferromagnetism. Certain elements such as iron, nickel, and cobalt are described as ferromagnetic since they exhibit the familiar properties of a magnet. These properties arise from the presence of a magnetic dipole in each atom of the element. Each pole of the atom repels like poles, but attracts oppositely charged poles. For this reason, the orientation of a particular atom depends on how its neighbouring atoms are oriented. The consequence of this dependence is that the entire population tends to assume either the ordered state (Fig. 1(a)) or the random state (Fig. 1(b)). This tendency of certain components of a system to assume either one or the other of two alternative states, depending on the states assumed by other components of the system, is the fundamental characteristic of co-operative phenomena.

With an increase of temperature, a magnet retains its permanent magnetism up to a certain point, but not beyond it. At this particular temperature, referred to as the lambda point, there is a co-operative transition from an orderly arrangement of atoms to a disorderly arrangement. The earliest reported lambda point was that for the ferromagnetic co-operative transition discovered by Curie; hence, this particular lambda point, and occasionally other lambda points, are known as the Curie-point.

Another well-known co-operative order–disorder transition is that which occurs in alloys. Thus, β-brass, an alloy of copper and zinc, can assume either an ordered state in which Cu and Zn atoms are arranged in an orderly and predictable fashion, or a disordered state in which they are distributed at random. The order–disorder transition of β-brass with increasing temperature is co-operative and has a lambda point. The β-brass transition is historically important because this co-operative system was first successfully treated using statistical methods by Bragg and Williams (1934), although an equivalent thermodynamic treatment was suggested by Gorsky (1928). For a further refinement of the statistical mechanical treatment, see Fowler and Guggenheim (1960); additional references can be found in Jost (1960).

Co-operative transitions, in contrast to ordinary phase transitions, have also been referred to as transitions of the second order. Thus, in co-operative transitions, both Gibbs free energy and entropy are continuous; it is the specific heat that is discontinuous. This quantity is related to the second order derivative of the Gibbs free energy with respect to temperature.

In the above section we have outlined the conventional distinctions between ordinary phase transitions and co-operative transitions. It should be pointed out that this distinction between the two types of transition partly owes its origin to the historical order in which these phenomena were understood; co-operative phenomena became understood long after the so-called ordinary phase transition had been explained. In reality, condensed systems of liquids and solids are all co-operative assemblies and thus most, if not all, transitions are co-operative.

B. EFFECTS OF TEMPERATURE ON THE STRUCTURE OF WATER

1. *The Structure of Water*

The question of whether liquid water possesses structure has a long history. Over half a century ago, Roentgen (1892) produced evidence in favour of the idea that water is a mixture of a denser species, $(H_2O)_d$, and a bulkier species, $(H_2O)_b$, and that they exist in equilibrium:

$$(H_2O)_d \leftrightarrows (H_2O)_b$$

Stewart (1930), from X-ray diffraction studies, unequivocally established the existence of short-range order in liquid water. Bernal and Fowler (1933), in an important comprehensive thesis, suggested that such short-range order arises from a quartz-like hydrogen bonded (H-bonded) structure which would then correspond to the bulkier species of Roentgen; water molecules not H-bonded would arrange themselves more like close-packing spheres and would thus correspond to the denser species.

The quartz-like structure of bulkier water postulated by Bernal and Fowler was not supported by X-ray data (Morgan and Warren, 1938) and was also rejected by Pauling (1959) on theoretical grounds. Pauling (1959) suggested, instead, a cage-like or "clathrate" dodecahedral complex consisting of 20 water molecules forming an H-bonded cage and one water molecule, not H-bonded, occupying the central void within the cage. Berendson (1962), employing model-building investigations, suggested another type of cage-like structure consisting of two stacked pentagonal parallel planes with another non-H-bonded water molecule inside the cage. Still other "bulkier" structures were proposed by Eck *et al.* (1958) and by Heemskerk (1962) (see Frank, 1965, for references to additional postulated water structures). Thus, there are many postulated structures for water, and it is clear that we have not yet reached a final understanding of this problem.

2. *The Theory of the Co-operative Structure of Water*

Frank (1958) pointed out that, in the liquid state, water molecules do not form rigid immutable bonds; rather they mutually polarize each other and form H-bonds of different strengths. Thus, as in ferromagnetic transition, the transition between a bulkier water structure like those postulated by Pauling (1959) and Berendson (1962) and a closer-packed, dense structure would be co-operative. When one water molecule forms a H-bond with another water molecule, the participating water molecules become a stronger proton-donor and proton-acceptor, respectively. This inductive effect intensifies the interaction of these water molecules with other neighbouring water molecules and a chain of such bonds is formed. Conversely, when a H-bond is broken by thermal motion, a chain of bonds will tend to be broken. In this view, a sample of liquid water is normally made up of "flickering clusters". This basic concept was developed in a more detailed statistical mechanical treatment by Némethy and Sheraga (1962).

A slightly different view is held by Lennard-Jones and Pople (1951) and also Pople (1951), who have put forward a modification of the Bernal-Fowler picture which disposes of the difficulties mentioned. Their model retains, in essence, the tetrahedral structure of water as postulated by Bernal and by Fowler with the addition of non-breaking, bending H-bonds. In their view, the bending accounts for the absorption of heat and entropy when ice melts.

Since Pople's model also predicts the co-operative structure of liquid water, the chief difference between the "flickering cluster" model and the "bending H-bond" model lies in the definition of the making and breaking of an H-bond. Frank (1965) very recently pointed out that, if one defines a true H-bond as one involving only the O—H...O bond the angle of which is practically straight, two species of water molecules can again be considered and the differences between the two models may be reconciled.

3. *Effect of Temperature on the Co-operative Structure of Water*

Magat (1935) reviewed the evidence for "kinks" in the temperature dependence of a large number of properties of liquid water. He suggested

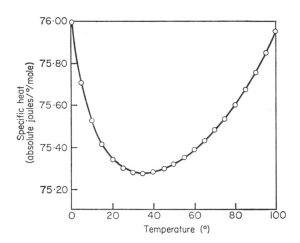

FIG. 2. A graph showing the specific heat of pure water at different temperatures and constant pressure (1 atm.). Note the distinct minimum at about 35°. From Ginnings and Furukawa (1953).

that these "kinks" are lambda points in the co-operative structural transitions of liquid water. Although not all of the evidence he quoted can be considered definitive, there is little question that more recent indisputable experimental findings do support this conclusion (see Feates and Ives, 1956). The data of Ginnings and Furukawa (1953) on the specific heat of pure water at different temperatures is reproduced in Fig. 2. There is a well-marked minimum near 35° in the heat capacity at constant pressure. Similar "kinks" are seen in a plot of the surface tension of pure water against temperature Fig. 3; Timmermans and Bodson, 1937). Thus, in general, these results indicate that the structure of liquid water is co-operative and that, with rising temperature, a crucial lambda point is reached at which a particular structure collapses.

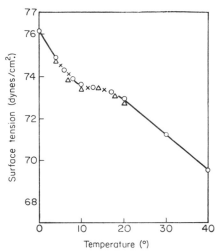

FIG. 3. Effect of temperature on the surface tension of water.   Circles represent data obtained by the capillary rise method; triangles, by the drop weight method; and crosses, by bubble pressure. From the data of Timmermans and Bodson (1937).

4. *Structural Effects of Solutes*

Frank (1965) has classified the general effects of different types of solutes on the structure of water (tabulated in Table I). The terms "structure-breaking" and "structure-making" refer to the structure of normal water. The structure-breaking effect of an ion, for example, does not signify the breaking down of all structure in the water, but rather that the ion tends to orient water in its own pattern, thus causing the breakdown of the overall water structure. Conventionally, the first layer of water molecules around each ion is called the "water of primary hydration" (Bochris, 1949). Water molecules beyond the first layer are often regarded as a different kind of hydration (secondary hydration); these molecules have certain translational freedom, but have lost considerable rotational freedom; they possess a certain structure dictated by the ion and the primary hydration layer. Another way of looking at the hydration of ions is to regard all the water molecules around the ion as being oriented in multilayers with restriction of all motion, and particularly rotational motion, falling off gradually as the water molecules are further removed from the ions. The structure-breaking effect of ions is seen in the larger number of water molecules immediately beyond the secondary hydration layer. In this region, the ordering influence of the ionic charge and the forces creating the structure of normal water annul one another, and so create an area of maximum disorder (Frank and Evans, 1945).

TABLE I. *Classification of Solute Effect on Water Structure* (*According to Frank, 1965*)

Type	A	B	C	D
Nature of solute	Ionic	H-bonding	Inert	Polyfunctional
Structural effect	Weakening	Little or none except urea (structure breaker)	Structure-making	Additive due to different functional groups

The structure-making ability of certain compounds is due to the formation of an "iceberg" or clathrate; once again, although there is still uncertainty as to the precise structure around, say, a saturated hydrocarbon chain, little doubt remains that such organized structures do exist (Frank, 1945).

5. *Structural Effects of Proteins*

In the introductory section to this chapter, reference was made to the growing evidence that proteins orient water molecules to a considerable depth in the surrounding solution. However, there is less certainty about precisely how such orientation is brought about. Protein molecules are, as a rule, polyfunctional. Clearly their effects on water structure would be multiple and complex as with polyfunctional small molecules (Table I). It is convenient to discuss the separate classes of functional groups according to Frank's classification of small molecules.

a. Ionic groups. These include β- and γ-carboxyl anionic groups and ϵ-amino and guanidyl cationic groups. Like all ions, potentially they can orient water molecules in multilayers to a greater or smaller degree. However, when these ionic groups are joined in salt linkages, the shielding effect as a rule greatly diminishes their effect on water structure.

b. Hydrogen-bonding groups. These include a number of side-chain functional groups such as the hydroxyl groups of serine and tryptophan and the amide groups of asparagine and glutamine. Much more important, however, are the backbone peptide groups (—NH—CO—). The fact that silk fibroin, which is practically free of ionic groups, can be dissolved in water (Harrington and Schellman, 1957), suggests an inter-action between the backbone —NH—CO— groups and water molecules. The study of the nuclear magnetic resonance of collagen-oriented water (Berendsen, 1962; see p. 17) has left little doubt that the backbone —NH—CO— groups can form H-bonds with, and thus polarize, water molecules.

c. *Inert groups*. Saturated hydrocarbon chains, such as those carried by valine and leucine, are structure-making. It is very likely that such chains create iceberg structures around parts of a protein surface under certain conditions. Extensive formation of strong ice-like sheaths around entire protein molecules, however, is not very likely. As pointed out by Némethy (1965), if such structures exist, they would result in instability and, hence, aggregation of macromolecules, analogous with the forma-tion of micelles. Although extensive ice-sheath formation is extremely unlikely in native proteins, under certain conditions (e.g. denatured protein), the hydrocarbon groups may be of importance in determining the protein structure. Carrying both hydrophobic and hydrophilic groups, proteins resemble soap; they differ from soap in that the fixed ionic groups are usually of opposite signs and approximately equal in number and that they also have both proton-accepting and proton-donating (H-bonding) groups. However, at extreme pH values, one species of charged group is usually neutralized. Under these conditions, there should be a pronounced tendency for the protein to assume a structure similar to soap micelles, exposing the ionic groups, and enclosing the hydrophobic groups in the interior.

6. *Effect of Temperature on Protein-Water Interactions*

a. *Effect of heat*. That heat denatures proteins has been known for a long time. Only recently, however, has denaturation been recognized as a co-operative phenomenon (Schellman, 1955; Zimm and Bragg, 1958; Gibbs and DiMarzio, 1958; Ling, 1962, 1964). As in all other co-operative phenomena, there is a sharp transition temperature corre-sponding to the lambda point. In native ribonuclease, for example, large sections of the molecule exist in an α-helical form. On heating in a near-neutral solution, the α-helical structure rather abruptly disappears between 60° and 70° (Fig. 4), and the denatured protein molecules assume a form often referred to as a random coil. If the pH value of the solution is decreased below the pK value of the β- and γ-carboxyl groups (4·6–4·7), the lambda point shifts to a much lower temperature. This indicates, in a general way, that salt linkages formed by the carboxyl groups with fixed cationic groups stabilize the α-helical structure.

As the α-helix is a fairly rigid structure, salt linkages can form between oppositely charged ionic groups only if they are within reach of each

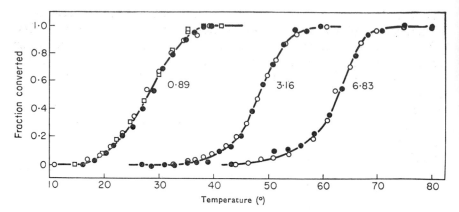

FIG. 4. Effect of temperature and pH value on conversion to the non-α-helical form during the reversible denaturation of ribonuclease. Values on the ordinate indicate the fraction converted to the non-α-helical form. pH values are given on the graphs. Open and closed symbols correspond to ultraviolet spectra and optical rotation measurements, respectively (Hermans and Scheraga, 1961).

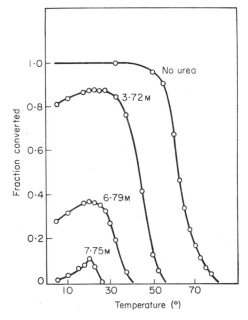

FIG. 5. Effect of temperature and urea concentration on the extent of hydrogen bonding in ribonuclease. Values on the ordinate indicate the fraction in the α-helical form, and are therefore opposite to those indicated on the ordinate in Fig. 4. The figures on the graphs indicate urea concentrations (Foss and Schellman, 1959).

other. Some ionic groups may not be able to form salt linkages; these may then be associated with counter-ions or be free, which means they associate with water molecules. Thus, each native protein must possess a specific complex water structure surrounding it. Once the protein is denatured, one may anticipate that the hydrophobic groups would tend to aggregate to form a core from which the hydrophilic groups are directed outward; the hydrophilic groups would include many of the backbone amide groups that maintain the α-helix in the native state.

Thus one can readily conclude that heat denaturation involves not just protein but the entire protein–water system, for, without water, protein cannot undergo denaturation. Any more precise general statement is precluded at this time by the complexity and great variability of protein structure illustrated by the fact that, as a rule, increasing the temperature causes denaturation of proteins (Fig. 4). In the presence of a high concentration of urea, however, and within a certain temperature range, an increase of temperature actually brings about an increase in the extent of the α-helical structure in ribonuclease (Fig. 5).

b. *Effect of freezing.* Highly purified water, completely freed from

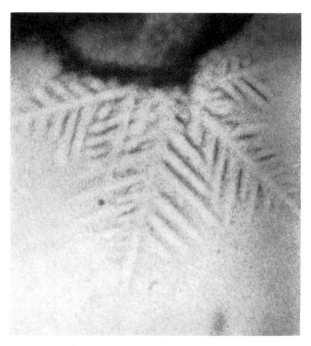

FIG. 6. Crystal growth in supercooled pure water initiated by the insertion of a single crystal at $-3.5°$. The dendrite follows the orientation of the nucleating crystal (Hallet, 1965).

small particles, can be supercooled to very low temperatures (−34°; Pruppacher and Neiburger, 1963). The introduction of a single ice crystal into water supercooled to above −5° brings about the rapid formation of thin hexagonal dendrites following the orientation of the nucleating crystals (Fig. 6). As a rule, solutes in water tend to slow down crystal growth (Walton and Brann, 1916), although a few hasten the process (Lindemeyer and Chalmer; quoted by Chalmer, 1961). Solutes also tend to distort the crystal structure of the ice formed (see Hallet,

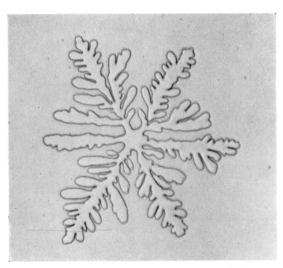

Fig. 7. Hexagonal ice formations obtained in myosin solutions, at high, sub-zero temperatures, illustrating club-shaped axial columns and branches. The concentration of myosin was 11·2%; the temperature, −3°; and the thickness of the protein solution layer approximately 0·01 mm. Magnification × 81. (Rapatz and Luyet, 1959).

1965). Figure 7 shows the pattern of ice formation in myosin solution as observed by Rapatz and Luyet (1959) at a temperature of −3°. Note that the hexagonal dendrites have become very irregular.

7. Inanimate Proteinaceous Fixed-Charge Systems

For proteins in solution, the half-lives of the oriented water molecules, especially those on the outer edge of the multilayer, are short because the protein molecules are themselves subject to Brownian motion. This tends to disarrange the more weakly oriented water molecules. On the other hand, when protein molecules are immobilized into a three-dimensional network, the half-life of the water structure is increased and the effective range of protein-oriented water structure also increases.

The water structure tends to be further stabilized if the adjacent protein chains are regularly spaced at close distances. Here, the orientation produced by the two adjacent protein surfaces tends to merge and thus be re-inforced.

There is a great deal of evidence that the water in proteinaceous fixed-charge systems possesses a high degree of orientation. Figure 8 shows how the water vapour sorption on collagen follows a theoretical adsorption isotherm derived by Bradley (1936), indicating that the water molecules are adsorbed in polarized multilayers. Water in sheep's wool follows the same isotherm. Berendson has shown, from nuclear

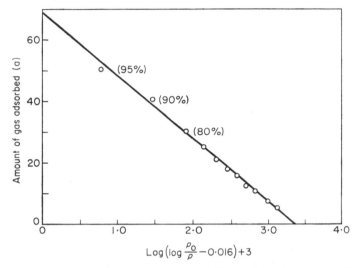

FIG. 8. Water vapour sorption on collagen (hide) at 25°, plotted according to the Bradley Isotherm for the multilayer adsorption of polarized molecules:

$$\log \frac{p_0}{p} = K_1 K_3^a + K_4$$

where a is the amount of gas adsorbed at pressure, p; and p_0 is the gas pressure at full saturation under the same condition. K_1, K_3 and K_4 are constants for a particular system under specified conditions. Data of Bull (1944); from Ling (1965).

magnetic resonance studies of partially dried collagen, that the backbone —NH—CO— groups do indeed orient water molecules, and cause them to lose freedom of rotation. As the temperature is increased, the anisotropic motion of this portion of water in collagen gradually becomes isotropic, like the remainder of the water present.

Further evidence that a portion of the water in fixed-charge systems is oriented is provided by the work of Moran (1926) with gelatin. Subjecting concentrated gelatin solutions to slow freezing at relatively high subzero temperatures, he found that the system separated into two phases, an ice phase and an unfrozen gelatin phase. At equilibrium (Fig. 9), the gelatin phase still contained 35% water. This internal water could not be frozen even at the temperature of liquid air, indicating that it must be strongly oriented by the protein molecules.

Another well-known property of water oriented in multilayers is that it tends to exclude solutes. Work in my own laboratory has shown that this exclusion is relative and varies with the molecular size and the number of H-bonds possessed by the solute. For ions, the water in sheep's wool at equilibrium accommodates only 10–20% of the Na^+ ion in the external medium. As an example, the relative exclusion

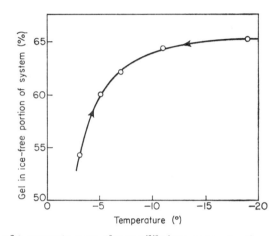

Fig. 9. Effect of temperature on the equilibrium concentration of non-freezable water in a gelatin–water gel. The ordinate indicates the percentage of gel in the ice-free portion of the system. The minimum non-freezable water content of the gel at equilibrium is 34–35%. Each point on the curve is the mean of eight separate analyses and represents a true equilibrium value. The values show no change over a number of days. Any point can be reached from either direction along the curve (Moran, 1926).

of solutes from an ion-exchange resin (sulphonate type; H-form) follows the order sucrose > xylose > glycerol > ethylene glycol > methanol. Sucrose exclusion at equilibrium is thus a simple means of determining the degree of orientation of the water within a fixed-charge system.

C. EFFECTS OF TEMPERATURE ON THE PHYSICAL STATE OF WATER IN THE LIVING CELL

Living protoplasm, as a rule, contains about 20% protein and 70–80% water in the form of a gel. In one extreme, such as skeletal molecules, the proteins are highly organized, show definite X-ray diffraction patterns, and possess elaborate repeating patterns in their ultra-structures (as revealed by electron microscopy); at the other extreme, the cytoplasm of an amoeba is transiently at least more like a sol than a gel. As in fixed-charge systems, there is considerable evidence that water in cells exists as polarized multilayers. Thus, ionic exclusion from water in frog muscle cells resembles ionic exclusion from wool water both qualitatively and quantitatively. Exclusion of alcohols and sugars in water of human red blood cells and muscle cells follows the sequence: sucrose > xylose > glycerol > ethylene glycol > methanol. This is exactly the same sequence of relative exclusion as already quoted for a sulphonate resin which, from our earlier discussion of ionic effects on water structure, must also contain water in polarized multilayers.

1. *Effect of Heating*

The data in Fig. 10 show the effect of temperature on the distribution of sucrose in the cell water of frog voluntary muscles. Below 30°, the concentration of sucrose in the cell water at equilibrium is only 30% of that in the external medium. Above 35°, the concentration rises abruptly, reaching 80% at 45°. Above 35°, these muscles also go into

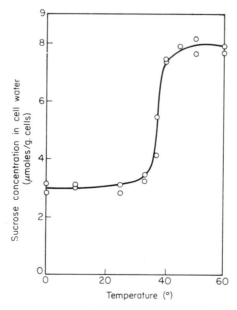

FIG. 10. Effect of temperature on the equilibrium distribution of sucrose between the external medium and the cell water in frog sartorius muscles. The equilibrium concentration of glucose was 8·4-mM. Unpublished data of G. N. Ling and P. Shannon.

heat rigour. The change may reasonably be ascribed to heat denaturation of the cell protein, resulting in a change in the multilayer water structure dictated by the native protein structure. In this system, the lambda point is about 37°; but, for rat muscles, a somewhat different picture was seen with the lambda point at a considerably higher temperature. This is clearly a physiological adaptation, since the body temperature for mammals is above 37°.

2. Effect of Cooling and Freezing

Cooling from body temperature to 0° or even below (but without freezing) brings about relatively small changes in living cells; these changes are, as a rule, reversible.

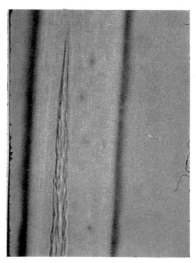

FIG. 11. A non-dehydrated single frog muscle fibre, showing the development of an ice spear. The freezing was at −2·5° (Rapatz and Luyet, 1959).

When the temperature is brought below freezing, ice formation begins in the extracellular fluid and spreads very rapidly. However, ice formation does not extend into the cells except those that are dead or injured. This led to the early recognition that the cell membrane acts as a barrier to ice formation. Intracellular freezing can be induced by further cooling or by seeding, e.g. touching a cut surface with an ice crystal or by inserting into the cell a micropipette with small ice crystals protruding from its tip.

The most instructive intracellular freezing studies were made with single frog muscle fibres (Chambers and Hale, 1932; Rapatz and Luyet, 1959). In these elongated cells, the ice crystals formed are in the shape of long spears (Fig. 11) and thus are quite different from the ice crystals

formed in pure water (Fig. 6) or in protein solutions (Fig. 7). Rapatz
and Luyet (1959) concluded that the spears represent the limbs of
irregular dendrites. The number of spears formed increases with
decreasing temperature. Chambers and Hale (1932) showed that the
direction of the propagation of ice formation, and hence the shape of

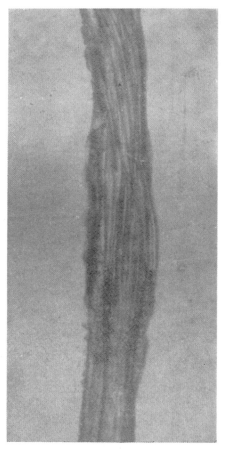

FIG. 12. Formation of ice spears in a single frog sartorius muscle fibre. The
twisting of the ice spears follows the twisting of the muscle fibre (Chambers and
Hale, 1932).

the spears, are dictated by the protein structure of the cell, and become
twisted when the muscle fibre is twisted (Fig. 12). The width of the
spears was small at low temperatures; at higher temperatures, the width
increased, but only one-twentieth as much as the lengthwise growth
rate of the spears (Rapatz and Luyet, 1959).

The fundamental structural elements determining the shape of ice
crystals in muscle fibres are the myofilaments. However, the space

between filaments is 200–300 Å, which is far narrower than the width of the ice spears shown in Figs. 11 and 12 (about 10^5 Å). This shows that, as the ice crystal grows, it must continually draw water from neighbouring spaces to which, however, the crystal cannot itself penetrate. Perhaps the most readily available water is that along the direction in which the ice spear is propagating. Thus, Chambers and Hale (1932) noted that, if the temperature was rather high and the propagation rate slow, the spear reaches only a certain length, due to dehydration in the region in front of the advancing spear.

Recalling Moran's (1926) conclusion that the water in a 65% gelatin solution cannot, under any conditions, be frozen (and there is no

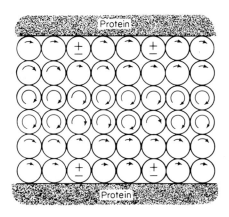

Fig. 13. Diagram of a possible configuration of the water in sheep's wool, collagen, and in living cells, showing multilayer adsorption and decreasing rotational restriction away from the protein surface (Ling, 1965).

question that muscle cytoplasm is in the form of a gel), one may safely conclude that the water–protein system of myofilaments cannot be frozen into ice. In other words, water molecules in the protein–water system are so strongly oriented that it is energetically very unfavourable for them to turn around and re-organize into the tridymite structure of ice.

The improbability of ice formation by the protein–water system in the cell offers a further understanding of the nature of the cell membrane. Thus, if one conceives of the cell membrane essentially as a protein matrix with channels of polarized water, there is no need to postulate the existence of a continuous lipid membrane surrounding the cell. The oriented water itself prevents ice crystal formation. The relative facility with which the water in the longitudinal channels can be crystallized, together with the non-crystallizability of water more closely associated with the muscle protein, reaffirms the conclusion that the cell water exists in polarized multilayers oriented by the structure of the cell protein (Fig. 13).

III. Acknowledgements

This investigation was supported by the National Science Foundation Research Grants GB-2637 and GB-3921, by the National Institutes of Health Research Grants 2RO1-GM11422-02 and 2RO1-GM11422-03, and by the Office of Naval Research Grant No. 4371(00)-105327. The investigator was also supported by Public Health Research Career Development Award K3-GM-19,032.

I thank Miss Patricia Shannon for her assistance with this work, and Dr. Margaret Neville for her critical reading of the manuscript.

References

Beeman, W. W. (1961). Quoted by Berendson (1962).
Berendson, H. J. C. (1962). Ph.D. Thesis: University of Groningen.
Bernal, J. D. and Fowler, R. H. (1933). *J. Chem. Phys.* **1**, 575.
Bochris, J. O'M. (1949). *Quart. Rev.* **3**, 173.
Bradley, S. (1936). *J. Amer. chem. Soc.* 1799.
Bragg, W. L. and Williams, E. J. (1934). *Proc. Roy. Soc. A* **145**, 699.
Bull, H. (1944). *J. Amer. chem. Soc.* **66**, 1499.
Chalmer, B. (1961). Edgar Marburg Lecture. Amer. Soc. Testing and Materials.
Chambers, R. and Hale, H. P. (1932). *Proc. Roy. Soc. B* **110**, 336.
van Eck, C. L. van P., Mendel, H. and Fahrenfort, J. (1958). *Proc. Roy. Soc. A* **247**, 472.
Ernst, E. (1928). *Pflüger Arch. ges. Physiol.* **220**, 672.
Feates, F. S. and Ives, D. J. G. (1956). *J. chem. Soc.* 2798.
Fischer, M. and Suer, W. (1938). *Arch. Pathol.* **25**, 51.
Forslind, E. (1952). Tekniska Hogskolam, Svenska Forskningsinstitute for Cement och Betong vid Kungl. No. 16. Hadlingar, Stockholm.
Foss, J. G. and Schellman, J. A. (1959). *J. phys. Chem.* **63**, 2007.
Fowler, R. H. and Guggenheim, E. A. (1960). "Statistical Thermodynamics". University Press, Cambridge.
Frank, H. S. (1945). *J. chem. Phys.* **13**, 378.
Frank, H. S. (1958). *Proc. Roy. Soc. A* **247**, 481.
Frank, H. S. (1965). *Fed. Proc.* **24**, S-1.
Frank, H. S. and Evans, M. W. (1945). *J. chem. Phys.* **13**, 507.
Gibbs, J. H. and DiMarzio, E. A. (1958). *J. chem. Phys.* **28**, 1247.
Ginnings, D. C. and Furukawa, G. T. (1953). *J. Amer. chem. Soc.* **75**, 522.
Gorsky, W. S. (1928). *Zeit. Physik.* **50**, 64.
Gortner, R. A. (1937). *In* "Selected Topics in Colloid Chemistry", Cornell University Press, Ithaca, N.Y.
Gortner, R. A. (1938). "Outlines of Biochemistry", 2nd edit. John Wiley & Sons, New York.
Hallett, J. (1965). *Fed. Proc.* **24**, S-34.

Harrington, F. W. and Schellman, J. A. (1957). *Compt. rend. trav. Lab. Carlsberg, Ser. Chim.* **30**, 167.

Hearst, J. E. and Vinograd, J. (1961). *Proc. nat. Acad. Sci., Wash.* **47**, 1005.

Heemskerk, J. (1962). *Rec. Trav. Chim.* **81**, 904.

Hermans, J. Jr. and Sheraga, H. A. (1961). *J. Amer. chem. Soc.* **83**, 3283.

Jacobson, B. (1953). *Nature, Lond.* **172**, 666.

Jacobson, B. (1955). *J. Amer. chem. Soc.* **77**, 2919.

Jost, W. (1960). "Diffusion in Solids, Liquids, Gases". Academic Press, New York.

Klotz, I. M. (1960). *Brookhaven Symp. Biol.* **13**, 25.

Klotz, I. M., Ayers, J., Ho, J. Y. C., Horowitz, M. G. and Heiney, R. E. (1958). *J. Amer. chem. Soc.* **80**, 2132.

Lennard-Jones, J. E. and Pople, J. A. (1951). *Proc. Roy. Soc. A* **205**, 155.

Ling, G. N. (1962). "A Physical Theory of the Living State". Blaisdell Publ. Co., New York.

Ling, G. N. (1964). *Biopolymers Symposia*, No. 1, p. 91.

Ling, G. N. (1965). *Ann. N.Y. Acad. Sci.* **125**, 401.

Magat, M. (1935). *J. de Physique et le Radium, ser.* 7, **6**, 179.

Moran, T. (1926). *Proc. Roy. Soc. A* **112**, 30.

Morgan, J. and Warren, B. E. (1938). *J. chem. Phys.* **6**, 666.

Nasonov, D. N. (1962). "Local Reaction of Protoplasm and Gradual Excitation". Office of Technical Services, Washington, D.C.

Némethy, G. (1965). *Fed. Proc.* **24**, S-38.

Némethy, G. and Sheraga, H. A. (1962). *J. chem. Phys.* **36**, 3382.

Pauling, L. (1959). *In* "Hydrogen Bonding", (D. Hadzi and H. W. Thompson, eds.), p. 1. Pergamon Press, London.

Pople, J. A. (1951). *Proc. Roy. Soc. A* **205**, 163.

Pruppacher, H. and Neiburger, M. (1963). *J. Atmos. Sci.* **20**, 376.

Rapatz, G. and Luyet, B. (1959). *Biodynamica* **8**, 121.

Ritland, H. N., Kaesberg, P. and Beeman, W. W. (1950). *J. chem. Phys.* **18**, 1237.

Roentgen, W. K. (1892). *Ann. Phys. Chem.* **45**, 91.

Schellman, J. A. (1955). *Compt. rend. trav. Lab. Carlsberg, Ser. Chim.* **29**, 15.

Stewart, G. W. (1930). *Phys. Rev.* **35**, 1426.

Szent-Györgyi, A. (1957). "Bioenergetics". Academic Press, New York.

Timmermans, J. and Bodson, H. (1937). *Compt. Rend.* **204**, 1804.

Troschin, A. S. (1958). "Das Problem der Zellpermeabilität". Fischer Publ. Co., Jena.

Walton, J. H. and Brann, A. (1916). *J. Amer. chem. Soc.* **38**, 317.

Zimm, B. H. and Bragg, J. K. (1958). *J. chem. Phys.* **28**, 1246.

Chapter 3

Heat Effects on Proteins and Enzymes

JOHN F. BRANDTS

Chemistry Department, University of Massachusetts, Amherst, Massachusetts, U.S.A.

I. Introduction

There has been a great deal of speculation through the years as to why native globular proteins assume their characteristic three-dimensional conformations. There are of course many different levels at which one might attempt to answer this question. It has been shown by Anfinsen and his coworkers (Epstein *et al.*, 1963; Goldberger *et al.*, 1964; Epstein and Goldberger, 1964) that certain native proteins can be unfolded in urea, that their disulphide bonds can be cleaved by mer-captoethanol or some other suitable reagent, and that these proteins will then assume a random coil conformation. If the urea is removed, and if solution conditions are adjusted so that reformation of the disulphide links can occur, the pairing of the disulphides will ultimately become identical to the pairing in the original native protein, and the overall three-dimensional conformation of the final product is, so far as can be judged by various physical properties and activity assays, identical with that of the original protein. This is adequate proof that the particular native conformation which these proteins assume is governed solely by the amino acid sequence of the protein and by the immediate

2+T.

solution conditions, and is independent of the past history of the protein. This might be stated somewhat differently by saying that the conformation of the globular protein is thermodynamically controlled, and that the particular conformation or conformations which have the lowest free energy under any particular set of solution conditions are those which will be present in the largest amounts from the spontaneous establishment of equilibrium.

Confirmation of the thermodynamic control of protein conformation comes from denaturation studies. The loss of the native conformation by an increase in temperature, or pressure, or by the addition of some denaturing agent, has been shown to be completely reversible for a number of different proteins and for many different denaturing agents (Brandts, 1964a, b, 1965). It should be pointed out, however, that in many instances solution conditions must be carefully controlled before a complete return to the native conformation can be observed. The extent of irreversibility for most conformational unfolding reactions increases as the concentration of the protein is increased, although there are some exceptions to this generalization. This would imply that the failure of the denatured protein to revert to the native conformation after denaturing conditions are removed is due to an aggregation reaction which occurs subsequent to the unimolecular unfolding reaction, i.e.

$$N \rightleftharpoons D \rightarrow \text{Aggregate}$$

the aggregation step being kinetically irreversible. One would presume therefore that the aggregation reaction can be prevented quite simply by lowering the protein concentration, and this has been demonstrated with some proteins such as chymotrypsinogen, ribonuclease and chymotrypsin for which complete reversibility can be demonstrated only at low protein concentrations. With other proteins, such as ovalbumin, the aggregation reaction is so favourable that it occurs even at very low concentrations, and good reversibility has never been demonstrated for this protein (Simpson and Kauzmann, 1953; Frensdorff et al., 1953; Schellman et al., 1953; Holme, 1963).

Accepting the ultimate thermodynamic basis of protein conformation, the detailed analysis of conformational stability as it applies to denaturation reactions becomes greatly simplified. In recent years, a great deal has been learned about the molecular basis of conformational stability, not only through experimental studies on proteins themselves but also through the study of low mol. wt. model compounds which in one way or another resemble the various parts of a large protein molecule (see, for example, Kauzmann, 1959; or Brandts, 1964b). These studies tend to place major emphasis on the different types of forces involved in the folding of a globular protein, and to show the tremendous role which the solvent plays in determining the thermodynamic behaviour of proteins.

In view of the intimate relation between enzyme conformation and physiological response, a thorough understanding of the general aspects of protein denaturation is the necessary first step toward the interpretation of biological activity, and the way in which this depends upon temperature, pressure and local solvent conditions. Section II of this chapter will be devoted to thermodynamic considerations for an ideal denaturation reaction which, hopefully, bears a strong resemblance to the actual process although certainly a number of the finer details are not included. It will be shown that, largely because of the participation of water molecules in the denaturation reaction, a number of unusual features of conformational stability are predicted and, if the ideal model has not led us too far astray, these features should be readily observed with native proteins. In Section III, most of the suitable data available on purified proteins, studied under carefully controlled experimental conditions, will be examined in order to ascertain the validity of the model conformational reaction and its application to real situations. Finally in Section IV we shall see if any of the features of the model and of simple protein systems are to be found in the more complex systems of living organisms. In this section, it will be shown that the analysis of biological activity, as exemplified by the treatment of Johnson *et al.* (1954), is no longer completely consistent with the existing facts regarding protein stability and must be modified if it is to provide useful information in the future.

II. Factors Affecting the Thermal Stability of Proteins

A. FORMULATION OF A MODEL FOR REVERSIBLE DENATURATION

There are numerous reports of loss in activity, colour change, aggregation, insolubility and other easily detectable changes that occur on heating proteins. Many of these denaturation reactions occur very abruptly with a change in temperature, and so have often been described as "all-or-none" processes. This description implies a discontinuity in state for the denaturation reactions such that only one state exists below the prevailing "transition temperature" and one above. Hence the term "two-state process" is also frequently used to describe these reactions. The latter term is actually more suitable since denaturation reactions do not involve a true discontinuity in state but only a very abrupt change, so that they are not, in the strictest sense of the word, all-or-none processes.

The concept of a two-state process, as it applies to conformational changes in proteins, is schematically illustrated in Fig. 1. The reader is referred to Hill, 1963 and 1964, for a detailed description of two-state processes in general. A more complete discussion of two-state protein transitions is found in Lumry *et al.*, 1966. At temperatures somewhat below the transition temperature (T_0), the overwhelming majority of protein molecules will be in the compact, well-folded native state. The native state will not consist merely of a single conformation assumed by

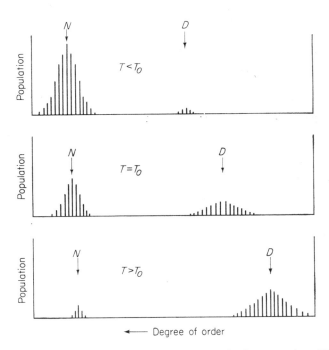

Fig. 1. A graphical illustration of a two-state protein denaturation. The ordinate indicates the relative population for the numerous microstates of the native (N) and denatured (D) distributions. The arrows indicate the average "degree of order" for the two thermodynamic states and demonstrate the temperature dependence of this property as the temperature is increased (top to bottom) through the transition region.

all molecules, but will be made up of a distribution of available conformations or microstates as shown in Fig. 1. These microstates may be classified with respect to their degree of order, a term which will be used here to signify both the extent of folding of the polypeptide chain and also the extent to which solvent molecules are ordered as a result of contact with protein groups. Thus, most native proteins can best be represented as a distribution centred about some relatively high degree of order, in keeping with their normally low entropy. The protein molecules may assume any of these available microstates, and will do so in a manner such that the time-average population of each microstate will be determined in accordance with its relative free energy.

Likewise, at high temperatures, all molecules will be in the denatured state, which again may be visualized as a distribution of available microstates, the populations of which will be thermodynamically controlled. All of these microstates will ordinarily be characterized by a relatively low degree of order compared to microstates of the native protein.

In a small but finite temperature range, i.e. in the transition range, there will be significant populations in both the native and denatured states and, at the transition temperature, by definition, the integrated total populations in the two states will be equal in size, as illustrated in Fig. 1. The most important effect of increasing temperature in terms of a two-state process is then merely to increase the total population of the denatured state at the expense of the native state. This shift in the relative sizes of the populations will usually occur over a comparatively small temperature range, and gives rise to the S-shaped transition curves typical of denaturation reactions. The precise temperature range over which the transition occurs will depend on pressure, pH value and other solution variables.

It is important to recognize, however, that there is a second somewhat more subtle effect as temperature is changed. This is concerned with changes in the native and denatured distributions themselves. Since the microstates in each distribution are characterized by different energies and entropies, their relative probabilities of occurrence will be altered with changing temperature. This might be viewed as a shift in the centre of mass of each distribution with changing temperature, as illustrated in Fig. 1. Thus, the *average* degree of order of the native state may be altered with changing temperature as will the *average* degree of order of the denatured state. These shifts in average conformational properties may also occur from other perturbations such as pressure changes and changes in solvent composition, as will be discussed later.

In this general sense, it is seen that a two-state process does not necessarily imply an equilibrium between two static conformations. In fact, it is highly unlikely that such a situation will ever occur for proteins. The large number of degrees of freedom involved in the folding of a long polypeptide chain would seem to preclude the possibility that a single conformation would be so energetically favourable as to rule out the existence of all others. Consequently, it is clear that thermodynamics gives information only about *average* properties and that these average properties will unquestionably change as solution conditions are altered. In the following account, we shall not always distinguish these dynamic aspects of the two-state process, but it should be understood that the differential thermodynamic variables which will be discussed (e.g. ΔF°, ΔS°, ΔH°) will always refer to average conformational differences and average solvation differences between native and denatured states under the particular solution conditions in which these parameters were evaluated. The extent to which these variables are altered by variations in solution conditions may then be used to obtain information about variations in conformation, or variations in the solvation properties of native and denatured states, as solution conditions change.

Assuming the existence of a two-state process, we need to find an expression for the difference in free energy (ΔF°) between the average

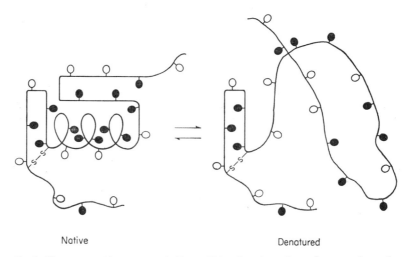

Native   Denatured

FIG. 2. A diagrammatic representation of the denaturation of a protein molecule. Hydrophobic side-chains (filled circles) are mostly buried in the molecule in the native state but are exposed to the solvent in the denatured state, while the polar and ionic side-chains (open circles) are largely solvated in both the native and denatured states.

native and average denatured conformations, and we will use this difference as a quantitative measure of stability. The denaturation process is illustrated schematically in Fig. 2, in which average conformational states are depicted. At the level of approximation necessitated by the complexity of the reaction, we shall concern ourselves only with the more important structural differences between these two states, since it is these which will make the largest contributions to the overall stability. The gross structural features of native and denatured proteins, illustrated schematically in Fig. 2, are well known and have been discussed at length by other authors (Kauzmann, 1954, 1959; Tanford, 1962; Kendrew, 1962; Scheraga, 1963; Schellman, 1964). Those aspects of structure with which we shall be especially concerned are listed in Table I.

TABLE I. *Important Structural Features which Contribute to the Difference in Free Energy between Native and Denatured States*

Native	Denatured	Contribution
1. Rigid structure with little rotational freedom	⇌ Flexible structure	$-pNT\overline{\Delta s_C}$
2. Peptide–peptide hydrogen bonds	⇌ Peptide–solvent hydrogen bonds	$pN\overline{\Delta h_H}$
3. Non-polar side-chains in protein interior	⇌ Non-polar side-chains exposed to solvent	$p \sum \Delta f_{sc}^t$
4. High charge density due to compactness	⇌ Low charge density in extended conformation	ΔF_{elec}
5. Ionizable side-chains with local interactions	⇌ Ionizable side-chains fully solvated	ΔF_{titr}°

Total: $\Delta F^{\circ} = pN\overline{\Delta h_H} - pNT\overline{\Delta s_C} + p \sum \Delta f_{sc}^t + \Delta F_{elec} + \Delta F_{titr}^{\circ}$

To a good approximation, the total free energy change for a co-operative two-state process may be represented as the algebraic sum of the contributions from each of the individual structural transitions which, together, constitute the overall process (Tanford, 1962; Kauzmann, 1959). Accordingly, the free energy contributions arising from the specific structural modifications listed in Table I may be regarded separately. For instance, as stated at the top of the table, there will be a contribution arising from the increased freedom of motion in the polypeptide chain associated with denaturation. Each residue in the folded regions of the polypeptide chain in the native state will be restricted in its rotational motion, and will be in a more or less rigid state due to interactions with adjacent groups. This same residue, if it is located in an unfolded region of the polypeptide chain in the denatured state, will have considerable rotational freedom since it will be well solvated and not restricted by intramolecular interactions. Consequently, such a residue will undergo an increase in conformational entropy during denaturation which can be symbolized as Δs_C. The total increase in conformational entropy for the entire protein will then be $pN\overline{\Delta s_C}$ where $\overline{\Delta s_C}$ is the average conformational entropy change for the unfolding of a single residue, N is the total number of residues in the protein, and p is that fraction of N which is actually unfolded during denaturation. In the general case, some particular residues may be in a folded region in both the native and denatured states while others may be in unfolded regions in both states, so that there may not be 100% participation in the unfolding process which occurs during denaturation. The p factor is intended to take this into account and pN should therefore be a measure of the true size of the co-operative unit which undergoes unfolding.

Secondly, most peptide groups in the native protein will be involved in intramolecular hydrogen bond formation. Peptide–peptide hydrogen bonds will form not only in helical regions of the native protein but in amorphously folded regions as well, as indicated by recent X-ray studies on proteins of low helical content (Phillips, 1965). In the present context, the precise three-dimensional structure of the protein is unimportant since it will only be assumed that any folded residue will have its hydrogen bonding valences satisfied intramolecularly, but whether this is best accomplished by the formation of a helical structure or by an amorphous folding of the polypeptide chain is immaterial. The peptide–peptide interactions in the well-folded native state will be replaced by peptide–solvent interactions in the unfolded state, so that the total contribution to $\Delta F°$ arising from this factor will be $pN\overline{\Delta h_H}$ where $\overline{\Delta h_H}$ is the average enthalpy change for the breaking of a single peptide hydrogen bond in the particular solvent.

Thirdly, most proteins contain a large number of non-polar and very slightly polar side-chains which, according to indirect evidence from solution studies (see, for example, Kauzmann, 1959; or Tanford, 1962) and direct evidence from X-ray work on hydrated protein crystals (Kendrew, 1962; Dickerson, 1964), will be largely buried in the interior of the native protein and out of contact with the solvent, as shown in Fig. 2. This represents the well-known hydrophobic bonding tendency which certainly must be one of the strongest stabilizing factors for native proteins. The hydrophobic bonding reaction, as it pertains to denaturation studies, involves the transition of a non-polar or slightly polar side-chain from its folded state in the protein interior, where its local environment will consist mostly of other non-polar groups and portions of the polypeptide backbone, to its unfolded state in water, i.e.

$$\text{Side-chain } i \text{ (protein interior)} \overset{\Delta f^i_{sc}}{\rightleftharpoons} \text{Side-chain } i \text{ (water)} \qquad (1)$$

where Δf^i_{sc} will be the free energy change for transferring side-chain i from the protein interior to contact with water. The total hydrophobic contribution to $\Delta F°$ will then be $p \sum \Delta f^i_{sc}$ where the sum is taken over all hydrophobic residues in the protein. The p factor will again take into account the proportion of such residues that take part in the unfolding reaction. Ordinarily, the contribution from reactions involving the transfer of polar and ionic side-chains will be small, since these hydrophilic groups will be located almost exclusively at the protein–solvent interface in the native state (Kendrew, 1962) and will therefore undergo no changes in solvation during unfolding.

The last two features listed in Table I are concerned with the general long-range electrostatic interactions (ΔF_{elec}), and the stronger short-range interactions ($\Delta F^{\circ}_{\text{titr}}$) of ionizable side-chains which give rise to "anomalous groups" that titrate with vastly different pK values in the native state as compared with the denatured state. Although these contributions are undoubtedly critical in so far as the pH dependence of stability is concerned, they have been shown to be of minor importance (Brandts, 1964a,b) with respect to the effect of temperature on protein stability. Consequently, although they will be carried along for the sake of completeness, a detailed consideration of these contributions will not be included, and the reader is referred to other sources (Kauzmann, 1954; Tanford, 1961; Brandts, 1964b) for further information concerning these contributions.

Finally, the total free energy difference between the native and denatured forms will be the algebraic sum of all of the individual contributions:

$$\Delta F^{\circ} = pN\overline{\Delta h_H} - pNT\overline{\Delta s_C} + p \sum \Delta f_{sc}^i + \Delta F_{\text{elec}} + \Delta F^{\circ}_{\text{titr}} \qquad (2)$$

B. THE IMPORTANCE OF HYDROPHOBIC BONDING

The contribution of hydrophobic bonding to the ΔF° value deserves particular attention since it is this contribution which gives rise to some unusual thermal effects associated with the conformational stability of proteins. The free energy change for transferring an amino acid side-chain from the protein interior to contact with water (Δf_{sc}^i in eqn. 1) can be estimated from the free energy change for model compound transfer reactions of the type:

$$\text{non-polar} \atop \text{solute} \left(\text{non-polar} \atop \text{solvent} \right) \rightleftharpoons \text{non-polar} \atop \text{solute} \text{(water)} \qquad (3)$$

where the non-polar (or slightly polar) solute is chosen so that it is physically similar to the amino acid side-chain of interest (e.g. one can use methane as a model for the alanyl side-chain) and where the non-polar solvent is intended as a representation of the hydrophobic environment in the protein interior (Kauzmann, 1959). An analogous, but slightly different, method of estimation from amino acid solubilities was proposed by Tanford (1962) and the application of this method shows (Brandts, 1964b) that the transfer free energy for hydrophobic side-chains can be derived from the expression:

$$\Delta f_{sc}^i = a^i T + b^i T^2 + c^i T^3 \qquad (4)$$

2*

where a^i, b^i, and c^i are temperature-independent constants which may be numerically evaluated for different hydrophobic side-chains. Actually, many of the hydrophobic side-chains show very similar values for Δf_{sc}^i so that, at the present level of approximation, it is convenient to divide all hydrophobic side-chains into three different groups the members of which can be considered to be identical. These groups are shown in Table II along with the characteristic values of the temperature-independent coefficients from eqn. 4. In an earlier publication (Brandts, 1964b), the tyrosyl side-chain was placed in a separate group so that four groups were used to classify the hydrophobic side-chains of amino acids. Since then, it has been found that the literature data used to determine the temperature-independent constants for tyrosine are

TABLE II. *Classification of the Hydrophobic Side-Chains of Amino Acid Residues and the Characteristic Values of the Temperature-Independent Constants for these Side-Chains*

Group	Members	a^i	Constants[a] $b^i \times 10^2$	$c^i \times 10^5$
I.	leucine, isoleucine, phenylalanine, proline, tryptophan, tyrosine	$-24{\cdot}906$	$20{\cdot}265$	$-31{\cdot}330$
II.	valine, methionine, lysine (non-polar portion)	$-25{\cdot}746$	$18{\cdot}394$	$-27{\cdot}354$
III.	alanine, arginine (non-polar portion)	$-19{\cdot}000$	$13{\cdot}258$	$-20{\cdot}790$

[a] See eqn. 4, p. 33.

inaccurate so that, until more accurate data are available, tyrosine has been placed in the group with other amino acids that have large hydrophobic side-chains. For most proteins this will not matter a great deal since the tyrosine content is normally low.

The curves in Fig. 3 show the values of Δf_{sc} for these different categories of hydrophobic side-chains, as the temperature is increased above $0°$. It is seen that the free energy of transfer from the protein interior to water is large and positive at all temperatures, but becomes decidedly more positive as the temperature is increased. At high temperatures (about $75°$ for the large side-chains in groups I and II, and $60°$ for the smaller side-chains in group III) the transfer free energies reach a maximum and decrease slowly with a further increase in temperature. Thus, the hydrophobic contribution will stabilize native proteins at all temperatures but considerably more so at high than at low temperatures.

It should be stated emphatically that the temperature dependence of the thermodynamics for the transfer reactions of these hydrophobic groups is very unusual when compared with similar reactions of highly polar molecules. The curves of Fig. 3 indicate that the entropic and enthalpic contributions to Δf_{sc} are very temperature-dependent, since a straight line relationship (i.e. from $\Delta f_{sc} = \Delta h_{sc} - T\Delta s_{sc}$) would result in the absence of a temperature dependence. For instance, the transfer enthalpy, Δh_{sc} (evaluated from eqn. 4 as $\Delta h_{sc} = d(\Delta f_{sc}/T)/d(1/T)$) for the side-chains of group I will be about -2400 cal. at $0°$ but will increase as the temperature is raised, becoming positive at about $50°$ and increasing above this temperature to a value of about 3300 cal. at $80°$. Likewise, the entropy of transfer (Δs_{sc}) is highly negative at low

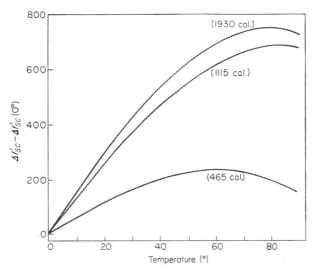

FIG. 3. The effect of temperature on the values of Δf_{sc}^i for the different hydrophobic groups of amino acid side-chains. The values of Δf_{sc}^i for each group at $0°$ are shown in parentheses. Redrawn from Brandts (1964b) by permission of the American Chemical Society.

temperatures (-17 e.u. for group I side-chains at $0°$), becomes less negative as the temperature is increased, and becomes positive at about $75°$. This temperature dependence of heat and entropy effects results from the existence of an anomalously high heat capacity of these non-polar side-chains in water. Thus ΔC_p (i.e. $\Delta C_p = d\Delta h_{sc}/dT$) is 30 cal./°/mole at $0°$ and increases to a value of 90 cal./°/mole at $80°$ for group I side-chains. This is an exceedingly large heat capacity change, and indicates that these non-polar groups have heat capacities in water which are as much as five-fold greater than the heat capacities of the same groups in less associated solvents or in the gas phase. Therefore the large heat capacity term involved in the hydrophobic transfer reaction appears to be associated with the unique features of water as a structured solvent.

It is seen then that, at low temperatures, the hydrophobic bonding tendency arises from a large negative entropy of solvation in water. The enthalpy term itself is negative and will therefore favour location in water rather than in the protein interior. It has been suggested on numerous occasions (Frank and Evans, 1945; Kauzmann, 1959; Némethy and Scheraga, 1962a,b,c) that the large negative entropy and the negative enthalpy of solvation in water arise from an ordering of solvent molecules into "iceberg" or "clathrate" structures which will encompass the hydrophobic group. This clathrating tendency evidently reflects an effort on the part of water molecules to maximize hydrogen bonding in the presence of a non-hydrogen bonding solute, but this can

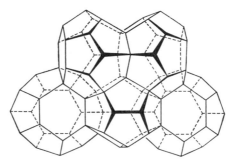

Fig. 4. The clathrate framework for chlorine hydrate. Oxygen atoms are located at each of the corners with hydrogen bonding valences along each edge. Reproduced from Pauling (1960) with the permission of Cornell University Press.

be accomplished only at a considerable cost in entropy necessary to achieve the proper orientation for maximum water–water interactions. The exact physical appearance of these solution clathrate structures has not been determined unambiguously. There have been suggestions (Masterson, 1954; Kauzmann, 1959) that they may be similar or identical in appearance to the clathrates which have been directly observed in the X-ray studies of crystalline gas hydrates which form from aqueous solutions of a number of non-polar gases under very high pressure. The structure of the gas hydrate of chlorine is shown in Fig. 4. Whether or not the identity between solution clathrates and the solid gas hydrates is a valid one remains to be seen, however, and, for the present, nothing will be assumed regarding the physical nature of solution clathrates other than the fact that they are highly ordered structures formed by the co-operation of a number of water molecules in the form of a hydrogen-bonded network.

Although the preferred mode of accommodation of hydrophobic side-chains in water at low temperatures is undoubtedly by clathrate formation, the exceedingly large heat capacity shows conclusively that the clathrate structures are only marginally stable and are disrupted as the temperature is increased. This leads to less negative, and eventually positive, values for the entropy and enthalpy of transfer as the temperature is increased. Consequently, the accommodation of hydrophobic side-chains of proteins in the denatured state must be viewed with respect to a solvent order–disorder transition which can be referred to as "clathrate melting". A schematic illustration of hydrophobic bonding in proteins, utilizing this concept, is shown in Fig. 5. According to

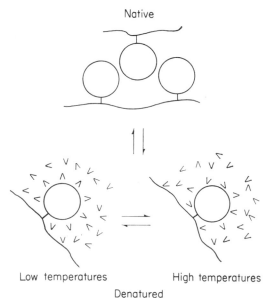

FIG. 5. A diagrammatic representation of the hydrophobic bonding reaction and the clathrate melting transition. Non-polar side-chains in the native state are surrounded locally by other non-polar groups. In the denatured state, the exposed non-polar groups will be accommodated by an ordered solvation shell of water molecules (represented as V's) at low temperatures (left) but by a disordered solvation shell at high temperatures (right).

this, the solvent assumes no importance for the native state since the local environment of the non-polar side-chain consists of other protein groups. In the denatured state, however, the solvent assumes the dominant role, particularly so in view of the clathrate melting transition which can be expected to impart unusual aspects to the thermal stability of proteins.

C. PERSPECTIVE

In the model denaturation reaction, the side-chain transfer terms for the hydrophobic groups can be evaluated from eqn. 4 and the appropriate constants, if the amino acid composition of the protein is known. The final form of the equation for the standard free energy change will then be:

$$\Delta F^\circ = pN\overline{\Delta h_H} - pNT\overline{\Delta s_C} + AT + BT^2 + CT^3 + \Delta F_{elec}$$
$$+ \Delta F^\circ_{titr} \qquad (5)$$

where

$$A = \sum_{\text{I–III}} a^i; \qquad B = \sum_{\text{I–III}} b^i; \qquad C = \sum_{\text{I–III}} c^i$$

and the sums will be taken over all hydrophobic side-chains in groups I–III for the particular protein.

Unfortunately, it is not possible to use eqn. 5 to calculate the conformational stability for any native protein. Model compound studies on various systems (Schellman, 1955; Klotz and Franzen, 1962; Wada, 1960; Miller and Nylund, 1965) suggest that the value of Δh_H should be 200–1500 cal. and that the Δs_C parameter probably lies in the range 2–6 e.u. (Peller, 1959; Kauzmann, 1959; Schellman, 1955; Miller and Nylund, 1965); but it is difficult to decide on precise values within these ranges. For a typical denaturation reaction involving 100 or more residues, an error of 100 cal. in the estimate for the $\overline{\Delta h_H}$ value, or 0·3 e.u. in the $\overline{\Delta s_C}$ value, will lead to an error of 10,000 cal. in the value for ΔF°, and this can mean the difference between a fairly stable or a fairly unstable native protein.

Experimentally it is observed that most native proteins are marginally stable or marginally unstable in the sense that the ΔF° value for denaturation is below about 10,000 cal. over the normal range of solution conditions. Thus, while the values of the terms for individual hydrogen bonding, hydrophobic bonding and conformational entropy contributions in eqn. 5 may each be well in excess of 100,000 cal. in absolute value for a typical transition, the resultant ΔF° value will be considerably smaller because of nearly complete cancellation of stabilizing and unstabilizing contributions. Therefore, even small contributions to the ΔF° value, which have been neglected in this treatment, may be quite important in determining the magnitude of the total free energy. Consequently, the use of eqn. 5 will be restricted to a consideration of changes in free energy resulting from various changes in solution conditions. Under these circumstances, small contributions which have been neglected will tend to cancel out in the subtraction process, and we may still be able to gain valuable insight into the nature of the forces that are important in controlling conformational stability and how these forces depend upon temperature, pressure and solvent composition.

III. Thermodynamic Studies on Purified Proteins

A. THE TEMPERATURE DEPENDENCE OF PROTEIN STABILITY

1. *Experimental Studies*

An experimental study of the thermodynamics of conformational transitions may utilize any solution property that is capable of distinguishing between the native and denatured states. If the transition is of the two-state type, then the equilibrium constant will be:

$$K = \frac{(D)}{(N)} = \left(\frac{\theta - \theta_N}{\theta_D - \theta}\right)$$

where θ_N and θ_D are the values of the solution parameter for the native and denatured states respectively, and θ is the value of the parameter in the transition region where an equilibrium mixture of the two states exists. In general, not only the value for θ but also those for θ_N and θ_D will depend on temperature to some extent due to small changes in microscopic distribution functions of each state with temperature; but this can ordinarily be taken into account (Brandts, 1964a). The standard free energy change may be obtained from the relation:

$$\Delta F° = -RT \ln K \tag{6}$$

and the derived parameters $\Delta H°$, $\Delta S°$, and ΔC_p can then be obtained from the $\Delta F°$ value using standard thermodynamic relations.

There is a vast amount of data in the literature on thermal denaturation reactions for a large number of purified proteins. Unfortunately, the great bulk of these studies were carried out under conditions in which reversibility was incomplete so that the data cannot be subjected to thermodynamic interpretation except in the most qualitative way. Even in those experiments in which reversibility was demonstrated, the data are not usually of sufficient accuracy to evaluate values for ΔC_p, which is very sensitive to small experimental errors. Consequently, the present discussion will focus on the rather small amount of experimental data which meet the desired standards, and the conclusions derived from these data will later be examined for their possible general application.

The data of Fig. 6 show typical transition curves for the thermal denaturation of ribonuclease A at different pH values, using data obtained from difference spectra. These curves illustrate rather well a troublesome experimental limitation in the study of protein denaturation. The large degree of co-operation exhibited by these conformational transitions necessitates that the transition region will be very narrow with regard to the perturbing variable (temperature in these experiments). The equilibrium constant can only be measured with high precision in the range from about 0·03 to 30, corresponding to $\Delta F°$ values from 2000 cal. to -2000 cal. With ribonuclease, this limits the thermodynamic data to a temperature span of about 15° for any single set of experimental conditions. For proteins of higher molecular weight, the available temperature span will be considerably smaller than this due to greater co-operation. This means that, under solution conditions in which the T_0 value is fairly high, there is no way of measuring directly the thermodynamic properties at low temperatures. This problem is general not only for temperature but also for pressure and

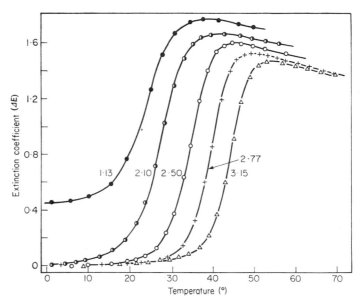

FIG. 6. The effect of temperature on the extinction coefficient at 287 mμ of a solution of ribonuclease at five different pH values. pH values are noted on the curves. From Brandts (1965), with the permission of the American Chemical Society.

solvent perturbations. This limitation greatly restricts our knowledge of the denaturation process since it is highly desirable to have available information on protein stability over wide ranges of solution conditions.

The problem can be overcome to some extent by using a method of extrapolation (Brandts, 1965). The free energy values from a single transition curve may be expressed in the form of a power series in absolute temperatures; i.e.

$$\Delta F° = E + FT + GT^2 + HT^3 \tag{7}$$

If very accurate data are available, reliable values of the temperature-independent constants may be determined by a statistical analysis of the experimental data in the transition region, using the method of least-squares fit. Assuming that these constants are also independent of temperature above and below the transition region in which experimental measurements cannot be made, eqn. 7 can then be used to give thermodynamic data over a wide temperature range.

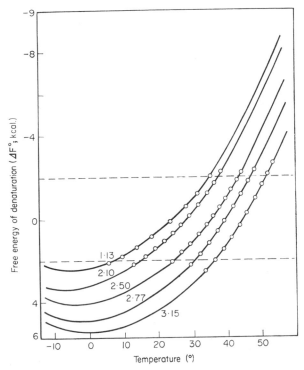

FIG. 7. The temperature dependence of the free energy of denaturation (ΔF°) for ribonuclease at different pH values. The horizontal dashed lines show the limits of the transition region where experimental points (circles) were measured directly. The extension of the curves outside this region was by the extrapolation of the free energy values from eqn. 7.

The results of treating the ribonuclease data in Fig. 6 by the above procedure are shown in Fig. 7. The experimental points obtained in the transition region are shown for each pH value. By applying eqn. 7 the curves were extended beyond the region, using the best values of the constants determined independently at each pH value. The advantages of the extrapolation are immediately obvious from the comparison of the five curves in Fig. 7. These curves show that the temperature dependence of free energy is not drastically altered as the pH value is varied since the curves at all pH values are very similar in shape. The principal effect of increasing acidity is simply to shift the entire free energy profile towards more negative values, and consequently to lower the transition temperature. It would be difficult to draw this conclusion without the benefit of extrapolation, since each transition covers a different temperature range so that a direct comparison could not be made.

The detailed analysis of the curves in Fig. 7 reveals several interesting features which earlier had been predicted from the approximate theoretical treatment of denaturation in Section II. At high temperatures, the temperature coefficient of free energy is very large, indicating large positive values for $\Delta H°$ and $\Delta S°$. There is a great deal of curvature in the plots, however, which arises from a large positive ΔC_p value. There is, therefore, a continuous decrease in the temperature coefficient

TABLE III. *Values of the Enthalpy, Entropy and Heat Capacity Changes for the Thermal Transition of Ribonuclease A at 0° and 60°*

| pH value | Temperature | | | | | |
| | 0° | | | 60° | | |
	$\Delta H°$ kcal.	$\Delta S°$ e.u.	ΔC_p cal.	$\Delta H°$ kcal.	$\Delta S°$ e.u.	ΔC_p cal.
1·13	11	32	1230	137	442	3050
2·10	15	44	1175	135	436	2920
2·50	10	23	1180	131	416	2925
2·77	8	12	1210	132	416	3005
3·15	6	1	1180	126	395	2930

until, at about 0° to −5° (depending somewhat on pH value), the free energy function goes through a positive maximum for ribonuclease, corresponding to $\Delta H°$ and $\Delta S°$ values of about zero. At this temperature (T_{max}), the native protein has maximum stability so that denaturation can, in principle, be accomplished by either raising or lowering the temperature from T_{max}. The extrapolation suggests that the free energy-temperature profile is nearly parabolic in nature with the vertex corresponding to the T_{max} value. This is distinctly different from the linear relationship between $\Delta F°$ and temperature which had been assumed frequently in the past on the basis of imprecise thermodynamic data and which appeared consistent with a temperature-independence for $\Delta H°$ and $\Delta S°$ values.

The temperature dependence of the derived thermodynamic parameters for the ribonuclease transition are shown more clearly in Table III. These values have been obtained from eqn. 7 using the best values of the temperature-independent constants at each pH value. There appears to be a systematic decrease in the magnitude of the entropy and enthalpy terms with increasing pH value, but this is a rather small change which probably arises from variations in electrostatic properties and titration properties associated with the ionization of side-chains. The heat capacity term, although exhibiting a large temperature dependence, shows no pH dependence within experimental error.

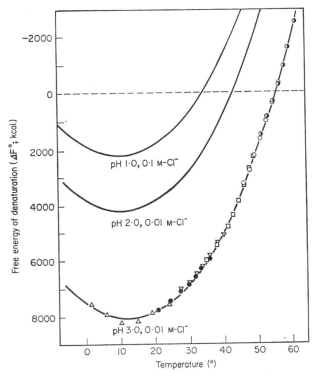

FIG. 8. The temperature dependence of the free energy of denaturation ($\Delta F°$) for chymotrypsinogen at different pH values and ionic strengths. Taken from Brandts (1965), with the permission of the American Chemical Society.

The essential features of the ribonuclease thermal transition are undoubtedly typical of most denaturation reactions. The curves in Fig. 8 show similar free energy profiles for the reversible transition of chymotrypsinogen, which were obtained in an analogous, although slightly different, manner as those for ribonuclease. The similarity in the two sets of data is apparent. The most striking difference is that the T_{max} value for the chymotrypsinogen transition is around 10–12°, or about 15° higher than that for the ribonuclease transition. The relationships between temperature and the derived thermodynamic parameters for

the chymotrypsinogen transition are shown in Fig. 9. The temperature
dependence is again exceedingly large as previously found for ribonuclease. At high temperatures, values for $\Delta H°$ and $\Delta S°$ are large and
positive, being about 180 kcal. and 550 e.u. respectively at 65°. As the
temperature is lowered, both values decrease abruptly and become zero
in the region of 10° and negative below this temperature. The heat
capacity term is about 1700 cal./mole/° at 0° and increases in an
approximately linear fashion to a value of 4100 at 60°. It should be

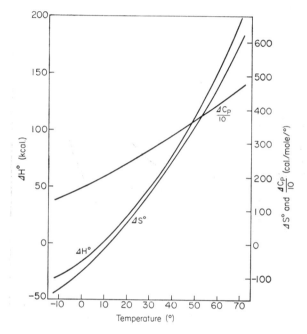

FIG. 9. The temperature dependence of the enthalpy ($\Delta H°$), entropy ($\Delta S°$), and
heat capacity (ΔC_p) of denaturation for chymotrypsinogen. Taken from Brandts
(1964a), with the permission of the American Chemical Society.

noted that the differential heat capacities associated with denaturation
reactions are undoubtedly the largest to be reported for any type of
unimolecular reaction.

Native chymotrypsinogen and native ribonuclease are both stable
proteins at low temperatures even in very acid solutions. Consequently,
it is very difficult to observe directly the low temperature denaturation
which is predicted on the basis of extrapolation of data from higher
temperatures. With ribonuclease there is an additional complication,
since the low temperature denaturation does not begin to occur until
below 0° in liquid water, under which conditions it is experimentally

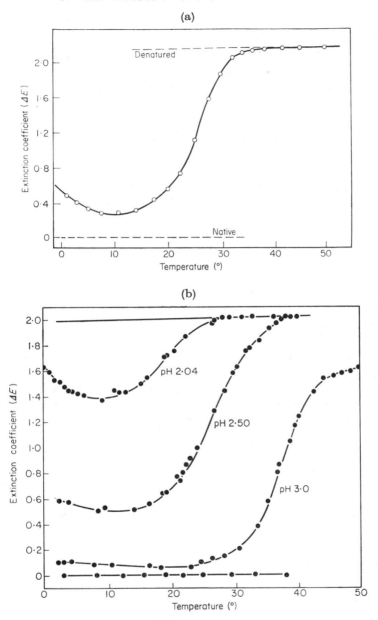

Fɪɢ. 10. The temperature dependence of the extinction coefficient at 293 mμ for (a) chymotrypsin at pH 1·47 (J. F. Brandts and Y. Ting, unpublished observations), and (b) dimethionine sulphoxide chymotrypsin at three different pH values (from Biltonen, 1965; reproduced by permission of the author). The dashed lines at the top and bottom on Fig. 10 (a) indicate the extinction coefficient for the denatured and native states respectively.

impossible to observe. There are other proteins, however, which are less stable so that the low temperature inversion in the free energy curve, which leads to "cold denaturation", can be observed directly in water. Chymotrypsin, for instance, is somewhat less stable than its zymogen so that a direct observation of thermodynamic parameters at low temperatures can be made, and this has been done independently in two laboratories (Biltonen and Lumry, 1965; J. F. Brandts and Y. Ting, (unpublished observations). The data in Fig. 10(a) show a representative transition curve for this protein under conditions of low stability. The overall similarity to the transitions of ribonuclease and chymotrypsinogen is unmistakable. The temperature of maximum stability for this protein (T_{max}) is about 12° which is virtually identical to the value found for chymotrypsinogen by extrapolation.

A chemical derivative of chymotrypsin, dimethionine sulphoxide chymotrypsin (which has methionine residues 179 and 191 oxidized to sulphoxides), is even less stable than chymotrypsin and can be almost completely denatured at low temperatures and moderate acidities. Typical transition curves for this protein are shown in Fig. 10(b). The low temperature transition is particularly apparent in the pH 2·04 curve, where it is seen that the temperature of maximum stability is close to 10° or about the same as for chymotrypsin and chymotrypsinogen.

There have now been numerous other examples of low temperature denaturations reported on other proteins on the basis of less extensive data than those reported above. In some instances, reversibility is virtually complete, but the common situation is only partial reversibility. Studies on the enzymic activity of lipase (Ayengar and Roberts, 1952), β-fructofuranosidase (Sizer and Josephson, 1942), α-glucan phosphorylase (Graves et al., 1965), mitochondrial ATP-ase (Pullman et al., 1960), pyruvate carboxylase (Scrutton and Utter, 1964), glutamate decarboxylase (Skukuya and Schwert, 1960), and trypsin (Adams and Whittaker, 1950) suggest that all of these proteins undergo cold denaturation between room temperature (18–22°) and 0°. Extinction coefficient measurements show that yeast phosphopyruvate hydratase (enolase) also undergoes a reversible conformational change at temperatures below 30° (Rosenberg and Lumry, 1964). Calorimetric measurements on the conformational transitions of serum albumin (Bro and Sturtevant, 1958) and ferrihaemoglobin (Forrest and Sturtevant, 1960) show clearly that these two transitions are characterized by heat capacity effects similar in magnitude to those reported for the chymotrypsin, chymotrypsinogen and ribonuclease transitions if the differences in molecular weight are taken into account. It appears too that native serum albumin and native ferrihaemoglobin exhibit maximum stability around room temperature.

In summary, there seems to be ample experimental evidence to conclude that most, if not all, denaturation reactions are affected by temperature in a manner very similar to that which has now been well characterized for chymotrypsinogen, ribonuclease and chymotrypsin. The generality of this behaviour suggests that it must be a fundamental manifestation dependent upon structural transitions common to all denaturation reactions. Indeed it will be recalled that the rather striking thermal effects associated with the above conformational transitions are exactly those which would be expected on the basis of a reaction involving the exposure of non-polar side-chains to aqueous solvent, and there can be little doubt that they arise predominantly from those aspects of water structure upon which hydrophobic bonding depends.

2. *Comparison of Experimental Data with the Theoretical Model*

It is instructive to analyse the available experimental data in terms of the approximate model for denaturation developed previously. In the following analysis, the electrostatic and titration free energy terms are neglected since their contributions to the temperature dependence of ΔF° are small. If a more exact treatment is desired, these terms can be calculated approximately from experimental data, as has been shown by Brandts (1964a,b). Neglecting these terms in eqn. 5, the expression for the free energy can be written as:

$$F^\circ = pN\overline{\Delta h}_H + (pA - pN\overline{\Delta s}_C)T + pBT^2 + pCT^3 \qquad (8)$$

A comparison of this theoretical expression with the corresponding expression for ΔF° given by eqn. 7 reveals that the two values will be equal at all temperatures if:

$$p = \frac{G}{B} = \frac{H}{C}$$

$$\overline{\Delta h}_H = \frac{EB}{NG} \qquad (9)$$

$$\overline{\Delta s}_C = \frac{A}{N} - \frac{FB}{NG}$$

Consequently, the theoretical model is capable of exactly reproducing the experimental free energy profiles at all temperatures with the choice of parameters indicated above. These structural parameters may then be evaluated for any protein, the amino acid composition of which is known and the denaturation thermodynamics of which have been accurately measured.

The result of this type of analysis of the ribonuclease data is shown in Table IV in which the estimates of p, $\overline{\Delta h}_H$ and $\overline{\Delta s}_C$ for five different pH values are shown. It is seen that, to a good approximation, these three parameters are independent of pH value and temperature. There is what appears to be a small systematic increase in the $\overline{\Delta s}_C$ term as the pH value is decreased. This might well result from our neglect of the electrostatic and titration contributions, since it can be argued that variation in these contributions with changing pH value will result largely from entropy effects in acid solutions (Brandts, 1964a,b). Nevertheless, the relative constancy of these parameters, particularly the p factor, strongly suggests that the co-operative unit in the ribonuclease molecule which undergoes reversible unfolding is the same at

TABLE IV. *Empirical Estimates of the Structural Parameters p, $\overline{\Delta h}_H$, and $\overline{\Delta s}_C$ for the Thermal Transition of Ribonuclease A*

pH value	p	$\overline{\Delta h}_H$	$\overline{\Delta s}_C$	Deviation from two-state model[a]
1·13	0·83	1020	5·50	0·15%
2·10	0·80	1060	5·60	0·20%
2·50	0·80	1010	5·40	0·10%
2·77	0·82	990	5·30	0·10%
3·15	0·80	970	5·20	0·15%

[a] These figures are the average root mean square deviation of the experimentally determined molar extinction coefficients, as compared with those calculated using eqn. 8.

all pH values. This is an important conclusion since it implies that the average conformation of the native state and the average conformation of the denatured state are relatively independent of pH value and that the unstabilization produced by increasing the acidity arises predominantly from varying the state of ionization of the existing native and denatured conformations.

The final column in Table IV gives some indication of the extent to which the two-state theory is obeyed for ribonuclease. This shows the average root mean square deviation of the experimentally determined extinction coefficients as compared with those calculated from the two-state equation (eqn. 8) using the best values of the structural parameters. This is expressed relative to the total difference in the molar extinction coefficient for the native and denatured states, i.e. $\epsilon_N - \epsilon_D$. Thus, deviations of the experimental data from the two-state approximation are always less than 0·2% of the total change in extinction coefficient for complete denaturation, and therefore well within the range of experimental error. This serves as experimental verification of the two-state assumption for the ribonuclease transition, since it has been shown that unfolding mechanisms not based on two-state distributions lead to transition curves that are markedly different from those with a two-state distribution, and that the extent of departure increases as the importance of intermediate states increases (Lumry et al., 1966).

It should be noted that Poland and Scheraga (1965) have arrived at the opposite conclusion, on the basis of molar extinction coefficient measurements of moderate precision (Hermans and Scheraga, 1961), that the ribonuclease transition deviates markedly from a two-state mechanism. However, the high precision of the data represented in Table IV would seem to discount any but the very smallest deviations from two-state behaviour, and it seems likely that the conclusion of Poland and Scheraga is in error.

TABLE V. *Estimates of the Structural Parameters for the Thermal Transitions of Ribonuclease, Chymotrypsinogen, Chymotrypsin, and Dimethionine Sulphoxide Chymotrypsin*

Protein	p	$\overline{\Delta h}_H$	$\overline{\Delta s}_C$	Reference
Ribonuclease	0·80	1000	5·4	Brandts, 1965
Chymotrypsinogen[a]	0.55	930	5·4	Brandts, 1964a,b
Chymotrypsin[a]	0·87	910	5·4	Biltonen and Lumry, 1965
Dimethionine sulph-oxide chymotrypsin[a]	0·51	920	5·5	Biltonen and Lumry, 1965

[a] The estimates of the structural parameters given here differ slightly from those given in the original references. This is due to the difference in the treatment of the contributions by tyrosine side-chains (see p. 34).

Of the four proteins which have been examined carefully, all show transitions consistent with the two-state description. The values of the structural parameters which have been found by analysis of their transition curves, in a manner analogous to that shown for ribonuclease, are summarized in Table V. It would be anticipated that, in so far as the model is correct, the parameters $\overline{\Delta h}_H$ and $\overline{\Delta s}_C$ should be of about the same magnitude for all proteins, since they are primarily a function of the peptide group content and should not vary appreciably with the amino acid composition or the size of the protein. To a good approximation, this appears to be true for the four proteins referred to in Table V. The values for the hydrogen bonding parameter are all close to 1000 cal./mole; this is within the limits of 200–1500 cal./residue which as we have seen had been delineated by independent estimates from the study of model compounds. The same conclusions may be made regarding the conformational entropy term. Values of Δs_C for these four proteins are all of comparable magnitude, around 5·5 e.u./residue, which is again within the expected range of 2–6 e.u./residue.

It is probably true that the estimate of $\overline{\Delta h}_H$ obtained in this manner must be regarded as an upper limit for the estimate of the peptide hydrogen bonding contribution. In the approximate treatment which has been used, other sources of enthalpy stabilization (such as London dispersion forces, side-chain hydrogen bonds and ion pair interactions) have been omitted from eqn. 8 so that these contributions, by default, will be included in the $\overline{\Delta h}_H$ term. Consequently, it seems likely that the correct estimate of the peptide hydrogen bonding contribution will be less than 1000 cal./mole residues. Somewhat the same situation holds true for the $\overline{\Delta s}_C$ term so that this must be considered to arise from rotational restrictions from side-chain interactions as well as from peptide interactions.

It is difficult to draw any conclusions regarding the estimates of the value of the p factor, since we would expect this to vary quite significantly from one protein to another, and since there is no reliable means of providing an independent estimate of this factor. It is somewhat reassuring that the estimates are larger than about 0·3 since it seems highly likely that a significant fraction of all residues participates in most major denaturation reactions (Tanford, 1963). Regarding chymotrypsin and chymotrypsinogen, it has previously been suggested (Rupley et al., 1955; Imahori et al., 1960) that the native enzyme is more highly folded than the native zymogen and, if this is correct, we would anticipate that the p factor for chymotrypsin might be significantly larger than that for chymotrypsinogen if the denatured forms for the two proteins are roughly equivalent (Biltonen, 1965). The present estimates of 87% participation for chymotrypsin and 55% participation for chymotrypsinogen serve to confirm this point of view.

The magnitude of the total contributions from hydrogen bonding, hydrophobic bonding and conformational entropy for the chymotrypsinogen transition, which is also representative of the other transitions, are shown in Fig. 11. Hydrogen bonding will contribute about 120,000 cal. of stabilizing free energy to native chymotrypsinogen according to this analysis. The contribution from hydrophobic bonding will be about 105,000 cal. at 0° and this will increase rapidly at low temperatures, level off at about 145,000 cal. at 75°, and decrease at higher temperatures. These two important contributions to the free energy are approximately balanced at all temperatures by the unstabilizing free energy arising from the increase in conformational entropy. Thus, although there may be well over 250,000 cal. of stabilizing free energy, the net free energy of denaturation will seldom exceed 10,000 cal. because of the delicate balance between stabilizing and unstabilizing factors. It is therefore apparent that, even though the contributions from factors such as anomalous groups or from electrostatic free energy are small in comparison with the total stabilizing and unstabilizing free energy, they will be large enough to control the free energy balance and seriously to alter the equilibrium as the pH value is changed under the usual conditions of marginal stability.

This type of analysis shows that the thermal stability of these proteins is quite clearly consistent with preconceived notions regarding the strength of intramolecular interactions which have arisen rather indirectly from studies on model compounds. Although the quantitative

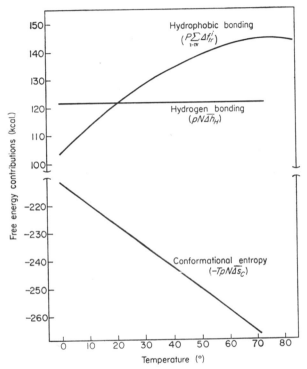

FIG. 11. Estimates of the effect of temperature on the total contributions to the stability of native chymotrypsinogen resulting from hydrogen bonding, hydrophobic bonding and conformational entropy. From Brandts (1964b), with the permission of the American Chemical Society.

agreement between the model reaction and various protein transitions is exceedingly good, the number of assumptions and omissions necessary to construct such a model necessitates that one must regard the values which emerge from this and similar treatments as being very tentative. However, there are certain qualitative conclusions which now seem to be more firmly established as a result of the demonstration of quantitative consistency.

First of all, it seems likely that the two-state approximation is probably a good one for many protein conformational transitions when temperature is the perturbing variable. This will not necessarily be the general case for all proteins nor will it necessarily be true for other perturbants such as pressure and solvent, but it will probably be the best first approximation to be used until contradictory experimental evidence arises.

Secondly, all major conformational transitions of proteins will undoubtedly be found to be characterized by rather unusual thermodynamic behaviour arising from the solvation of hydrophobic side-chains in the denatured state. The highly ordered clathrate structures, which form about these groups at low temperatures, tend to melt as the temperature is increased, and give rise to an anomalously large ΔC_p term for the conformational transition. This leads to a marked curvature in the free energy-temperature profile and ultimately, at low temperatures, to an inversion in the temperature dependence of free energy such that proteins can be expected to show a cold denaturation as well as a heat denaturation. In view of the lack of any pronounced temperature dependence of the p factors for the four transitions examined, it appears that the low temperature- and high temperature-denatured forms have roughly the same time-average conformation in the polypeptide chain. Although this must be regarded as a very approximate conclusion at the present time, it does seem likely that the principal difference between the two denatured forms is in the mode of accommodation of the hydrophobic side-chains in the solvent phase.

The value of the stability maximum (T_{max}) on the temperature scale will depend on several factors. It will in general occur at that temperature at which the value for $\Delta S°$ (i.e. $\Delta S° = -(d\Delta F°/dT)$) is zero. As suggested above, the total entropy change can be regarded as arising principally from two sources: (a) a conformational entropy which will be large and positive at all temperatures; (b) an entropy contribution arising from the solvation of hydrophobic groups which will be large and negative at low temperatures but which will become less negative as the temperature is increased. It is at T_{max} that these two contributions will be equal in absolute value so that $\Delta S° = 0$. We would then expect that those proteins with a high relative content of the large non-polar side-chains will exhibit maximum stability at a higher temperature than those proteins with a low content. For the proteins which have thus far been examined carefully, ribonuclease has the smallest proportion of hydrophobic groups and was also observed to have the lowest value for T_{max}. The amino acid composition of chymotrypsinogen, chymotrypsin, and dimethionine sulphoxide chymotrypsin are almost identical and all were observed to have about the same values for T_{max}. There are, of course, other less important entropy sources which might also influence the value for T_{max} to some extent, but it does seem fairly certain that, even for those proteins with the largest proportion of hydrophobic groups, the upper limit for T_{max} should be about 25–30°.

In terms of the distribution of microstates, it is then obvious that the average degree of order of the denatured distribution is actually greater than that of the native distribution at low temperatures since the ordering effect of clathrate formation more than compensates for the disordering that arises from the unfolding of the polypeptide chain. On the other hand, at high temperatures the opposite situation, which is the one shown in Fig. 1, is true. Thus, one of the principal differences between the native and denatured distributions is that the average properties of the denatured distribution are much more sensitive to temperature variations because of the clathrate melting transition. This should hold true not only for temperature variations but also for pressure and solvent variations.

B. THE RELATION BETWEEN TEMPERATURE AND PRESSURE EFFECTS

The dependence of free energy on pressure for a two-state denaturation reaction will always obey the expression:

$$\Delta V°(T, P) = \left(\frac{d\Delta F°}{dP}\right)_T \tag{10}$$

where $\Delta V°(T, P)$ is the difference in partial molar volume between the average native and average denatured species at the temperature T and the particular pressure at which the derivative is evaluated. As with temperature variations, there are two obvious effects of pressure in perturbing a macromolecular equilibrium situation. An increase in pressure (other conditions being constant) will always act to increase the population for the state of low volume and, accordingly, decrease the population for the state of high volume, as implied in eqn. 10. In addition, since we must regard the native and denatured states as each consisting of a collection of microstates with thermodynamic population distributions, pressure will act to alter these distributions and thereby change the average conformational and solvation properties of the two states. This change in distributions will introduce a pressure dependence into the $\Delta V°$ term. For small to moderate pressures (up to 1000 atm.), the second effect is undoubtedly very small and we shall neglect it in this discussion.

With this simplification, we need be concerned only with the temperature dependence of the volume change, which can now be written approximately as:

$$\Delta V°(T) = \Delta V°(T_0) + \int_{T_0}^{T} \bar{V}_N(\alpha_D - \alpha_N) \, dT \tag{11}$$

where $\Delta V°(T_0)$ is the volume change at some standard temperature (T_0) and α_N and α_D are the thermal coefficients of expansion of the native and denatured forms defined in the usual way as:

$$\alpha_N = \frac{1}{\overline{V}_N}\left(\frac{\partial \overline{V}_N}{\partial T}\right)_P$$
$$\alpha_D = \frac{1}{\overline{V}_D}\left(\frac{\partial \overline{V}_D}{\partial T}\right)_P \tag{12}$$

where $\overline{V}_N$ and $\overline{V}_D$ are the respective partial molar volumes.

There are two main sources of volume change during the unfolding of a protein molecule. Firstly, void volume may be created or destroyed during the unfolding process as a result of changes in the packing of residues and solvent molecules. Secondly, solvation changes and concommitant volume changes will result when groups which are buried in

TABLE VI. *Volume Changes in the Transfer of Hydrocarbons from Non-polar Solvents to Water at 25°[a]*

Process	ΔV (ml./mole)
CH_4 in hexane $\rightarrow$ CH_4 in H_2O	$-22\cdot7$
C_2H_6 in hexane $\rightarrow$ C_2H_6 in H_2O	$-18\cdot1$
C_3H_8, pure liquid $\rightarrow$ C_3H_8 in H_2O at 10 atm.	-21
C_6H_6, pure liquid $\rightarrow$ C_6H_6 in H_2O	$-6\cdot2$

[a] Taken from Kauzmann (1959).

the native state become exposed to solvent in the denatured state. At the present time, it is not known what the relative importance of these two effects might be. It seems certain that the most important single contribution to volume change arising from solvation changes will result from the exposure of non-polar side-chains. The data in Table VI show volume changes for model compound reactions which are analogous to the hydrophobic transfer reactions for denaturation. It is evident that these hydrophobic molecules have an anomalously low volume in water as compared with their volume in other less associated solvents. These same qualitative effects are observed with numerous other small molecules which might serve as models for the non-polar side-chains of proteins (Kauzmann, 1959). It has been suggested previously (Masterson, 1954; Kauzmann, 1959), and it is undoubtedly true, that these low volumes result from the formation of dense clathrate structures when these non-polar molecules are dissolved in water at low or moderate temperatures.

This again serves to emphasize the importance of the clathrate melting transition in so far as the thermal properties of proteins are concerned. Since the small partial molar volume of solvated hydrophobic groups in water is apparently associated with the clathrate structure, it would be anticipated that the shift from clathrate accommodation to random accommodation as the temperature is increased will tend to normalize the volume. In other words, we should expect these groups to exhibit an anomalously large thermal coefficient of expansion. The highly accurate density data of Masterson (1954) on aqueous solutions of methane, ethane and propane show that this is indeed true. The

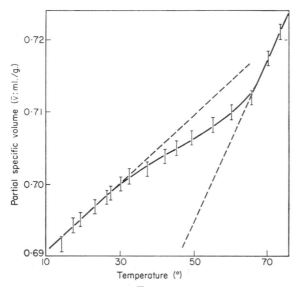

FIG. 12. The partial specific volume ($\bar{V}$) of ribonuclease measured in the temperature region of thermal denaturation. The extrapolated lines (- - -) from values at high and low temperatures indicate the expected dependence for the denatured and native states, respectively. From Holcombe and van Holde (1962), with the permission of the American Chemical Society.

thermal coefficient of expansion of these non-polar molecules in water is approximately $10^{-2}/°$ at low temperatures. This is to be compared with various polar molecules, such as methanol or formamide, or ionic solutes, such as ammonium formate, in water for which the coefficients of expansion are usually between 10^{-4} and $10^{-3}/°$. Thus, the coefficients of expansion associated with non-polar groups in water are an order of magnitude greater than those for polar and ionic groups, and this in all likelihood results from the thermal disruption of the clathrate structures.

To the extent that the hydrophobic contribution controls the magnitude of the total $\Delta V°(T)$ value for denaturation reactions, we should expect these same effects to be observed. Although there are little suitable experimental data available, what there are tend to substantiate this conclusion. Holcomb and van Holde (1962) have measured the partial specific volume of ribonuclease (dilatometrically) and their results are shown in Fig. 12. Under the conditions of their experiment, the transition temperature for the thermal denaturation was about 50°. The dashed line, extrapolated from the values at low temperatures, indicates the approximate temperature dependence of the volume for the native protein, while the extrapolated line from the high temperature values bears the same relation to the denatured protein. The slopes of these lines will be very nearly proportional to α_N and α_D, respectively. Thus, the value for α_N is of the order of $5 \times 10^{-4}/°$ which is a small value consistent with a structure, the polar and ionic groups of which are solvated but in which the non-polar groups are for the most part buried. During denaturation there is a three-fold increase in the coefficient of expansion (*i.e.* α_D $1 \cdot 5 = \times 10^{-3}/°$) undoubtedly arising in great measure from the additional exposure of the non-polar side-chains. Therefore, the value for $\Delta V°(T)$, (which is proportional to the distance between the two dashed lines in Fig. 12) is negative at low temperatures but, due to the large difference in the coefficients of expansion, becomes less negative as the temperature is raised and will eventually become positive at about 70° for the ribonuclease transition.

Since this is precisely the type of behaviour expected from fundamental arguments, it seems likely that other denaturation reactions will be similar to that observed with ribonuclease in the temperature dependence of the volume parameter. In general the precise temperature at which $\overline{V}_N$ and $\overline{V}_D$ become equal will depend to a great extent on the amino acid composition, precise conformation, and the amount of void volume of the protein so that it would be expected that other proteins would exhibit the inversion in the sign of the value for $\Delta V°(T)$ at temperatures which may be considerably higher or lower than 70°. With chymotrypsinogen denaturation, for instance, it has been observed (Brandts and Lumry, 1963) that the value for $\Delta V°(T)$ is positive at 45° so that the inversion point must occur below this temperature.

In accordance with their effect on volume changes, moderately high pressures should act by unstabilizing native proteins at low temperatures and by stabilizing these same proteins against reversible denaturation at high temperatures. Preliminary studies in this laboratory on the effects of increased pressures on the reversible denaturations of ribonuclease and chymotrypsinogen confirm this expectation and demonstrate the strong temperature dependence of the volume parameter.

It appears that most proteins, if subjected to very high pressures, will ultimately be denatured irrespective of the temperature at which the pressure is applied (Johnson *et al.*, 1954; Miyagawa and Suzuki, 1963; Suzuki and Miyosawa, 1965). This is very seldom a reversible process, however, and it is frequently accompanied by precipitation so that it seems possible that the conformational changes involved may be quite different from those that occur at low and moderate pressures. It is conceivable, however, that it is basically the same process that occurs at low pressures, which would suggest that the coefficient of compressibility for denatured proteins is much larger than for native proteins.

C. RELATION BETWEEN TEMPERATURE AND SOLVENT COMPOSITION

The alterations in the stability of native proteins which arise from the addition of a second solvent component to an aqueous protein solution might conceivably result from changes in the magnitude of any of the contributions included in eqn. 5 or from changes in less important contributions that have been omitted from this equation. However, the most striking relation between temperature and solvent composition in terms of their mutual effects on protein stability arise, predictably, from the effects of hydrophobic bonding. The importance of these effects of hydrophobic bonding can be demonstrated rather convincingly on appropriate model compounds, purified proteins and, as noted in Section IV (p. 62), certain biological systems.

Although the exact physical nature of solution clathrates is not known, it seems certain that their existence depends to a very great extent on the nearly tetrahedral arrangement of the four hydrogen bonding valences of water. This permits, as shown in the gas hydrate structure depicted in Fig. 4, the formation of a regular three-dimensional hydrogen-bonded framework which will include a relatively large number of lattice sites. Structures of this sort will certainly be co-operative to a high degree. The relative free energy of any single molecule in the framework will depend upon its having all of its hydrogen bonds to neighbouring sites intact. Consequently, the result of removing a water molecule from a single site in the clathrate lattice, and its replacement with a different type of solvent molecule which does not meet the specific hydrogen bonding requirements of the clathrate, may be the sequential disruption of the entire framework. Although it is probably an exaggeration to imply perfect co-operation of this sort, there will certainly be a strong tendency for this situation to occur because of the interdependence of all sites necessitated by the hydrogen bond network.

The consequences of this situation can be illustrated by referring to Fig. 13. At *low temperature*, the best way of accommodating non-polar groups in water is by clathrate formation. As a second solvent component, which cannot fit into the clathrate framework, is added, the initial effect will be to decrease the stability of the clathrate simply by

3 + T.

decreasing the availability of water molecules necessary to form the clathrate. As the activity of the second component is further increased, it becomes entropically favourable (and perhaps energetically favourable) for these molecules to enter the solvation sphere. The only way in which this can be accomplished is by a co-operative, isothermal "melting" of the clathrate structures to give a random accommodation sphere in which both solvent components can participate. Since the non-polar solute molecule (or the non-polar side-chain) is hydrophobic,

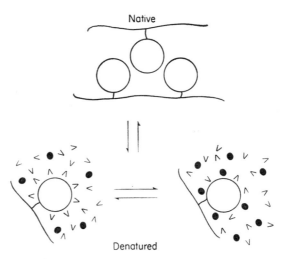

FIG. 13. A diagram illustrating the relation between hydrophobic bonding and the clathrate melting transition in binary solvents. In accommodating a non-polar group (bottom left) into the clathrate, only water molecules (V's) will be in the solvation shell while, in random accommodation (bottom right), both water and the non-aqueous solvent component (circles) will be in the solvation shell, with the non-aqueous component usually providing preferential solvation.

it will probably be true that, for most aqueous binary solvents, the non-polar group will be preferentially solvated by the non-aqueous solvent component once clathrate melting has taken place. Consequently, we should expect to see two effects as a second solvent component is added. At low concentrations, the non-polar group should be unstabilized due to the disruption of the stable clathrates. Once this disruption is complete, the effect of further additions of the non-aqueous solvent component should be to stabilize the non-polar group by preferential solvation. On the other hand, at *high temperatures*, the situation is less complex since the thermodynamically-favoured form of accommodation, even in pure water, is by random solvation so that the only observable effect upon addition of a second solvent component should be the preferential solvation effect which will exert a stabilizing influence on the non-polar group at all concentrations.

The thermodynamics of argon, which is a good model compound analogue for studies on non-polar side-chains, in binary solvents have been extensively studied (Ben-Naim and Moran, 1965; Ben-Naim and Baer, 1964) and illustrate the differences in the high- and low-temperature behaviour noted above. The experimental results, which are summarized in Fig. 14, show that, at low temperature (5°), the initial effect of adding dioxan to aqueous solutions of argon is to increase its free energy until a mole fraction of about 0·1 is reached, whereupon further additions of dioxan decrease the relative free energy of argon.

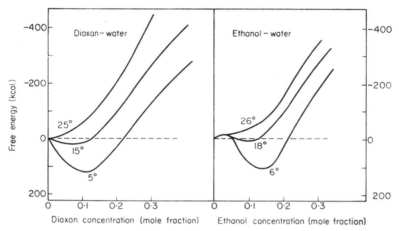

FIG. 14. The relative free energy of argon in binary solvents at different temperatures. The curves summarize the solubility data of Ben-Naim and Baer (1964) (using ethanol-water) and Ben-Naim and Moran (1965) (using dioxan-water). For each temperature, the free energy of argon in pure water has been assigned an arbitrary free energy of zero.

As the temperature is increased to 15° and to 25°, the initial increase in free energy at low dioxan concentrations, which is attributed to isothermal clathrate melting, becomes less pronounced since more of the clathrate melting has been accomplished thermally, and the predominant effect of adding dioxan at 25° appears to be the preferential solvation effect.

The data on the free energy of argon in aqueous ethanol solutions, also shown in Fig. 14, are similar to those for dioxan except that, at low temperatures, there is an initial small decrease in free energy as the ethanol concentration is changed from 0 to 0·02 mole fraction, and this has no counterpart in the dioxan-water solvent. The reason for this is not clear although a tentative explanation has been suggested by Ben-Naim (1965). Nevertheless, it is clear from the comparison of the two sets of curves in Fig. 14 that the same qualitative thermal effects are observed for the two binary solutions indicating the importance of the common component (i.e. water) in determining these effects.

If these effects are attributable to fundamental aspects of the solvation of non-polar groups in water, they should occur during protein denaturation reactions in binary solvents. Since the non-polar side-chains in the native state will be out of contact with the solvent for the most part, the variation in the standard free energy of denaturation (i.e. $\Delta(\Delta F^\circ)$) upon the addition of a second solvent component will depend principally upon variations in the free energy of the exposed non-polar groups in the denatured state. Consequently, to the extent that the total variations in the value for ΔF° are controlled by hydrophobic bonding, we should expect $\Delta(\Delta F^\circ)$ to show a behaviour similar to that depicted in Fig. 14 for the model hydrophobic compound. There are sufficient data available (J. F. Brandts, unpublished observations) on the ribonuclease denaturation to demonstrate that this is indeed so. These data are summarized in Fig. 15 which shows the effect of ethanol concentration on the relative free energy of denaturation (referred again to pure water at the same temperature as the standard state). A comparison of these protein data with the model compound data in Fig. 14 show unmistakably that it is the hydrophobic bonding which must control the effect of ethanol on the conformational stability of ribonuclease, and therefore support the previous suggestions regarding the importance of the clathrate melting transition.

On this basis, we might expect that there would be a number of organic reagents, similar to ethanol, which would stabilize native proteins at low temperatures (and at low concentrations) but would unstabilize or denature them at high temperatures. In the past, it has always been implicitly assumed that the action of these agents was a denaturing one at all temperatures. This impression has arisen however from high temperature studies, and from low temperature studies in the presence of *high* concentrations of the reagent, when the effect would be expected to be an unstabilizing one (Fig. 15). There have been very few studies on the effects of low concentrations of reagents at low temperatures. What data there are seem to support the contention that the observed effects of ethanol on ribonuclease may be typical for other proteins and for other reagents. For instance, Graves *et al.* (1965) have studied the effect of low temperatures on the stability of α-glucan phosphorylase and found that, at pH 6·0 and 0°, the protein was 70% denatured as judged by activity assays. However, the addition of 10% methanol, 10% propylene glycol or 10% dimethyl sulphoxide at this low temperature, restored the protein almost completely to the native state. Skukuya and Schwert (1960) found that, for the reversible transition of glutamate decarboxylase, small concentrations of ethanol stabilized the native form at 0° but denatured the protein to a small extent at 25°.

Urea acts as a denaturing agent for native ribonuclease at all concentrations and all temperatures (J. F. Brandts, unpublished observation; Foss and Schellman, 1959) and the same is true for its effect on chymotrypsinogen (Brandts, 1964a), although with this enzyme it is a much better denaturing agent at high temperatures than at low

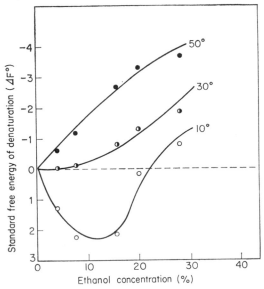

FIG. 15. The effect of ethanol concentration on the change in standard free energy of denaturation for ribonuclease at three different temperatures. The results show stabilization of the native protein at 10° and low concentrations of ethanol, and an unstabilization at 30° and 50° at any concentration of ethanol.

temperatures. As regards its effects on model compounds, the addition of urea to aqueous solutions of methane and ethane has been observed to decrease the solubility of the gases below 20°, and to increase their solubility above this temperature (Wetlaufer *et al.*, 1964). This is qualitatively the same effect as observed for dioxan and ethanol on the solubility of argon (Fig. 14). The inability to observe a stabilizing effect of urea on proteins at low temperatures probably indicates that the "hydrophobic effect", although important, is obscured to some extent because of other effects which urea has on proteins. One of these other effects may be a decrease in the hydrogen bonding contribution ($\overline{\Delta h_H}$) (Kauzmann, 1959).

There are numerous ionic compounds, the effects of which on hydrophobic bonding may be of secondary importance. The effects of protons and hydroxyl ions are probably best understood in terms of changes in electrostatic properties and in terms of the titration of anomalous groups (Brandts, 1964b). As shown earlier, there is a very small temperature coefficient involved in their effects.

The studies of von Hippel and Wong (1965) on the effects of salts on the thermal stability of ribonuclease show that there are certain cations and anions which stabilize, and others which unstabilize, the native conformation under otherwise identical conditions. The relative effectiveness of the various ions apparently follows very closely the classical Hofmeister series. They have observed the same order of effectiveness on the collagen–gelatin phase transition (von Hippel and Wong, 1962, 1963) and conclude that the effects arise indirectly from variations in solvent structure upon the addition of salts. Specifically, they point out that any ion which tends to disrupt the ordered solvation shell about the non-polar side-chains in the denatured state should act to denature the protein. This is incorrect reasoning, however, since the disruption of the ordered solvation shell, under conditions where it is the thermodynamically favoured mode of accommodation of non-polar side-chains, will tend rather to stabilize the native protein unless the ordered accommodation shell which is lost can be replaced by a better (i.e. thermodynamically more stable) mode of accommodation in the salt solution. This need not always be so as was shown previously in relation to the effects of uncharged solutes on model compounds and proteins at low temperatures (Figs. 14 and 15).

An alternative interpretation of the effects of salts on proteins has been suggested (Robinson and Jencks, 1965; Nagy and Jencks, 1965). These workers have shown, using appropriate model compounds, that the net effects of salts on protein stability correlate more closely with their effects on the peptide and amide groups of proteins than with their effects on the hydrophobic groups. It seems likely, however, that both effects are important to a significant extent.

IV. Analogies in the Heat Responses of Living Organisms

The various explanations put forth in the past to explain the importance of protein denaturation in reversible biological processes are now seen to be incomplete since they neglected to consider the thermodynamic consequences arising from the participation of solvent molecules in the denaturation reaction. These effects become so important at low temperatures that they lead to an inversion in the temperature dependence of free energy, and to some interesting relationships between temperature and pressure and also between solvent composition and temperature. These thermodynamic phenomena must have biological significance in terms of regulation and control of metabolism but the implications have not yet been systematically explored. Although it is outside the major objective of this chapter, and outside the area of competence of the author, to provide a detailed discussion of the biological implications arising from the discussion of the previous sections, it is perhaps worth while to point out some of the more obvious manifestations at the organism level which appear to illustrate concepts developed earlier in relation to model compounds and purified proteins under well controlled solution conditions.

What is usually observed in biological systems is not the denaturation equilibrium directly but rather the rate of some particular reaction which is catalysed by the enzyme of interest whenever that enzyme is in its native form. Thus, in addition to the equilibrium:

$$N \rightleftharpoons D; \qquad (D)/(N) = e^{-\Delta F^\circ /RT}$$

we must also concern ourselves with the rate process:

$$S \xrightarrow{N} P; \qquad \text{Rate} = (N)C\, e^{-\Delta E_a /RT}$$

where C is a constant which depends upon the concentration of reactant (which can ordinarily be assumed to be constant in an open ended biological system), the concentration of cofactors or other secondary catalysts (e.g. protons) and the Arrhenius frequency factor. The Arrhenius activation energy for the rate process is ΔE_a. Combining the above two equations gives:

$$\text{Rate} = \frac{C\, e^{-\Delta E_a /RT}}{1 + e^{-\Delta F^\circ /RT}} \tag{13}$$

Finally, in order to apply eqn. 13 to biological systems, it has always been assumed that ΔF° may be expressed as a two-term power series in absolute temperature:

$$\Delta F^\circ = \Delta H^\circ - T\Delta S^\circ \tag{14}$$

where ΔH° and ΔS° are treated as temperature-independent constants and may be identified with the enthalpic and entropic contributions to the free energy of denaturation when this assumption is correct.

Certain inconsistencies have arisen when attempting to interpret experimental data in terms of eqns. 13 and 14. Specifically, as low temperatures are approached, it is frequently observed that the Arrhenius plot of eqn. 13 shows large deviations from the linear relation between the logarithm of the rate and the reciprocal of the absolute temperature which is expected if the values for $\Delta H°$ and $\Delta S°$ are nearly temperature-independent. Also, when average slopes are calculated from the data at low temperature, the apparent values of the activation energies are frequently of the order of 30–100 kcal./mole, which are unrealistically high values for enzyme-catalysed reactions. These low-temperature deviations have been so frequently and systematically observed that they have led Kavanau (1950) and Hultin (1955) to suggest that there may be a second denaturation process which occurs

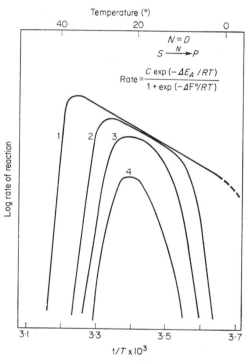

FIG. 16. Arrhenius plots for the reaction $S \rightarrow P$ catalysed by an enzyme (N) which is assumed to have different heat stabilities. See text for explanation.

at low temperatures for many enzymes. They treated the low temperature and the high temperature denaturations as completely distinct and different processes, since there was no basis, at that time, for doing otherwise.

From the recent results reported in this chapter, it is apparent that eqn. 14 gives a very poor approximation for $\Delta F°$ (i.e. if the values for $\Delta H°$ and $\Delta S°$ are considered to be temperature-independent), and it should be abandoned in favour of a more exact representation (e.g. eqn. 7) which contains sufficient parameters to specify the heat capacity contribution that gives rise to the inversion in the free energy profile which leads to the low-temperature denaturation. With this modification, eqn. 13 will then adequately account for many of the low temperature anomalies noted previously.

For instance, the curves in Fig. 16 are typical Arrhenius plots assuming a normal activation energy (about 10 kcal./mole) and a temperature dependence of the $\Delta F°$ value in keeping with that determined previously for purified proteins (Figs. 7 and 8). The temperature of maximum stability (T_{max}) for this hypothetical enzyme happens to be about 20°. Curve 1 (Fig. 16) then shows the expected behaviour for a reaction catalysed by a rather stable enzyme which has a transition temperature for high temperature denaturation of about 40°. The region of linear decrease in the logarithm of the rate from 0° to 40° corresponds to a temperature range in which the native enzyme is very stable and is present to the extent of nearly 100%, so that the slope of the curve will be $-\Delta E_a/R$, in accordance with eqn. 13. Because this enzyme is very stable, the low temperature denaturation, manifested as a sharp decrease in rate, will not be observed until the temperature falls below 0°, as indicated in Fig. 16; ordinarily it would not be experimentally observable. Consequently, the general appearance of the Arrhenius plot for a stable enzyme would be qualitatively similar to that expected using the classical treatment (i.e. eqns. 13 and 14) since the low temperature denaturation does not manifest itself in the available temperature range.

Curve 2 in Fig. 16 shows the expected behaviour for a similar but less stable enzyme. The high temperature denaturation begins to occur at about 30° and the linear portion of the Arrhenius plot covers a much shorter temperature range. The onset of the low temperature denaturation is now observed as the temperature is lowered below about 15° as indicated by the sharp change in slope.

The remaining curves (3 and 4) in Fig. 16 show the Arrhenius plots expected from reactions catalysed by enzymes that are even less stable and show how the high and low temperature parts of the denaturation curve tend to merge. The most obvious indication of this is that the curves tend to become more symmetrical on the high and low temperature sides of the maxima, although they will never become completely symmetrical since the high temperature denaturation always occurs more abruptly with changing temperature than does the low temperature denaturation. It should be noted that, in curves 3 and 4, the enzyme is so unstable that there is never 100% native protein at any temperature and, consequently, the maximum in the rate does not coincide with the linear portion in curves 1 and 2. Under these circumstances, there is no way of measuring ΔE_a accurately.

3*

It is instructive to examine several real systems to illustrate the relationships observed in Fig. 16. The curve in Fig. 17, for instance, shows the Arrhenius plot for the reduction of methylene blue by the bacterium *Rhizobium trifolii* (Koffler *et al.*, 1947). This reaction evidently is catalysed by an enzyme of high stability, as indicated by the fact that the high temperature denaturation does not begin to occur until above 40°. Consequently, the linear portion of this curve covers a very broad temperature span and, even at 15°, there is no evidence of low temperature denaturation. The activation energy indicated in the linear region is 13 kcal./mole, which is comparable to the values commonly observed for reactions catalysed by enzymes *in vitro*.

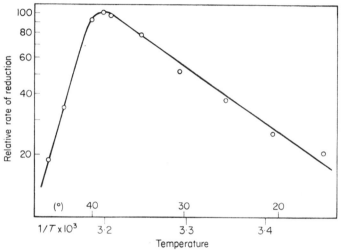

FIG. 17. An Arrhenius plot for the reduction of methylene blue by *Rhizobium trifolii*. Redrawn from Koffler *et al.* (1947), with the permission of the American Chemical Society.

A different type of temperature optimum is observed in Fig. 18 for the growth of the protozoon *Tetrahymena pyriformis* in media containing different concentrations of D_2O. It appears that the enzyme catalysing the rate-determining reaction for the growth of this organism is only moderately stable since the high temperature denaturation begins below 30°. It is comparable then to the hypothetical case shown in curve 2 of Fig. 16. The linear portion of the curves in Fig. 18 indicates activation energies of about 20 kcal./mole. With these data, there is a clear indication of the low-temperature denaturation which begins to occur below 17°. The value of T_{max} for this enzyme would then be about 20–22°.

The decrease in growth rate with an increase in the concentration of

D_2O (Fig. 18) might at first glance be interpreted in terms of an un-stabilization of the native enzyme. This is probably incorrect, however, since the sequence of curves expected for this situation would be similar to curves 2, 3, and 4 of Fig. 16. In Fig. 18, the temperature region of linearity, (17–27°) is unchanged following an increase in the D_2O concentration, implying that the stability of the enzyme is virtually

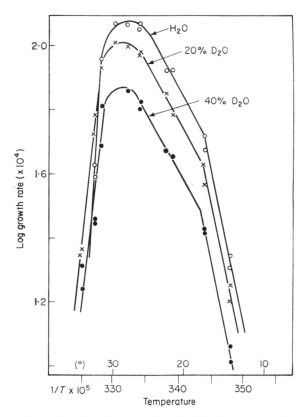

FIG. 18. Arrhenius plots for the growth of *Tetrahymena pyriformis* in media containing different concentrations of D_2O. Unpublished observations; reproduced by courtesy of Dr. John G. Moner.

unaffected. This is in keeping with studies on purified proteins in which it has usually been found that the presence of D_2O has only a small effect on the stability of the protein (Hermans and Scheraga, 1959; Maybury and Katz, 1956; Berns, 1965). Thus, the predominant effect of D_2O must be on the rate parameters in eqn. 13.

There are also numerous reversible physiological processes which exhibit more symmetrical temperature optima characteristic of more unstable enzyme systems and similar in appearance to those illustrated in curves 3 and 4 of Fig. 16. Perhaps the most extensively studied processes of this type are the reactions involved in the production of visible radiation by certain bacteria. The data in Fig. 19 show Arrhenius plots for the intensity of luminescence by *Photobacterium phosphoreum* at three different hydrostatic pressures, and it is evident that, under the conditions of these experiments, the linear region of the Arrhenius plot corresponding to 100% native enzyme is absent. Thus it would appear that the production of visible radiation by this bacterium involves one or more reactions catalysed by an enzyme that is partially denatured at

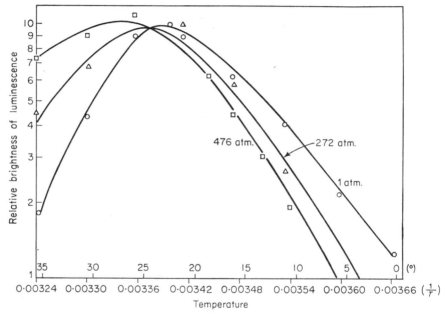

Fig. 19. Arrhenius plots of the intensity of luminescence produced by *Photobacterium phosphoreum* at three different hydrostatic pressures. From Johnson *et al.* (1954) with the permission of John Wiley & Sons.

all temperatures but less so at T_{max} (about 23° at 1 atm. pressure) than at higher or lower temperatures.

The effects of pressure shown in the data in Fig. 19 are also interesting and appear to illustrate a point brought out earlier in connection with model compounds and purified proteins. If the volume change for activation ($\Delta V \ddagger$) for the reaction $S \xrightarrow{N} P$ can be assumed to be small for this process, as it is for most enzyme-catalysed reactions *in vitro* (Johnson *et al.*, 1954), then the effects of pressure shown in Fig. 19 must result predominantly from a shift in the denaturation equilibrium due to the difference in volume ($\Delta V°$) between the native and denatured enzyme. Consequently, below 24° (the intersection point of the three curves in Fig. 19) pressure would appear to unstabilize while, above 24°, it would appear to stabilize the native form. The denatured form must therefore be the form of lowest volume at low temperatures and also the form of greatest volume at high temperatures. This illustrates a possible biological manifestation of the previous conclusion that denatured proteins will have a much larger thermal coefficient of expansion than

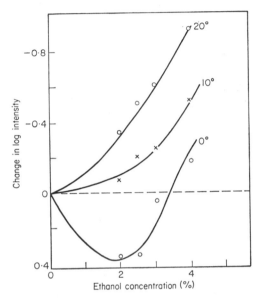

FIG. 20. The effect of ethanol concentration on the luminescent intensity of *Photobacterium phosphoreum* at three different temperatures. From data reported by Johnson *et al.* (1945).

native proteins due to the clathrate melting about exposed hydrophobic groups. There are other systems which exhibit an analogous relationship between temperature and pressure effects (Johnson *et al.*, 1954) when the perturbing pressures are small, so that this behaviour may be somewhat general.

The effect of ethanol on the reversible reaction involved in the luminescence of *P. phosphoreum* has also been carefully studied by Johnson *et al.* (1945). The results they obtained are summarized in Fig. 20. At low temperature (0°), the addition of small amounts of ethanol leads to an initial increase in the luminescent intensity and this is followed by a decrease in intensity as more ethanol is added at this temperature. At higher temperatures, the initial enhancement seen at

$0°$ is no longer present so that the only effect of adding ethanol is a loss in luminescent activity. If the effects of ethanol are primarily upon the denaturation equilibria and not upon the rate parameters in eqn. 13, then this suggests that ethanol stabilizes the native enzyme at low temperatures and low concentrations and unstabilizes the enzyme at higher concentrations and higher temperatures. It also suggests that the hydrophobic effect, described previously in connection with model compounds and purified proteins (Figs. 14 and 15), may be the controlling factor in determining luminescent intensity following the addition of ethanol. Qualitatively similar behaviour to that shown in Fig. 20 has been observed for the effect of urethan on *P. phosphoreum* (Johnson *et al.*, 1945) and on *Vibrio phosphorescens* (Johnson *et al.*, 1943) where a loss in luminescent activity was observed at high temperatures but where urethan had either no significant effect or brought about an enhancement in activity at low temperatures and low urethan concentrations.

Although this discussion is too incomplete to permit broad generalizations to be made, it nevertheless serves to illustrate the possible importance of the effects of thermal energy on protein stability, particularly those effects which arise from solvent accommodation of hydrophobic side-chains, in relation to the control of biological processes. The generally poor control of variables in these systems, and the numerous possibilities for complications which would render simple interpretations meaningless, necessitate that one exercises a certain amount of caution in drawing analogies between complex biological systems and well controlled protein systems studied *in vitro*. Obtaining more extensive experimental data on both types of systems seems desirable in order to establish the proper perspective. Nevertheless, it does seem obvious that, at least for certain simple systems, the inversion in the relation between biological activity and temperature, pressure and solvent variations, which occurs as these systems are taken from high to low temperatures, must be closely related to the same phenomena which have been observed in well controlled systems and serves to emphasize the rather unique role played by water in biological processes.

References

Adams, D. H. and Whittaker, V. P. (1950). *Biochim. biophys. Acta* **4**, 543.
Ayengar, P. and Roberts, E. (1952). *J. biol. Chem.* **197**, 453.
Ben-Naim, A. (1965). *J. phys. Chem.* **69**, 3420, 3245.
Ben-Naim, A. and Baer, S. (1964). *Trans. Far. Soc.* **60**, 1736.
Ben-Naim, A. and Moran, G. (1965). *Trans. Far. Soc.* **61**, 821.
Berns, D. S. (1965). *Biochemistry* **2**, 1377.
Biltonen, R. (1965). Ph.D. Thesis: University of Minnesota, Minneapolis Minnesota, U.S.A.

Biltonen, R. and Lumry, R. (1965). *J. Amer. chem. Soc.* **87**, 4208.

Brandts, J. F. (1964a). *J. Amer. chem. Soc.* **86**, 4291.

Brandts, J. F. (1964b). *J. Amer. chem. Soc.* **86**, 4302.

Brandts, J. F. (1965). *J. Amer. chem. Soc.* **87**, 2759.

Brandts, J. F. and Lumry, R. (1963). *J. phys. Chem.* **67**, 1484.

Bro, P. and Sturtevant, J. M. (1958). *J. Amer. chem. Soc.* **80**, 1789.

Dickerson, R. E. (1964). *In* "The Proteins", Vol. II, 2nd edit. (H. Neurath, Ed.). Academic Press, New York.

Epstein, C. J. and Goldberger, R. F. (1964). *J. biol. Chem.* **239**, 1087.

Epstein, C. J., Goldberger, R. F. and Anfinsen, C. B. (1963). *Cold Spr. Harb. Symp. quant. Biol.* **28**, 439.

Forrest, W. W. and Sturtevant, J. M. (1960). *J. Amer. chem. Soc.* **82**, 585.

Foss, J. G. and Schellman, J. A. (1959). *J. phys. Chem.* **63**, 2007.

Frank, H. S. and Evans, M. W. (1945). *J. chem. Phys.* **13**, 507.

Frensdorff, H. K., Watson, M. T. and Kauzmann, W. (1953). *J. Amer. chem. Soc.* **75**, 5157.

Goldberger, R., Epstein, C. J. and Anfinsen, C. B. (1964). *J. biol. Chem.* **239**, 1406.

Graves, D. J., Sealock, R. W. and Wang, J. H. (1965). *Biochemistry* **4**, 290.

Hermans, J., Jr. and Scheraga, H. A. (1959). *Biochim. biophys. Acta* **36**, 534.

Hermans, J. Jr. and Scheraga, H. A. (1961). *J. Amer. chem. Soc.* **83**, 3283.

Hill, T. L. (1963). "Thermodynamics of Small Systems". Part 1. Benjamin, New York.

Hill, T. L. (1964). "Thermodynamics of Small Systems". Part 2. Benjamin, New York.

von Hippel, P. H. and Wong, K. (1962). *Biochemistry* **1**, 664.

von Hippel, P. H. and Wong, K. (1963). *Biochemistry* **2**, 1387.

von Hippel, P. H. and Wong, K. (1965). *J. biol. Chem.* **240**, 3909.

Holcomb, D. N. and van Holde, K. E. (1962). *J. phys. Chem.* **66**, 1999.

Holme, J. (1963). *J. phys. Chem.* **67**, 782.

Hultin, E. (1955). *Acta Chem. Scand.* **9**, 1700.

Imahori, K., Yoshida, A. and Hashisume, H. (1960). *Biochim. biophys. Acta* **45**, 380.

Johnson, F. H., Eyring, H. and Kearns, W. (1943). *Arch. Biochem.* **3**, 1.

Johnson, F. H., Eyring, H., Steblay, R., Chaplin, H., Huber, C. and Gherardi, G. (1945). *J. gen. Physiol.* **28**, 463.

Johnson, F. H., Eyring, H. and Polissar, M. J. (1954). "The Kinetic Basis of Molecular Biology". John Wiley & Sons, New York.

Kauzmann, W. (1954). *In* "The Mechanism of Enzyme Action", (W. D. McElroy and B. Glass, Eds.). Johns Hopkins University Press, Baltimore.

Kauzmann, W. (1959). *Advanc. protein Chem.* **14**, 1.

Kavanau, J. L. (1950). *J. gen. Phys.* **34**, 193.

Kendrew, J. C. (1962). *Brookhaven Symp. Biol.* **15**, 216.

Klotz, I. M. and Franzen, J. (1962). *J. Amer. chem. Soc.* **84**, 3461.

Koffler, H., Johnson, F. H. and Wilson, P. W. (1947). *J. Amer. chem. Soc.* **69**, 1113.

Lumry, R., Biltonen, R. and Brandts, J. F. (1966). *Biopolymers* **4**, 917.

Masterson, W. L. (1954). *J. chem. Phys.* **22**, 1830.

Maybury, R. H. and Katz, J. (1956). *Nature, Lond.* **177**, 629.

Miller, W. G. and Nylund, R. E. (1965). *J. Amer. chem. Soc.* **87**, 3542.

Miyagawa, K. and Suzuki, K. (1963). *Rev. Phys. Chem. Japan* **32**, 43, 51.

Nagy, B. and Jencks, W. P. (1965). *J. Amer. chem. Soc.* **87**, 2480.

Némethy, G. and Scheraga, H. A. (1962a). *J. chem. Phys.* **36**, 3382.

Némethy, G. and Scheraga, H. A. (1962b). *J. chem. Phys.* **36**, 3401.

Némethy, G. and Scheraga, H. A. (1962c). *J. phys. Chem.* **66**, 1773.

Pauling, L. (1960). "The Nature of the Chemical Bond", 3rd edit. Cornell University Press, Ithaca, New York.

Peller, L. (1959). *J. phys. Chem.* **63**, 1194, 1199.

Phillips, D. C. (1965). *Abstr. 49th Ann. Meeting Fed. Amer. Soc. exp. Biol.*, p. 114.

Poland, D. and Scheraga, H. A. (1965). *Biopolymers* **3**, 401.

Pullman, M. E., Penefsky, H. S., Datta, A. and Racker, E. (1960). *J. biol. Chem.* **235**, 3322.

Robinson, D. R. and Jencks, W. P. (1965). *J. Amer. chem. Soc.* **87**, 2470.

Rosenberg, A. and Lumry, R. (1964). *Biochemistry* **3**, 1055.

Rupley, J., Dreyer, W. and Neurath, H. (1955). *Biochim. biophys. Acta* **18**, 162.

Schellman, J. A. (1955). *Compt. rend. trav. lab. Carlsberg. Ser. chim.* **29**, 223.

Schellman, J. A. (1964). *In* "The Proteins", Vol. II, 2nd edit. (H. Neurath, Ed.). Academic Press, New York.

Schellman, J. A., Simpson, R. B. and Kauzmann, W. (1953). *J. Amer. Chem. Soc.* **75**, 5152.

Scheraga, H. A. (1963). *In* "The Proteins", Vol. I, 2nd edit. (H. Neurath, Ed.). Academic Press, New York.

Scrutton, M. C. and Utter, M. F. (1964). *Fed. Proc.* **23**, 162.

Simpson, R. B. and Kauzmann, W. (1953). *J. Amer. chem. Soc.* **75**, 5139.

Sizer, I. W. and Josephson, E. S. (1942). *Food Res.* **7**, 201.

Skukuya, R. and Schwert, G. (1960). *J. biol. Chem.* **235**, 1658.

Suzuki, K. and Miyosawa, Y. (1965). *J. Biochem. (Tokyo)* **57**, 116.

Tanford, C. (1961). "Physical Chemistry of Macromolecules". John Wiley & Sons, New York.

Tanford, C. (1962). *J. Amer. chem. Soc.* **84**, 4240.

Tanford, C. (1963). *J. Amer. chem. Soc.* **86**, 2050.

Wada, A. (1960). *Mol. Phys.* **3**, 409.

Wetlaufer, D. B., Malik, S. K., Stoller, L. and Coffin, R. (1964). *J. Amer. chem. Soc.* **86**, 508.

Chapter 4

Effects of Elevated Temperatures on DNA and on Some Polynucleotides: Denaturation, Renaturation and Cleavage of Glycosidic and Phosphate Ester Bonds

Waclaw Szybalski

*McArdle Laboratory, University of Wisconsin,
Madison, Wisconsin, U.S.A.*

I. Introduction

The principal effect of elevated temperature on any compound in general, and on nucleic acids in particular, is to supply enough kinetic energy to disrupt the bonds between atoms and molecules. It is necessary, therefore, to ask which of the bonds are responsible for maintaining the three-dimensional structure of the nucleic acids, and which of them are most susceptible to the effects of temperature, depending obviously on the nature of the solvent (environment). The major part of this review pertains to native, double-stranded DNA and to several synthetic double-stranded polydeoxynucleotides. Single-stranded DNA, RNA* and some synthetic polyribonucleotides will be discussed only

* Abbreviations: DNA, deoxyribonucleic acid; RNA, ribonucleic acid; A, adenine: C, cytosine; G, guanine; T, thymine; U, uracil; BU, 5-bromouracil; CU,

briefly. This review does not attempt to cover exhaustively the voluminous and amorphous literature on the heat degradation and denaturation of DNA. For earlier references the reader is referred to the reviews
and papers of Eigner (1960), Geiduschek and Holtzer (1958), Inman and
Jordan (1960a,b,c), Jordan (1960), Josse and Eigner (1966), Lanyi
(1963), Mahler and Cordes (1966), Marmur *et al.* (1963b), Michelson
(1963), Peacocke and Walker (1962), Rownd (1963), Singh (1965), and
Steiner and Beers (1961), and to the papers of Gulland *et al.* (1947),
Thomas (1954), Rice and Doty (1957), Rice *et al.* (1958) and Sturtevant
et al. (1958), who apparently were among the first to recognize the
nature of DNA denaturation. It is interesting to note, however, that the
general notions of the thermal denaturation of DNA were still vague
only a decade ago (Chargaff and Davidson, 1955) and were not even
included in the 1960 volume of this standard compendium on nucleic
acids (Chargaff and Davidson, 1960).

II. Structure of DNA as Related to Heat Stability

The structure of DNA is depicted in Fig. 1. Two complementary
polydeoxynucleotide strands are held together with non-covalent bonds
consisting mainly of (1) hydrogen bonding between adenine (A) and
thymine (T) or guanine (G) and cytosine (C), and (2) stacking forces
between the interacting π electrons of the purine and pyrimidine bases,
including "hydrophobic" and London dispersion forces together with
dipole-dipole interactions. These bonds hold the native DNA in the
form of a double-stranded helix, usually with 10 base pairs per turn of
34 Å length (Watson, 1965). The stacking free energy for bonds of type
(2) corresponds to about 7 kcal., whereas the hydrogen bonds provide
2 kcal. (A—T)–3 kcal. (G—C) of free energy per mole of base pairs.
Thus, the principal forces which hold the polynucleotide chain together
come from the stacking free energy, acting from one base pair to the
next, while the hydrogen bonds between the members of a base pair,
while contributing only a minor amount of stabilization, take the role of
discriminators in permitting only the canonical base pairs to form with-

5-chlorouracil; FU, 5-flourouracil; meC, 5-methylcytosine; r, ribose; d, deoxyribose. The abbreviations for the polynucleotides are essentially identical to those
proposed by Inman and Baldwin (1962) and used by Chamberlin (1965) and Riley
et al. (1966) e.g., dAT:dAT symbolizes a double-stranded helix, each strand
consisting of a perfectly alternating copolymer of deoxythymidylate and de-
oxyadenylate residues; dI:dI:dI symbolizes a triple-stranded helix of polyino-
sinic homopolymers; (dA:dT)rU symbolizes a 3-stranded complex prepared by
mixing dA:dT with rU, and rA(d)U:rA(d)U a double-stranded helix, each strand
consisting of a perfectly alternating copolymer of adenylate and deoxyuridylate
(Chamberlin, 1966). T_m, melting temperature of DNA (Fig. 4); T_t, temperature
(midpoint) of final strand separation (Fig. 4).

out paying a price in broken bonds to water. The net free energy, which stabilizes one base pair with respect to separation, was estimated to be approximately − 1 kcal., which is made up of − 2 to − 3 kcal. of free energy of hydrogen binding, − 7 kcal. of stacking free energy, and contributions from other unresolved sources amounting to the remainder, about 8–9 kcal. (quoted from Crothers and Zimm, 1964). On the other hand, the heat of the transition from coil to helix amounts to

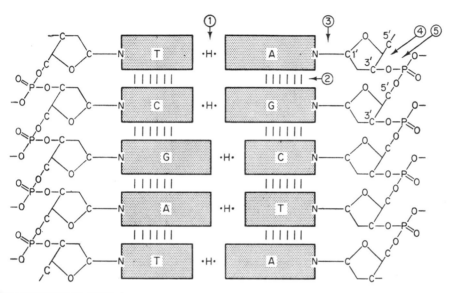

FIG. 1. Diagrammatic representation of a fragment of a double-stranded (native) DNA molecule. The bonds which are most sensitive to elevated temperatures include (1) hydrogen bonds between the complementary bases, adenine (A) and thymine (T), or guanine (G) and cytosine (C); (2) stacking interaction between the bases, moderated by the supporting water envelope; (3) N-glycosidic bonds; (4) C(3′)-O and C(5′)-O bonds; and (5)O-(3′)P and O-(5′)P phosphate ester bonds.

nearly 7 kcal. of released heat per mole of base pairs (Sturtevant et al., 1958; Rawitscher et al., 1963). The main subject of this chapter will be the stability of bonds of types (1) and (2) as a function of temperature.

III. Denaturation

A. GENERAL FEATURES

Denaturation is not a well-defined term and usually indicates a change in some readily perceptible property of a polymer as a result of a physical or chemical treatment. When discussing the thermal denaturation of DNA, the equilibrium:

$$\text{native DNA} \rightleftharpoons \text{denatured DNA}$$

and the conditions affecting this equilibrium should be taken into consideration. The dynamic aspects of this equilibrium could be described as the alternative opening and closing of short segments of the double helix ("breathing"). At room temperature, in neutral aqueous solvents, the equilibrium is predominately shifted toward the

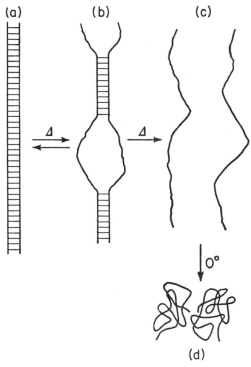

FIG. 2. Thermal denaturation of (a) double-stranded, native DNA proceeding through state (b) of partial strand dissociation at temperatures within the B to M range (Fig.4), and state (c) complete separation at temperatures above point M. Upon rapid cooling, completely denatured DNA (c) collapses into structure (d).

native state. Raising the temperature, decreasing the salt concentration, protonation or deprotonation of bases by extreme shifts of pH value, or modifying the hydrophobic interactions between bases by replacing water with organic solvents, results in shifts of the equilibrium toward the denatured state.

Denaturation of native, double-stranded DNA consists usually of three overlapping steps: (i) *collapse* of the hydrogen-bonded, double-helical structnre, (ii) *collapse* of base stacking, and (iii) *dissociation* or complete *separation* of the complementary strands. Thus, DNA in the *native, double-stranded* form (2 nucleotides per 3·4 Å of strand length) would, upon denaturation and depending on the conditions, assume either the *intermediate* form with the strands more or less dissociated but still in the helical, base-stacked configuration (one nucleotide per 3·2–3·8 Å of strand length) or would collapse completely into a *random coil* form, with the strands completely or incompletely untangled.

Evidence for the intermediate form, which might include several states of DNA, is derived from the small-angle X-ray scattering data of Luzzati *et al.* (1964) and the circular dichroism experiments of Brahms and Mommaerts (1964). The hypochromicity of poly A, at neutral or slightly alkaline pH values where no double- or triple-stranded helices are observed, also seems to indicate the presence of the intermediate form characterized by non-co-operative stacked structures (Barszcz and Shugar, 1964; Leng and Felsenfeld, 1966; Brahms *et al.*, 1966). Depending on the relative orientation of the induced transition dipoles (Tinoco, 1960) in the polynucleotides or in the intermediary form of denatured DNA, a large part of the hypochromicity is retained ("alkaline" poly A; Barszcz and Shugar, 1964) or practically complete hyperchromicity develops (DNA in organic solvents; Luzzati *et al.*, 1964).

As mentioned earlier, the cleavage of hydrogen bonds at elevated temperatures is often a gradual process with A—T bonds and solitary G—C bonds melting out first, leading to the formation of still other types of intermediate structures (conformation b in Fig. 2). This gradual melting-out reaction, which at low temperatures is responsible for hydrogen exchange in the hydrogen bonds of such a "breathing" DNA (Printz and von Hippel, 1965), is in principle fully and rapidly reversible even upon rapid cooling of the heated DNA. However, with some particular base sequences, as in the alternating dAT:dAT copolymer, the DNA can be re-arranged into a new "metastable" structure (b in Fig. 3) even when only partially denatured (Inman and Baldwin, 1962, 1964).

The denatured conformation becomes stable to rapid cooling when all of the interstrand bonds collapse with resulting complete strand dissociation and/or linear shift, so that no complementary regions are any longer situated opposite to each other and in register. The possible reversibility of reaction b → c (Fig. 2) will be considered (p. 106).

These considerations indicate that the first reaction (a ↔ b; Fig. 2) can be studied best at the ambient temperature, whereas the irreversible all-or-none reaction (b → c; Fig. 2) can be assayed even after cooling of the DNA solution. Alternatively, reaction a → b can be studied even after cooling, but only under conditions which block the reverse reaction b → a, e.g., in the presence of formaldehyde.

The rate of DNA denaturation and strand separation seems to depend on the "persistence length" of the particular DNA sequences, on the length of the uninterrupted DNA strands and on the temperature.

Thermally induced strand separation was found to be a rather slow process (3 sec.), its rate depending inversely on the G + C content of the DNA (Takashima and Arnolds, 1965). The conformational transition of DNA is associated with a heat absorption of approximately 8000 cal./mole of base pairs (Bunville *et al.*, 1965).

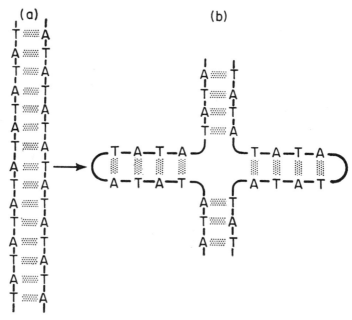

FIG. 3. Structural re-arrangement ("folding") of a dAT copolymer exposed to temperatures below the melting region. This diagrammatic representation does not take into account the fact that three or more bases must be unpaired at the tip of the hairpin turn.

The theory of unwinding, and the kinetics and the thermodynamics of denaturation are discussed by Bunville *et al.* (1965), Crothers *et al.* (1965), Crothers and Zimm (1964), Fixman (1963), Flory and Miller (1966), Fong (1964a,b), Freese and Freese (1963), Jordan (1960), Kawai *et al.* (1965), Kit (1960b), Kotin (1963), Kuhn (1957, 1961), Levinthal and Crane (1956), Lewin and Munroe (1966), Longuet-Higgins and Zimm (1960), Mahler and Cordes (1966), Rice *et al.* (1958), Schildkraut and Lifson (1965), Sturtevant *et al.* (1958), and Zimm (1960).

B. ASSAY

The most common assays used in nucleic acid denaturation are physicochemical, chemical and biological. The first two can detect both the first and the second reaction, whereas the biological assays detect in most cases only the irreversible reaction (b → c; Fig. 2), since they cannot be carried out at elevated temperatures or in solvents strongly favouring the cleavage of hydrogen and "hydrophobic" bonds.

In general, the DNA solution is heated either by a stationary or circulating water bath in conjunction with spacers surrounding the DNA-containing vessel, or by an electrical heater. The temperature is controlled either manually or by a programmer, as described by Szybalski and Mennigmann (1962). High frequency electrical heating has been used by Takashima and Arnolds (1965), and this permitted higher rates of heating. A temperature jump method was adopted by Reinert (1964) and by Spatz and Baldwin (1965).

1. Physicochemical Assays: Spectral Properties of DNA

a. *Extinction change assay* is the most commonly used method applicable to reactions a ↔ b and b → c (Fig. 2). One of the earliest papers describing this assay was that of Thomas (1954). When a solution of native double-stranded DNA is heated in a quartz cuvette, and the extinction at the wavelength of 260 mμ (O.D.$_{260}$) is simultaneously measured, one obtains a curve (R) of the type shown in Fig. 4. This curve indicates that the extinction of the DNA solution increases as the secondary structure gradually collapses and the interaction between the π electrons in the stacked bases is eliminated. Not until the edge of the plateau (M) is reached are all the interstrand bonds disrupted, assuming that we are dealing with a homogeneous population of identical DNA molecules, e.g. DNA gently released from a small bacteriophage such as coliphage T7. Point M corresponds to the temperature of irreversible denaturation (b → c; Fig. 2).

Co-inciding with point M is the sharp increase in extinction of DNA samples heated to the ambient temperatures and rapidly cooled (curve I, Fig. 4). Temperature T_i denotes the temperature at which the reaction b → c proceeds rapidly. For a homogeneous population of DNA molecules, curve I should exhibit a very sharp, almost vertical, transition at temperature T_i. The shape of curve R will depend on the gross inhomogeneities of the base composition in the DNA molecule, with long clusters of GC pairs shifting point M to the right, and long clusters of AT pairs shifting point B (the beginning of melting) to the left. The DNA of coliphage λ is a good example of a homogeneous population of molecules with a sharp T_i transition, but with an inhomogeneity of the base composition (half the molecule having an average of 10% more G + C pairs than the other half) and thus showing a broad transition (10° distance between points B and M, Fig. 4; Hershey *et al.*, 1962). The melting temperature, T_m, is defined as the midpoint on the transition curve R, as shown in Fig. 4. With heterogeneous DNA populations, both the R and I curves may exhibit broad, skewed or multistep (Pivec *et al.*, 1964) transitions, with some molecular species "melting out" earlier and others at much higher temperatures. Base

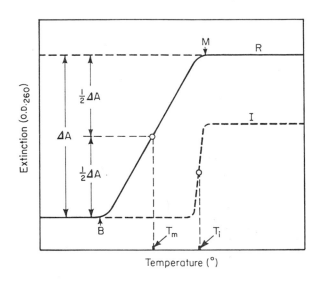

Temperature (°)

FIG. 4. An idealized graph showing the effect of temperature on the extinction of a solution of native DNA composed of a homogeneous population of molecules all of the same length and composition. Curve R ("reversible" denaturation) represents the extinction measured at the indicated (ambient) temperature. The midpoint of this transition is designated the melting temperature, T_m. Curve I ("irreversible" denaturation) represents the extinction of the DNA solution heated to the indicated temperature and rapidly cooled in ice. The extinction was then determined either at 0° or at room temperature. The midpoint transition of curve I is designated T_i. The breadth (M–B) of the transition for curve R indicates non-co-operative melting of the DNA, which takes its origin in the inhomogeneities of the linear sequence of base pairs or in the clusters of alternating base pairs, and is modulated by the ionic strength and composition of the solvent. For a homogeneous population of the DNA molecules, transition I should be quite steep, and its breadth not dependent upon the distribution of bases but governed only by statistical considerations.

composition, chemical modifications of the DNA, and the nature of the solvent can have pronounced effects on the transition temperatures (T_m and T_i) and on the profile of the transition curves R and I, as discussed in later sections. The heterogeneity of DNA samples is assessed by comparing the thermal transition profiles (Kit, 1960a).

The equipment for measuring the melting profiles of DNA consists of an ultraviolet spectrophotometer equipped with a cuvette compartment, the temperature of which can be both controlled and measured. The temperature can be regulated manually, or stepwise, with the instrument recording the R curves, as with the "recording thermo-spectrophotometer" developed by Szybalski and Mennigmann (1962).

It should be stressed that the hypochromicity is not a direct indicator of the double-stranded state, and that single-stranded oligonucleotides and polynucleotides exhibit some hypochromicity, depending on the induced transition dipole interactions between stacked bases held together by phosphate ester bonds.

The increase in extinction upon heating a solution of DNA is a measure of the extent and the type of base stacking (Applequist, 1961b). The u.v. spectra of native and heat-denatured DNA were measured in detail by Falk (1964). From the measurement of extinction changes at different wavelengths during the thermal transition, it is possible to deduce information on the base composition and distribution in the helical regions of DNA and RNA (Boublik *et al.*, 1965; Felsenfeld and Sandeen, 1962; Felsenfeld and Cantoni, 1964; Fresco, 1963; Mahler *et al.*, 1964). The theory of hypochromism has been discussed by Bolton and Weiss (1962), Devoe and Tinoco (1962), Michelson (1962), Nesbet (1964), Sinanoglu(1963), Tinoco (1960), Weiss (1963) and Ladik and Appel (1966).

b. Other optical methods which can be used to measure the thermal transition as a function of temperature include infrared and nuclear magnetic resonance (NMR) spectroscopy (Howard *et al.*, 1966), fluorescence polarization (Millar and Steiner, 1965), assays of optical rotation and rotatory dispersion (Ts'o *et al.*, 1962b; Samejima and Yang, 1965; Ulbricht *et al.*, 1966), circular dichroism (Brahms and Mommaerts, 1964), refractivity, light scattering (Rice and Doty, 1957; Geiduschek and Holtzer, 1958), small-angle X-ray scattering (Luzzati *et al.*, 1964, 1966), and any other parameter which changes with the denaturation of DNA. No changes visible to the naked eye occur during the denaturation of dilute solutions of DNA.

Electron microscopy reveals the changes in native DNA produced by heat denaturation. Rigid well-defined rods of double-stranded DNA collapse upon denaturation into amorphous "puddles" (Beer and Thomas, 1961; Bartl and Boublik, 1965), or can be extended and made visible as faint thin lines when "fixed" with formaldehyde (Freifelder *et al.*, 1964). Quantitative electron microscopic studies on preferential melting of only a part of each phage λ DNA molecule, of lower G + C content, have been carried out by Inman (1966).

2. *Physicochemical Assays: Hydrodynamic Properties of DNA*

a. Viscosity is another property of DNA which is strongly affected by denaturation (Zamenhof *et al.*, 1954; Rice and Doty, 1957; Eigner, 1960) since the rigid double-stranded molecules exhibit higher viscosity, especially at higher salt concentrations, than the collapsed denatured

molecules. Viscosity measurements can also reveal early structural re-
arrangements like those depicted in Fig. 3, since the folding of DNA or
DNA-like polymers decreases the viscosity at temperatures far below
point B (Fig. 4), where hardly any changes in extinction are perceptible
(Inman and Baldwin, 1962; Freund and Bernardi, 1963; Tikchonenko
et al., 1963; Aksenova *et al.*, 1964). There is no appreciable difference in
extinction between solutions of forms a and b (Fig. 3). Viscosity changes
might also indicate some disaggregation of native DNA molecules at temperatures much below the melting transition (Bartl and Boublik, 1965).

b. Sedimentation behaviour of DNA in 1 *M*-NaCl changes drastically
upon denaturation, since the collapsed denatured molecules sediment
about three times more rapidly than the native molecules (Studier,
1965). This assay is also quite sensitive to predenaturation conformational changes in DNA, such as those shown in Fig. 3. The method also
permits the physical separation of the native from the denatured molecules, especially by employing band centrifugation (Vinograd *et al.*, 1963)
or preparative zone centrifugation in preformed gradients.

c. Buoyant density of DNA in CsCl (Meselson *et al.*, 1957) or Cs_2SO_4
(Erikson and Szybalski, 1964) gradients increases by 10–25 mg./cm.³
upon denaturation, and this permits not only the detection but also the
physical separation of the native from the denatured molecules. Formaldehyde at concentrations below 1% increases this separation between
native and denatured DNA (Freifelder and Davison, 1962; Opara-
Kubinska *et al.*, 1963), as do Ag^+ or Hg^{2+} ions, which react preferentially with denatured DNA (Davidson *et al.*, 1965).

3. *Other Physicochemical and Chemical Techniques*

Other techniques which enable one to distinguish and/or separate the
native from the denatured DNA molecules include various chromatographic techniques, such as chromatography on methyl-esterified
albumin deposited on kieselguhr (Mandell and Hershey, 1960; Sueoka
and Cheng, 1962a), on hydroxyapatite (Bernardi, 1965) and on other
media (Rosenkranz and Bendich, 1959), adsorption on nitrocellulose
membranes (Nygaard and Hall, 1964), and the liquid–liquid extraction
method between two aqueous phases (Albertsson, 1965; Kidson and
Kirby, 1964) or one aqueous and one non-aqueous phase (Piechowska
and Shugar, 1963, 1965). In addition, there are electrophoretic mobility
(Olivera *et al.*, 1964; Costantino *et al.*, 1964), conductivity measurements
(Inman and Jordan, 1960a; Felsenfeld *et al.*, 1963), determination of dielectric properties (Mesnard and Vasilescu, 1964), electric birefringence
(Jakabhazy and Fleming, 1966), and oscillopolarographic behaviour
(Paleček, 1961, 1965; Boháček and Paleček, 1965). Denatured DNA can
also be distinguished from native DNA by its reactivity with formalde-

hyde or Pb^{2+} (Sinsheimer, 1959) and other ions (Aldridge, 1962), by its staining properties (Stone and Bradley, 1961; Nash and Plaut, 1964), and by the displacement of the titration curves (Peacocke and Walker, 1962).

4. Biological Assays

The irreversible denaturation of DNA can be followed by the loss of its transforming or infectious activity. Upon denaturation, transforming

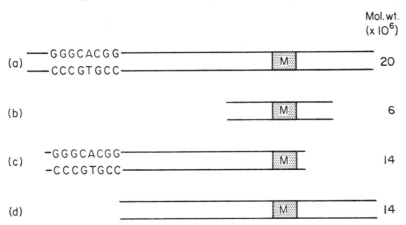

FIG. 5. Diagrammatic representation of fragments of a transforming DNA molecule, all containing the genetic marker M, but all of different sizes and base composition. The temperature of critical thermal inactivation ("melting") of marker M would be highest when M was located on fragment (a) because of the high mol. wt. (20×10^6) and presence of a GC-rich region. This region would also impart higher thermal resistance to fragment (c) when compared with fragment (d), although both are of the same size (mol. wt. 14×10^6). Marker M on the shortest (mol. wt. 6×10^6) fragment (b) would irreversibly denature at the lowest temperature.

DNA loses 90–99·9% of its biological activity, since collapsed DNA is taken up only with low efficiency by the receptor cells (Lerman and Tolmach, 1959). The inactivation profile (a plot of the loss of transforming activity versus temperature for a 3–10 min. heating followed by rapid chilling) corresponds roughly to curve I (Fig. 4) of irreversible DNA denaturation. Since the typical transforming DNA contains a mixture of various DNA fragments, each marker usually shows a different inactivation profile (Canner and Spizizen, 1965; Ganesan, 1963; Roger and Hotchkiss, 1961; Zamenhof, 1961; Zamenhof et al., 1953, 1956), often rather broad and consisting of several steps. This result indicates that denaturation is not the property of the genetic marker, but of the DNA fragment on which a given marker happens to be located

(Geiduschek, 1962; Opara-Kubinska and Szybalski, 1962; Guild, 1963; Szybalski and Opara-Kubinska, 1965b). On the average, a marker associated with longer DNA fragments (a, Fig. 5) has a higher temperature of irreversible denaturation (T_i, which corresponds to the inactivation temperature) than the same marker associated with shorter DNA fragments (b or d, Fig. 5) since, in longer fragments, there is a greater chance to encounter a longer GC-rich region which forms the residual link holding the complementary strands together up to comparatively high temperatures. However, even two molecules of the same size (c and d, Fig. 5) might be inactivated at various temperatures, depending upon whether the fragment includes both the marker M and the GC-rich region (c) or only the marker M (d). Other biological assay methods measure the effect of temperature on the infectivity of extracted bacteriophage DNA (Fiers and Sinsheimer, 1962), on the ability of DNA to serve as a template for enzymic DNA or RNA synthesis, sensitivity to specific exo- or endonucleases attacking only denatured DNA (Lehman, 1963), antigenic activity (Levine et al., 1963) and several other biological or radiobiological properties of DNA.

C. FRACTIONATION OF PARTIALLY DENATURED DNA

In DNA preparations consisting of heterogeneous populations of molecules with various base compositions and sequences, so-called partial denaturation (heating to temperatures between points B and M, Fig. 4) followed by chilling would result in the complete collapse of some molecules and little conformational change in others. This approach may be used as the basis of a fractionation of heterogeneous DNA, since the collapsed, denatured fragments can be separated from the native-like molecule by a variety of methods, including CsCl density gradient centrifugation, as attempted by Doty et al. (1959b), and methyl-esterified albumin column chromatography (Roger et al., 1966b). Miyazawa and Thomas (1965) carried out such a fractionation of sonicated DNA fragments on a heated hydroxyapatite column. The general principles of these methods as applied to the fractionation of transforming DNA were discussed in the previous section (III. B. 4 p. 83) and in the contributions of Szybalski and Opara-Kubinska (1965b) and Roger et al. (1966b).

D. MODIFICATION OF DNA SUSCEPTIBILITY TO THERMAL DENATURATION

1. Effect of Solvent

Solvents which modify the melting temperature of DNA either form bonds with DNA or interact with the water envelope surrounding the DNA double helix. In this section, only solvents which are known not to form strong bonds with DNA are discussed, although it should be realized that, since there is no clear demarcation line between strong and weak bonds, some overlapping between this and the following sections is unavoidable. Only aqueous and water-miscible organic solvents will be discussed here. It does not seem to matter whether normal (H_2O) or heavy water (D_2O) is employed, since the thermal transition of DNA extinction is not affected (Crespi and Katz, 1962; Mahler et al., 1963). However, using viscosity change or elution pattern from a hydroxy-apatite column as the criterion of DNA denaturation, Grechko et al. (1964) and Maslova and Varshavsky (1966) claimed that the melting temperature of DNA is 2–5° higher in D_2O than in H_2O.

a. Salts. The stability of DNA to denaturation usually increases with increasing ionic strength of the solvent (Dove and Davidson, 1962a,b; Marmur and Doty, 1962; Colvill and Jordan, 1963; Ts'o et al., 1963; Schildkraut and Lifson, 1965). Figure 6 depicts the increase in the melting temperature (T_m) of DNA as a function of the Na^+ concentration. This stabilization, which decreases somewhat with increasing ionic radius (Li, Na, K, Rb, Cs; Zimmer and Venner, 1962), is based mainly on the electrostatic neutralization of the repulsive negative charges on the phosphate groups.

As expected from the above data, divalent cations, such as Mg^{2+}, Co^{2+}, Ba^{2+}, Mn^{2+}, Ni^{2+}, Zn^{2+}, used in moderate concentrations have, on the average, a stronger stabilizing effect than monovalent cations (Eichhorn, 1962). At high concentrations, however, there is either little further effect of salts on the T_m value, or, with some salts such as $NaClO_4$, CCl_3COONa, CF_3COONa or KCNS (Hamaguchi and Geiduschek, 1962, Geiduschek, 1962) which are known to disrupt strongly the structure of the water envelope, there is a sharp drop in the temperature of the melting transition of DNA (Fig. 6). Moreover, such a good stabilizing salt as $MgCl_2$ seems to lose partly its protective effect on $Mg \cdot DNA$ salt at concentrations above 10^{-3} M (Lyons and Kotin, 1965), and to lower somewhat the T_m value of DNA at high NaCl concentrations (Dove and Davidson, 1962a).

The breadth of the thermal transition of many natural DNAs generally increases with a decrease in ionic strength (Dove and Davidson, 1962a,b), indicating a loss of the co-operative effects between the AT and GC regions. If this explanation is correct, one could predict that the breadth of the thermal transition should be ionic strength-independent for polymers containing only one kind of base pair, such as the dI:dC, dA:dT, or monotonous structures like dTC:dGA or dTG:dCA. This hypothesis was experimentally confirmed by Inman and Baldwin (1964), Riley et al. (1966), and Wells et al. (1965). It is possible also to widen artificially the breadth of the thermal transition by the addition of a limited amount of divalent cations (e.g., Mg^{2+}) which, having a preferential affinity for the native form of DNA, accumulate on and stabilize the remaining native regions during the melting process (Dove and Davidson, 1962a).

In a special case, such as that of the alternating dAT:dAT polymer, the breadth of the thermal transition actually increases with increasing ionic strength, which indicates an intermediate folding reaction (Fig. 3;

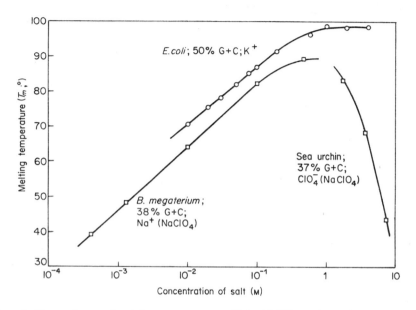

FIG. 6. Dependence of melting temperature (T_m) of DNA on the molar concentration of KCl or NaClO$_4$, plotted on the basis of the published data for *Escherichia coli* K-12 DNA in KCl (Marmur and Doty, 1962; Schildkraut and Lifson, 1965), *Bacillus megaterium* DNA in As(CH$_3$)$_2$O$_2^-$-buffered NaClO$_4$, pH = 7 (Dove and Davidson, 1962a), and sea urchin DNA in NaClO$_4$ + 0·1 M-EDTA, pH = 7 (Hamaguchi and Geiduschek, 1962).

a → b) that is favoured at higher salt concentrations (Inman and Baldwin, 1962, 1964). Melting of such folded loops is not co-operative and therefore spans a wide temperature range. Theoretical treatment of the variation in T_m value with salt concentration is presented by Kotin (1963) and Schildkraut and Lifson (1965).

b. Organic solvents and related organic compounds. If the water structure and the supporting effect of intra-water hydrogen bonding have an important effect on the stability of the DNA helix (Hamaguchi and Geiduschek, 1962; Lewin, 1964; Gordon *et al.*, 1965), one should expect that water-miscible organic solvents would profoundly affect the melting temperature. In general it was found that most organic solvents depress the melting temperature of DNA and, at high enough concentration, force the collapse of the helix even at room temperature.

Organic solvents which were studied rather extensively include alcohols such as methanol, ethanol, propanols, higher aliphatic, thio-, and cyclic alcohols (Herskovits et al., 1961; Szybalski and Mennigmann, 1962; Levine et al., 1963; Mahler and Dutton, 1964); ethylene glycol, glycerol (Duggan, 1961; Eliasson et al., 1963), formamide, N,N'-dimethyl formamide, and dimethylsulphoxide (Marmur and Ts'o, 1961; Herskovits, 1962, 1963; Aubel-Sadron et al., 1964; Subirana, 1965, 1966; Subirana and Doty, 1966; Helmkamp and Ts'o, 1961; Ts'o and Helmkamp, 1961; Ts'o et al., 1962b, 1963). An especially extensive survey of these solvents and of other organic compounds, including urea, di- and tetra-methylurea, and other urea derivatives, cyclic compounds, amides, carbamates and many other compounds, was published by Levine et al. (1963) and Herskovits (1963). The effects of N-methylpyrrolidone were studied by Kurihara et al. (1963).

These results indicate that, by choosing a proper solvent, it is possible to compare the melting profiles of various DNA samples at almost any desired temperature and ionic strength. Since melting temperature measurements are more convenient in the range of 30–50° than in the higher ranges (80° to over 100°) normally encountered with the commonly employed SSC solvent (0.15 M-NaCl + 0.02 M-sodium citrate; pH 7.5–7.8), three types of solvents are frequently used in this and other laboratories. A low melting temperature can be achieved either by using (i) aqueous buffer of very low ionic strength, (ii) the addition of an organic solvent, or (iii) a very high concentration of a salt such as sodium perchlorate (7.2 M-NaClO$_4$). Solvent (iii) is convenient since it gives a steep gradient when T_m values are plotted against G + C content (Fig. 7), and since small amounts of contaminating salts carried over with the DNA sample do not affect significantly the melting temperature, as often could be the case with solvents of type (i) or type (ii).

On the other hand, the effect of several agents which are suspected of interacting with DNA, as, e.g. acridine and antibiotic dyes (Kersten et al., 1966) can be studied only in solvents of type (i). Solvents of type (ii) are sometimes very helpful to promote the solubility of water-insoluble agents, e.g. polycyclic hydrocarbons (Kersten et al., 1966) or sterols, if the interaction between these agents and DNA is being studied.

2. Presence of Reactive Chemicals in the Solvent

Reactive chemicals present in the solvent can either stabilize the DNA structure by stabilizing the AT or GC bonds, or destabilize the DNA by reacting with the sites involved in the hydrogen bonding. They can also neutralize the negative charges on the phosphate groups, thereby decreasing the repulsive forces between the DNA strands.

a. Amines and basic proteins. Positively charged aliphatic polyamines such as spermine, spermidine, and cadaverine, raise the melting temperature of DNA (Tabor and Tabor, 1964). In this respect, their action is quite similar to that of cations such as Na^+ or Mg^{2+}, which also stabilize the secondary DNA structure by neutralizing the repulsive charges on the phosphate groups. However, the polyamines are more active on a molar basis, their activity depending on the distance between their amino groups (Mahler and Mehrota, 1963). Spermine and spermidine are

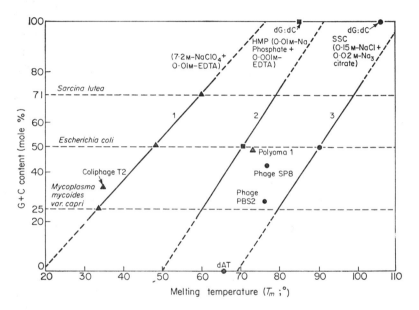

FIG. 7. Relationship between the melting temperature, T_m, and the guanine plus cytosine (G + C) content of various samples of DNA containing the usual four bases (adenine, guanine, cytosine, and thymine). The T_m values for the synthetic polydeoxynucleotides (e.g. poly dAT and poly dG:dC) and natural DNAs with a twisted ring configuration (e.g. polyoma virus) or containing exotic bases (e.g. *Bacillus subtilis* phages PBS2 and SP8) and glucose residues (e.g. coliphage T2) deviate from the linear relationship. Curve 1 (7·2 M-NaClO$_4$ + 0·01 M-EDTA; pH = 7·6–7·8) is based on the data obtained in this laboratory, and is in good agreement with the data of Hamaguchi and Geiduschek (1962) and Geiduschek (1962) obtained in 7·2 M-NaClO$_4$ + 0·1 M-EDTA (pH = 7). The T_m value for the twisted double ring of polyoma virus DNA (polyoma I) is reported by Lebowitz *et al.* (1966). The T_m value for a similar DNA ring with single strand break (polyoma II) falls very near to the curve 1. Curve 2 (0·001 M-Na$_2$HPO$_4$ + NaH$_2$PO$_4$ + 0·001 M-EDTA; pH = 7) and curve 3 (0·15 M-NaCl + 0·02 M-trisodium citrate; pH = 7) are based on the data of Marmur and Doty (1962), Takahashi and Marmur (1963), and Kallen *et al.* (1962).

the most effective of all the polyamines in raising the melting temperature of DNA, assayed also by its transforming activity (Tabor, 1961, 1962). The relative increase in melting temperature upon the addition of $2mM$-spermine or other diamines is inversely proportional to the G + C content of the DNA (Mandel, 1962; Mahler and Mehrota, 1962). Stabilization of DNA by diamines is somewhat greater in pure aqueous buffers than in buffers containing organic solvents (Mehrota and Mahler, 1964). Cyclobuxine, a steroidal diamine, has a biphasic effect on the melting of DNA, in that it increases the T_m value at low concentrations and destabilizes DNA at concentrations above $10^{-3} M$ (Mahler and Dutton, 1964). Ammonium ions and aliphatic monoamines depress slightly the melting temperature of DNA (Venner et al., 1963).

Polyamines raise the temperature of thermal transition of poly rT and poly U, the polynucleotides known to form helical structures, but are without effect on poly C or poly A, which at neutral pH values are not in a helical configuration (Szer, 1966a,b). In this respect, the effect of polyamines is similar to substitution with 5-methyl groups (Szer, 1965).

Some proteins (e.g. chymotrypsinogen; Bobb, 1966), and nuclear proteins, such as histones or protamines, also elevate significantly the melting temperature of DNA (Bonner and Ts'o, 1964; Lee et al., 1963; Huang et al., 1964; von Hahn, 1965; Walker, 1965; Savitsky, 1964). Lysine-rich histones were found to be more active in this respect than arginine-rich nucleohistones (Hnilica and Billen, 1964). The addition of polylysine to DNA or to poly I:poly C resulted in two-step thermal transition curves. The first step (at a lower temperature) corresponded to the melting of the free DNA or polynucleotide double-helix, and the second step (at a higher temperature) to the melting of the polylysine-containing complex (Tsuboi et al., 1966). It is difficult to reconcile these well-documented data with the claims of Zimmermann (1965), who stated that the addition of protamine seems to destabilize the resulting nucleoprotein to heat, as assessed by the determination of the melting temperatures of DNA from the viscosity versus temperature plots.

The polypeptide antibiotic, phleomycin, increases the T_m value of poly dAT. When Mg^{2+} and the antibiotic are present, the T_m value is less affected, but the breadth of the transition is increased, indicating that under these conditions the melting of poly dAT is less co-operative. With other DNA samples, the main effect of phleomycin is to broaden the transition curve as long as the T_m value is below 80°, since, beyond this temperature, the DNA-antibiotic complex does not seem to be stable (Falaschi and Kornberg, 1964).

Denaturation of DNA has even been studied in intact nucleoprotein structures, including spermatozoa (Chamberlain and Walker, 1965) and chromosomes in situ (Nash and Plant, 1964). Some proteins such as

4+T.

ribonuclease, which show preferential affinity for A—T pairs, can have a destabilizing effect on DNA (Felsenfeld *et al.*, 1963), or under different conditions increase the melting temperature (Kopylova-Sviridova, 1964). Histones, at the extreme 25:1 ratio of histone:DNA, were claimed to depress the melting temperature of DNA (Šormova, 1962).

b. Actinomycins, acridines and related compounds. Actinomycins react principally with guanine residues in the native DNA configuration and stabilize preferentially the G—C bonds (Haselkorn, 1964; Reich and Goldberg, 1964; Permogorov and Lazurkin, 1965). This interaction results in a shift of point M (Fig. 4) towards higher temperatures with a resulting increase in T_m value and a large increase in the value for T_i (Haselkorn, 1964; Kersten *et al.*, 1966). Actinomycin does seem to intercalate (Crothers, 1966) between the planes of the complementary purine–pyrimidine pairs, introducing, however, additional distortions not observed with acridine dyes (Lerman 1964), chlorpromazine (Ohnishi and McConnell, 1965), ethidium bromide (Waring, 1965) and the anthracycline antibiotics. All these intercalating compounds raise the melting temperature of DNA (Gersch and Jordan, 1965; Walker, 1965; Kersten *et al.*, 1966) with a relatively higher effect observed for DNA with a high A + T content (Kleinwächter and Koudelka, 1964; Bhuyan and Smith, 1965; Ward *et al.*, 1965). Miracil D (Weinstein *et al.*, 1965) and chloroquine (Allison *et al.*, 1965) also increase the melting temperature of DNA. Only under special conditions do the antibiotics chromomycin, olivomycin and mithramycin have an effect on the T_m value of DNA (Kersten *et al.*, 1966).

c. Cupric and silver ions. Cu^{2+} ions react preferentially with the G—C pairs of the DNA in the *denatured* configuration (Eichhorn and Clark, 1965; Coates *et al.*, 1965), thus decreasing the melting temperature of the DNA. Also the differences between the T_m and T_i values (Fig. 4) become smaller, and the T_m values decrease with increasing G + C content of the DNA, a relationship which is opposite to that in the absence of Cu^{2+} ions (Venner and Zimmer, 1964, 1966; Hiai, 1965). Silver ions also react preferentially with the G—C pairs, but this interaction results in thermal stabilization of the DNA, RNA and polynucleotides (Jensen, 1965; Daume *et al.*, 1966).

d. Agents which react principally with A—T pairs. Depending on whether an agent has preferential affinity for the AT pairs in the native DNA configuration or in the non-hydrogen bonded state, it will have respectively a stabilizing or a destabilizing effect. The former effect would increase the T_m value and diminish the difference between the T_m and T_i values, while the latter would decrease the T_m value, broaden the thermal transition curve and widen the difference between the T_m and T_i values. For example, Hg^{2+} ions react preferentially with non-hydrogen bonded thymine residues, and force a "denaturation" in the form of a small lateral displacement of DNA strands with a simultaneous bridging between the opposite thymine residues (Katz, 1962). On the other hand, nogalamycin, which seems to bind preferentially to the A—T pairs in the native DNA configuration, stabilizes DNA towards thermal denaturation (Bhuyan and Smith, 1965; Kersten *et al.*, 1966).

e. *Formaldehyde* is a widely used agent, which reacts with the amino groups of the A, C and G bases when these are not in the paired, hydrogen-bonded configuration. This agent therefore lowers somewhat the T_m value (Grossman *et al.*, 1961) but, of more importance, it renders reaction a → b (Fig. 2) irreversible, and fixes the DNA in a partially or completely denatured state (Stollar and Grossman, 1962). The latter property earned formaldehyde the informal name of the "chaperoning" agent (Thomas and Berns, 1962). Formaldehyde is experimentally very useful in preserving the denatured amino-hydrogen bond-free configuration of DNA (Inman, 1966), but it must be used in moderate concentrations and for a short time, since its secondary reactions include the crosslinking of the complementary DNA strands (Freifelder and Davison, 1962). Formaldehyde (3·63%) was found to react slowly with DNA heated to submelting temperatures (60°; 10^{-2} M-phosphate buffer), causing denaturation of the DNA at a rate highly dependent on the A + T content of the DNA, and increasing 13-fold with the change from 27% to 57% A + T (Aleinikova and Poverennyi, 1964).

f. *pH value.* The pH value of the solvent within 2 or 3 units of neutrality has little effect on the melting profile of natural DNAs (Zimmer and Venner, 1963, 1965). However, the T_m values of some polymers are very pH-dependent even in the neutral range, since pH controls the charge state of the polynucleotides. For example, in 0·1 M-Na$^+$ the T_m value of the dC:dC (actually dC·H$^+$:dC) helix varies from 97° (pH = 5·0) through 73° (pH = 6) to 49° (pH = 7·0) with a still more precipitous drop above pH = 7 (Inman, 1964a; Table 1), since, in this pH range, the dC·H$^+$ strand becomes deprotonated. Very low or very high pH values decrease profoundly the melting temperature of natural DNAs (Lewin and Pepper, 1965; Mora, 1965) or, in other words, cause the collapse of the secondary structure even at very low temperatures, because certain hydrogen bonds between base pairs are broken by the addition or removal of protons (Gulland *et al.*, 1947; Dove and Davidson, 1962a,b). The breadth of the thermal melting transition narrows at low pH values (Zimmer and Venner, 1964). The threshold values of the change, which results in the denaturation of DNA, depend on the G + C content, temperature and ionic strength, and amount to approximately 0·55 charge units per base pair relative to pH = 6 for 37% G + C, and 0·78 for 64% G + C, at 25° in 0·1 M-NaCl (Bunville *et al.*, 1965).

TABLE I. *Melting Temperatures of Synthetic Polynucleotides in Various Solvents*

Polynucleotide	MELTING TEMPERATURES (°)				
	SOLVENTS				
	Na$^+$(pH 7·0)			SSC[35]	Other Solvents
	10^{-2}M	10^{-1}M	M		
rA:rA					pH = 5·05; 0·2 M-Na$^+$: 50[2]
					pH = 4·5; 0·15 M-Na$^+$:∼85[1]
rA	36[27]			36[27]	
dA					no secondary helical structure[2]
r6̄meA					no secondary helical structure[2]
r6̄dimeA					no secondary helical structure[2]
rU:rU					10^{-2}M-Mg^{2+}:8·5[5, 23, 25]
dU:dU					10^{-2}M-Mg^{2+}:35[5]
rT:rT				29[23]	10^{-2}M-Mg^{2+}:36[21, 23, 25]
r̄meT					no secondary helical structure[2]
dT					no secondary helical structure[2]
r$\overline{FU}$:r$\overline{FU}$				2·5[22]	
r$\overline{CU}$:r$\overline{CU}$					0·1M-Mg^{2+},0·05M-Na$^+$: < 1[32]
r$\overline{BU}$:r$\overline{BU}$					0·1M-Mg^{2+},0·05M-Na$^+$:18·5[3]
r$\overline{IU}$:r$\overline{IU}$					0·1M-Mg^{2+},0·05M-Na$^+$:14·5[3]
r$\overline{\psi U}$:r$\overline{\psi U}$					0·1M-Mg^{2+},0·05M-Na$^+$:61[34]
dA:rU					not identified; converted to dA:rU:rU at all concentrations tested[1, 26]
dA:rU:rU	15[1]	45·5[1]	75·5[1]		
dA:dT	48[1]	68·5[1]	86·2[1]		3·8 M-Na$^+$:97·5[1]; 0·15-M-Na
dA:dT:dT		24·5[1]		85·5[1]	:78[32]
(dA:dT)rU		27[1]		72[1]	0·15M-Na$^+$:70[32]
rA:rU	38[1, 10]	57[1]	75[1]	59[23]	0·5 M-Na$^+$:69·5[1]
		59[5]	81[13]	61[3]	1/10 SSC:43[22]
rA:rU:rU	20[1, 10]	50·5[1]	84[10]	60[30]	0·5 M-Na$^+$:72[1]
		56[10]			
(rA:dT)rU					0·5 M-Na$^+$:74[1]
rA:dT	46[1]	64[1]	76[1]		0·5 M-Na$^+$:81[1]
rA:dT:dT					0·5 M-Na$^+$:78[1]
rA:rT		72[2]		79[5, 23]	1/10 SSC:63[22]
rA:r$\overline{FU}$				55[22]	1/10 SSC:40[22]
rA:r$\overline{BU}$					1/10 SSC:69[22]
rA:r$\overline{FU}$:r$\overline{FU}$					0·15M-Na$^+$:50[32]
rA:r$\overline{CU}$:r$\overline{CU}$				82[22]	0·15M-Na$^+$:86[32]
rA:r$\overline{BU}$:r$\overline{BU}$				87[22]	0·5 M-Na$^+$:95[32]
rA:r$\overline{IU}$:r$\overline{IU}$					0·5 M-Na$^+$:95[32]
r6̄meA:rU					pH 7·4; 0·08 M-Na$^+$:∼13[29]
r6̄dimeA:rU					no secondary helical structure[2]
rAU:rAU	47·5[4]	66[3]			

TABLE I.—(contd.)

Polynucleotide	Na$^+$(pH 7·0)			SSC[35]	Other Solvents
	$10^{-2}M$	$10^{-1}M$	M		
rAT:rAT		(72)[5]			
rABU:rABU	67·3[4]	79[3]			
rA(d)U:rA(d)U	18·4[4]				
dAU:dAU	37·2[9]	58[9]			
dAT:dAT	39·9[9]	61[7,9]	74[7,9]	66[15]	
dABU:dABU	49·5[9]	65[9]	73[9]		
rI:rI:rI				43·5[6,13]	
rI:rI:rA		39[20,31]	51[13]		
dI:dI		18[6,7]	49[6,7]		
rG:rG	(75)[16]				0·002 M-Na$^+$:100[14,17]
dG:dG					no data available
rmeC:rmeC					pH 4, 0·1 M-Na$^+$:79[21] pH 4, 0·1 M-Na$^+$:82[21]
rC:rC					0·15 M-Na$^+$ pH$\Big\}$ 3·5 4·4 5 5·5[19] 61 73 57 24
rBC:rBC					no secondary helical structure[32]
dC:dC					0·1 M-Na$^+$ pH$\Big\}$ 5 6 7[7] 97 74 49 0·4 M-Na$^+$ pH$\Big\}$ 5 6 6·9 7[7] 90 65 44 37
dBC:dBC					0·4 M-Na$^+$; pH 6·9:33[19]
dI:dI:dBC		26[8]			
dI:dBC	53[9]	72[8,9]	91[8]		
dI:dC	27·5[6]	46·1[6]	55[6]		
dI:rC	10·1[6]	35·4[6]	52·6[6]		
rI:dC	34·8[6]	52·3[6]	64·3[6]		
rI:rC	41·5[6]	58[31] 60·2[6] 62[28]	75·3[6]	69[13]	M-Na$^+$$\begin{cases}0·02 0·11 0·15 0·2 ^{21,28,32}\\52·5 61 63 66·5\end{cases}$
rI:rmeC		78[28]			M-Na$^+$ $\begin{cases}0·02 0·11 0·2^{21,2}\\68·5 79 83\end{cases}$
r7meI:rC					0·15M-Na$^+$:39[33]
r7meI:rBC					0·15M-Na$^+$:56[33]
rI:rBC					0·15M-Na$^+$:89[33]
dG:dC	82[9]	102[9]		106[15]	10^{-4} M-Na$^+$ + EDTA:63·5[4]
dG:rC					10^{-4} M-Na$^+$ + EDTA:70·5[4]

(TABLE I.—*contd.*)

Polynucleotide	MELTING TEMPERATURES (°)				
	SOLVENTS				
	Na⁺(pH 7·0)			SSC[35]	Other Solvents
	$10^{-2}M$	$10^{-1}M$	M		
rG:dC					10^{-4} M-Na⁺ + EDTA:90[4]
					10^{-4} M-Na⁺ + EDTA:97[4]
rG:rC					80% CH_3OH;
					10^{-3} M-Na⁺:89[17]
rG:r$\overline{BC}$					80% CH_3OH;
					10^{-3} M-Na⁺:100[17]
dTC:dGA				84[24]	1/10 SSC:68[24]
dTG:dCA				91·5[24]	1/10 SSC:76[24]
DNA (50% G + C)				90·5[15]	

[1] Riley *et al.* (1966)
[2] Shugar and Szer (1962) (calculated by Riley *et al.*, 1966)
[3] Chamberlin *et al.* (1963)
[4] Chamberlin (1965, 1966)
[5] Swierkowski, Szer and Shugar (1965)
[6] Chamberlin and Patterson (1965)
[7] Inman (1964a)
[8] Inman (1964b)
[9] Inman and Baldwin (1964)
[10] Massoulié *et al.* (1964)
[11] Ross and Sturtevant (1962)
[12] Stevens and Felsenfeld (1964)
[13] Doty *et al.* (1959a)
[14] Fresco and Massoulié (1963)
[15] Marmur and Doty (1962)
[16] Hayashi and Egami (1963)
[17] Pochon and Michelson (1965)
[18] Van Holde *et al.* (1965)
[19] Hartman and Rich (1965)
[20] Sarkar and Yang (1965)
[21] Szer (1965)
[22] Szer and Shugar (1963)
[23] Szer *et al.* (1963)
[24] Wells *et al.* (1965) and R. D. Wells (personal communications)

[25] There is no evidence that rT:rT, rU:rU and rFU:rFU are twin stranded complexes (D. Shugar, personal communication)
[26] M. J. Chamberlin (personal communication)
[27] Barszcz and Shugar (1964); 0·2 M-Na⁺ was chosen to depress the melting temperature, since heating of poly A to temperatures above 75° results in cleavage of the polynucleotide chain at pH 5 or lower, rendering the melting curves irreversible. At pH 7, poly A does not form the double-stranded helical structure, but still develops considerable hyperchromicity upon heating; such a thermal transition does not seem to depend on the ionic strength.
[28] Szer and Shugar (1966)
[29] Griffin *et al.* (1964)
[30] Fresco (1963) claims that a 1:1 mixture of poly A and poly U forms a triple helix rA:rU:rU in SSC, with some free poly A remaining in solution. The phase diagram relating the T_m values for rA:rU and for rA:rU:rU to the Na⁺ concentration is presented in this reference (p. 127)
[31] Sigler *et al.* (1962)
[32] Massoulié *et al.* (1966)
[33] Michelson and Pochon (1966)
[34] Michelson (1965)
[35] 0·15M-NaCl+0·02M-Na₃·citrate, pH7·5

g. Other agents. Several compounds known to exhibit various biological activities have been examined for their effect on the thermal transition of DNA. These compounds included carcinogens, mutagens or related substances such as urethan (ethyl carbamate) and methylcarbamate (Kaye, 1962), 2-naphthylamine derivatives, β-propiolactone, hydroxylamine (Troll *et al.*, 1963, and personal communication), butter yellow (Singh, 1965) and caffeine (T'so *et al.*, 1962a) which depress the melting temperature, and carcinogenic hydrocarbons (Kersten *et al.*, 1966) which have no effect. In addition, several purines and pyrimidines depress the melting temperature of DNA and of other polynucleotides, indicating the presence of competitive stacking interactions between the polynucleotides and these monomers (Ts'o *et al.*, 1962a). The effect of purines seems to be specific for nucleic acids (Akinrimisi and Ts'o, 1964). Oestrone and related hormones were reported to be still more specific in lowering the melting transition only of human placental DNA, but not of bacterial DNA or of poly dAT and poly dGdC (Goldberg and Atchley, 1966).

3. Modifications of the Chemical and Physical Structure of DNA

a. Base composition. Since interstrand interactions within G—C pairs seem to be stronger than within A—T pairs, the melting temperature depends strongly on the GC content of DNA (Marmur and Doty, 1959, 1962; Doty *et al.*, 1959b; Doty, 1961; Marmur *et al.*, 1962: the legend does not match Fig. 4 in this paper (Marmur *et al.*, 1962) and should be replaced by Fig. 4 of Marmur and Doty (1962)). Conversely, it is possible to predict the GC content of a DNA from determination of the T_m values, which offer a simple and convenient method for the rapid survey of the base composition of DNA derived from different sources. This has proved to be an important criterion in taxomomic studies (Marmur *et al.*, 1963a; Falkow *et al.*, 1962; Colwell *et al.*, 1965). The relationship between the melting temperature and the G + C content for three commonly used solvents is presented in Fig. 7. The effect of the base composition on the melting temperature in these and other solvents, including SSC and HMP (0·0025 M-disodium phosphate + 0·050 M-monosodium phosphate + 0·001 M-EDTA; pH = 6·8; Lanyi, 1963), PE buffer (10^{-3} M-Na$_2$HPO$_4$, 10^{-4} M-EDTA; pH = 7·6; Kersten *et al.*, 1966), 7·2 M-NaClO$_4$, 6·5 M-CF$_3$COONa, and 51% methanol (Geiduschek, 1962; Hamaguchi and Geiduschek, 1962) is discussed in the above mentioned references.

As seen in Fig. 7, the melting temperatures of synthetic DNA-like polymers with 0% (poly dAT) or 100% G + C content (poly dG:dC) do not wholly conform to the linear relationship established for the natural DNAs. This is not surprising in view of the special features of their very uniform structure; for example, re-arrangements of the type depicted in Fig. 3 could play a very major role only in a polymer such as poly dAT. Other types of complex re-arrangements were observed by Inman (1964 a,b) during heating of the dI:dC polymer, which was converted to a mixture of dI:dI and dC:dC. In the presence of d$\overline{BC}$ the following reaction takes place: dI:dC + d$\overline{BC}$ → dI:d$\overline{BC}$ + dC.

The stability of DNA as related to the sequence of the neighbouring bases was discussed by DeVoe and Tinoco (1962).

b. Role of the sugar residues. The melting temperatures of several other DNA- or RNA-like polymers are summarized in Table I. Double helices of two polyribonucleotides are usually more thermostable than those composed of polydeoxyribonucleotides. Hydrogen bonds potentially supplied by the 2'-hydroxyl groups seem to provide additional thermal stability for ribose-containing polymers, although the mechanism of this phenomenon is not understood. Double helices composed of ribo- and deoxyribonucleotide strands generally exhibit intermediate stability, with the ribopurines supplying more heat resistance than the ribopyrimidines. On the other hand, the stability of an alternating double-stranded polymer, which contains only purine residues in one strand and only pyrimidine residues in the other (dTC:dGA), is lower ($T_m = 84°$) than that of the DNA-like polymer with purine and pyrimidine residues evenly distributed among the strands (dTG:dCA; $T_m = 91·5°$; Wells et al., 1965). The T_m of the latter polymer (91·5°) resembles closely that of natural DNA of 50% G + C content ($T_m = 90·5°$; Table I).

The study of these polymers is further complicated by the capacity of some of them to form stable triple-stranded helices, such as a helix containing two strands of poly U and one poly A strand (Stevens and Felsenfeld, 1964; Lipsett, 1964; Lipsett et al., 1961; Riley et al., 1966; Massoulié et al., 1964; Fresco, 1963; Blake and Fresco, 1966; Rich, 1960). The thermal transition of mixed poly AB:poly U double and triple helices (where B denotes any purine or pyrimidine) was studied by Bautz and Bautz (1964). Poly A:poly U interactions were extensively studied by Warner (1963), who was one of the first to recognize the true nature of the thermal collapse of such double-helical complementary structures. Reduction of poly U decreases its affinity for poly A (Cerutti et al., 1966). Poly G (low to moderate mol. wt.) seems to exhibit a pronounced hypochromicity with a sharp thermal transition at temperatures above 100° (Fresco and Massoulié, 1963; Pochon and Michelson, 1965; Table I). This relatively high melting temperature indicates a marked stability of the secondary poly G structure. The properties of complexes between poly G and poly C (1:1) are discussed by Fresco (1963), Chamberlin (1965), Riley et al. (1966), Pochon and Michelson (1965), and Ulbricht et al. (1966). At slightly acid pH values, poly A or poly C forms helical structures and shows a rather abrupt thermal transition, whereas at neutral pH value poly rA changes extinction only gradually during heating (Fasman et al., 1964; Fresco and Klemperer, 1959), and poly rU does not exhibit any thermal transition above 10° (Singer et al., 1962; Table I). A helical complex between poly I and protonated poly C (poly $C·H^+$) is more stable than a similar complex with non-protonated poly C (Giannoni and Rich, 1964). The melting temperature of poly rT, and its various complexes with poly A and poly U, were studied in detail by Świerkowski et al. (1965) and Naylor and Gilham (1966). Other papers pertaining to the thermal behaviour of ribo- or deoxyribopolymers include Chamberlin et al. (1963),

Chamberlin (1965), Inman (1964a,b), Riley et al. (1966), Brahms (1965), Pochon and Michelson (1965), Van Holde et al. (1965), Hartman and Rich (1965), Szer (1965), Wells et al. (1965), Michelson et al. (1966), and Byrd et al. (1965). High melting temperatures were reported for double-stranded RNA, as for example that of wound tumour and reoviruses (Gomatos and Tamm, 1963), and for the replicative form of single-stranded RNA phages or viruses (Erikson and Franklin, 1966). Melting of the complementary DNA: mRNA complexes derived from Escherichia coli and coliphage T2 was studied by Khesin and Shemiakin (1962).

c. *Single-stranded DNA and RNA* show a considerable rise in extinction upon heating, although this transition is usually more gradual (Doty et al., 1959a) than that observed for double-helical molecules (Fig. 4). This hypochromicity existing at lower temperatures indicates some degree of intra- or intermolecular hydrogen bonding between the complementary bases together with stacking of the bases. A broad thermal transition indicates a lack of a co-operative effect between these individual helical regions, which were postulated to exist in several hairpin-like turns (Fresco et al., 1960; Doty, 1961). These and other authors (Bielka et al., 1964a,b) have discussed the calculation of the degree of helicity in DNA as determined on the basis of thermal hypochromicity. Complex changes in the s-RNA conformation upon heating, followed by the denaturation of the helical regions, were recently described by Henley et al. (1966). Thermal interconversion of s-RNA between two forms, stabilized by Mg^{2+}, was described by Lindahl et al. (1966) and by Gartland and Sueoka (1966). As with DNA, many mono- and divalent ions, including Na^+, Mg^{2+}, and Ni^{2+}, shift the thermal transition of RNA towards higher temperatures (Doty et al., 1959a; Fuwa et al., 1960; Boedtker, 1960; Cox and Littauer, 1962). However, Mg^{2+}, which by itself is 25,000 times more effective than Na^+, stabilizes RNA at much higher Na^+ concentrations (Boedtker, 1960; Goldberg, 1966) than is the case with DNA (Dove and Davidson, 1962a). These results point to some specific interactions between Mg^{2+} ions and the 2'-hydroxyl groups.

Non-specific intermolecular interactions, in the presence of Mg^{2+} or at high salt concentrations, were observed with ribosomal- and m-RNA (Hayes et al., 1966a; Marcot-Queiroz and Monier, 1965; Kubinski et al., 1966). These interactions were most probably caused by the formation of double- or triple-stranded complexes between the short sequences of complementary bases in a manner similar to that reported for dC-rich sequences in denaturated DNA and G-rich sequences in r-RNA or poly IG (Opara-Kubinska et al., 1964; Kubinski et al., 1966). Poly C forms complexes with 16S and 23S r-RNA at salt concentrations above 0·1 M (Hayes et al., 1966b; Kubinski et al., 1966). In the presence of poly U or poly C, purines, purine ribosides and nucleotides

4*

were shown to form stacked, helical base-paired structures (Howard *et al.*, 1964, 1966; Huang and T'so 1966). These structures, which seem to be triple-stranded at the lower and double-stranded at the higher temperatures, exhibit definite melting transitions, usually within the 0-40° range. No analogous complexes were observed between the pyrimidine monomers and purine polynucleotides.

Even in the absence of polynucleotides, some association between dinucleotides (Chan *et al.*, 1966) or monomers was observed, as for instance the formation of helical structures (gels) by GMP (Gellert *et al.*, 1962; Howard and Miles, 1965), and other purine-purine or complementary purine-pyrimidine hydrogen-bonding interactions (Katz and Penman, 1966; Schweitzer *et al.*, 1965; Pullman *et al.*, 1965; Van de Vorst and Pullman, 1965; Shoup *et al.*, 1966). Another indication of the interactions between bases or nucleosides and polynucleotides or DNA is the lowering of the temperature of helix-coil transition by purine and pyrimidine derivatives (T'so *et al.*, 1962a).

d. Base substitutions. In several naturally occurring DNAs, the pyrimidine base cytosine is replaced by 5-hydroxymethylcytosine in glucose-free or in glucosylated forms (T-even coliphages), whereas thymine is replaced either by 5-hydroxymethyluracil (SP-8 and related *Bacillus subtilis* phages; Kallen *et al.*, 1962) or by uracil (PBS1 and PBS2 *B. subtilis* phages; Takahashi and Marmur, 1963). All of these DNAs have T_m values lower than those predicted from their G + C contents. The thymine in DNA can also be artificially replaced by 5-chloro, 5-bromo-, or 5-iodouracil, a change which increases the thermal stability but decreases the alkali denaturation stability of native DNA (Szybalski, 1961; Kit and Hsu, 1961; Szybalski and Mennigmann, 1962; Baldwin and Shooter, 1963), as could be predicted from comparison of the pK_a of thymine with that of its halogenated analogues. On the other hand, the replacement of thymine by 5-trifluoromethyluracil decreases the T_m value of DNA (Szybalski *et al.*, 1963a; Gottschling and Heidelberger, 1963). Replacement of uracil by 5-fluorouracil in single-stranded phage RNA has little effect on its thermal transition (Shimura *et al.*, 1965), whereas incorporation of 8-azaguanine destabilizes RNA and decreases hypochromicity (Levin and Litt, 1965).

Substitution of uracil in position C-5 modifies the melting transition of the corresponding polyribonucleotides (order of stability: IU > BrU > U > ClU > FU) and their heterocomplexes with poly A (IU ∼ BrU > ClU > U > FU) as reported by Massoulié *et al.* (1966). This paper and the communication of Michelson and Pochon (1966) discuss the effect of halogenation and N-1, N-6 or N-7 methylation on the melting of poly I:poly C helices and of homopolynucleotides.

e. Crosslinking of DNA. Exposure of DNA to certain bifunctionally acting chemicals, including mustards (Geiduschek, 1961), formaldehyde (Freifelder and Davison, 1962), and reduced mitomycin (Szybalski and Iyer, 1964), results in covalent links being formed between the complementary DNA strands. Ultraviolet irradiation (Marmur *et al.*, 1961a; Marmur and Grossman, 1961; Opara-Kubinska *et al.*, 1963), exposure to HNO_2 (Geiduschek, 1961; Becker *et al.*, 1964) or to solutions of low pH (Freese and Cashel, 1964) can also result in DNA crosslinking. If the number of crosslinks in each molecule is low, the melting behaviour of the DNA, as measured by the a → b transition (Fig. 2), is hardly affected, but complete strand separation (reaction b → c) becomes impossible, and such crosslinked DNA heated beyond point M (Fig. 4) returns to the native configuration even upon rapid chilling.

f. Shearing of DNA. The length of the complementary sequences in comparatively short, double-stranded oligomers dictates their thermal stability, because of the additive effects of the hydrogen bonding and stacking forces. Thus, shearing of DNA resulting in fragments less than a few hundred nucleotide pairs long should decrease the melting temperature. The denaturation of short DNA fragments should also become an irreversible process, since the rate of unsnarling and of complete dissociation of such short strands should be higher than for high mol. wt. DNA.

Closely spaced single-strand breaks on one of the DNA strands could result in the excision-like loss of short single-strand fragments much below the average melting temperature. This was observed with coliphage T5 DNA (known to possess single-strand interruption) exposed to submelting temperatures. This process of "partial denaturation" (i.e. a loss of single-strand fragments) was further accelerated by subcritical shearing forces (Hershey *et al.*, 1963; Sternglanz and Doty, 1966).

Formation of complementary double-stranded helices and the "melting out" of such structures was observed between oligonucleotides composed of only a few bases, and even for mononucleotides, which stack along a single strand of the complementary polynucleotide when the temperature is low enough and the solvent conducive for such an interaction (Ts'o *et al.*, 1962a; Schweizer *et al.*, 1965; Howard *et al.*, 1966; Huang and Ts'o, 1966; Singer *et al.*, 1962).

g. Other effects. Increased hydrostatic pressures seem to stabilize the secondary structure of DNA, since the T_m increases by 6° at 2700 atmospheres pressure (Hedén *et al.*, 1964). Ultraviolet or X-ray irradiation decreases T_m, hypochromicity, and the renaturability of DNA (Marmur *et al.*, 1961a; Boháček and Blažiček, 1965; Ekert and Tisne, 1966; Harriman and Zachau, 1966; Hagen and Wellstein, 1965).

4. Spontaneous Renaturation of DNA

Some natural DNAs can return to a native-like conformation following seemingly complete thermal denaturation and rapid cooling, and in this respect they resemble artificially crosslinked DNA.

a. *High molecular weight DNA.* A small fraction (5–10%) of almost any high mol. wt. DNA renatures spontaneously following heat denaturation and rapid cooling (Rownd, 1963; Szybalski et al., 1963b; Szybalski, 1964; Alberts, 1965; Subirana, 1965). Such a DNA fraction seems to contain interstrand crosslinks which are terminally located and might be a by-product of the shearing reaction during the DNA extraction. However, further shearing does not produce many more such crosslinks (Alberts, 1965). Residual protein has also been claimed to account for such crosslinks (Subirana, 1965). One may wonder whether this phenomenon is related to the observation of Yoshikawa (1966) on the stable DNA-protein complex.

Spontaneous renaturation of a small fraction of DNA is closely related to the origin of the residual transforming activity in denatured DNA (Lerman and Tolmach, 1959; Marmur and Lane, 1960; Ginoza and Zimm, 1961; Roger and Hotchkiss, 1961). Although earlier papers indicated that the residual biological activity might be the property of the denatured molecules (Guild, 1961; Rownd et al., 1961), later data suggested that the small native-like fractions might carry most of this residual transforming activity (Rownd, 1963; Marmur et al., 1963b; Lanyi, 1963; Barnhart and Herriott, 1962; Szybalski et al., 1963b; Szybalski, 1964; Chevallier and Bernardi, 1965). It might depend on the surface properties of the recipient cells, and whether they could (Pneumococci?) or could not take up the denatured DNA. For example, *Escherichia coli* protoplasts could be infected either by single-stranded or double-stranded φX-174 phage DNA, but with higher efficiency for the single-stranded DNA which must be in a circular form. Only double-stranded λ phage DNA is infectious to the *E. coli* host, with the additional requirement of short terminal single-stranded, cohesive regions (Strack and Kaiser, 1965).

b. *Enzymically synthesized DNA* is fully renaturable, since its structure consists of many loops with two complementary sequences folded upon each other (Schildkraut et al., 1964). Each such loop could be formally considered as a terminally crosslinked DNA segment, with the terminal phosphate ester bond equivalent to the crosslink.

c. *Natural poly dAT.* The DNA of some crabs contains up to 30% of a poly dAT-like polymer (Sueoka and Cheng, 1962a,b) which is almost completely renaturable upon heating and rapid cooling, since the separated poly dAT strands can either come into register in any linear alignment or can form double-stranded structures when folding upon themselves. Such renatured poly dAT-like material, however, has a structure resembling more that outlined in Fig. 3b than the original linear double helix (Davidson *et al.*, 1965). The presence of the long dAT sequences is suspected also in the high A + T fraction of mouse DNA which renatures spontaneously (Walker and McLaren, 1965).

d. Circular DNA. Circularity in double-stranded DNA, with no interruptions in either strand, imposes severe restrictions on strand unsnarling and lateral shift. Therefore, such DNA, which is found in some oncogenic viruses such as polyoma virus (Vinograd *et al.*, 1965), in mitochondria (Borst and Ruttenberg, 1966), or as the replicative form of phage ϕX-174 (Kleinschmidt *et al.*, 1963), renatures spontaneously upon heating and rapid cooling, unless single-strand breaks occur as a side reaction during the thermal treatment. Also, the denaturation, as measured by u.v. extinction changes, is shifted to higher temperatures for a perfect double ring ($T_m = 73°$ in $7 \cdot 2$ M-NaClO$_4$) as compared with an open ring ($T_m = 40°$; Lebowitz *et al.*, 1966).

Two more phenomena are observed during thermal (or alkali) denaturation of circular DNA, which reveal another feature of its tertiary conformation. The circular molecule has an additional supertwist with an orientation the same as that of the helicity of DNA. During inception of the denaturation process, the supertwist disappears, and is compensated by the unwinding of the double helix. Further unwinding of the complementary strands twists the circle in the opposite direction, ultimately forming a very compact twisted structure with an anomalously high sedimentation constant and buoyant density (Vinograd *et al.*, 1965; Vinograd and Lebowitz, 1966).

Two more types of circular DNA have been studied from the point of view of thermal denaturation and renaturation. DNA released from λ coliphages can assume a circular configuration because of the cohesion of its complementary, single-stranded ends (Hershey *et al.*, 1963). Many other phage DNAs could acquire such cohesive ends by limited treatment with an exonuclease (Thomas, 1966). The kinetics of cohesion and thermal dissociation of λ DNA-circles was studied by Wang and Davidson (1966). Their data indicate that approximately 10 nucleotide pairs constitute the cohesive junction in the λ DNA, and that the joining of the cohesive ends is an identical process for cyclization and for the association of two half-molecules. The latter result indicates that large DNA molecules are hydrodynamically equivalent to a random coil. The circular permutation of T-even coliphage DNA permits an artificial formation of circular molecules by thermal annealing of denatured DNA (Thomas and McHattie, 1964).

e. Reversibly denatured DNA. DNA molecules heated below the temperature of complete dissociation of the strands (point M; Fig. 4) would renature spontaneously even upon rapid cooling. In some water-miscible organic solvents, e.g. methanol or formamide, point M is apparently not reached at room temperatures for DNA with long G + C sequences, which are prevalent in some species such as bacilli (Opara-Kubinska *et al.*, 1964), and such DNAs therefore renature upon dilution or removal of the organic solvent by dialysis. Such an incomplete DNA denaturation or dissociation of DNA strands was studied extensively by Geiduschek and Herskovits (1961) and by Geiduschek (1962).

E. PROOF OF THE DOUBLE-STRANDED NATURE OF DNA

Native DNA has been shown to consist of two subunits of equal mass which need not be subdivided again in further replication, and which can be separated on heating (Meselson and Stahl, 1958). The results of these experiments, and of others reviewed by Baldwin (1964), are consistent with a semiconservative model for DNA replication, in which the two subunits are identified as two complementary polydeoxynucleotide strands of the DNA double helix. The attempts of other workers (Cavalieri and Rosenberg, 1962, 1963) to provide evidence for a conservative mode of DNA replication were not convincing; their views were discussed and experimentally refuted by Baldwin and Shooter (1963), Baldwin (1964) and Chamberlin (1965). The preparative separation of the individual complementary DNA strands of several phages (Cordes *et al.*, 1961; Marmur and Greenspan, 1963; Tocchini-Valentini *et al.*, 1963; Aurisicchio *et al.*, 1964; Kubinski *et al.*, 1966) and bacteria (using either the affinity of one strand to poly G, Opara-Kubinska *et al.*, 1964; chromatography on a denatured DNA agar column saturated with RNA, Doskočil and Hochmannová, 1965; or alkaline CsCl gradient or chromatographic fractionation, Guild and Robison, 1963; Roger *et al.*, 1966a) provides further and conclusive evidence that thermal denaturation effectively and completely separates the strands, contrary to the notions of the proponents of the conservative mode of DNA replication (Cavalieri *et al.*, 1962) who suggested that heating results only in the collapse of the hydrogen-bonded structure and leaves the original complementary strands still firmly entangled. The available experimental evidence therefore strongly favours a semiconservative mode of replication of double-stranded DNAs. Dispersion of DNA fragments among the progeny could be accounted for by genetic recombination-like phenomena (Meselson and Weigle, 1961; Kozinski and Kozinski, 1963). Single-stranded DNAs of some phages seem not to be transmitted to the progeny (Sinsheimer, 1961).

IV. Depuration and Phosphate Ester Bond Breakage

Depurination, an acid-catalysed reaction, is greatly accelerated by elevated temperatures (Tamm *et al.*, 1952; Brown and Todd, *in* Chargaff and Davidson, 1955). Its rate seems to increase at temperatures approaching the melting temperature of DNA (Ginoza and Zimm, 1961), although a two-fold greater loss of guanine as compared with adenine is not consistent with the higher thermal resistance of the hydrogen-bonded configuration in the GC as compared with the AT pairs. The mechanism of depurination is not known at the present time, but is believed to be initiated by the protonation of the ring oxygen in deoxyribose, breaking of this ring, and the formation of a highly reactive $C(1') = N(9)$ double bond, which is easily hydrolysed (Kenner, 1957;

DEPURINATION (H^+—catalysed)

Micheel and Heesing, 1961). This explanation was preferred to that involving the quaternization of the purine nitrogen, because of the greater acid stability of trimethylammonium glucoside as compared with dimethylammonium glucoside (Kenner, 1957). Thus protonation of the purine or pyrimidine ring, a reaction which occurs at lower pH values than the protonation of the ring oxygen in deoxyribose, should stabilize the N-glycosidic bond and interfere with the second protonation. The latter interference might account for the stability of the pyrimidine-deoxyribose bond, whereas in the purine ring the protonation charge would be more evenly distributed and interfere less with the protonation of the deoxyribose ring oxygen (Dekker, 1960). Glycosides are in general more stable than 2-deoxyglycosides, due probably to the inductive effect of the 2'-hydroxyl group, and this accounts for the stability of RNA to depurination.

Depurination of DNA by heating, either in solution or in the dry form, was studied in detail by Greer and Zamenhof (1962). This paper also contains a complete list of references to earlier work on the effect of heat on transforming DNA. The loss of guanine was twice as great as the loss of adenine, and there was no splitting of pyrimidines. The data on breakage of the glycosidic linkages in the free deoxyribosides did not parallel the results obtained with DNA. Estimation of the activation energy for depurination varied from 28 (Greer and Zamenhof, 1962) to 34–35 kcal./mole (Ginoza and Zimm, 1961; Fiers and Sinsheimer, 1962).

Following depurination and opening of the sugar ring, the adjoining 3'-phosphate ester bond becomes sensitive to heat and to alkali, since the presence of a free aldehyde group on the deoxyribose favours a β-elimination reaction (Tamm et al., 1953; Brown and Todd in Chargaff

(β) ELIMINATION REACTION (OH⁻—catalysed)

and Davidson, 1955; Brown, 1963; Michelson, 1963). Single-strand breaks were found to be associated with the thermal treatment of DNA but it is possible that some of these breaks are produced by contaminating DNases (Ginoza and Guild, 1961).

Released purines could be determined by chemical, radiochemical or microbiological methods, the last method being extremely sensitive (Bramwell et al., 1966). Single-strand breaks can be measured with even greater precision by employing sedimentation techniques, thermal transition measurements or sensitivity to exonucleases, in conjunction with the denaturation process (Strauss and Wahl, 1964; Davison et al., 1964; Summers and Szybalski, 1965).

During *subcritical* heating below the melting temperature, transforming DNA gradually loses its biological activity (Ginoza and Guild, 1961; Roger and Hotchkiss, 1961). Whereas removal of a single purine base is sufficient to inactivate the infectivity of single-stranded ϕX-174 DNA (Fiers and Sinsheimer, 1962) and might result in inactivation of the transforming capacity of DNA (Ginoza and Zimm, 1961), the results of van Sluis and Stuy (1962) indicated a dominant role for strand breakage in the subcritical inactivation of transforming DNA with "unlinking" of the linked marker similar to that observed during DNase treatment. The slow kinetics of this process are quite different from the abrupt loss of activity experienced by DNA during denaturation (*critical* heating). Also this subcritical inactivation, which is fully irreversible, interferes with the thermal renaturation process. 5-Bromouracil-labelled transforming DNA is more sensitive to subcritical thermal inactivation than the control DNA (Szybalski and Opara-Kubinska, 1965a). Thermal inactivation of the biological activity (infectivity) of single-stranded RNA has been studied by Ginoza (1958), Papaevangelou and Youngner (1961), Eigner *et al.* (1961), Gordon and Huff (1962), and Gordon *et al.* (1963), and inactivation of single-stranded circular DNA by Fiers and Sinheimer (1962). In the last of these studies, the depurination step, which results in a loss of infectivity, can be clearly distinguished from the subsequent chain scission assayed by the change in sedimentation behaviour and susceptibility to exonuclease. Ginoza *et al.* (1964), in their comparative study on the subcritical thermal inactivation of single-stranded ϕX-174 phage DNA and RNA extracted from tobacco mosaic virus and R17 phage, found that, at 37°, the infectivity of the RNA was about 30 times more rapidly inactivated than that of the single-stranded DNA of the same size. Estimates of the rate of RNA and of double- and single-stranded DNA degradation between 5° and 100° are tabulated by Eigner *et al.* (1961). The half life for single-stranded DNA (one phosphate ester bond break per 10,000 nucleotides), as determined by sedimentation and viscosity measurements, corresponded to 1160 days (5°), 10 days (37°) and 15 min. (100°). At these temperatures, the half life for RNA was 23 days, 15 hr. and 5 min. Native DNA was estimated to be degraded 10 times more slowly than denatured DNA. Adamiec and Shugar (1959) have studied in detail the thermal degradation of apurinic DNA, and Barszcz and Shugar (1964) the degradation of poly A. The theory of the thermal degradation of DNA was discussed by Applequist (1961a).

V. Renaturation and "Partially" Denatured States

Once two complementary single DNA strands are completely separated, reformation of the original double helix becomes a rather improbable, kinetically controlled reaction. To initiate renaturation, the complementary regions on the two strands have to collide in the proper steric orientation, forming a hydrogen-bonded, stacked "nucleation" centre. Once such an event occurs, the "zipping up" of the remaining portions of the DNA will proceed on either side of the nucleation centre, since partially dissociated DNA, in the form depicted in Fig. 2b (p. 76), could exist only in a very narrow range of the critical conditions between points B and M of Fig. 4 (p. 80). Thus denaturation and renaturation in principle are all-or-none reactions. *Partially denatured* (or *partially renatured*) DNA, often referred to in the literature, comprises either (i) different types of *damaged* DNA, in which a fragment of a complementary strand was lost (Fig. 8a) or some of the hydrogen bond-forming amino groups were selectively formylated (Fig. 8b) or chemically modified in some other manner; or (ii) *metastable* states of DNA caused by a mismatching between the repetitive sequences on the DNA strands, with resulting loop formation (Fig. 8c), or by the conformation analogous to that shown on Fig. 3b (p. 78). Both of the latter metastable forms (Figs. 8c and 3b) should return to thermodynamically more stable regular double helices when exposed for a sufficiently long time to renaturation conditions. Similarly form (a) (Fig. 8) can renature to an almost perfect double helix (d) when it encounters the missing fragment.

Synthetic DNA-like polymers, such as poly dA:dT, should renature perfectly whenever two complementary strands encounter each other. Some lengthwise alignment is, however, necessary if the single-stranded free end is to become converted to a double-stranded structure. These could also be paired with another complementary strand, extending in this way the length of the molecule. Thus renaturation of a mixture of poly dA and poly dT strands can produce a double-stranded product of high molecular weight but with many single-strand interruptions.

An alternating poly dAT copolymer would produce, during denaturation and renaturation, many terminal and interstitial folded structures (Fig. 3b). Incomplete renaturation is especially pronounced in natural poly dAT containing approximately 3% G + C pairs, which would become mismatched during rapid quenching (Sueoka and Cheng, 1962b; Davidson *et al.*, 1965; Pochon *et al.*, 1965). One may conclude that, although the renaturation of these polymers seems to be almost perfect if the criterion of hypochromicity is employed, the renatured structures differ in their conformation from the original (native) molecules.

Obviously all of these phenomena play important roles during the denaturation and renaturation of natural DNA, since short nucleotide sequences of the dG:dC, dA:dT or dAT:dAT type could exist in such DNAs (Kubinski *et al.*, 1966). Interaction between several single DNA strands, of the type already discussed for poly dA:dT, will result in large aggregates in renatured DNA (May, 1964), especially with a homogeneous DNA preparation derived from small phages and if the concentration of DNA during renaturation is quite high (Kozinski and Beer, 1962).

A. CONDITIONS FOR THERMAL RENATURATION

Previous considerations indicate that the conditions for successful and rapid renaturation are: (1) elevated temperatures, which increase the

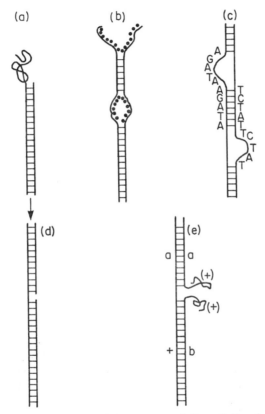

FIG. 8. A diagram showing various types of "partially denatured" DNA molecules, (a) depicts a molecule with a missing fragment of one complementary strand; (b) a molecule "fixed" in the partially denatured configuration by a reaction of the denatured regions with formaldehyde (dots indicate the bases, the amino groups of which reacted with formaldehyde); (c) a metastable configuration resulting from mispairing between repetitive regions; (d) a double-stranded molecule with a single-strand break, derived from renaturation between the molecule (a) and the missing single-stranded fragment; (e) a product of renaturation between two genetically marked DNA molecules, one $a+$ and another $+b$. One of the renaturation products is molecule (e), which is composed of one intact $a+$ strand and two complementary fragments, $a+$ and $+b$. Markers a and b on such a molecule behave as if they were genetically linked.

mobility of single strands and favour their unfolded elongated conformation, but still lie below point B on the melting curve (Fig. 4); (2) an optimum concentration of the complementary strands, leading to frequent bimolecular encounters but not to multimolecular aggregations; and (3) moderately high salt concentrations (e.g. $0.3–0.5$ M-NaCl), which neutralize the negative charge on the phosphate groups and decrease the electrostatic repulsion between the strands. It was possible to renature DNA even at low temperatures, if the extended state of the strands was maintained by using a high concentration of $NaClO_4$ (7.2 M, 35°; Geiduschek, 1962) or a pH in the neighbourhood of 10.5 (Hogness, 1966), providing conditions (2) and (3) were maintained. Marmur and T'so (1961) did not succeed in renaturing denatured DNA by slowly diminishing the formamide concentration or slow neutralization of acid-denatured DNA, but the ionic strength during the attempted renaturation was not specified by these authors.

Renaturation was realized for many DNA species, including biologically active transforming DNA, as first shown by Marmur and Lane (1960). Renaturation is also inadvertently observed during a slow second heating of denatured double-stranded DNA from phages and bacteria. The extinction versus temperature curve first rises, indicating the breakage of weak non-co-operative bonds, drops again, indicating renaturation, and then rises sharply at the original melting temperature (Grossman et al., 1961). Such composite curves are not observed with isolated noncomplementary DNA strands (Marmur and Cordes, 1963). Renaturation of DNA denatured in the presence of Cu^{2+} ions was claimed to be an extremely efficient process (Suzuki and Moriguchi, 1965), most probably since strand separation was incomplete.

Many theoretical and practical aspects of DNA renaturation, and the kinetics of this reaction, were discussed by Doty (1961), Marmur and Doty (1961), Marmur et al. (1963b), Wada and Yamagami (1964), Subirana (1966), Subirana and Doty (1966), and Thrower and Peacocke (1966). The various models for the formation of hybrid transforming units by thermal renaturation of the DNA mixture derived from two genetically marked strains, and the problem of genetic transcription from a unique-versus-any strand of transforming DNA, are discussed by Herriott (1961a,b; 1963; 1965), Marmur et al. (1963b), Rownd (1963), Lanyi (1963), Bresler et al. (1964a,b), and Zaleska and Pakula (1964); model (e) or (d) (Fig. 8) is currently preferred over others (Herriott, 1965).

B. RENATURATION AS A MEASURE OF HOMOLOGY

1. *Caesium Chloride Gradient Techniques*

The denatured molecule of DNA should renature perfectly, barring accidents of the type discussed in previous sections. Thus perfect renaturation is a sign of complete homology between the complementary base sequences. This is conceptually easiest to detect when working with a homogenous population of DNA, in which all of the molecules are identical as to length and base composition, e.g. DNA derived from coliphage T7 (Schildkraut et al., 1962). When such DNA is prelabelled with heavy isotopes ^{2}H or ^{15}N, or with 5-bromodeoxyuridine (or a naturally dense label such as glucose in T-even phage DNA; Erikson and Szybalski, 1964), combined with unlabelled DNA and centrifuged in the CsCl gradient, two well separated bands are obtained. Similarly, two bands are observed if each of these DNAs is separately denatured, renatured, treated with *Escherichia coli* exonuclease I to remove non-renatured regions, and then banded together in the CsCl gradient. However, if renaturation is carried out on the mixture of denatured molecules, not two but *three* bands are obtained, with the new intermediate density band containing hybrid duplex molecules with one strand derived from the originally non-labelled ("light") and the second strand from the labelled ("heavy") molecules. The ratio of the "heavy" to "hybrid" to "light" material should be 1:2:1. The amount of material in the hybrid band is a rough measure of the homology, both intramolecular and intermolecular. Intermolecular heterology has to be considered with all materials of molecular weight larger than the DNA of small phages, since the DNA is then composed of many non-identical molecules or molecular fragments of various lengths, base compositions and sequences. The lower the degree of homology, the smaller the amount of material that appears in the hybrid band, either since it does not form a stable hybrid or because its nonhomologous regions are digested by the exonuclease used for selective removal of the single-stranded unpaired regions.

Exonuclease is an important tool in this type of hybridization experiment, since otherwise five poorly defined instead of three sharp peaks appear in the CsCl gradient upon successful hybridization; these correspond in order of increasing density to (1) renatured "light" DNA, (2) denatured or only partially renatured "light" DNA, (3) a broad band of renatured and imperfectly paired "hybrid" DNA, (4) renatured "heavy" DNA, and (5) denatured or only partially renatured "heavy" DNA. Upon treatment with a nuclease specific only for single-stranded I NA, peaks (2) and (5) disappear and the double-stranded regions of the partially renatured DNA shift to peaks (1), (3) and (4).

With extremely heterogeneous DNA samples, such as those derived from mammalian sources, efficient renaturation is almost impossible, since it is difficult to achieve a high enough concentration of homologous DNA molecules and not to increase the total DNA concentration to values that are impractical because of interfering viscosity. Renaturation of mammalian DNA could, however, be performed on fractionated DNA (e.g. on the basis of its G + C content), since a given fraction attains a much higher degree of homogeneity. The detection of DNA homologies by the CsCl density centrifugation method, and its genetic and taxonomic implications, were discussed in detail by Marmur and Schildkraut (1963), Marmur et al. (1961b, 1962, 1963a,b), and Schildkraut et al. (1961a, 1962). A similar technique has been used in studying homologies and complementarities between DNA and RNA or RNA-like polymers (Rich, 1960; Schildkraut et al., 1961b).

2. Adsorption and Entrapment Techniques

The CsCl density gradient technique requires that a dense label be attached to one of the DNA partners. Techniques described in this section do not require this rather cumbersome density labelling, but instead use radioactive DNA. One of the DNA partners (high mol. wt.) is immobilized in a column material, and the other (low mol. wt.) is filtered through this immobilized DNA phase under renaturing, denaturing or neutral conditions. The methods of nucleic acid immobilization include non-covalent (Walker and McCallum, 1966) or covalent chemical binding to the column material (Adler and Rich, 1962; Bautz and Hall, 1962; Britten, 1963; Gilham, 1964), trapping of high mol. wt. DNA in agar granules (Bolton and McCarthy, 1962) or, the adsorbing of denatured DNA on nitrocellulose discs, without (Nygaard and Hall, 1964) or with thermal fixation (Gillespie and Spiegelman, 1965; Denhardt, 1966). The amount of labelled DNA or RNA specifically bound by such immobilized DNA, under conditions of thermal renaturation, and eluted under conditions of dissociation of the hybrids, is considered to be a measure of the molecular homology between the various DNAs. This technique was used widely for the detection of genetic and taxonomic relationships between DNAs of various species and tissues or between DNA and its transcription products, mRNA, rRNA and sRNA (Attardi et al., 1965a,b; Bautz and Hall, 1962; Goodman and Rich, 1962; Hayashi et al., 1965; Hoyer et al., 1965; Humm and Humm, 1966; Martin and Hoyer, 1966; Oishi and Sueoka, 1965; Ritossa and Spiegelman, 1965; Spiegelman and Yankofsky, 1965; Tocchini-Valentini et al., 1963; Yankofsky and Spiegelman, 1962a,b). In the latter case, it is important to eliminate specific binding between the G-rich regions in RNA and the dC-rich regions in DNA, by using post-treatment with T_1RNase and annealing in the presence of competing poly C (Opara-Kubinska et al., 1964; Kubinski et al., 1966).

The minimum sizes of RNA fragments which would still hybridize with denatured DNA are 50 nucleotides at 67°, 32 nucleotides at 55°, 17 nucleotides at 44°, and somewhat over 6 nucleotides at 23° and 37°

(Gillespie and Spiegelman, 1966). The variation in the degree of methylation of the r-RNA did not seem to have any effect on its hybridization with denatured DNA (McConkey and Dubin, 1966).

VI. Conclusions and Summary

Elevated temperatures have two principal effects on nucleic acids: (1) disruption of the secondary structure held together by non-covalent bonds, including hydrogen bonds, and a variety of stacking forces, and (2) cleavage of the N-glycosidic and of phosphate ester bonds.

(1) The first effect leads to a very abrupt change in the conformation of double-stranded native DNA with a disruption of the double helix and dissociation of the individual complementary strands. Within a narrow range of temperatures, this reaction is rapidly reversible, but it becomes irreversible upon rapid cooling, as soon as the last hydrogen bond is broken (between the G—C clusters) and the strands become fully separated. Such completely denatured DNA does not regain the helical double-stranded configuration upon cooling, and assumes a random coil structure. Thus, thermal denaturation of helical DNA followed by chilling is, in principal, an all-or-none phenomenon; the DNA either regains its native helical configuration or collapses into the denatured form. Some exceptional cases of stable "partially denatured" states are discussed in the text.

Denatured or single-stranded DNA or RNA is not entirely devoid of quasihelical, base-stacked, and nonspecifically hydrogen-bonded regions. The extent of these regions depends on the temperature and on the solvent. Thus, heating of such a DNA or RNA results in a "melting" process heralded by a slow increase in extinction. However, this gradual unfolding of randomly coiled DNA or RNA is different from the abrupt co-operative "melting" process observed for double-stranded DNA.

(2) Temperature-induced and proton-catalysed cleavage of N-glycosidic bonds is of practical importance only for the purine deoxynucleotides in DNA. This reaction, and breakage of the phosphate ester bonds which is caused by a base-catalysed β-elimination reaction (and also by a proton-catalysed reaction) as a sequel to the depurination, are the chief reasons for the loss of biological activity by nuclease-free DNA at temperatures below the thermal denaturation range. Thermal inactivation of nuclease-free RNA is caused by the cleavage of the phosphate ester bonds, but the chemical mechanism, which depends on the formation of cyclic 2'-3' phosphates, is quite different from that for DNA. Although single-stranded RNA is resistant to depurination, its biological activity (infectivity) is 30 times more sensitive to thermal inactivation

than that of single-stranded DNA. It should be stressed that, with impure DNA and RNA preparations, the omnipresent nucleases are the main cause of the degradation and inactivation, and that this enzymic reaction is also temperature-dependent.

No thermal treatment can reverse the damage to the covalent bonds in DNA, although enzymic repair systems present in the cells may reunite the broken phosphate bonds and replace missing or modified bases in double-stranded DNA, using the complementary undamaged strand as a template. On the other hand, denatured but otherwise undamaged DNA can regain its original helical double-stranded structure when subjected to thermal treatment at submelting temperatures in appropriate solvents. This purely physical, non-enzymic renaturation process is a bimolecular reaction. In the first rate-determining step, two complementary strands must collide in the proper alignment and form the first "nucleation" centre between the complementary base sequences. "Zipping up" of the whole double helix then follows as the second, rapid and inevitable step.

As usual in nature, many complications and idiosyncrasies are observed with these basically simple processes. Many of these secondary phenomena are discussed in this review.

VII. Acknowledgements

I wish to thank Dr. E. P. Geiduschek, of the University of Chicago, Dr. M. J. Chamberlin of the University of California, and my colleagues at the University of Wisconsin, Drs. W. F. Dove, A. Guha, P. Sheldrick, and R. D. Wells for critical reading of parts of the manuscript and for many helpful comments and additions. I am also grateful to the many investigators who have authorized the references to unpublished material and supplied us with their manuscripts. For that and for many stimulating discussions, helpful criticism and exchange of pertinent correspondence I am especially obliged to Drs. B. M. Alberts, R. L. Baldwin, H. Boedtker, P. Brookes, D. M. Brown, K. Burton, A. Dipple, J. Eigner, R. L. Erikson, J. R. Fresco, D. Hayes, R. B. Inman, S. Lewin, G. N. Ling, H. R. Mahler, J. Marmur, A. M. Michelson, H. T. Miles, A. Rich, M. Riley, D. Shugar, R. F. Steiner, I. Tinoco, Jr., W. Troll, P. O. P. T'so, H. Venner, J. Vinograd, R. C. Warner, and B. H. Zimm.

Thanks are also due to Dr. Elizabeth H. Szybalski for her editorial assistance, and for the far more than routine editorial help of Dr. A. H. Rose. Support for writing this review came from grants from the National Science Foundation (B-14976), the National Cancer Institute (CA-07175) and the Alexander and Margaret Stewart Trust Fund.

References

Adamiec, A. and Shugar, D. (1959). *Acta Biochim. Polonica* **6**, 425.

Adler, D. J. and Rich, A. (1962). *J. Amer. chem. Soc.* **84**, 3977.

Akinrimisi, E. O. and Ts'o, P. O. P. (1964). *Biochemistry* **3**, 619.

Aksenova, N. N., Vorobyev, V. I. and Kushner, V. P. (1964). *Biochimia* **29**, 161.

Alberts, B. M. (1965). Ph.D. Thesis: Harvard University, Cambridge, Mass., U.S.A.

Albertsson, P. A. (1965). *Biochim. biophys. Acta* **103**, 1.

Aleinikova, T. L. and Poverennyi, A. M. (1964). *Biochimia* **29**, 945.

Aldridge, W. G. (1962). *Nature, Lond.* **195**, 284.

Allison, J. L., O'Brien, R. L. and Hahn, F. E. (1965). *Science* **149**, 1111.

Applequist, J. (1961a). *Arch. Biochem. Biophys.* **95**, 42.

Applequist, J. (1961b). *J. Amer. chem. Soc.* **83**, 3158.

Attardi, G., Huang, P. C. and Kabat, S. (1965a). *Proc. nat. Acad. Sci. Wash.* **53**, 1490.

Attardi, G., Huang, P. C. and Kabat, S. (1965b). *Proc. nat. Acad. Sci. Wash.* **54**, 185.

Aubel-Sadron, G., Beck, G. and Ebel, J. P. (1964). *Biochim. biophys. Acta* **80**, 448.

Aurisicchio, S., Dore, E., Frontali, C., Gaeta, F. and Toschi, G. (1964). *Biochim. biophys. Acta* **80**, 514.

Baldwin, R. L. (1964). *In* "The Bacteria", (I. C. Gunsalus and R. Y. Stanier, Eds.), Vol. 5, pp. 327–372. Academic Press, New York.

Baldwin, R. L. and Shooter, E. M. (1963). *J. molec. Biol.* **7**, 511.

Barnhart, J. and Herriott, R. M. (1962). *Fed. Proc.* **21**, 374.

Barszcz, D. and Shugar, D. (1964). *Acta Biochim. Polonica* **11**, 481.

Bartl, P. and Boublik, M. (1965). *Biochim. biophys. Acta* **103**, 678.

Bautz, E. K. F. and Bautz, F. A. (1964). *Proc. nat. Acad. Sci. Wash.* **52**, 1476.

Bautz, E. K. F. and Hall, B. D. (1962). *Proc. nat. Acad. Sci. Wash.* **48**, 400.

Becker, Jr., E. F., Zimmerman, B. K. and Geiduschek, E. P. (1964). *J. molec. Biol.* **8**, 377.

Beer, M. and Thomas, Jr., C. A. (1961). *J. molec. Biol.* **3**, 699.

Bernardi, G. (1965). *Nature, Lond.* **206**, 779.

Bhuyan, B. K. and Smith, C. G. (1965). *Proc. nat. Acad. Sci. Wash.* **54**, 566.

Bielka, H., Schneiders, I. and Henske, A. (1964a). *Acta biol. med. german* **13**, 13.

Bielka, H., Junghahn, I. and Schneiders, I. (1964b). *Z. f. Naturforsch.* **19b**, 1121.

Blake, R. and Fresco, J. (1966). *J. molec. Biol.* **19**, 145.

Bobb, D. (1966). *Biochim. biophys. Acta* **119**, 639.

Boedtker, H. (1960). *J. molec. Biol.* **2**, 171.

Boháček, J. and Blažiček, G. (1965). *Biophysik* **2**, 233.

Boháček, J. and Paleček, E. (1965). *Coll. Czech. Chem. Comm.* **30**, 3455.

Bolton, E. T. and McCarthy, B. J. (1962). *Proc. nat. Acad. Sci. Wash.* **48**, 1390.

Bolton, H. C. and Weiss, J. J. (1962). *Nature, Lond.* **195**, 666.

Bonner, J. and Ts'o, P. O. P., Eds. (1964). "The Nucleohistones", p. 398. Holden-Day, Inc., San Francisco.

Borst, P. and Ruttenberg, G. J. C. M. (1966). *Biochim. biophys. Acta* **114**, 645.

Boublik, M., Pivec, L., Šponar, J. and Šormova, Z. (1965). *Coll. Czech. Chem. Comm.* **30**, 2645.

Brahms, J. (1965). *J. molec. Biol.* **11**, 785.

Brahms, J. and Mommaerts, W. F. H. M. (1964). *J. molec. Biol.* **10**, 73.

Brahms, J., Michelson, A. M. and Van Holde, K. E. (1966). *J. molec. Biol.* **15**, 467.

114   WACLAW SZYBALSKI

Bramwell, J., Nichols, B. and Ginoza, W. (1966). *Abstr. Biophys. Soc.* p. 68.
Bresler, S. E., Kreneva, R. A., Kushev, V. V. and Mosevitskii, M. I. (1964a). *J. molec. Biol.* **8**, 79.
Bresler, S. E., Kreneva, R. A., Kushev, V. V. and Mosevitskii, M. I. (1964b). *Z. Vererbungsl.* **95**, 288.
Britten, R. J. (1963). *Science* **142**, 963.
Brown, D. M. (1963). *In* "Comprehensive Biochemistry", (M. Florkin and E. H. Stotz, Eds.) Vol. 8B, pp. 209–269. Elsevier, Amsterdam.
Bunville, L. G., Geiduschek, E. P., Rawitscher, M. A. and Sturtevant, J. M. (1965). *Biopolymers*, **3**, 213.
Byrd, C., Ohtsuka, E., Moon, M. W. and Khorana, H. G. (1965). *Proc. nat. Acad. Sci. Wash.* **53**, 79.
Canner, M. K. and Spizizen, J. (1965). *J. Bact.* **80**, 915.
Cavalieri, L. F. and Rosenberg, B. H. (1962) *In* "The Molecular Basis of Neoplasia", pp. 44–58, Univ. of Texas Press, Austin, Texas.
Cavalieri, L. F. and Rosenberg, B. H. (1963). *Progr. nucleic acid Res.* **2**, 1.
Cavalieri, L. F., Small, T. and Sarkar, N. (1962). *Biophys. J.* **2**, 339.
Cerutti, P., Miles, H. T. and Frazier, J. (1966). *Biochem. Biophys. res. Commun.* **22**, 466.
Chamberlin, M. J. (1965). *Fed. Proc.* **24**, 1446.
Chamberlin, M. J. (1966) *In* "Procedures in Nucleic Acid Research", (G. L. Cantoni and D. R. Davies, Eds.), pp. 513–519, Harper and Row, New York.
Chamberlin, M. J., Baldwin, R. L. and Berg, P. (1963). *J. molec. Biol.* **7**, 334.
Chamberlin, M. J. and Patterson, D. L. (1965). *J. molec. Biol.* **12**, 410.
Chamberlain, P. J. and Walker, P. M. B. (1965). *J. molec. Biol.* **11**, 1.
Chan, S. I., Bangerter, B. W., and Peter, H. H. (1966). *Proc. nat. Acad. Sci. Wash.* **55**, 720.
Chargaff, E. and Davidson, J. N. (1955). "The Nucleic Acids", Vol. 1, 692 pp. and vol. 2, 576 pp. Academic Press, New York.
Chargaff, E. and Davidson, J. N. (1960). "The Nucleic Acids", Vol. 3, 588 pp. Academic Press, New York.
Chevallier, M.-R. and Bernardi, G. (1965). *J. molec. Biol.* **11**, 658.
Coates, J. H., Jordan, D. O. and Srivastava, V. K. (1965). *Biochem. Biophys. res. Commun.* **20**, 611.
Colwell, R. R., Citarella, R. V. and Ryman, I. (1965). *J. Bact.* **90**, 1148.
Colvill, A. J. E. and Jordan, D. O. (1963). *J. molec. Biol.* **1**, 700.
Cordes, S., Epstein, H. T. and Marmur, J. (1961). *Nature, Lond.* **191**, 1097.
Costantino, L., Liquori, A. M. and Vitagliano, V. (1964). *Biopolymers* **2**, 1.
Cox, R. A. and Littauer, U. Z. (1962). *Biochim. biophys. Acta* **61**, 197.
Crespi, H. L. and Katz, J. J. (1962). *J. molec. Biol.* **4**, 65.
Crothers, D. M. (1966). *40th. Nat. Colloid Symp.* Madison, Wis., U.S.A.
Crothers, D. M., Kallenbach, N. R. and Zimm, B. H. (1965). *J. molec. Biol.* **11**, 802.
Crothers, D. M. and Zimm, B. H. (1964). *J. molec. Biol.* **9**, 1.
Daume, M., Dekker, C. A. and Schachman, H. K. (1966). *Biopolymers* **4**, 51.
Davidson, N., Widholm, J., Nandi, U. S., Jensen, R., Olivera, B. M. and Wang, J. C. (1965). *Proc. nat. Acad. Sci. Wash.* **53**, 111.
Davison, P. F., Freifelder, D. and Holloway, B. W. (1964). *J. molec. Biol.* **8**, 1.
Dekker, C. A. (1960). *Annu. Rev. Biochem.* **29**, 453.
Denhardt, D. T. (1966). *Biochem. Biophys. res. Commun.* **23**, 641.
DeVoe, H. and Tinoco, Jr., I. (1962). *J. molec. Biol.* **4**, 500.
Doskočil, J. and Hochmannová, J. (1965). *Biochim. biophys. Acta.* **108**, 504.

Doty, P. (1961). *Harvey Lectures* **55**, 103.
Doty, P., Boedtker, H., Fresco, J. R., Haselkorn, R. and Litt, M. (1959a). *Proc. nat. Acad. Sci. Wash.* **45**, 482.
Doty, P., Marmur, J. and Sueoka, N. (1959b). *Brookhaven Symp. Biol. No.* **12**, 1.
Dove, W. F. and Davidson, N. (1962a). *J. molec. Biol.* **5**, 467.
Dove, W. F. and Davidson, N. (1962b). *J. molec. Biol.* **5**, 479.
Duggan, E. L. (1961). *Biochem. Biophys. res. Commun.* **6**, 93.
Eichhorn, G. L. (1962). *Nature, Lond.* **194**, 474.
Eichhorn, G. L. and Clark, P. (1965). *Proc. nat. Acad. Sci. Wash.* **53**, 586.
Eigner, J. (1960). Ph.D. Thesis: Harvard University, Cambridge, Mass., U.S.A.
Eigner, J., Boedtker, H. and Michaels, G. (1961). *Biochim. biophys Acta* **51**, 165.
Ekert, B. and Tisne, M. R. (1966). *Biochim. biophys. Acta* **114**, 481.
Eliasson, R., Hammarsten, E., Lindahl, T., Björk, I. and Laurent, T. C. (1963). *Biochim. biophys. Acta* **68**, 234.
Erikson, R. L. and Franklin, R. M. (1966). *Bact. Rev.* **30**, 267.
Erikson, R. L. and Szybalski, W. (1964). *Virology* **22**, 111.
Falaschi, A. and Kornberg, A. (1964). *Fed. Proc.* **23**, 940.
Falk, M. (1964). *J. Amer. chem. Soc.* **86**, 1226.
Falkow, S., Ryman, I. R. and Washington, O. (1962). *J. Bact.* **83**, 1318.
Fasman, G. D., Lindblow, C. and Grossman, L. (1964). *Biochemistry* **3**, 1015.
Felsenfeld, G. and Cantoni, G. L. (1964). *Proc. nat. Acad. Sci. Wash.* **51**, 818.
Felsenfeld, G. and Sandeen, G. (1962). *J. molec. Biol.* **5**, 587.
Felsenfeld, G., Sandeen, G. and von Hippel, P. H. (1963). *Proc. nat. Acad. Sci. Wash.* **50**, 644.
Fiers, W. and Sinsheimer, R. L. (1962). *J. molec. Biol.* **5**, 420.
Fixman, M. (1963). *J. molec. Biol.* **6**, 39.
Flory, P. J. and Miller, W. G. (1966). *J. molec. Biol.* **15**, 284.
Fong, P. (1964a). *Proc. nat. Acad. Sci. Wash.* **52**, 239.
Fong, P. (1964b). *Proc. nat. Acad. Sci. Wash.* **52**, 641.
Freese, E. and Cashel, M. (1964). *Biochim. biophys. Acta* **91**, 67.
Freese, E. B. and Freese, E. (1963). *Biochemistry* **2**, 707.
Freifelder, D. and Davison, P. F. (1962). *Biophys. J.* **2**, 249.
Freifelder, D., Kleinschmidt, A. K. and Sinsheimer, R. L. (1964). *Science* **146**, 254.
Fresco, J. R. (1963). In "Informational Macromolecules", (H. J. Vogel, V. Bryson, and J. O. Lampen, Eds.) pp. 121–148. Academic Press, New York.
Fresco, J. R., Alberts, B. M. and Doty, P. (1960). *Nature, Lond.* **188**, 98.
Fresco, J. R. and Klemperer, E. (1959). *Ann. N. Y. Acad. Sci.* **81**, 730.
Fresco, J. R. and Massoulié, J. (1963). *J. Amer. chem. Soc.* **85**, 1352.
Freund, A.-M. and Bernardi, G. (1963). *Nature, Lond.* **200**, 1318.
Fuwa, K., Wacker, W. E. C., Druyan, R., Bartholomay, A. F. and Vallee, B. L. (1960). *Proc. nat. Acad. Sci. Wash.* **46**, 1298.
Ganesan, A. T. (1963). Ph.D. Thesis: Stanford University, California, U.S.A.
Gartland, W. J. and Sueoka, N. (1966). *Proc. nat. Acad. Sci. Wash.* **55**, 948.
Geiduschek, E. P. (1961). *Proc. nat. Acad. Sci. Wash.* **47**, 950.
Geiduschek, E. P. (1962). *J. molec. Biol.* **4**, 467.
Geiduschek, E. P. and Herskovits, T. T. (1961). *Arch. Biochem. Biophys.* **95**, 114.
Geiduschek, E. P. and Holtzer, A. (1958). *Advanc. biol. med. Physics* **6**, 469.
Gellert, M., Lipsett, M. N. and Davies, D. R. (1962). *Proc. nat. Acad. Sci. Wash.* **48**, 2013.
Gersch, N. F. and Jordan, D. O. (1965). *J. molec. Biol.* **13**, 138.
Giannoni, G. and Rich, A. (1964). *Biopolymers* **2**, 399.
Gilham, P. T. (1964). *J. Amer. chem. Soc.* **86**, 4982.

Gillespie, D. and Spiegelman S. (1965). *J. molec. Biol.* **12**, 829.
Gillespie, D. and Spiegelman, S. (1966). *Bact. Proc.* 34.
Ginoza, W. (1958). *Nature, Lond.* **181**, 958.
Ginoza, W. and Guild, W. R. (1961). *Proc. nat. Acad. Sci. Wash.* **47**, 633.
Ginoza, W. and Zimm, B. H. (1961). *Proc. nat. Acad. Sci. Wash.* **47**, 639.
Ginoza, W., Hoelle, C. J., Vessey, K. B. and Carmack, C. (1964). *Nature, Lond.* **203**, 606.
Goldberg, A. (1966). *J. molec. Biol.* **15**, 663.
Goldberg, M. L. and Atchley, W. A. (1966). *Proc. nat. Acad. Sci. Wash.* **55**, 989.
Gomatos, P. J. and Tamm, I. (1963). *Proc. nat. Acad. Sci. Wash.* **50**, 878.
Goodman, H. M. and Rich, A. (1962). *Proc. nat. Acad. Sci. Wash.* **48**, 2101.
Gordon, D. E., Curnutte, Jr., B. and Lark, K. G. (1965). *J. molec. Biol.* **13**, 571.
Gordon, M. P. and Huff, J. W. (1962). *Biochemistry* **1**, 481.
Gordon, M. P., Huff, J. W. and Holland, J. J. (1963). *Virology* **19**, 416.
Gottschling, H. and Heidelberger, C. (1963). *J. molec. Biol.* **1**, 541.
Grechko, V., Maslova, R., Shkarenkova, L. and Varshavsky, J. (1964). *Abhandl. Deutsch. Acad. Wiss. Berlin. Klasse Med. No.* 6, 295.
Greer, S. and Zamenhof, S. (1962). *J. molec. Biol.* **4**, 123.
Griffin, B. E., Haslam, W. J. and Reese, C. B. (1964). *J. molec. Biol.* **10**, 353.
Grossman, L., Stollar, D. and Herrington, K. (1961). *J. Chim. Phys.* **58**, 1078.
Guild, W. R. (1961). *Proc. nat. Acad. Sci. Wash.* **47**, 1560.
Guild, W. R. (1963). *J. molec. Biol.* **6**, 214.
Guild, W. R. and Robison, M. (1963). *Proc. nat. Acad. Sci. Wash.* **50**, 106.
Gulland, J. M., Jordan, D. O. and Taylor, H. F. W. (1947). *J. chem. Soc.* 1131.
Hagen, U. and Wellstein, H. (1965). *Strahlentherapie* **128**, 37.
von Hahn, H. P. (1965). *Experientia* **21**, 90.
Hamaguchi, K. and Geiduschek, E. P. (1962). *J. Amer. chem. Soc.* **84**, 1329.
Harriman, P. D. and Zachau, H. G. (1966). *J. molec. Biol.* **16**, 387.
Hartman, Jr., K. A. and Rich, A. (1965). *J. Amer. chem. Soc.* **87**, 2033.
Haselkorn, R. (1964). *Science* **143**, 682.
Hayashi, H. and Egami, F. (1963). *J. Biochem. Tokyo* **53**, 176.
Hayashi, M. N., Hayashi, M., and Spiegelman, S. (1965). *Biophys. J.* **5**, 231.
Hayes, D. H., Hayes, F. and Guérin, M. (1966a). *J. molec. Biol.* **18**, 499.
Hayes, D. H., Grunberg-Manago, M. and Guérin, M. (1966b). *J. molec. Biol.* **18**, 477.
Hedén, C.-G., Lindahl, T. and Toplin, I. (1964). *Acta Chem. Scand.* **18**, 1150.
Helmkamp, G. K. and Ts'o, P. O. P. (1961). *J. Amer. chem. Soc.* **83**, 138.
Henley, D. D., Lindahl, T. and Fresco, J. R. (1966). *Proc. nat. Acad. Sci. Wash.* **55**, 191.
Herriott, R. M. (1961a). *Proc. nat. Acad. Sci. Wash.* **47**, 146.
Herriott, R. M. (1961b). *J. Chim. Phys.* **58**, 1103.
Herriott, R. M. (1963). *Biochem. Z.* **338**, 179.
Herriott, R. M. (1965). *Genetics* **52**, 1235.
Hershey, A. D., Burgi, E., Frankel, F., Goldberg, E. and Ingraham, L., (1962). *Carnegie Inst. Wash. Year Book* 61, 443.
Hershey, A. D., Burgi, E. and Ingraham, L. (1963a). *Proc. nat. Acad. Sci. Wash.* **49**, 748.
Hershey, A. D., Goldberg, E., Burgi, E. and Ingraham, L. (1963b). *J. molec. Biol.* **6**, 230.
Herskovits, T. T. (1962). *Arch. Biochem. Biophys.* **97**, 474.
Herskovits, T. T. (1963). *Biochemistry* **2**, 335.

Herskovits, T. T., Singer, S. J. and Geiduschek, E. P. (1961). *Arch. Biochem. Biophys.* **94**, 99.

Hiai, S. (1965). *J. molec. Biol.* **11**, 672.

Hnilica, L. S. and Billen, D. (1964). *Biochim. biophys. Acta* **91**, 271.

Hogness, D. S. (1966). *J. gen. Physiol.* **49**, 29.

Howard, F. B. and Miles, H. T. (1965). *J. biol. Chem.* **240**, 801.

Howard, F. B., Frazier, J., Lipsett, M. N. and Miles, H. T. (1964). *Biochem. Biophys. res. Commun.* **17**, 93.

Howard, F. B., Frazier, J., Singer, M. F. and Miles, H. T. (1966). *J. molec. Biol.* **16**, 415.

Hoyer, B. H., Bolton, E. T., McCarthy, B. J. and Roberts, R. B. (1965). *In* "Evolving Genes and Proteins", (V. Bryson and H. J. Vogel, Eds.) pp. 581–590. Academic Press, New York.

Huang, W. M. and T'so, P. O. P. (1966). *J. molec. Biol.* **16**, 523.

Huang, R. C. C., Bonner, J. and Murray, K. (1964). *J. molec. Biol.* **8**, 54.

Humm, D. G. and Humm, J. H. (1966). *Proc. nat. Acad. Sci. Wash.* **55**, 114.

Inman, R. B. (1964a). *J. molec. Biol.* **9**, 624.

Inman, R. B. (1964b). *J. molec. Biol.* **10**, 137.

Inman, R. B. (1966). *J. molec. Biol.* **18**, 464.

Inman, R. B. and Baldwin, R. L. (1962). *J. molec. Biol.* **5**, 172.

Inman, R. B. and Baldwin, R. L. (1964). *J. molec. Biol.* **8**, 452.

Inman, R. B. and Jordan, D. O. (1960a). *Biochim. biophys. Acta* **42**, 421.

Inman, R. B. and Jordan, D. O. (1960b). *Biochim. biophys. Acta* **43**, 9.

Inman, R. B. and Jordan, D. O. (1960c). *Biochim. biophys. Acta* **43**, 206.

Jakabhazy, S. Z. and Fleming, S. W. (1966). *Biopolymers* **4**, 793.

Jensen, R. H. (1965). Ph.D. Thesis: Calif. Inst. of Technol., Pasadena, Calif., U.S.A.

Jordan, D. O. (1960). "The Chemistry of Nucleic Acids", 358 pp. Butterworths, London.

Josse, J. and Eigner, J. (1966). *Annu. Rev. Biochem.* **35**, 789.

Kallen, R. G., Simon, M. and Marmur J. (1962). *J. molec. Biol.* **5**, 248.

Katz, L. and Penman, S. (1966). *J. molec. Biol.* **15**, 220.

Katz, S. (1962). *Nature, Lond.* **195**, 997.

Kawai, Y., Ozaki, M., Tanaka, M. and Teramoto, E. (1965). *J. phys. Soc. Japan* **20**, 1457.

Kaye, A. M. (1962). *Biochim. biophys. Acta* **61**, 615.

Kenner, G. W. (1957). *In* "Symposium on the Chemistry and Biology of Purines", (G. E. W. Wolstenholme and C. M. O'Connor, Eds). pp. 312–314. Churchill, London.

Kersten, W., Kersten, H. and Szybalski, W. (1966). *Biochemistry* **5**, 236.

Khesin, R. B. and Shemiakin, M. F. (1962). *Biochimia* **27**, 761.

Kidson, C. and Kirby, K. S. (1964). *Biochim. biophys. Acta* **91**, 627.

Kit, S. (1960a). *Biochem. Biophys. res. Commun.* **3**, 361.

Kit, S. (1960b). *Biochem. Biophys. res. Commun.* **3**, 377.

Kit, S. and Hsu, T. C. (1961). *Biochem. Biophys. res. Commun.* **5**, 120.

Kleinschmidt, A. K., Burton, A. and Sinsheimer, R. L. (1963). *Science*, **142**, 961.

Kleinwächter, V. and Koudelka, J. (1964). *Biochim. biophys. Acta* **91**, 539.

Kopylova-Sviridova, T. N. (1964). *Biofizika* **9**, 13.

Kotin, L. (1963). *J. molec. Biol.* **1**, 309.

Kozinski, A. W. and Beer, M. (1962). *Biophys. J.* **2**, 129.

Kozinski, A. W. and Kozinski, P. B. (1963). *Virology* **20**, 213.

Kubinski, H., Opara-Kubinska, Z. and Szybalski, W., (1966) *J. molec. Biol.* **20**, 313.

Kuhn, W. (1957). *Experientia* **13**, 301.

Kuhn, W. (1961). *J. molec. Biol.* **3**, 473.

Kurihara, K., Hachimori, Y. and Shibata, K. (1963). *Biochim. biophys. Acta* **68**, 434.

Ladik, J. and Appel, K. (1966). *Theoret. chim. Acta* **4**, 132.

Lanyi, J. (1963). Ph.D. Thesis: Harvard Univ., Cambridge, Mass., U.S.A.

Lebowitz, J., Watson, R. and Vinograd, J. (1966). *Abstr. Biophys. Soc.* p. 108.

Lee, M. F., Walker, I. P. and Peacocke, A. R. (1963). *Biochim. biophys. Acta* **72**, 310.

Lehman, I. R. (1963). *Progr. nucleic acid Res.* **2**, 83.

Leng, M. and Felsenfeld, G. (1966). *J. molec. Biol.* **15**, 455.

Lerman, L. S. (1964). *J. cell. comp. Physiol.* **64**, Suppl. 1, 1.

Lerman, L. S. and Tolmach, L. J. (1959). *Biochim. biophys. Acta* **33**, 371.

Levin, D. H. and Litt, M. (1965). *J. molec. Biol.* **14**, 506.

Levine, L., Gordon, J. A. and Jencks, W. P. (1963). *Biochemistry* **2**, 168.

Levinthal, C. and Crane, H. R. (1956). *Proc. nat. Acad. Sci. Wash.* **42**, 436.

Lewin, S. (1964). *Biochem. J.* **93**, 16P.

Lewin, S. and Munroe, D. P. (1966). *Biochim. biophys. Acta* **114**, 637.

Lewin, S. and Pepper, D. S. (1965). *Arch. Biochem. Biophys.* **109**, 192.

Lindahl, T., Adams, A. and Fresco, J. R. (1966). *Proc. nat. Acad. Sci. Wash.* **55**, 941.

Lipsett, M. N. (1964). *J. biol. Chem.* **239**, 1256.

Lipsett, M. N., Heppel, L. A. and Bradley, D. F. (1961). *J. biol. Chem.* **236**, 857.

Longuet-Higgins, H. C. and Zimm, B. H. (1960). *J. molec. Biol.* **2**, 1.

Luzzati, V., Mathis, A., Masson, F. and Witz, J. (1964). *J. molec. Biol.* **10**, 28.

Luzzati, W., Witz, J. and Mathis, A. (1966). *Proc. 3rd. Meeting Europ. Biochem. Soc. Warsaw* (in press).

Lyons, J. W. and Kotin, L. (1965). *J. Amer. chem. Soc.* **87**, 1781.

Mahler, H. R. and Cordes, E. C. (1966) *In* "Biological Chemistry", pp. 124–188, Harper and Row, New York.

Mahler, H. R. and Dutton, G. (1964). *J. molec. Biol.* **10**, 157.

Mahler, H. R. and Mehrota, B. D. (1962). *Biochim. biophys. Acta* **55**, 252.

Mahler, H. R. and Mehrota, B. D. (1963). *Biochim. biophys. Acta* **68**, 211.

Mahler, H. R., Dutton, G. and Mehrota, B. O. (1963). *Biochim. biophys. Acta* **68**, 199.

Mahler H. R., Kline, B. and Mehrota, B. D. (1964). *J. molec. Biol.* **9**, 801.

Mandel, M. (1962). *J. molec. Biol.* **5**, 435.

Mandell, J. D. and Hershey, A. D. (1960). *Anal. Biochem.* **1**, 66.

Marcot-Queiroz, J. and Monier, R. (1965). *Bull. Soc. Chim. Biol.* **47**, 1627.

Marmur, J. and Cordes, S. (1963) *In* "Symposium on Informational Macromolecules", (H. J. Vogel, V. Bryson and J. O. Lampen, Eds.), pp. 79–87. Academic Press, New York.

Marmur, J. and Doty, P. (1959). *Nature, Lond.* **183**, 1427.

Marmur, J. and Doty, P. (1961). *J. molec. Biol.* **3**, 588.

Marmur, J. and Doty, P. (1962). *J. molec. Biol.* **5**, 109.

Marmur, J. and Greenspan, C. M. (1963). *Science* **142**, 387.

Marmur, J. and Grossman, L. (1961). *Proc. nat. Acad. Sci. Wash.* **47**, 778.

Marmur, J. and Lane, D. (1960). *Proc. nat. Acad. Sci. Wash.* **46**, 453.

Marmur, J. and Schildkraut, C. L. (1963). *Proc. Fifth Int. Congr. Biochem.* **1**, 232.

Marmur, J. and Ts'o, P. O. P. (1961). *Biochim. biophys. Acta* **51**, 32.

Marmur, J., Anderson, W. F., Matthews, L., Berns, K., Gajewska, E., Lane, D. and Doty, P. (1961a). *J. cell. comp. Physiol.* **58**, Suppl. 1, 33.

Marmur, J., Schildkraut, C. L. and Doty, P. (1961b). *J. Chim. Phys.* **58**, 945.

Marmur, J., Schildkraut, C. L. and Doty, P. (1962). In "Molecular Basis of Neoplasia", pp. 9–43. Univ. of Texas Press, Austin, Texas.

Marmur, J., Falkow, S. and Mandel, M. (1963a). Annu. Rev. Microbiol. 17, 329.

Marmur, J., Rownd, R. and Schildkraut, C. L. (1963b). Progr. nucleic acid Res. 1, 231.

Martin, M. A. and Hoyer, B. H. (1966). Biochemistry 5, 2706.

Maslova, R. N. and Varshavsky, Ya. M. (1966). Biochim. biophys. Acta 119, 633.

Massoulie, J., Blake, R., Klotz, L. and Fresco, J. (1964). Compt. rend. Acad. Sci. 259, 3104.

Massoulié, J., Michelson, A. M. and Pochon, F. (1966). Biochim. biophys. Acta 114, 16.

May, P. (1964). J. molec. Biol. 9, 263.

McConkey, E. H. and Dubin, D. T. (1966). J. molec. Biol. 15, 102.

Mehrota, B. D. and Mahler, H. R. (1964). Biochim. biophys. Acta 91, 78.

Meselson, M. and Stahl, F. W. (1958). Proc. nat. Acad. Sci. Wash. 44, 671.

Meselson, M. and Weigle, J. J. (1961). Proc. nat. Acad. Sci. Wash. 47, 857.

Meselson, M., Stahl, F. W. and Vinograd, J. (1957). Proc. nat. Acad. Sci. Wash. 43, 581.

Mesnard, G. and Vasilescu, D. (1964). Biochim. biophys. Acta 91, 531.

Micheel, F. and Heesing, A. (1961). Chem. Berichte 94, 1814.

Michelson, A. M. (1962). Biochim. biophys. Acta 55, 841.

Michelson, A. M. (1963). "The Chemistry of Nucleosides and Nucleotides", 622 pp. Academic Press, London.

Michelson, A. M. (1965) Bull. Soc. Chim. Biol. 47, 1553.

Michelson, A. M. and Pochon, F. (1966). Biochim. biophys. Acta 114, 469.

Michelson, A. M., Massoulié, J. and Guschlbauer, W. (1966). Progr. nucleic acid Res. (in press).

Millar, D. B. S. and Steiner, R. F. (1965). Biochim. biophys. Acta 102, 571.

Miyazawa, Y. and Thomas, Jr., C. A. (1965). J. molec. Biol. 11, 223.

Mora, P. T. (1965). Biochim. biophys. Acta 109, 568.

Nash, D. and Plaut, W. (1964). Proc. nat. Acad. Sci. Wash. 51, 731.

Naylor, R. and Gilham, P. T. (1966). Biochemistry 5, 2722.

Nesbet, R. K. (1964). Biopolymers Symposia No. 1, 129.

Nygaard, A. P. and Hall, B. D. (1964). J. molec. Biol. 9, 125.

Ohnishi, S. O. and McConnell, H. M. (1965). J. Amer. chem. Soc. 87, 2293.

Oishi, M. and Sueoka, N. (1965). Proc. nat. Acad. Sci. Wash. 54, 483.

Olivera, B. M., Baine, P. and Davidson, N. (1964). Biopolymers 2, 245.

Opara-Kubinska, Z. and Szybalski, W. (1962). Abstr. Biophys. Soc., p. WA8.

Opara-Kubinska, Z., Borowska, Z. K. and Szybalski, W. (1963). Biochim. biophys. Acta 72, 298.

Opara-Kubinska, Z., Kubinski, H. and Szybalski, W. (1964). Proc. nat. Acad. Sci. Wash. 52, 923.

Paleček, E. (1961). Biochim. biophys. Acta 51, 1.

Paleček, E. (1965). J. molec. Biol. 11, 839.

Papaevangelou, G. J. and Youngner, J. S. (1961). Virology 15, 509.

Peacocke, A. R. and Walker, I. O. (1962). J. molec. Biol. 5, 550.

Permogorov, V. I. and Lazurkin, Yu. S. (1965). Biofizyka 10, 17.

Piechowska, M. and Shugar, D. (1963). Acta Biochim. Polonica 10, 263.

Piechowska, M. and Shugar, D. (1965). Acta Biochim. Polonica 12, 11.

Pivec, L., Šponar, J. and Šormova, Z. (1964). Biochim. biophys. Acta 91, 357.

Pochon, F. and Michelson, M. (1965). Proc. nat. Acad. Sci. Wash. 53, 1425.

Pochon, F., Massoulié, J. and Michelson, M. (1965). Compt. rend. Acad. Sci. 260, 2937.

Printz, M. P. and von Hippel, P. H. (1965). Proc. nat. Acad. Sci. Wash. 53, 363.

Pullman, B., Claverie, P. and Caillet, J. (1965). *Compt. rend. Acad. Sci.* **260**, 5387.

Rawitscher, M. A., Rows, P. D. and Sturtevant, J. M. (1963). *J. Amer. chem. Soc.* **85**, 1915.

Reich, E. and Goldberg, I. H. (1964). *Progr. nucleic acid Res.* **3**, 183.

Reinert, K. E. (1964). *Abhand. Deutch. Akad. Wiss. Berlin, Klasse Med.*, No. 6, 27.

Rich, A. (1960). *Proc. nat. Acad. Sci. Wash.* **46**, 1044.

Rice, S. A. and Doty, P. (1957). *J. Amer. chem. Soc.* **79**, 3937.

Rice, S. A., Wada, A. W. and Geiduschek, E. P. (1958). *Faraday Soc. Discussions* No. 25, **130**.

Riley, M., Maling, B. and Chamberlin, M. J. (1966). *J. molec. Biol.* **20**, 359.

Ritossa, F. M. and Spiegelman, S. (1965). *Proc. nat. Acad. Sci. Wash.* **53**, 737.

Roger, M. and Hotchkiss, R. D. (1961). *Proc. nat. Acad. Sci. Wash.* **47**, 653.

Roger, M., Beckman, C. O. and Hotchkiss, R. D. (1966a). *J. molec. Biol.* **18**, 174.

Roger, M., Beckman, C. O. and Hotchkiss, R. D. (1966b). *J. molec. Biol.* **18**, 156.

Ross, P. D. and Sturtevant, J. M. (1962). *J. Amer. chem. Soc.* **84**, 4503.

Rownd, R. H. (1963). Ph.D. Thesis: Harvard University, Cambridge, Mass., U.S.A.

Rownd, R., Lanyi, J. and Doty, P. (1961) *Biochim. biophys. Acta* **53**, 225.

Rozenkranz, H. S. and Bendich, A. (1959). *J. Amer. chem. Soc.* **81**, 6255.

Samejima, T. and Yang, J. T. (1965). *J. biol. Chem.* **240**, 2094.

Sarkar, P. K. and Yang, J. T. (1965). *Biochemistry* **4**, 1238.

Savitsky, J. P. (1964). *Biochim. biophys. Acta* **80**, 183.

Schildkraut, C. and Lifson, S. (1965). *Biopolymers* **3**, 195.

Schildkraut, C. L., Marmur, J. and Doty, P. (1961a). *J. molec. Biol.* **3**, 595.

Schildkraut, C. L., Marmur, J., Fresco, J. R. and Doty, P. (1961b). *J. biol. Chem.* **236**, PC3.

Schildkraut, C. L., Richardson, C. C. and Kornberg, A. (1964). *J. molec. Biol.* **9**, 24.

Schildkraut, C. L., Wierzchowski, K. L., Marmur, J., Green, D. M. and Doty, P. (1962). *Virology* **18**, 43.

Schweitzer, M. P., Chan, S. I. and Ts'o, P. O. P. (1965). *J. Amer. chem. Soc.* **87**, 5241.

Shimura, Y., Moses, R. E. and Nathans, D. (1965). *J. molec. Biol.* **12**, 266.

Shoup, R. R., Miles, H. T. and Becker, E. D. (1966). *Biochem. Biophys. res. Commun.* **23**, 194.

Shugar, D. and Szer, W. (1962). *J. molec. Biol.* **5**, 580.

Sigler, P. B., Davies, D. R. and Miles, H. T. (1962). *J. molec. Biol.* **5**, 709.

Sinanoglu, O. (1963). *Rad. Res.* **20**, 149.

Singer, M. F., Heppel, L. A., Rushizky, G. W. and Sober, H. A. (1962). *Biochim. biophys. Acta* **61**, 474.

Singh, H. S. (1965). Ph.D. Thesis: Banaras Hindu University, Varanasi, India.

Sinsheimer, R. L. (1959). *J. molec. Biol.* **1**, 43.

Sinsheimer, R. L. (1961). *Fed. Proc.* **20**, 661.

Šormova, Z. (1962). *Coll. Czech. Chem. Comm.* **27**, 1743.

Spatz, H. C. and Baldwin, R. L. (1965). *J. molec. Biol.* **11**, 213.

Spiegelman, S. and Yankofsky, S. A. (1965). *In* "Evolving Genes and Proteins", (V. Bryson and H. J. Vogel, Eds.) pp. 537–579, Academic Press, New York.

Steiner, R. F. and Beers, Jr. R. F. (1961). "Polynucleotides", 444 pp. Elsevier Publ. Co., Amsterdam.

Sternglanz, R. and Doty, P. (1966). *40th. Nat. Colloid Symp.* Madison, Wis., U.S.A.

Stevens, C. L. and Felsenfeld, G. (1964). *Biopolymers* **2**, 293.

Stollar, D. and Grossman, L. (1962). *J. molec. Biol.* **4**, 31.

Stone, A. L. and Bradley, D. F. (1961). *J. Amer. chem. Soc.* **83**, 3627.

Strack, H. B. and Kaiser, A. D. (1965). *J. molec. Biol.* **12**, 36.

Strauss, B. S. and Wahl, R. (1964). *Biochim. biophys. Acta* **80**, 116.

Studier, F. W. (1965). *J. molec. Biol.* **11**, 373.

Sturtevant, J. M., Rice, S. A. and Geiduschek, E. P. (1958). *Faraday Soc. Discussions No.* 25, 138.

Subirana, J. A. (1965). *Biochim. biophys. Acta* **103**, 13.

Subirana, J. A. (1966). *Biopolymers* **4**, 189.

Subirana, J. A. and Doty, P. (1966). *Biopolymers* **4**, 171.

Sueoka, N. and Cheng, T.-Y. (1962a). *J. molec. Biol.* **4**, 161.

Sueoka, N. and Cheng, T.-Y. (1962b). *Proc. nat. Acad. Sci. Wash.* **48**, 1851.

Summers, W. C. and Szybalski, W. (1965). *Rad. Research* **25**, 246.

Suzuki, K. and Moriguchi, E. (1965). *J. molec. Biol.* **11**, 690.

Świerkowski, M., Szer, W. and Shugar, D. (1965). *Biochem. Z.* **342**, 429.

Szer, W. (1965). *Biochem. Biophys. res. Commun.* **20**, 182.

Szer, W. (1966a). *Biochem. Biophys. res. Commun.* **22**, 559.

Szer, W. (1966b). *J. molec. Biol.* **16**, 585.

Szer, W. and Shugar, D. (1963). *Acta Biochim. Polonica* **10**, 219.

Szer, W. and Shugar, D. (1966). *J. molec. Biol.* **17**, 174.

Szer, W., Świerkowski, W. and Shugar, D. (1963). *Acta Biochim. Polonica* **10**, 87.

Szybalski, W. (1961). *In* "Progress in Photobiology", (B. C. Christensen and B. Buchmann, Eds.) pp. 542–545. Elsevier Publ. Co., Amsterdam.

Szybalski, W. (1964). *Abhandl. Deutsch. Acad. Wiss. Berlin, Klasse Med., No.* 4, 1.

Szybalski, W., Cohn, N. K. and Heidelberger, C. (1963a). *Fed. Proc.* **22**, 532.

Szybalski, W., Erikson, R. L., Gentry, G. A., Gafford, L. G. and Randall, C. C. (1963b). *Virology* **19**, 586.

Szybalski, W. and Iyer, U. N. (1964). *Fed. Proc.* **23**, 946.

Szybalski, W. and Mennigmann, H.-D. (1962). *Anal. Biochem.* **3**, 267.

Szybalski, W. and Opara-Kubinska, Z. (1965a). *In* "Cellular Radiation Biology", pp. 223–240, William & Wilkins Co., Baltimore.

Szybalski, W. and Opara-Kubinska, Z. (1965b). *Symp. Biol. Hungarica* **6**, 43.

Tabor, H. (1961). *Biochem. Biophys. res. Commun.* **4**, 228.

Tabor, H. (1962). *Biochemistry* **1**, 496.

Tabor, H. and Tabor, C. W. (1964). *Pharmacol. Rev.* **16**, 245.

Takahashi, I. and Marmur, J. (1963). *Nature, Lond.* **197**, 794.

Takashima, S. and Arnolds, E. A. (1965). *Biochim. biophys. Acta* **94**, 546.

Tamm, C., Hodes, E. and Chargaff, E. (1952). *J. biol. Chem.* **195**, 49.

Tamm, C., Shapiro, H. S., Lipshitz, R. and Chargaff, E. (1953). *J. biol. Chem.*, **203**, 673.

Thomas, Jr., C. A. (1966). *J. gen. Physiol.* **49**, 143.

Thomas, Jr., C. A. and Berns, K. I. (1962). *J. molec. Biol.* **4**, 309.

Thomas, Jr., C. A. and McHattie, L. A. (1964). *Proc. nat. Acad. Sci. Wash.* **52**, 1297.

Thomas, R. (1954). *Biochim. biophys. Acta* **14**, 231.

Thrower, K. J. and Peacocke, A. R. (1966). *Biochim. biophys. Acta* **119**, 652.

Tikchonenko, T. I., Perevertajlo, G. A. and Dobrov, E. (1963). *Biochim. biophys. Acta* **68**, 500.

Tinoco, Jr., I. (1960). *J. Amer. chem. Soc.* **82**, 4785.

Tocchini-Valentini, G. P., Stodolsky, M., Aurisicchio, A., Sarnat, M., Graziosi, F., Weiss, S. B. and Geiduschek, E. P. (1963). *Proc. nat. Acad. Sci. Wash.* **50**, 935.

Troll, W., Belman, S. and Levine, E. (1963). *Cancer Res.* **23**, 841.

Ts'o, P. O. P. and Helmkamp, G. (1961). *Tetrahedron* **13**, 198.

Ts'o, P. O. P., Helmkamp, G. and Sander, C. (1962a). *Proc. nat. Acad. Sci. Wash,* **48**, 686.

Ts'o, P. O. P., Helmkamp, G. and Sander, C. (1962b). *Biochim. biophys. Acta* **55**, 584.

Ts'o, P. O. P., Helmkamp, G., Sander, C. and Studier, F. W. (1963). *Biochim. biophys. Acta* **76**, 54.

5 + T.

Tsuboi, M., Matsuo, K. and T'so, P. O. P. (1966). *J. molec. Biol.* **15**, 256.

Ulbricht, T. L. V., Swan, R. J. and Michelson, A. M. (1966). *Chem. Comm.* 63.

Van de Vorst, A. and Pullman, A. (1965). *Compt. rend. Acad. Sci. Paris*, **261**, 827.

van Holde, K. E., Brahms, J. and Michelson, A. M. (1965). *J. molec. Biol.* **12**, 726.

van Sluis, C. A. and Stuy, J. H. (1962). *Biochim. Biophys. res. Commun.* **7**, 213.

Venner, H. and Zimmer, C. (1964). *Naturwiss*, **51**, 173.

Venner, H. and Zimmer, C. (1966) *Biopolymers* **4**, 321.

Venner, H., Zimmer, C. and Schröder, S. (1963). *Biochim. biophys. Acta* **76**, 312.

Vinograd, J. and Lebowitz, J. (1966). *J. gen. Physiol.* **49**, 103.

Vinograd, J., Bruner, R., Kent, R. and Weigle, J. (1963). *Proc. nat. Acad. Sci. Wash.* **49**, 902.

Vinograd, J., Lebowitz, J., Radloff, R., Watson, R. and Laipis, P. (1965). *Proc. nat. Acad. Sci. Wash.* **53**, 1104.

Wada, A. and Yamagami, H. (1964). *Biopolymers* **2**, 445.

Walker, I. O. (1965). *Biochim. biophys. Acta* **109**, 585.

Walker, P. M. B. and McCallum, M. (1966). *J. molec. Biol.* **18**, 215.

Walker, P. M. B. and McLaren, A. (1965). *Nature, Lond.* **208**, 1175.

Wang, J. C. and Davidson, N. (1966). *J. molec. Biol.* **15**, 111.

Ward, D., Reich, E. and Goldberg, I. H. (1965). *Science* **149**, 1259.

Waring, M. J. (1965). *J. molec. Biol.* **13**, 269.

Warner, R. C. (1963). *In* "Informational Molecules", (H. J. Vogel, V. Bryson and J. O. Lampen, Eds). pp. 111–120, Academic Press, New York.

Watson, J. (1965). "Molecular Biology of the Gene", 494 pp. W. A. Benjamin, Inc., New York.

Weinstein, I. B., Chermoff, R., Finkelstein, I. and Hirschberg, E. (1965). *Molec. Pharmacol.* **1**, 297.

Weiss, J. J. (1963). *Nature, Lond.* **197**, 1296.

Wells, R. D., Ohtsuka, E. and Khorana, H. G. (1965). *J. molec. Biol.* **14**, 221.

Yankofsky, S. A. and Spiegelman, S. (1962a). *Proc. nat. Acad. Sci. Wash.* **48**, 1069.

Yankofsky, S. A. and Spiegelman, S. (1962b). *Proc. nat. Acad. Sci. Wash.* **48**, 1466.

Yoshikawa, H. (1966). *Abst. Biophys. Soc.* 10*th. Ann. Meet.* p. 103.

Zaleska, H. and Pakula, R. (1964). *Acta Biochim. Polonica* **11**, 139.

Zamenhof, S. (1961). *J. Bact.* **81**, 111.

Zamenhof, S., Alexander, H. E. and Leidy, G. (1953). *J. exp. Med.* **98**, 373.

Zamenhof, S., Griboff, G. and Marullo, N. (1954). *Biochim. biophys. Acta* **13**, 459.

Zamenhof, S., Leidy, G., Hahn, E. and Alexander, H. E. (1956). *J. Bact.* **72**, 1.

Zimm, B. H. (1960). *J. chem. Phys.* **33**, 1349.

Zimmer, C. and Venner, H. (1962). *Naturwiss.* **49**, 86.

Zimmer, C. and Venner, H. (1963). *J. molec. Biol.* **7**, 603.

Zimmer, C. and Venner, H. (1964). *Abh. Deutsch. Acad. Wiss. Berlin, Klasse Med.* No. 6, 287.

Zimmer, C. and Venner, H. (1965). *Monatsberichte Deutsch. Akad. Wissenschaft. Berlin* **7**, 883.

Zimmermann, E. (1965). *Biochem. Z.* **341**, 129.

Chapter 5

The Effect of Heat on Membranes and Membrane Constituents

D. Chapman

Molecular Biophysics Unit, Unilever Research Laboratory,
The Frythe, Welwyn, Herts., England

I. Introduction

A. THE CONCEPT OF A MEMBRANE

In order to discuss the effect of heat on membranes and their constituents, it is necessary for us first to discuss what is at present known about biological membranes. It should be pointed out at once that the concept of a cell membrane is at present receiving considerable attention and is still in a stage of development. There is a lack of definite information on the subject and, because of this, there are a number of rather different attitudes to the definition of a cell membrane, dependent upon the degree of speculation involved (Danielli and Davson, 1943; Kavanau, 1965) and the degree of sophistication demanded.

As the present picture of a biological membrane is somewhat diffuse, we must expect that our understanding of the detailed membrane processes which may be affected by heat will also be somewhat uncertain. By comparing the properties of the individual constituents of biological membranes with the effects observed with natural tissue, we may, however, obtain some insight into the processes which can occur.

For many years the concept of a cell membrane was demanded by physiological experiments which showed that there is a barrier to diffusion between the interior of the cell and its surroundings. The barrier was called a membrane because it was thought to be a thin layer completely enclosing the cytoplasm, providing an effective barrier against uncontrolled exchange of molecules between the cytoplasm and its surroundings. The barrier, therefore, had to have certain definite mechanical and physical properties. The introduction of the electron microscope with its powerful resolving power has developed this concept of a membrane, and clearly defined layered structures can be seen at the borders of cell territories in electron micrographs. These structures are associated with membranes. They are observed not only at the surfaces of cells but in a variety of internal structures within the cell. Inside the cell the mitochondria and lysosomes are seen to be bounded by membranes, and the interior of cells contains paired membranes called endoplasmic reticulum. Membrane-type structures are also observed in the chloroplasts of plant cells and in the rods and cones of the eye. However, the necessary treatment required of the material prior to electron microscope examination, i.e. fixing, dehydrating, embedding and sectioning, causes some caution to be aroused about the validity of the structures observed (Bangham and Horne, 1964).

Although cell membranes are considered to have considerable functional diversity, the electron micrographs show little differentiation. The typical appearance, as indicated in the electron micrograph, is of a single black line of about 75 Å gross thickness which, under certain conditions, can be seen to be trilaminar, the outer layers taking up heavy metal stains, e.g. osmium tetroxide, more strongly than the inner lamina. Each lamina is about 25 Å thick. There has been considerable discussion concerning the interpretation of the electron micrographs, particularly with respect to the position of the osmium-stained material in fixed material (Stoeckenius, 1962; Hayes et al., 1963). After permanganate fixation, a fairly uniform result is obtained, and a triple-layered structure, about 75 Å thick, is always seen. This led Robertson (1959) to propose the term "unit membrane" for cell membranes in general. Thus one concept of a cell membrane is that it is a semipermeable barrier of about 100 Å thickness.

B. MEMBRANE CONSTITUENTS

The electron microscope provides evidence for the existence of a membrane, but there is some uncertainty regarding the constituents of membranes. The isolation and analysis of membranes is a difficult process and has been carried out with only a few types of cells. The membrane of the erythrocyte or red blood cell is the one which has received most attention. The erythrocyte is first converted to a ghost by careful haemolysis, and it is thought that a carefully prepared ghost contains all of the membrane material (Parpart and Ballentine, 1952). The major constituents of this membrane have been found to be lipid and protein, but it is not certain that the protein is definitely part of the membrane, and it is suggested that some of the protein could originate in the interior of the cell. The protein is considered to consist of several fractions, one of which is called stromatin (Jorpes, 1932). Other proteins are known as elenin, reticulin and S-protein.

Several classes of lipids are found in the lipid fraction which, depending upon the way the ghosts are prepared, amounts to 20–40% of the dry weight of the membrane. The most important lipids are cholesterol and phospholipids, e.g. phosphatidylcholine (lecithin), phosphatidylethanolamine (cephalin) and sphingomyelin (see Fig. 1). Modern analyses on the relative amounts of these lipids in human and bovine red cell membranes have been carried out by Turner et al. (1958) and Hanahan et al. (1960) and confirmed by Kögl et al. (1960), de Gier (1960) and de Gier and van Deenen (1961). Phospholipids account for about 60% of the total lipid material present in all animal red cell membranes. Marked differences are observed between the various classes of phospholipids in the ghosts from different animal erythrocytes, e.g. sheep, ox, pig, man, rabbit and rat. Thus the lecithin content is greatest in the rat and lowest in the sheep membrane. The fatty acids associated with the total lipid also show species differences (see Fig. 2). In the series of animals sheep, ox, pig, man, rabbit and rat, there is an increase in the ratio of palmitic acid:oleic acid, an increase in the arachidonic acid content as well as an increase in lecithin content in that order, which can be correlated with an increase in permeability of the red cells to polar substances. The number of double bonds in the fatty acid residues of the membrane lipids of the various animal species remains fairly constant.

It is generally assumed that other cells have cell membranes containing protein and lipids of the same type as those found in red blood cells. Blood plasma, liver and heart tissues contain significant quantities of phospholipid. The brain is remarkably rich in membrane material and also possesses a very high phospholipid content, probably due to its myelin component, which is the fatty sheath surrounding the axons. All analyses show that the lecithin class of phospholipids predominates in biological tissues. Phospholipids are high in content in the nervous system of vertebrates and lower in invertebrates. Some authors have suggested that phospholipids occur in all biological membranes, and it is

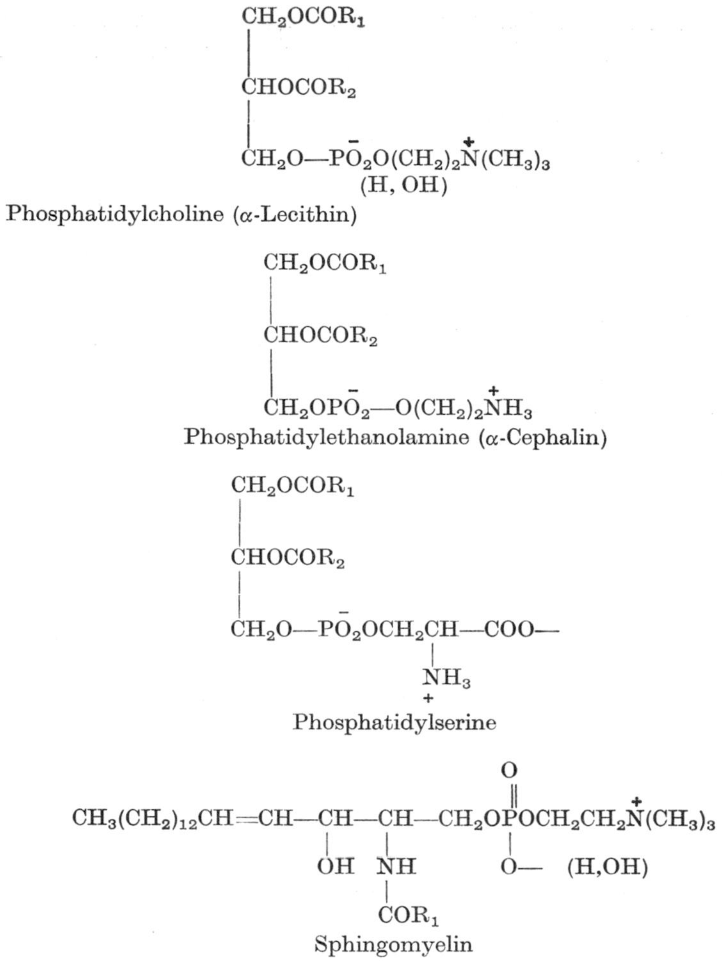

$$CH_2OCOR_1$$
$$|$$
$$CHOCOR_2$$
$$|$$
$$CH_2O\!-\!P\bar{O}_2O(CH_2)_2\overset{+}{N}(CH_3)_3$$
$$(H, OH)$$

Phosphatidylcholine (α-Lecithin)

$$CH_2OCOR_1$$
$$|$$
$$CHOCOR_2$$
$$|$$
$$CH_2OP\bar{O}_2\!-\!O(CH_2)_2\overset{+}{N}H_3$$

Phosphatidylethanolamine (α-Cephalin)

$$CH_2OCOR_1$$
$$|$$
$$CHOCOR_2$$
$$|$$
$$CH_2O\!-\!P\bar{O}_2OCH_2CH\!-\!COO\!-$$
$$|$$
$$\underset{+}{NH_3}$$

Phosphatidylserine

$$\overset{\textstyle O}{\overset{\|}{CH_3(CH_2)_{12}CH\!=\!CH\!-\!\underset{|}{\underset{OH}{CH}}\!-\!\underset{|}{\underset{NH}{CH}}\!-\!CH_2OPOCH_2CH_2\overset{+}{N}(CH_3)_3}}$$
$$\underset{|}{\underset{O-\ \ (H,OH)}{}}$$
$$COR_1$$

Sphingomyelin

Fig. 1. Structural formulae of three phospholipids commonly found in biological membranes.

speculated further that perhaps only biological membranes contain phospholipids. The one outstanding exception to this generalization appears to be with the serum lipoproteins, which contain neutral lipid and phospholipid.

As lipids, particularly phospholipids, are constituents of cell membranes, models have been proposed using these molecules as the basic building bricks. These models have been influenced by the ideas of Hardy (1913) and Langmuir (1917) on the way in which long chain polar molecules form monolayers and are oriented at the air–water interface. Gorter and Grendel (1925) found that the total lipid which could be extracted from erythrocyte ghosts was sufficient to cover twice the surface area of the erythrocyte. This has led to the concept of a double layer of lipids forming the basic structure of cell membranes. Because

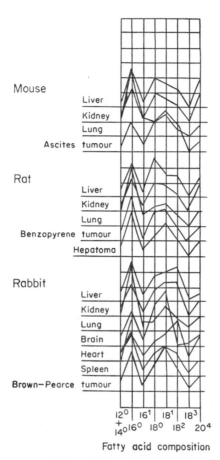

Fatty acid composition

FIG. 2. The fatty acid compositions of phospholipids from tissues of three different animal species. On the abscissa, the fatty acid compositions are indicated by the number of carbon atoms and (as superscripts) by the number of double bonds. On the ordinate, the weight percentages of fatty acid methyl esters are plotted. The distance between two horizontal lines corresponds to 10% fatty acid. (After van Deenen, 1965.)

the surface tension at the surface of the cell was found to be very low, this concept was later modified to include protein interaction (Danielli, 1952). The protein layer was thought to be adsorbed on the polar groups of the lipid molecules (Fig. 3). Kavanau (1963) has suggested that membranes can shift between two extreme arrangements termed open and closed configurations. In the open arrangement it is suggested that the lipids are in cylindrical micelles, 180–200 Å thick, attached at each end to external protein monolayers 10–15 Å thick, and the pillars are separated and arranged hexagonally with aqueous regions between. Other arrangements have been suggested by Green and Fleischer (1963). Bungenberg de Jong (1949) and Booij and Bungenberg de Jong (1956) suggested that the biological membrane involved a tricomplex system which included phospholipids, proteins and cations. Various suggestions have been made as to the arrangement of cholesterol in the membrane (Finean, 1953), but there is little definite evidence regarding its precise organization. In addition to their function in maintaining an interface, membranes are also involved in active transport and metabolic activity. The metabolic activity is thought to involve a continuous renewal of certain of its structural compounds.

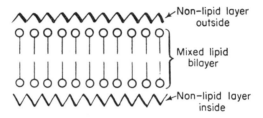

FIG. 3. Generalized structure of the unit membrane.

To summarize, our picture of the cell membrane is that it is not a static system, such as a rigid film, but a dynamic system, one in which a turnover in fatty acid and phospholipid composition occurs, and in which phase transitions from lamellar to some other phase, either spherical, micellar or hexagonal phase, may occur. The cell membrane is also associated with a variety of phenomena that involve ion and molecule transport as well as probably providing a quasi-catalytic surface for the activation of chemical or enzymic reactions.

II. The Effects of Heat on Natural and Model Membranes

The previous section described the present-day concepts of the biological membrane and how these are still in an active state of development. In this section, consideration will be given to the effects of heat or cold on cells and tissues in so far as the observed effects are probably related to phenomena occurring in or at the cell membranes.

A. LOW TEMPERATURE EFFECTS

The effects of low temperatures on tissues have been studied since the 18th century. It was soon evident that there is a remarkable species variation in sensitivity, some organisms having a capacity for withstanding extreme cold whereas others are killed or damaged at temperatures little below the freezing temperature of water (Luyet and Gehenio, 1940). As long ago as 1897, Brown and Escombe (1897) observed that the germinative power of seeds was not affected by slow cooling to, and storage for 11 hours at, $-182°$ in liquid air. Later, Macfadyen and Rowland (1900) showed that bacteria retained unimpaired vitality and their enzymes remained active after exposure to, or storage in, liquid air and liquid hydrogen.

It has been known for some time that a sudden fall in temperature to a value above $0°$ has a harmful or lethal effect on a variety of living cells to which a gradual temperature change over the same range, or maintenance at the low temperature, is innocuous. The effect is common in higher plants and also occurs in simple organisms, such as algae (Kylin, 1917). Certain bacteria (Hegarty and Weeks, 1940) are extremely sensitive to cold; for example, cultures of *Escherichia coli*, during their logarithmic growth phase, show great sensitivity to rapid cooling from $37°$ to $0°$. The majority of mammalian cells are susceptible to cold shock and the susceptibility can be increased or decreased by altering the composition of the medium.

Lovelock (1957) has suggested that some of these effects may arise from the action of the cold stress on cell membranes. Freezing can cause profound changes in the physical environment of the cell which are sufficient to denature the lipoprotein of the membrane. Although the crushing effect of ice crystal growth has been considered to be the major effect, there are other important effects which can also take place. The dilute aqueous medium surrounding the cell is affected on freezing the cell. The ice can separate while the solutes and cells are concentrated between the ice crystals. This concentrating effect increases the electrolyte concentration and raises the ionic strength of the suspending medium as well as affecting the pH value. There are a number of examples of the effect of lowering the temperature of lipoproteins which illustrate this behaviour: (a) Membranes of human red cells, on freezing to $0°$ in different concentrations of sodium chloride, are observed to lose phospholipid and cholesterol. The loss of phospholipid makes the cell permeable to cations so that it swells and, ultimately, bursts. The red blood cell membranes of other animals (e.g. rat, rabbit and ox) behave in a similar way; (b) Egg yolk and its principal lipoprotein, lipovitellin, also appear to denature on freezing, as indicated by

5*

the loss of solubility in sodium chloride solution, or the release of lipid from the complex. The rate of damage is slower at $-20°$ than at $-3°$; (c) The human plasma β-lipoprotein also becomes denatured on freezing in sodium chloride solution to temperatures between $-18°$ and $-55°$. The damage is slow to occur and does not commence until $-20°$ is reached. It is suggested that not only the cell membranes but also the internal membranes of the cell can suffer irreversible damage during freezing. The effect of freezing is known to be inhibited by the presence of glycerol.

The potential and current thresholds of the squid axon membrane are affected by temperature. Hodgkin and Katz (1949) have shown that the propagating spike of this axon increases in amplitude and duration with a decrease of temperature. The rate constants of the conductances used by Hodgkin and Huxley (1945) decrease by a factor of three for a $10°$ decrease in temperature. Recent studies by Guttman (1962) indicate that the overall effect of temperature on the threshold value is first shown by the membrane potential response for a current stimulus. As the temperature decreases the responses become slower and larger. Cooling has been found invariably and reversibly to decrease the threshold current in the axons over a range of temperature from $5°$ to $25°$.

B. HIGH TEMPERATURE EFFECTS

At temperatures in the region of 40–45° most animals die within a few hours, and this applies to both hot- and cold-blooded animals. The cause of death by heat and the mechanism of heat injury at temperatures below those at which a visible destruction of the tissue (e.g. coagulation of protein) has taken place has led to speculation and discussion over many years. In the older literature, death by heat was attributed to the coagulation of protein, destruction of enzymes, and asphyxiation, but a "lipoid liberation" theory has also been put forward. In this theory heat injury, whether reversible or irreversible, is attributed to the melting of lipid constituents in the cell or in the cell membranes. This idea is linked with the observation that lipid formed by living organisms at high temperatures is more solid than the lipid formed at lower temperatures.

There are a number of examples in which the iodine numbers of lipids (a value which is related to the number of double bonds in the molecule) have been shown to change with the temperature at which the organisms are grown. Studies of the lipids of poikilothermic organisms show that they vary with the temperature of growth. Plants (Howell and Collins, 1957), insects, blow fly larvae (Fraenkel and Hopf, 1940) and micro-organisms (Terroine et al., 1930; Gaughran, 1947) all appear to contain increased proportions of unsaturated fatty acids or more highly unsaturated fatty acids if they are grown at low temperatures. House *et al.* (1958) have shown that the resistance of larvae of *Pseudosarcophaga affinis* (Fall) to a high temperature is affected by the diet on which they are reared. Insects fed diets containing higher saturated fatty acids had a greater resistance to mortality at a temperature of 45° than did those fed with unsaturated fatty acids. Homeothermic organisms also contain a greater proportion of unsaturated fatty acids in the surface lipids if the environmental temperature is low. This led to the idea that the composition of the lipid may set the limits of temperature for growth of micro-organisms. Gaughran (1947) investigated the lipid composition of steno- and eurithermophilic bacteria and suggested that cells cannot grow at temperatures below the solidification point of their lipids, i.e. the temperature at which the lipids solidify is the minimum temperature for growth. On the other hand, it has been suggested (Heilbrunn, 1924; Bělehrádek, 1931) that the melting of lipids at high temperatures destroys essential structures of the cell, i.e. the temperature at which the lipid melts is the maximum temperature for growth. Recently, Marr and Ingraham (1962) showed that the proportion of unsaturated fatty acids in *Escherichia coli* decreases continuously as the growth temperature is increased. The fatty acids in bacteria are mainly contained in phospholipids. Recently a study has been made of the brain lipid fatty acids of goldfish acclimatized to various temperatures (Johnston and Roots, 1964). This showed that with decreasing acclimatization temperatures (a) the total amount of lipid increased, and (b) there was an overall tendency for the degree of unsaturation of the fatty acids to increase. Gas–liquid chromatographic (GLC) analysis showed that the major changes in the brain involved the polyunsaturated fatty acids of twenty carbon atoms or more. It was suggested that acclimatization involves the ability to control the degree of unsaturation of cellular lipids to maintain a specific liquid-crystalline state of cell membranes.

X-ray studies of the myelin in the frog sciatic nerve (Elkes and Finean, 1953) showed that maximum changes occur in the diffraction pattern of fresh nerve between 0° and −2° and between 58° and 61°. The patterns of dried nerve and total lipid extract showed wide variations in the relative intensities of the 43·0 ± 1·0 Å and 60·0 ± 1·0 Å lines. Freezing appeared to cause the separation of a labile lipid component from the complex and produced an irreversible change. Some differential thermal analysis (DTA) studies have been carried out with human peripheral and central nervous system myelin (Chapman, 1965; unpublished observations). These show endothermic transitions at temperatures of about 33° and 48° respectively.

The rate of haemolysis in 0·303 M-glycerol has been determined as a function of temperature for erythrocytes from nine different species of animals (J. de Gier, L. L. M. van Deenen and K. van Senden, personal communication). Red cells of one group (rat, man, rabbit and guinea pig) exhibit rapid haemolysis which is rather independent of the temperature; those of the second group (pig, dog, cat, sheep and ox) exhibit slight haemolysis to show a significant increase in permeability at elevated temperatures. At 37°, or at higher temperatures, the differences between the two groups are less pronounced. These results are shown in Fig. 4. When the pH value of the environment is lowered from 7·8 to 5·0, the time for complete haemolysis of a suspension of rabbit red cells is increased, giving it a temperature dependence similar

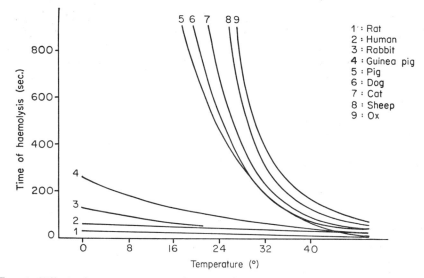

FIG. 4. Effect of temperature on the rate of haemolysis in isosmotic glycerol of erythrocytes from different mammals (J. de Gier, L. L. M. van Deenen and K. van Senden, unpublished observations).

to that of the erythrocytes of the second group. In general, the erythrocytes that lyse at low temperatures are highly permeable to glycerol, and appear to contain a high percentage of lecithin. But no simple correlation between the time of haemolysis and the type of phospholipid in the membrane has yet been reported.

C. MODEL MEMBRANES

Recent attempts have been made to prepare model membranes with a variety of phospholipids using 0·1-M sodium chloride solutions (Mueller et al., 1962, 1963; Huang et al., 1964). To form a membrane, a small droplet of lipid is dissolved in chloroform–methanol solvent and applied with a very fine sable brush to a 2 mm. diameter aperture in a polyethylene cup. A film of about 100 μ thickness rapidly forms across the aperture as the chloroform and methanol diffuse into the aqueous phase surrounding the cup. Continued loss of solvent to the aqueous phase results in a gradual thinning of the film in the aperture to a thickness of about 1000 Å. At this point, small regions of the film can be observed to undergo an abrupt transition to a much thinner structure, determined to be about 61 Å thick. This film might be considered to be analogous to the lamellar type structure of a membrane as put forward by Gorter and Grendel (1925).

The formation of model membranes is apparently affected by temperature (Huang *et al.*, 1964), and this has been investigated in the range from 16° to 45°. At a temperature of 36°, the membrane is formed in the system in about 4 min. As the temperature is lowered, the time for membrane formation increases and is about 30 min. at 20°. Below this temperature membrane formation is never observed although colour films are formed slowly. At temperatures above 39° the time for membrane formation decreases to less than 1 min. but the membranes formed under these conditions are not stable. The membrane materials used in these temperature experiments were made with egg yolk phosphatidylcholine and n-tetradecane (Thompson, 1964).

The resistance of these model membranes is also reported to be affected by temperature (Huang *et al.*, 1964). At a temperature of 36°, the resistance of 1 cm.^{2} of membrane is $3 \cdot 7 \times 10^6$ ohms. As the temperature is lowered, the resistance increases linearly until, at 29°, there is an abrupt decrease in resistance to $4 \cdot 1 \times 10^6$ ohm/cm.^{2}. This is followed again by an increase in resistance and a second abrupt decrease at about 22°. Thus there are two temperature-dependent transitions for these model membrane systems. It is suggested that these changes in resistance are due to phase changes occurring in the lipid film at the different temperatures. However, other studies on model membranes of this type have not shown similar resistance changes with temperature (van den Berg, 1965).

III. The Effects of Heat on Membrane Constituents

A. PHOSPHOLIPIDS

The major constituents of cell membranes are phospholipids, sphingolipids and cholesterol but, because of the difficulty of synthesizing pure phospholipids, very few studies on the effect of heat on these constituents have until recently been reported. The various physical techniques which have recently been applied to pure anhydrous phospholipids, such as the phosphatidylethanolamines and phosphatidylcholines, have shown that marked transitions occur at temperatures well below the capillary melting point of the phospholipid.

1. *Infrared Spectroscopic Studies*

The individual bonds in the infrared absorption spectrum of a compound in solution arise from vibrations often associated predominantly with functional groups such as —OH and $>$C$=$O groupings. With a molecule in a crystalline state, however, additional bands can arise from interactions between the vibrations of molecules in the unit cell so that different crystallographic forms can show marked differences in their infrared spectra (Chapman, 1965). An additional effect is shown by chain molecules. This is because of the possibility of rotational isomerism occurring in the liquid state or in solution as a result of the $>$CH$_2$ groups of the chain twisting and flexing. This gives rise to broad smeared-out bands in certain regions of the spectrum. In the solid state usually only one isomer occurs and the chains lie in the all-planar *trans* configuration. The spectrum of a crystalline long chain compound shows considerable fine structure, and often a regular series of bands occur in the 1250 cm.$^{-1}$ region, the number of bands being related directly to the chain length.

Infrared spectroscopic studies of pure phospholipids (Byrne and Chapman, 1964) first showed clearly the detailed mechanism of the marked transition which occurs on heating phospholipids. The infrared absorption spectra of a fully saturated phospholipid, such as 2,3-dilauroyl-DL-phosphatidylethanolamine, at room temperature shows considerable fine structure associated with the absorption bands that are usually observed with a molecule present in a crystalline condition. On cooling the phospholipid to liquid nitrogen temperatures, there is an increase in the fine structure in the spectra and many bands, which are single in studies done at room temperature, are observed to be split into doublets at the lower temperature. This shows that the phospholipid, although crystalline, has some degree of mobility even at room temperature, the mobility being probably associated with the hydrocarbon chain of the molecule. The absorption band associated with the $>$CH$_2$ rocking mode at 720 cm.$^{-1}$, which is apparently single at room temperature, shows considerable splitting. This doublet is probably associated with orthorhombic O$\perp$ chain packing. On heating the phospholipid, especially to temperatures above 120°, all of the fine structure in the spectrum is replaced by broad diffuse bands. Thus, the spectrum becomes similar to that which is normally observed with a long chain molecule in the liquid condition, and it is clear that the hydrocarbon chains of the phospholipids are undergoing considerable molecular motion. Nevertheless, this is some 80° below the published capillary

melting point of the phospholipid (Fig. 5). A similar effect was observed
some years ago with anhydrous sodium soaps (Chapman, 1958).

With unsaturated phospholipids, such as the 2,3-dioleoyl-DL-phos-
phatidylethanolamines, the infrared absorption spectrum at room

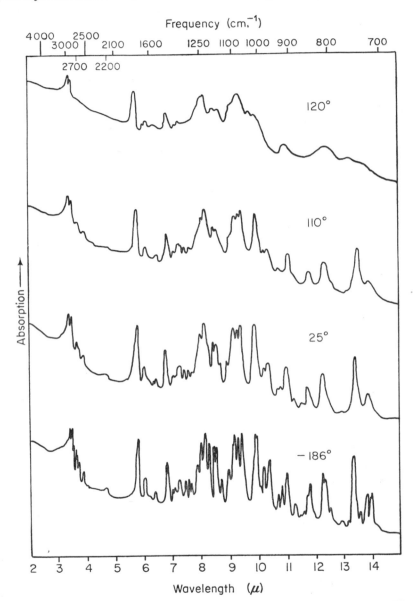

FIG. 5. Infrared spectra of 2,3-dilauroylphosphatidylethanolamine at different
temperatures (Chapman *et al.*, 1966a).

temperature is similar to that of a liquid. Cooling unsaturated phospholipids, such as 2-oleoyl-3-stearoyl-phosphatidylcholine (lecithin) to lower temperatures gives rise to crystalline-type spectra. This shows that the temperature for crystalline-to-liquid crystalline transitions occurs at lower temperatures with unsaturated than with saturated phospholipids. When lecithin is heated to about 40°, this spectrum is replaced by one in which all of the fine structure vanishes and the spectrum is typical of that observed with a liquid.

2. *Differential Thermal Analysis Studies*

Studies using differential thermal analysis (DTA) of pure anhydrous phospholipids (Chapman and Collin, 1965) show the existence of more

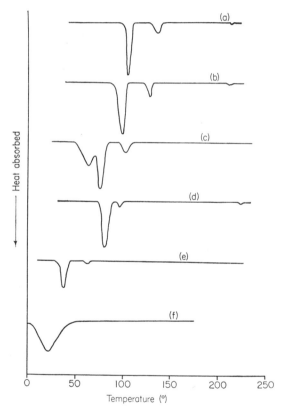

FIG. 6. Differential thermal analysis (DTA) heating curves for different phospholipids: (a) 2,3-dimyristoyl-DL-1-phosphatidylethanolamine; (b) 2,3-dielaidoyl-DL-1-phosphatidylethanolamine; (c) 2-oleoyl-3-stearoyl-DL-1-phosphatidylethanolamine; (d) 2,3-distearoyl-DL-1-phosphatidylcholine; (e) 2-oleoyl-3-stearoyl-DL-1-phosphatidylcholine; (f) Egg yolk lecithin.

than one thermal transition when a phospholipid is heated. An example of this is given by 2,3-dimyristoylphosphatidylethanolamine which shows a marked endothermic transition at about 120°, and a smaller endothermic transition at about 135°. The major thermal transition is not immediately reversible, and even keeping the compound at room temperature for some days does not produce complete reversion to the original form. When one of the chains is unsaturated, e.g. with a phospholipid such as 3-stearoyl-2-oleoylphosphatidylethanolamine, the large endothermic transition occurs at a lower temperature (about 70°), whilst the corresponding phosphatidylcholines also show endothermic transitions but at still lower temperatures. Very little heat change is observed at the temperature corresponding to the capillary melting point, and it is presumed that this temperature corresponds to the breakdown of the ionic sheets of the molecule. Other phospholipids, such as sphingomyelins, phosphatidylserines and natural lipid molecules, also show marked endothermic transitions. Natural phospholipid mixtures have been examined and egg yolk lecithin shows a marked endothermic transition at a temperature of about 20°. A number of DTA curves of phospholipids are shown in Fig. 6. Differential thermal analysis has also shown that these marked endothermic transitions occur at lower temperatures when the phospholipid is in the presence of water. The fully saturated phosphatidylethanolamines undergo an endothermic transition at about 80° when water is present, a temperature which is some 40° below the temperature for the anhydrous material. An exothermic peak is also observed with the phosphatidylethanolamines prior to the endothermic transition.

3. X-ray Studies

Although, as yet, no single crystal X-ray studies of phospholipids are available, a number of studies using X-ray methods have been carried out (Finean, 1953; Finean and Millington, 1955; Chapman et al., 1966a). These studies show that phospholipids can exist in more than one crystallographic form so that they exhibit the phenomenon of polymorphism. The spacings on the X-ray powder photographs obtained with long chain crystals fall into two types, known as long and short spacings. This division into two types of spacing arises from the considerable difference which exists between the length of the molecules and their width. For a particular polymorphic form, the X-ray short-spacings are similar from one homologue to another and are found to be similar to those which occur with other long-chain crystals, such as fatty acids, esters and glycerides. The long-spacings are known to vary with the length of the molecule, and the molecules can be at different angles to the crystallographic planes. By plotting the long-spacings as a function of chain length of a number of homologues, it is possible to deduce the angle of tilt of the molecules in the unit cell. The effect of heat on phospholipids, such as the 2,3-dimyristoyl-DL-phosphatidyl-ethanolamines, is to produce, at 120°, a considerable diminution in the long-spacing; further heating to about 140° produces another, but smaller, decrease. This decrease in long-spacing occurs with phospholipids containing unsaturated chains at lower temperatures and, significantly, at temperatures corresponding to those determined by

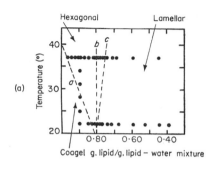

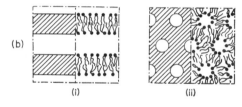

FIG. 7. (a) Phase diagram of a phospholipid-water system, showing the positions of the experimental points; (b) Structure of the liquid-crystalline phases of the phospholipid water system: (i) Lamellar, (ii) Hexagonal. (From data of Luzzati and Husson, 1962. Reprinted by permission of The Rockefeller Institute Press from J. Cell Biol. (1962) 12, 207.)

differential thermal analysis. By plotting the decrease in long-spacings as a function of carbon number for a number of homologues, it has been possible to show that the spacing taken up by the polar groups in the phospholipid remains unchanged in length so that the diminution in spacing is related to the hydrocarbon chains. At the temperature at which this diminution occurs, the short-spacings also show a marked change. In general, the new short-spacing is a diffuse line at about 4·6 Å, and is similar to the spacing observed with liquid long-chain hydrocarbons. The higher unsaturated phospholipids show this diffuse short-spacing at room temperature.

X-ray studies have been made with natural phospholipid mixtures in water. Luzzati and Husson (1962) examined a brain extract, containing 52% phosphatidylethanolamine, 35% phosphatidylcholine and 13% phosphoinositide, using X-ray scattering techniques. The phase diagram was explored as a function of concentration at two temperatures, 22° and 37°, and several X-ray patterns were taken with one sample ($c = 0.9$) as a function of temperature. The resultant phase diagram is shown in Fig. 7. Three main phases can be identified, namely the coagel, the hexagonal and the lamellar. Above the dotted line (Fig. 7), the behaviour is characteristic of liquid–crystalline structures. This material shows a few sharp lines at a small angle, and a broad band at 4·5 Å. Two phases exist, the lamellar and the hexagonal, which can be in equilibrium. With the lamellar phase, the structure is built up of alternate lipid and water layers; in the hexagonal phase, the water is in the interior of the cylinders and the lipid molecules fill the gaps between the cylinders.

4. Nuclear Magnetic Resonance Studies

Nuclear magnetic resonance spectroscopy has also been used in studying the effects of heat on pure phospholipids (Chapman et al., 1965a; Chapman and Salsbury, 1966). Due to magnetic dipole interactions between the magnetic nuclei of a solid, the resonance usually occurs over a broad region of magnetic field and, therefore, a broad absorption band is observed. As molecular motion increases, the interactions between the magnetic nuclei average out and, providing the frequency of the motion exceeds a certain value, the resulting absorption band is narrowed. From the narrowing of the line, it is possible to deduce the degree of molecular motion concerned. The studies of the proton resonance spectrum of pure anhydrous phospholipids show that, with a fully saturated phospholipid such as 2,3-dimyristoyl-DL-phosphatidylethanolamine, the line width at liquid nitrogen temperature is about 15 gauss and decreases with increasing temperature, showing that some molecular motion of the chains is occurring. As the temperature approaches 120°, the line width falls at a considerably increased rate giving rise to a very narrow line about 0·09 gauss wide. This line is sufficiently narrow to be observed with high resolution nuclear resonance techniques. As the resonance spectrum is being produced by the hydrogen nuclei in the phospholipid molecule, this indicates a very high degree of molecular motion of the hydrocarbon chains of the phospholipid. As shown by other physical techniques, this liquid–crystalline transition occurs at lower temperatures with unsaturated phospholipids.

5. *Electron Microscope Studies*

Electron microscope studies of phospholipids have been made by many investigators but, in general, the material used has been natural phospholipid and, particularly, egg yolk phosphatidylcholine. Some recent studies have been made on pure phospholipids (Chapman and Fluck, 1966). Fully saturated phospholipids show no interaction with the compounds commonly used for staining purposes (e.g. osmium tetroxide), and they are, in general, crystalline at room temperature.

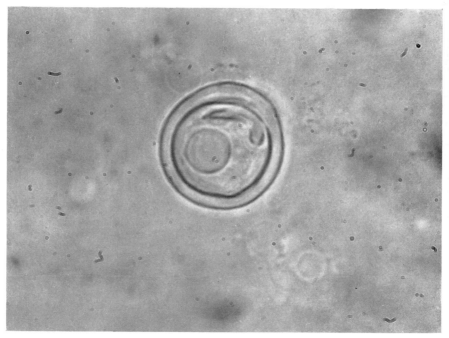

Fig. 8. Myelin tube formation observed with 2,3-distearoyl-DL-phosphatidylcholine on heating in water to 60° (Chapman and Fluck, 1966).

But, if the phospholipid is heated to the endothermic transition temperature of 80° in the presence of water, myelin tubes are formed (Fig. 8) and it is possible to stain these with osmium tetroxide. The lines seen in the electron micrograph are similar to those observed with egg yolk lecithin and with biological tissues which have been fixed at room temperature. Electron microscope studies have also been made on brain phospholipid. By choosing the temperature of fixing to match the different phases that are known to exist, using X-ray techniques, and carrying out the dehydration and embedding at room temperature, micrographs were obtained of both lamellar and hexagonal phases (Stoeckenius, 1962).

6. *Monolayer Studies*

Monolayer studies of phospholipids have been carried out for a number of years. In general this work has been done with natural phospholipid mixtures and, in the vast majority of experiments, with egg yolk phosphatidylcholine. In recent years a few studies have been made with pure synthetic phospholipids (Anderson and Pethica, 1956; van Deenen *et al.*, 1962). These show that the fully saturated phospholipids show much more condensed monolayers than the unsaturated phospholipids containing *cis* hydrocarbon chains. Phospholipids containing *trans* unsaturated chains give monolayers which are much more similar to the fully saturated phospholipids than are those of the unsaturated phospholipids (Chapman *et al.*, 1965b). The monolayers obtained with phosphatidylcholines are much more expanded than are those for the corresponding phosphatidylethanolamines. It is interesting to compare these results with the differential thermal analysis (DTA) results. A high transition temperature for liquid crystal formation is, in general, correlated with a condensed film, and a low transition temperature with an expanded film. The DTA transition temperatures are higher for the phosphatidylethanolamines than for the corresponding phosphatidylcholines. It will be appreciated that, if there is a high degree of molecular motion of the hydrocarbon chains in the solid material in the liquid–crystalline state, at the same temperature there will be at least as much motion when the phospholipid is in a monolayer.

Studies on model mixtures of phospholipids, such as egg yolk lecithin with cholesterol, show that the presence of cholesterol, in definite molar ratios with the phospholipid, causes a condensing effect to occur, so that a monolayer of mixed phospholipid–cholesterol content is more condensed than is the phospholipid itself. The monolayers of the saturated phospholipids, on the other hand, show no condensing effect in the presence of cholesterol; also *trans*-phosphatidylethanolamines show little, if any, condensing effect due to the presence of cholesterol. The effect of heat on the monolayers of a given phospholipid is, in general, to cause the monolayer to become more expanded, and phase changes can occur.

To summarize the information available on the effects of heat on pure phospholipids, it can be stated that they all undergo a transition from crystalline to the liquid–crystalline phase many degrees below the capillary melting point. In the liquid–crystalline phase, the hydrocarbon chains are in a very fluid condition. In the presence of water this transition temperature is lowered. At this temperature, myelin tube formation occurs and the phospholipids can be more easily dispersed. The temperature at which the change from lamellar to hexagonal phases occurs is also related to this temperature. There may also be changes in acid dissociation constants with temperature which need not be monotonic or of the same sign.

B. CHOLESTEROL

Studies have been made on crystalline cholesterol and it has been shown by X-ray and differential thermal analysis that a transition occurs near 40° (H. L. Spier and K. G. van Senden, personal communication). Studies on the effect of heat on cholesterol–phospholipid complexes are at present in progress but, as yet, information is rather limited. It is known that cholesterol and cetyl alcohol form a mixed liquid crystal which dissociates on heating into its two separate components. Relatively high temperatures are said to be required to expand cholesterol-stabilized lipid phases (Adam, 1941).

C. PROTEINS

The effect of heat on proteins is discussed in detail in Chapter 3 of this book. In general, the physical properties of pure proteins at low temperatures vary reversibly but, as the temperature is increased, irreversible changes may occur. This irreversible change in properties is termed denaturation and it is associated with an unfolding of the secondary and tertiary structure of the protein. Denaturation has been shown with the polypeptide insulin using optical rotation measurements (Schellman, 1958). The process usually begins between 50 and 60° and proceeds rapidly above 70°. Proteins are also known to show very high thermal expansion both in the dry state and in solution (Pollard, 1959), and it is thought that this process corresponds to an enlarging of the secondary and tertiary structures. As indicated in the earlier discussion, the role of protein in membrane structure is still somewhat unclear and it is not possible, therefore, to relate these physical changes directly to alterations in membrane structure and function.

D. WATER

Water is considered to be a major component of membrane systems, comprising 30–50% of the total system. It has been suggested that the water in the membrane must be highly ordered in relation to the polar groups of the protein and the phospholipid components. The type of organization suggested includes an ice-like or crystal hydrate lattice as an integral component of the membrane system. As yet there is no detailed information on the organization of the water molecules in membranes. However, studies have been made of water itself and of water in the presence of ions. Infrared studies have shown that there is a substantial change in the OH absorption band of water in the region of 1·4–1·5 μ as the temperature is altered (Klotz, 1965). This shows, and is consistent with other reports that, as the temperature of the water is increased, its degree of organization is decreased. On the other hand, it is suggested that the ordering of water molecules around weakly hydrated ions increases with an increase in temperature, whilst the fraction of hydrogen bonds that are unbroken in the first layer of water around the aliphatic hydrated solute has been calculated to decrease from 63·2–59·3% as the temperature increases from 10–20° (Némethy and Scheraga, 1962). Temperature may also affect the rate of proton interchange along membrane interfaces.

IV. Conclusions and Questions

This chapter has dealt with the temperature effects which can occur with natural biological membranes and with their constituents. In this final section, an attempt will be made to draw some connection between these observations. It is clear that this must be done cautiously because of the many uncertainties still associated with our knowledge of the biological membrane.

There are certain generalizations available which can be made and which are largely independent of the detailed molecular arrangement of phospholipids in biological membranes. One fact which has quite definitely been established from studies of pure phospholipids is that a thermotropic transition occurs from a crystalline to a liquid–crystalline phase at temperatures which are related to the degree of unsaturation in the hydrocarbon chains and also to the type of phospholipid present. This phenomenon must be important in relation to the behaviour of phospholipids in biological membranes. It is also established that lyotropic transitions from a lamellar to a hexagonal phase in water are related to temperature, as are dispersability and myelin tube formation. These phenomena will probably be seen to have some biological relevance.

The possible relationship of these generalizations about phospholipids to the behaviour of biological membranes can be seen from the following observations:

(a) Model membrane formation with egg yolk lecithin is rapid at 36° but does not occur at 20° (see p. 133). The DTA heating and cooling curves of egg yolk lecithin show that the latter temperature is the one at which the crystalline to liquid–crystalline transition occurs, so that model membrane formation appears to be directly related to hydrocarbon chain fluidity. It should be mentioned that the egg yolk lecithin model membrane is considered to be a good analogue of cell membranes.

(b) It is likely that one of the functions of the various distributions of fatty acid residues in membrane phospholipids is to provide the correct hydrocarbon chain fluidity at a particular environmental temperature to match the required diffusion rate or rate of metabolism. In tissues where these processes are required to be rapid, as in mitochondria, the transition temperature for hydrocarbon chain fluidity will be low compared with the environmental temperature. In membranes where these processes are slow, as in the myelin sheath of the central nervous system, this transition temperature may be close to the environmental temperature. Consistent with this, the phospholipids of mitochondrial membranes are known to be more unsaturated than those of the myelin sheath membranes (Green and Fleischer 1963, J. S. O'Brien and E. L. Sampson, personal communication). Cooling a membrane will then be expected to decrease hydrocarbon chain fluidity, and myelin tube and membrane formation, and affect cell growth, whilst heating a membrane will increase hydrocarbon chain fluidity and increase myelin tube and membrane formation. Diffusion and metabolic processes will also be affected and delicate lipid–protein interactions disturbed. Considerable supercooling can occur with some pure phospholipids below the liquid crystalline-to-crystal phase and this phenomenon may also occur in some membranes so that effects due to cooling need not necessarily be sharp. Poikilothermic organisms and bacteria appear to have a feedback mechanism which enables the composition of the fatty acid residues of the phospholipids to be altered so as to keep the hydrocarbon chain fluidity fairly constant, despite fluctuations in environmental temperature.

(c) If we envisage the hydrocarbon chains of the phospholipids of all biological membranes to be in a fluid condition, does this immediately rule out the lipoid liberation theory of heat damage? The answer to this must be: not necessarily so. It is known that, in the myelin sheath of the central nervous system, the hydrocarbon chains are less unsaturated than in other membranes so that their mobility may be considerably less than in other membranes. The organization of the lipids with cholesterol and protein could be considerably disturbed and even destroyed if this mobility were violently increased by an increase of temperature. This answer is, however, rather speculative and other mechanisms, such as water loss from tissues, could be involved.

(d) It seems possible that the liquid–crystalline transitions of some phospholipids will be affected by the interaction of different metal ions with the phospholipid polar groups. This interaction may play a part in processes such as the ion pump mechanism or the triggering of nerve impulses. Temperature effects on the bonding of metal ions to phospholipids would then be expected to affect these processes. As yet, however, there is insufficient evidence to be more definite about this suggestion.

References

Adam, N. K. (1941). *In* "The Physics and Chemistry of Surfaces". University Press, Oxford.

Anderson, P. J. and Pethica, B. A. (1956). *In* "Biochemical Problems of Lipids". Butterworths, London.

Bangham, A. D. and Horne, R. W. (1964). *J. molec. Biol.* **8**, 660.

Bělehrádek, J. (1931). *Protoplasma* **12**, 405.

Booij, H. L. and Bungenberg de Jong, H. G. (1956). *Protoplasmatologia* I (2).

Brown, H. T. and Escombe, F. (1897). *Proc. Roy. Soc.* **62**, 160.

Bungenberg de Jong, H. G. (1949). *In* "Colloid Science", (H. R. Kruyt, Ed.), Vol. II. Elsevier, Amsterdam.

Byrne, P. and Chapman, D. (1964). *Nature, Lond.* **202**, 987.

Chapman, D. (1958). *J. chem. Soc.* 784.

Chapman, D. (1965). "The Structure of Lipids". Methuen, London.

Chapman, D. and Collin, D. T. (1965). *Nature, Lond.* **206**, 189.

Chapman, D. and Fluck, D. J. (1966). *J. cell Biol.* **30**, 1.

Chapman, D. and Salsbury, N. J. (1966). *Trans. Farad. Soc.* **62**, 2607.

Chapman, D., Byrne, P. and Shipley, G. G. (1966a). *Proc. Roy. Soc.* A, **290**, 115.

Chapman, D., Owens, N. F. and Walker, D. A. (1966b). *Biochim. biophys. Acta* **120**, 148.

Danielli, J. F. (1952). *In* "Cytology and Cell Physiology", (G. Bourne, Ed.), p. 150. University Press, Oxford.

Danielli, J. F. and Davson, H. (1943). *In* "Permeability of Natural Membranes", p. 60. University Press, Cambridge.

de Gier, J. (1960). Ph.D. Thesis: University of Utrecht.

de Gier, J. and van Deenen, L. L. M. (1961). *Biochim. biophys. Acta* **49**, 286.

Elkes, J. and Finean, J. B. (1953). *Exp. Cell Res.* **4**, 69.

Finean, J. B. (1953). *Biochim. biophys. Acta* **10**, 371.

Finean, J. B. and Millington, P. F. (1955). *Trans. Farad. Soc.* **51**, 1008.

Fraenkel, G. and Hopf, H. S. (1940). *Biochem. J.* **34**, 1085.

Gaughran, E. R. L. (1947). *J. Bact.* **53**, 506.

Gorter, E. F. and Grendel, F. (1925). *J. exp. Med.* **41**, 439.

Green, D. E. and Fleischer, S. (1963). *Biochim. biophys. Acta* **70**, 554.

Guttman, R. (1962). *J. gen. Physiol.* **46**, 257.

Hanahan, D. J., Watts, R. M. and Pappajohn, D. (1960). *J. Lipid Res.* **1**, 421.

Hardy, W. B. (1913). *Proc. Roy. Soc.* A, **88**, 313.

Hayes, T. L., Lindgren, F. T. and Gofman, J. W. (1963). *J. cell Biol.* **19**, 251.

Hegarty, C. P. and Weeks, O. B. (1940). *J. Bact.* **39**, 475.

Heilbrunn, L. V. (1924). *Amer. J. Physiol.* **69**, 190.

Hodgkin, A. L. and Huxley, A. F. (1945). *J. Physiol.* **104**, 176.

Hodgkin, A. L. and Katz, B. (1949). *J. Physiol.* **108**, 37.

House, H. L., Riordan, D. F. and Barlow, J. S. (1958). *Canad. J. Zool.* **36**, 629.

Howell, R. and Collins, F. I. (1957). *Agron. J.* **49**, 593.

Huang, C., Wheeldon, L. and Thompson, T. E. (1964). *J. molec. Biol.* **8**, 148.

Johnston, P. V. and Roots, B. I. (1964). *Comp. Biochem. Physiol.* **11**, 303.

Jorpes, F. (1932). *Biochem. J.* **26**, 1488.

Kavanau, J. L. (1963). *Nature, Lond.* **198**, 525.

Kavanau, J. L. (1965). *In* "Structure and Function in Biological Membranes", Vol. 1. Holden–Day Inc., San Francisco.

Klotz, I. M. (1965). *Fed. Proc.* **24**, S24.

Kögl, F., de Gier, J., Mulder, I. and van Deenen, L. L. M. (1960). *Biochim. biophys. Acta* **43**, 95.

Kylin, H. (1917). *Ber. deut. botan. Ges.* **35**, 370.

Langmuir, I. (1917). *J. Amer. chem. Soc.* **37**, 1848.

Lovelock, J. E. (1957). *Proc. Roy. Soc.* **B 147**, 427.

Luyet, B. J. and Gehenio, P. M. (1940). *Biodynamica* **3**, 33.

Luzzati, V. and Husson, F. (1962). *J. cell Biol.* **12**, 207.

Macfadyen, A. and Rowland, S. (1900). *Proc. Roy. Soc.* **66**, 339.

Marr, A. G. and Ingraham, J. L. (1962). *J. Bact.* **74**, 1260.

Mueller, P., Rudin, D. O., Tien, H. T. and Wescott, W. C. (1962). *Circulation* **26**, 1167.

Mueller, P., Rudin, D. O., Tien, H. T. and Wescott, W. C. (1963). *J. phys. Chem.* **67**, 534.

Némethy, G. and Scheraga, H. A. (1962). *J. chem. Phys.* **36**, 3401.

Parpart, A. K. and Ballentine, R. (1952). *In* "Modern Trends in Physiology and Biochemistry", Academic Press, New York.

Pollard, E. (1959). Biophysical Society Meeting Abstracts.

Robertson, J. D. (1959). *Biochem. Soc. Symp.* **16**, 1.

Schellman, J. A. (1958). *Compt. rend. trav. Lab. Carlsberg, Ser. Chim.* **30**, 395.

Stoeckenius, W. (1962). *J. cell Biol.* **12**, 221.

Terroine, E. F., Hatterer, C. and Roehrig, P. (1930). *Bull. Soc. Chim. Biol.* **12**, 682.

Thompson, T. E. (1964). *In* "Cellular Membranes in Development", (M. Locke, Ed.). Academic Press, New York.

Turner, J. C., Anderson, H. M. and Gandal, C. P. (1958). *Biochim. biophys. Acta*, **30**, 130.

van Deenen, L. L. M. (1965). *In* "Progress in the Chemistry of Fats and Other Lipids", (R. T. Holman, Ed.), VIII. Part 1. Pergamon Press, Oxford.

van Deenen, L. L. M., Houtsmuller, U. M. T., de Haas, G. H. and Mulder, E. (1962). *J. Pharm. Pharmacol.* **14**, 429.

van den Berg, H. J. (1965). *J. molec. Biol.* **12**, 290.

Chapter 6

Temperature Effects on Micro-organisms

JUDITH FARRELL AND A. H. ROSE

Department of Microbiology,
University of Newcastle Upon Tyne, England

I. Introduction

The activities of living cells are the result of an intricately co-ordinated series of chemical reactions each of which is catalysed by a specific protein or enzyme. In order that these enzyme-catalysed, or metabolic, reactions can proceed at a rate that will permit the organism to grow and reproduce with continuity, it is essential that the organism be supplied with heat or thermal energy, which is needed to activate the molecules participating in the enzymic reactions. A small fraction of the heat requirement of living organisms comes from the organism itself which dissipates a portion of its metabolic energy in this form. However, the main source of heat for living organisms is the environment. It is important to note, nevertheless, that the amount supplied by the environment must not fall outside a certain critical range if growth and reproduction are to take place. On the one hand, the amount supplied must exceed a certain value in order that the metabolic reactions can take place at a reasonable speed. On the other hand, it must not be so great that the molecules (particularly enzymes, nucleic acids and lipids) that go to make up the living cell are inactivated or destroyed. The purpose of the present chapter is to describe the responses of micro-organisms, particularly the unicellular forms, to temperature.

Any account of the effects of temperature on micro-organisms differs in at least three important respects from accounts dealing with other groups of living organisms. Firstly, because of the ease and speed with which micro-organisms can be cultivated in the laboratory, the effects of temperature on these organisms have, on the whole, been studied far more extensively than with any other group of organisms, with the result that the available data are quite voluminous. Nevertheless, as will become apparent while reading this chapter, there are still sizeable gaps in our knowledge. A second important consideration is that the comparative biological simplicity of micro-organisms, in particular that of the unicellular forms which show a minimum of differentiation, has allowed microbiologists to study the effects of temperature on these organisms quite intensively. Consequently, our understanding of the effects of temperature, in molecular terms, is far more advanced for micro-organisms than for any other group of organisms. So much so, that many of the tentative generalizations that have been made regarding the overall effects of temperature on living cells have originated from observations made on micro-organisms. A third factor, which is perhaps more significant than either of those already mentioned, is that the effects of temperature on micro-organisms are of very considerable commercial and economic importance. The development of microbiology as a scientific discipline depended in no small way upon the discovery of suitable methods of freeing laboratory apparatus and growth media from unwanted micro-organisms. Following the pioneer work of Pasteur and Koch, the heat sterilization of perishable materials, which had been practised unwittingly for many centuries, quickly became a subject of active study. In the early years of this century, it was found that foodstuffs, and similar materials that are prone to microbial attack, could also be protected from microbial invasion by cooling to a temperature below the minimum for growth of potential spoilage organisms. Since freezing and cooling allowed the organoleptic qualities of foods to be retained, they soon began to be preferred to heat sterilization, which often causes some loss in taste and flavour. As a result of this commercial application of heat sterilization and of freezing and cooling, the microbiologist has been obliged to give almost as much attention to the behaviour of micro-organisms at temperatures outside the limits for growth as he has to temperatures within the growth range.

The first part of this chapter deals with the effects of temperature on various microbial activities, and the second part is devoted to a review of the economic importance of the temperature relationships of micro-organisms. In the past, fundamental studies on the effects of temperature on micro-organisms have tended to be divorced from the applied aspects of the subject. Microbiologists who are interested in the fundamental aspects of the temperature responses of micro-organisms usually strive for explanations of these responses in molecular terms. The applied microbiologist, on the other hand, frequently adopts a more empirical and pragmatic approach to the subject, and is concerned mainly with the problems that arise as a result of the development of microbial activity in materials that have been either heat sterilized or preserved by freezing or cooling.

This division of interest among microbiologists who are concerned with the effects of temperature on micro-organisms is reflected in the contents of review articles that have appeared on the subject. The physiological and biochemical aspects of the temperature responses of micro-organisms have been dealt with by Ingraham and Stokes (1959) and by Ingraham (1962), while the reviews by Witter (1961), Borgstrom (1955), and Elliott and Michener (1960) have emphasized the applied aspects of the subject. In a recent review, we dealt with both aspects (Farrell and Rose, 1965).

II. Effects of Temperature on Micro-organisms and Microbial Activities

It is well established that temperature profoundly affects all activities of micro-organisms. When an examination is made of the effects of temperature on various microbial activities, it is usually found that there are reasonably well-defined optimum, maximum and minimum temperatures for each activity, and that the optimum (or maximum or minimum) temperature for one activity does not necessarily coincide with those for other activities. A useful way of expressing quantitatively the effect of temperature on a microbial activity is in the form of the temperature co-efficient or Q_{10} value, examples of which are given in the texts by Johnson et al. (1954) and Thimann (1963). The main disadvantage in using temperature co-efficients in any detailed study of the effects of temperature on biological processes and reactions is that the values for any one process vary with the temperature span over which the rates are measured.

A generalized, and far more sophisticated, method of expressing quantitatively the effects of temperature on biological systems is by applying the Arrhenius equation. Over 75 years ago, Arrhenius (1889) derived the following equation to describe the effects of temperature on the rates of chemical reactions:

$$k = Ae^{-E/RT}$$

In this equation, k is the velocity constant for the particular reaction, and T the temperature in degrees Absolute. The pre-exponential term in the equation (A) was originally a constant of integration, but when it was realized that the rate of a reaction might be the product of the number of activated molecules and their frequency of collision (Lewis, 1918), the term was modified to include the collision number and a probability factor. Arrhenius initially considered E to represent the energy difference between the reactants and the activated species of the reacting molecules but, as students of chemical kinetics now envisage activated species as having structures transitional between those of the reactants and the products, E is now considered to be the minimum energy difference between the reactants and the transitional state. Some years later, Arrhenius (1908) extended his formula to the influence of temperature on the rates of biological processes and reactions and, in this modified form, he replaced E by the term μ, which is referred to as the *temperature characteristic* of the process.

Since the terms A and E (or μ) are usually assumed to be constants for a particular reaction, a plot of log k against $1/T$ should give a straight line with a slope of $-E/2 \cdot 303R$. This relationship has been shown to hold for a wide range of chemical reactions. However, several types of reactions are known not to give a straight line on this plot; these deviations from the Arrhenius reaction have been reviewed by Hulett (1964). Biological processes, including microbial growth and enzymic reactions studied *in vivo* or *in vitro*, characteristically give non-linear plots; some examples are given on p. 177. Several attempts have been made to explain the non-linearity of the Arrhenius plot for enzymic activity; these explanations have been discussed by Farrell and Rose (1965) and are further examined in Chapter 3 (p. 25) and in Section IID (p. 198) of this chapter. In our present state of ignorance concerning the roles of individual molecules in such complex biological processes as growth, it is clearly very difficult to explain the non-linearity of the Arrhenius plots for such phenomena. Nevertheless, the Arrhenius plot is still extremely useful for comparing the effects of temperature on different physiological processes, so long as no attempt is made to explain the observed responses on the basis of a similarity with the behaviour shown by enzymes studied *in vitro*.

A. GROWTH

The abilities to grow and to reproduce are the most commonly observed properties of micro-organisms, and this explains why so much interest has been shown in the effects of temperature on microbial growth.

1. *General Effects of Temperature on Growth*

Growth of a culture of micro-organisms is usually divided into three major phases, namely the lag, exponential and stationary phases. The duration of the lag phase, the rate of exponential growth and the yield of organisms are all affected by temperature. By far the greatest number of experiments have been designed to investigate the effects of temperature on growth rate, and we shall deal with this in detail before returning briefly to the effects on the duration of the lag phase and on the yield of organisms.

a. Growth rate. The exponential rate of growth of a micro-organism is most conveniently expressed as the specific growth rate (k) which can be calculated from the turbidity readings on a liquid culture of unicellular organisms using the expression:

$$k = \frac{2 \cdot 303(\log x_2 - \log x_1)}{t_2 - t_1}$$

in which x_2 and x_1 are the turbidity readings at times t_2 and t_1. When values for k (in hr.$^{-1}$) are determined for growth at several different temperatures, it is found that the value is greatest over a fairly narrow range, the mean of which is referred to as the *optimum temperature* for growth. The lowest value below the optimum at which growth just takes place ($k \simeq 0$) is called the *minimum temperature* for growth, while the maximum temperature for growth (again where $k \simeq 0$) is defined as the highest temperature above the optimum at which growth takes place.

The minimum, optimum and maximum temperatures for growth of micro-organisms have acquired a cardinal, indeed almost mystic, importance in microbiology. Nevertheless, it is well to remember that the values for these temperatures, for any one micro-organism, may vary depending upon the chemical and physical properties of the environment. Information on the extent to which environmental factors can affect the optimum, maximum and minimum temperatures for growth of different micro-organisms is meagre, and it is a subject which deserves more detailed study.

Already, some unusual effects of the environment on the cardinal temperatures for growth of micro-organisms have been reported. For example, Mitchell and Houlahan (1946) studied a *Neurospora crassa* mutant which synthesized riboflavin at a rate approaching that of the wild type up to 28°, but required exogenous riboflavin at temperatures above 28°. In media containing suboptimum concentrations of riboflavin, the mould showed two optimum temperatures for growth (25° and 37°), although in media containing an optimum concentration of the vitamin, the optimum temperature for growth was 32°, the same as for the wild type. In addition, an unnamed sulphate-reducing bacterium, which was probably a clostridium, was reported by Oppenheimer and Drost-Hansen (1960) to show optima for growth at 11°, 25° and 39°, and minima near 16°, 31° and 43°. They attributed this atypical behaviour to the abrupt changes that occur in certain properties of water (such as viscosity) as the temperature is increased from 0° to 60°. These changes occur within a rather narrow temperature range ($\pm 2°$) near 15°, 30°, 45° and 60°, and are believed to be caused by structural changes in the water (see Chapter 2, p. 5). A similar phenomenon has been reported by Sieburth (1964), who worked with an arthrobacter in which the temperature affected not only the rates of growth but also the morphology of the bacterium. The most recent report of this unusual type of behaviour was by Davey et al. (1966), who observed multiple optimum temperatures for growth of a strain of Streptococcus faecalis. We describe these reports as unusual if only because they have never been reported by other workers who for years have been studying the effects of temperature on the rate of growth of micro-organisms.

Another important reservation regarding the values for the optimum, maximum and minimum temperatures for growth is that these values are not sharply defined and frequently cannot be quoted accurately as single figures. This is mainly because of the technical difficulties, at least in many microbiological laboratories, of measuring growth rates at a sufficiently large number of temperatures. Such measurements require the availability of numerous incubators or constant temperature water baths, facilities which few laboratories can call upon. The problem has been solved in some laboratories by using temperature-gradient incubators. A number of different designs have been described, but they usually consist basically of bars of heavy gauge metal at one end of which heat is applied. This heat is dissipated along the length of the bar so that a temperature gradient is formed. It is possible to regulate the magnitude of the gradient by controlling the amount of heat applied, by varying the efficiency of the insulating material surrounding the bars, and by controlling the ambient temperature. An interesting development in the design of temperature-gradient incubators has been reported by Nakae (1966) who has constructed an apparatus in which a temperature gradient is maintained by heat conduction in a liquid. With certain types of temperature-gradient apparatus, it is possible to incubate microbial cultures at temperatures differing by as little as 0·2°. Temperature-gradient incubators have so far been used for studying the effects of temperature on the growth of bacteria (Oppenheimer and Drost-Hansen, 1960; Cannefax, 1962; Landman *et al.*, 1962; Elliott and Heiniger, 1965; Dimmick, 1965a) and algae (Halldal and French, 1958). They have the disadvantage that they can often be used only with

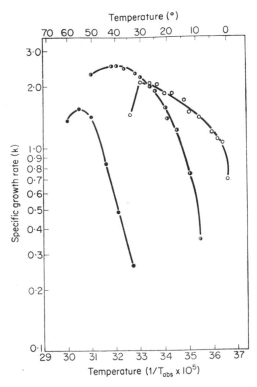

FIG. 1. Arrhenius plots of the specific growth rates of a psychrophilic pseudomonad (○), a mesophilic strain of *Escherichia coli* (◑), and a thermophilic strain of *Bacillus circulans* (●). Data for the psychrophil and the mesophil were replotted from those of Ingraham (1958). The thermophil data are from Allen (1953).

organisms growing on solid media, although modifications have been made to some instruments so that they can be used with liquid cultures (Landman *et al.*, 1962).

Despite these reservations concerning the cardinal temperatures for growth of micro-organisms, microbiologists have used them to separate micro-organisms into categories known as psychrophils, mesophils and thermophils. The data in Fig. 1 show Arrhenius plots for the growth rates of typical examples of psychrophilic, mesophilic and thermophilic bacteria. These are quite useful divisions of the microbial world if, as Ingraham (1962) has pointed out, one asks no more of them than that they refer to micro-organisms that grow best at low temperatures (psychrophils), intermediate temperatures (mesophils) and high temperatures (thermophils). Unfortunately, microbiologists have tried to make the demarcations more precise by fixing the ranges of temperature over which the growth rate is affected for each category, with the result that each of the three terms has come to have many different meanings to microbiologists.

Mesophilic micro-organisms. The majority of micro-organisms that have so far been isolated grow most rapidly at temperatures between about 25° and 40°; these organisms are described as mesophilic. Their optimum temperatures for growth usually correlate with the temperatures that prevail in their natural habitats. For example, micro-organisms which are pathogenic or saprophytic on man, usually grow best around 37°; the majority of fungi, which on the whole are found in relatively cool habitats, have optimum temperatures around 25°–30° (Cochrane, 1958). At temperatures above the optimum, the growth rate of mesophils usually declines very rapidly, and the maximum temperature for growth is often only 5°–10° above the optimum. Using their temperature-gradient incubator, Elliott and Heiniger (1965) showed that the maximum temperatures for growth of 34 representative strains of *Salmonella* (optimum temperature about 37°) lay between 43·2 and 46·2°. The growth rate declines much less rapidly at temperatures below the optimum for growth (Fig. 1). The majority of mesophilic micro-organisms that have been studied have minimum temperatures for growth of 5°–10°. However, some mesophils have higher minimum temperatures for growth. Strains of *Corynebacterium xerosis*, for example, are unable to grow at temperatures below about 20° (Stanley and Rose, 1967a).

At temperatures above the optimum for growth, some mesophilic micro-organisms become auxotrophic for compounds that do not need to be supplied exogenously at or below the optimum temperature, with the result that these organisms have higher maximum temperatures for growth in nutritionally complex media than in simple chemically defined media. Ingraham (1962) and Langridge (1963) have compiled useful lists of micro-organisms that show increased nutritional demands at temperatures above the optimum for growth. An interesting example of this effect of medium composition on the maximum temperature for growth of mesophils has been reported by Lichstein and Begue (1959) who showed that several strains of *Saccharomyces* are unable to grow in a glucose-salts medium at 38° although they are capable of growth at this temperature in a more complex glucose-casitone-yeast extract medium. The inability to grow at 38° was traced to an additional demand by the yeasts for pantothenate although, at 30°, the yeast gave abundant growth in pantothenate-free medium.

Reports of the minimum temperature for growth of micro-organisms being affected by the chemical composition of the medium are much rarer. O'Donovan and Ingraham (1965) have reported a mutant strain of *Escherichia coli* for which the minimum temperature for growth about 8°) is much lower in minimal glucose-salts medium supplemented with histidine than in unsupplemented minimal medium (20°). We shall return later to this question of the effect of incubation temperature on the nutritional requirements of micro-organisms, since these data give important clues regarding the effects of temperature on the metabolic processes of micro-organisms.

Thermophilic micro-organisms. Since the early nineteenth century, microbiologists have recognized the existence of organisms that can tolerate, and even prefer, temperatures above the maximum usually found for mesophilic micro-organisms. These have been called thermophilic micro-organisms, and representatives have been recorded among the algae, bacteria, and fungi.

Probably the first group of thermophilic micro-organisms to be recognized were the thermophilic algae which have been isolated from guysers and hot springs in Yellowstone National Park in Wyoming, U.S.A., and from similar sources in New Zealand, Iceland and Japan. These algae are almost all members of the Cyanophyta (blue-green algae) and include species of *Oscillatoria* and *Synechococcus* (Fogg, 1961). Many thermophilic algae grow best between 50° and 70° (Brock and Brock, 1966). There are claims that their maximum temperatures for growth may be as high as 89°, but some recent re-investigations of the problem have shown that the maximum is probably nearer 75° Kempner, 1963). It is worth noting in this context that, at the elevation of Yellowstone National Park where many of these thermophilic algae have been isolated, water boils at a temperature of 93°. For additional information on thermophilic algae, the reviews by Copeland (1936) and Gessner (1955) should be perused.

The first report of a thermophilic bacterium appeared in 1888 when Miquel described the isolation of one from the River Seine, a source scarcely thought to be favourable for the development of a bacterium which can grow at 73° and is incapable of growing at low temperatures. Since then, many more thermophilic bacteria have been isolated, and a considerable amount of attention has been given to them principally because these organisms can be important spoilage organisms in canned and processed foods (see Section IIIB, p. 207). The majority of thermophilic bacteria are aerobic spore-formers, members of the genus *Bacillus*,

6+T.

although thermophilic representatives have been found among the clostridia, sarcinae, spirochaetes, staphylococci and streptococci. The subject of aerobic, spore-forming thermophilic bacteria was exhaustively reviewed by Allen (1953), and readers are recommended to turn to her review in order to familiarize themselves with the earlier literature on these organisms. It seems that thermophilic variants of almost any mesophilic strain of *Bacillus* are likely to be encountered. Although thermophilic bacteria have been isolated from tropical soils and desert sands, they are not peculiarly indigenous to hot environments and have been isolated from temperate soils, sea water, ocean mud, sewage, and even freshly fallen snow. With the exception of the areas around fumaroles, thermophilic bacteria have not so far been reported to occur in the Antarctic.

Thermophilic strains of actinomycetes have been recognized for many years; they too are commonly found in soils and also in compost heaps. These actinomycetes usually have an optimum temperature for growth of 40–50° and were orginally grouped together as *Actinomyces thermophilus*. However, their manner of spore formation suggests that they should be classified as members of the genera *Micromonospora* and *Thermoactinomyces* (Waksman and Corke, 1953). Certain strains of *Streptomyces* have also been reported to be thermophilic, and some isolates of *Nocardia sebivorans* and other pathogenic aerobic actinomycetes are on record as having withstood a temperature of 90° for 10 min. (Erikson, 1955).

The first reference to a thermophilic fungus was made by Lindt (1886) However, until recently, these organisms were blatantly neglected, and even as late as 1963 only about six thermophilic fungi had been described. But it is now clear that these fungi are more numerous than the few reports would suggest. In a delightfully produced monograph by Cooney and Emerson (1964), there is an account of researches, which extended over several years, on the thermophilic fungi isolated from retted guayacule shrub and other materials. The work of these authors has considerably extended the list of known thermophilic fungi, which are defined by them as fungi with a maximum temperature for growth at or above 50° and a minimum temperature for growth above 20°. Fungi such as *Aspergillus fumigatus* and *Absidia ramosa*, with maxima near 50° but minima well below 20°, were considered to be *thermotolerant*. Cooney and Emerson concluded that the thermophilic habit is not particularly strongly expressed in any one of the three main classes of fungi, although no thermophilic basidiomycetes have yet been reported (Fig. 2). The studies of Cooney and Emerson should stimulate further research on thermophilic fungi, and the number of reports concerning these organisms will probably increase in the near future.

So far in this account, only occasional reference has been made to a definition of thermophilic micro-organisms, mainly because the term has come to mean many things to many workers. However, it is likely that few microbiologists would demur if the term were reserved for micro-organisms that are capable of growing at 55°. But as soon as attempts are made to specify further the characteristics of thermophils, disagreements arise among microbiologists. It is clear, for example, that

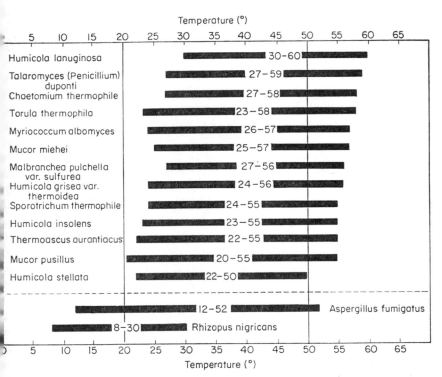

Fig. 2. Ranges of temperature for growth of certain thermophilic fungi. Data for *Rhizopus nigricans*, a common mesophil, and for *Aspergillus fumigatus*, one of the most temperature-tolerant mesophils, are included for comparison. From Cooney and Emerson (1964).

the effects of temperature on the growth rate of many enteric bacteria (e.g. *Escherichia coli*) and of certain thermophilic fungi are not very different; yet *E. coli* is usually regarded as a classical example of a mesophilic bacterium. Readers who wish to amuse themselves with the semantic problems that have arisen with regard to the definition of thermophilism in micro-organisms should turn to the introductory chapter in Cooney and Emerson's (1964) monograph.

Psychrophilic micro-organisms. The existence of micro-organisms which grow well at near-zero temperatures (0–5°) has been recognized for many years. Forster (1887) is generally credited with being the first to report bacterial growth at 0°, a priority which he jealously defended five years later (Forster, 1892). The term "psychrophil" (Gr. cold-loving) was coined by Schmidt-Nielsen (1902) to describe these organisms, and the term is now firmly established in the literature.

In the early years of this century, large numbers of psychrophilic micro-organisms were described, and their optimum, maximum and minimum temperatures for growth determined, albeit only very approximately with many of the organisms. It quickly became clear that they are ubiquitous. Large numbers of psychrophilic micro-organisms have been found in lakes and rivers and in soils. But they are not confined to cold environments and have been reported to occur in relatively warm habitats (Fell, 1961). Psychrophilic representatives occur in all of the major groups of micro-organisms. Psychrophilic bacteria are usually members of the genera *Achromobacter*, *Alcaligenes*, *Flavobacterium*, *Proteus*, *Pseudomonas* and *Serratia*, with the greatest representation in the genus *Pseudomonas* (Brown and Weidemann, 1958; Ingraham and Stokes, 1959). *Pseudomonas geniculata* is probably the most frequently isolated psychrophilic bacterium (Frank, 1962). There are also reports of obligatorily anaerobic psychrophilic bacteria, all of which have been grouped in the genus *Clostridium* (Sinclair and Stokes, 1964). Haines (1931) has reported the existence of psychrophilic actinomycetes, although very little further work has been done with these organisms.

This neglect has extended also to psychrophilic fungi, several of which have been described. For example, Brooks and Hansford (1923) found that some strains of *Cladosporium herbarum* were able to grow at − 6°. Psychrophilic moulds are commonly found as contaminants in cold rooms at even lower temperatures. It would appear, moreover, that the psychrophilic habit is fairly widely distributed among fungal genera. Not so, however, with psychrophilic yeasts, which are usually members of the genus *Candida* (Lawrence *et al.*, 1959), although psychrophilic cryptococci have also been described (Hagen and Rose, 1961).

The best known psychrophilic algae are those which grow on the surface of snow and are a common sight in the polar regions and on mountains. These algae include species of *Scotiella* and *Raphidonema*, and *Ancyclonema nordenskioldii*, *A. meridionale*, *Chlamydomonas nivolis* and *Ch. flavo-virens* (Marrè, 1962). One presumes that the psychrophilic habit must be fairly widespread among marine algae which exist in seas at temperatures that rarely rise above 5°. Little has, however, been published on the temperature characteristics of marine algae, although

Zobell (1962) has reported the isolation of a marine diatom with an optimum temperature for growth of 10°–12°.

Once a large number of psychrophilic micro-organisms had been described, microbiologists began to consider more deeply the problem of defining these organisms. At first, it was suggested that they be defined as organisms with an optimum temperature for growth below 20° (sometimes the limit was placed even lower), and this definition has wormed its way into several microbiological texts. But a careful scrutiny of the temperature characteristics of micro-organisms has shown quite clearly that only a small number of the organisms so far described could, according to this definition, be considered to be psychrophilic. A few such organisms have been reported although rarely in any detail. Some of the bacteria isolated from frozen soil by Lochhead (1926) had optimum temperatures for growth below 20°, as did certain strains of Candida isolated from refrigerated grape juice by Lawrence et al. (1959). One of the lowest optimum temperatures recorded is for a psychrophilic strain of Serratia marcescens which K. Eimhjellen, working in Trondheim, Norway, isolated from flounder eggs. Kates and Hagen (1964) showed that this bacterium grew optimally around 5°. These reports suggest that micro-organisms with low optimum temperatures for growth are rare. It is quite possible, however, that this is a false impression, since the conventional methods for examining material in the microbiological laboratory would lead to the death of such organisms, especially if they have maximum temperatures for growth only a few degrees above their optimum. Our colleague S. O. Stanley recently collected samples from lakes on Deception Island in Antarctica (maximum summer temperature around 5°) and took particular care to ensure that samples never encountered a temperature greater than 10° before and during the isolation of the organisms. Of the isolates obtained, well over half had optimum temperatures for growth in the range 15°–20° (Stanley and Rose, 1967b). These data suggest that micro-organisms with optimum temperatures below 20° may indeed be much more widespread than has hitherto been suspected.

Adaptation to a new temperature range. In view of the significance attached to the range of temperatures over which micro-organisms can grow, it was natural that microbiologists should want to know how readily a micro-organism can be adapted to grow at temperatures above or below its maximum and minimum (Ingraham, 1962). Adaptation of micro-organisms to growth over different temperature ranges has been studied by several workers, and their data show that, with the exception of one group of organisms, the temperature range for most micro-organisms growing under normal environmental or laboratory conditions is not readily altered. The ability of certain mesophilic bacteria to lose the capacity to grow rapidly at higher temperatures in the growth range, after several weeks of subculture at a low temperature in the growth range, was studied by Jennison (1935). Strains of *Aerobacter aerogenes*, *Chromobacter violaceum*, *Escherichia coli* and *Serratia marcescens* were cultured for several weeks at 22°, and the generation times of these bacteria at 22°, 27°, 32°, 37° and 42° were compared with the generation times of bacteria that had been subcultured at one of these four temperatures for several months. However, no significant changes in the generation times could be detected as a result of culturing at 22°.

An exception to the generalization made above has been reported with certain mesophilic bacteria which can often acquire the ability to grow at temperatures above their maximum for growth, and therefore become essentially thermophilic. The early experiments on this adaptation from the mesophilic to the thermophilic habit have been well reviewed by Allen (1953). Kluyver and Baars (1932) were among the first to report evidence for this adaptation when they showed that strains of the mesophil, *Desulphovibrio desulphuricans*, can acquire the thermophilic habit after culturing at high temperatures. But probably the most compelling evidence has come from Allen (1953). She reported that mesophilic strains of *Bacillus subtilis*, *B. cereus*, *B. megaterium*, and *B. circulans* consistently yielded thermophilic variants; the one strain of *B. pumilus* that she tested also gave a thermophilic variant, but the strains of *B. macerans* never did. Mefferd and Campbell (1952) have also reported a thermophilic variant of *B. globigii*. This capacity of mesophilic bacteria to give rise to thermophilic variants is not widespread and could not be demonstrated with strains of *Aerobacter*, *Escherichia*, *Mycobacterium*, *Pseudomonas* or *Streptococcus*, or with actinomycetes. It is also worth noting that facultative thermophilic bacilli growing in the mesophilic range require a brief period of adaptation at intermediate temperatures before gaining the capacity to initiate growth at thermophilic temperatures (Bausum and Matney, 1965).

Now that the technique for studying genetic transformation in bacilli has been established, it is possible to investigate the transfer of genetic characters that determine thermophily. McDonald and Matney (1963) showed that, when mesophilic strains of *B. subtilis* (which are unable to grow at 55°) were grown in the presence of DNA extracted from thermophilic strains of this bacterium (which had the ability to grow at 55°), the mesophils were transformed at the rate of about one organism in 10^4 for the ability to grow at 55°. The character controlling this ability appeared to be closely linked to the single-step high-level streptomycin-resistant locus. It would seem, therefore, that the acquisition of the thermophilic habit by these mesophilic bacilli involves a relatively small change in the metabolism of the bacteria.

The artificial production of mutant strains of micro-organisms with the ability to grow over a different temperature range from that of the parent is a comparatively easy task now that chemical mutagens such as ethylmethane sulphonate (EMS) are being used. Mutant strains with a lower maximum temperature for growth as compared with the parent, have been known for some time. Maas and Davis (1952), for example, obtained a mutant strain of *Escherichia coli* which, unlike the parent strain, was unable to grow in a glucose-salts medium at temperatures above 30°. Mutant strains of *Pseudomonas aeruginosa*, which have a lower minimum temperature for growth as compared with the parent, and are therefore psychrophilic, have been described by Azuma *et al.* (1962). In Ingraham's laboratory, chemical mutagens have been used successfully to produce mutants of *Escherichia coli* ML30 with higher minimum temperatures for growth (around 20°) than the parent strain which has a minimum temperature of about 8° (O'Donovan *et al.*, 1965), and also mesophilic mutants from psychrophilic strains of pseudomonads (S. Conden and J. L. Ingraham, unpublished observations). The use that is being made of these mutant strains of bacteria in studies on the biochemical bases of the minimum temperatures for growth is described in Section IIA.2 (p. 168).

b. Lag phase of growth. The effect of temperature on the rate of growth of micro-organisms is usually studied by inoculating portions of medium with organisms that have been grown at or near the optimum temperature for growth of the organism being tested, and observing growth after incubation at different temperatures. These experiments show that, not only is the rate of growth affected by the temperature of incubation, but that, as the temperature is lowered below the optimum for growth, the duration of the lag phase of growth is increased (Fig. 3). At temperatures above the optimum but below the maximum for growth, this phenomenon is not usually observed. The data in Fig. 4 are for growth of a psychrophilic Candida at 0°, using inoculum organisms that were grown at different temperatures, and show that the further the temperature of incubation of the inoculum organisms is removed from 0°, the longer is the lag phase of growth when these organisms are inoculated in media and the cultures incubated at 0°. Similar data have been reported for other micro-organisms, and they suggest that, during the lag phase of growth at any particular temperature, a micro-organism carries out metabolic processes (if necessary) that enable that organism to start growing at the rate characteristic for that temperature. If micro-organisms in cultures that have been grown at a particular temperature are harvested and re-inoculated into fresh medium and the

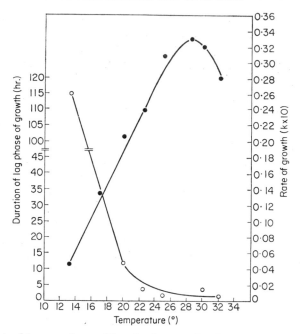

FIG. 3. Effect of temperature of incubation on the duration of the lag phase of growth (○) and on the specific growth rate (k; ●) of *Euglena gracilis*. Inoculum organisms were grown at 25°. Plotted from data of Buetow (1962).

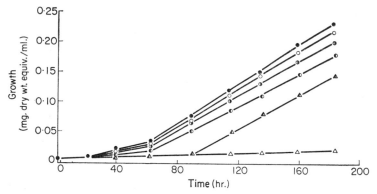

FIG. 4. Effect of incubation time on growth of a psychrophilic Candida at 0°. Inoculum organisms were grown at different temperatures. Organisms in the mid-exponential phase of growth were harvested and washed at the temperature at which they had been grown. The organisms were suspended in 0·89% (w/v) NaCl to a standard density, and the suspensions used to inoculate portions of medium precooled to 0°. Growth temperatures of inoculum organisms were: ●, 0°; ○, 5°; ◑, 10°; ◐, 15°; △, 20°. ▲ indicates the growth of inoculum organisms from agar slope cultures grown at 10°. The Candida was strain A3E-2 described by Rose and Evison (1965). Data from Evison (1966).

cultures incubated at the same temperature, which may be any temperature on the growth range, then the lag phase disappears or is of very short duration.

A more rigorous examination of the effect of shifts in incubation temperature on the growth of *E. coli* ML 30 was made by Ng *et al.* (1962). They showed that, if exponentially growing cultures of this bacterium were grown at one temperature in the range over which the value of μ is constant (Fig. 1), and then transferred to another temperature also in this range of constant μ, exponential growth resumed immediately at the new temperature at a rate characteristic of this temperature. But if the shifts were made to or from temperatures below the range of constant μ, there was a lag phase of growth and the initial rate of growth was intermediate between the rate for the initial and that for the final

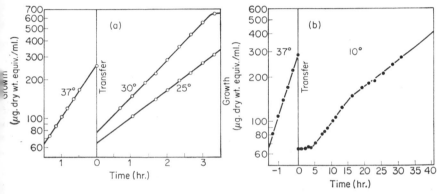

FIG. 5. Effect on the growth of *Escherichia coli* ML 30 of a shift in incubation temperature from 37° to (a) 30° or 25°, and (b) 10°. From Ng *et al.* (1962).

temperature (Fig. 5). The possible significance of these findings in relation to the effects of low temperatures on the metabolic processes of micro-organisms are discussed in Section IIA.2 (p. 168).

c. Yield. The temperature at which a micro-organism grows most rapidly in batch culture is frequently several degrees higher than the temperature at which the greatest crop of organisms is formed. Hess (1934) showed that, although a strain of *Pseudomonas fluorescens* grew most rapidly at 20°, the largest cell crops were obtained in cultures incubated at 5°. Furthermore, with *Streptococcus lactis*, the rate of growth was found to be greatest at 34° which is a temperature some 9° above that at which the largest crops of cells were produced. Similar observations have been reported with other micro-organisms. Sinclair and Stokes (1963) have attributed this effect to the greater solubility, and therefore availability to the organisms, of oxygen at low tempera-

6*

tures, and they showed that equally large cell crops can be obtained at higher temperatures when the batch cultures are vigorously aerated.

Recently, Ng (1965) has reported experiments on effects of tempera ture on the cell yield of *Escherichia coli* ML 30, the yield in these experiments being defined as the number of grams dry weight of organ ism formed from each gram of glucose utilized. Using batch cultures grown to low cell densities by glucose limitation, Ng showed that the yield of bacteria at 13° was about 92% of that at 30° but, when the temperature was decreased to 10°, the yield decreased to about 70% of that at 30°. Since the generation time at 13° was about 8–10 times longer than that at 30°, and that at 10° was approximately 15–20 times the value at 30°, the yield at 10° was clearly decreased disproportion ately to the decrease in the growth rate. Ng was unable to demonstrate a greater accumulation of metabolic end products in cultures grown at 10° as compared with those grown at higher temperatures. There would appear to be a need to examine the effect of temperature on cell yield still more rigorously, preferably using continuously grown cultures, since the effect is a very important factor in the food chains that operate in natural environments such as soils and oceans.

d. Cell size and morphology. Temperature is known to affect cell size and morphology of some micro-organisms, but the effects are not well documented, and few of the reports on the subject consist of more than the most superficial observations. On the whole, greater emphasis has been given to the effect of low temperatures in the growth range. For example, the flagellate *Chilomonas paramecium* showed a marked increase in cell size when the organism was grown at low temperatures in its growth range (Mučibabić, 1956; Johnson and James, 1960), but this was not accompanied by an increase in the dry weight of the cells. It would seem that, with this organism, the greater cell size at low temperatures is almost certainly caused by an increase in the amount of intracellular water. Maclean and Munson (1961) observed a decrease in the percentage of long cells in continuously grown cultures of *Escherichia coli* as the temperature was lowered, but the average cell length was independent of the growth rate. Unfortunately, these workers made no attempt to correlate the altered cell size with the dry weight of the cells. Similar results were reported by Schaechter *et al.* (1958), who showed that, in a given medium, the cell mass of *Salmonella typhimurium* was independent of the growth rate when this was varied by changing the incubation temperature. The yeast–mycelium transformation in yeasts and fungi is influenced by temperature. In general, the change from the typical yeast form to the mycelial form in yeasts is favoured by lowering the temperature (Scherr and Weaver, 1953). Also, the fungus *Ophiostoma multiannulatum* grows on solid media as hyphae at low temperatures out in the conidial phase at higher temperatures (von Hofsten and von Hofsten, 1958). Sieburth (1964), who studied the morphological changes undergone by a marine species of the bacterium *Arthrobacter*, claimed that certain morphological forms were characteristic of particular temperatures.

There are also reports that some bacteria tend to form filaments when grown at temperatures above the optimum for growth. Filaments are formed by *Escherichia coli* at temperatures above 40° (Hoffman and Frank, 1963) and by *Clostridium acidiurici* when grown at 44° (Terry *et al.*, 1966). Filament formation in the clostridium was shown to be due to an inability of the bacterium to synthesize cross walls at 44°. When organisms that had been incubated at 44° were transferred to 37°, cross walls were formed within 30 minutes.

2. *Induction of synchronous growth.* An exponential-phase batch culture contains micro-organisms at all stages in the division cycle. Several different methods have been described for inducing the micro-organisms in such a culture to divide more or less simultaneously, that is, within a very short period compared with the generation time. These are known as synchronously dividing cultures. The main reason for the interest in inducing synchronous growth in cultures is that, by analysing samples from such cultures, it is possible to follow the pattern of synthesis of cell constituents during the division cycle. There are three main ways of inducing synchronous growth of micro-organisms, namely by (a) mechanical selection of cells of a particular size, (b) manipulating the environment or the composition of the growth medium, and (c) subjecting the cultures to regimes of shifts in incubation temperature. Temperature shifts have long been used, particularly by students of tissue culture, to get a large number of cells in division. It has to be admitted, however, that the use of temperature shifts to induce synchronous growth of micro-organisms is in many ways the least suitable of the methods, since the division cycles induced by these shifts are thought to differ from the normal division cycle in certain respects (Maaløe, 1962).

Techniques for using temperature shifts to induce synchronous growth are of two types: (a) use of a prior temperature treatment which usually involves the application of one short low or high temperature shock to a population of cells, (b) periodic or multi-shift temperature treatments which involve the application of many cycles of temperature change. Both types of technique have been applied to micro-organisms, including bacteria (Hotchkiss, 1954; Maaløe, 1962), yeasts (Williamson and Scopes, 1961), and protozoa (Zeuthen and Scherbaum, 1954). The results of using periodic shifts in incubation to obtain synchronous growth in a culture of *Salmonella typhimurium* are shown in Fig. 6; Maaløe and Lark, 1954). Several general reviews have appeared dealing with the use of temperature shifts to induce synchronous growth of micro-organisms, and those by Zeuthen (1958), Scherbaum (1960) and Burns (1962) are recommended to readers. Numerous attempts have been made to explain the biochemical basis of the induction of synchronous growth using temperature shifts, but it is generally agreed that the phenomenon has a very complex and as yet unknown physiological basis. The reader might wish to peruse Scherbaum's (1960) review for some interesting speculations on the possible mechanisms involved.

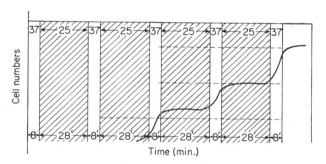

FIG. 6. Synchronous growth of *Salmonella typhimurium* after subjecting the culture to repeated shifts in incubation temperature from 37° (8 min.) to 25° (28 min.). From Maaløe and Lark (1954).

f. Growth of phages. Specific phages have been described for many species of micro-organisms, particularly strains of bacteria. Phages are known to infect psychrophilic, mesophilic and thermophilic bacteria. It has been established, moreover, that certain phages can invade psychrophilic bacteria when these organisms are growing at near-zero temperatures, and that others can invade thermophilic bacteria at temperatures near the upper limit of the temperature range of the host organisms. Both temperate (Thompson and Shafia, 1962; Shafia and Thompson, 1964a, b; Welker and Campbell, 1965a, b) and virulent (Adant, 1928; Koser, 1926; White *et al.*, 1954, 1955) strains of thermophilic bacteriophage have been reported. There are fewer reports of phages that invade psychrophils growing near the lower limit of their temperature range, although Spencer (1963) has reported that marine bacteria can be lysed by phages in sea water at 0°–2°. It would appear, therefore, that there exist psychrophilic, mesophilic and thermophilic bacteriophages.

The majority of experiments on the effect of temperature on phage growth have been done with virulent phages, and usually in the range of temperatures in which the host bacterium grows. Very little has been reported on the ability of phages to invade bacteria at temperatures below the minimum (but see Adams, 1955) or above the maximum for growth of the host bacterium.

The responses of phages to temperatures within the growth range of the host bacterium show many different patterns; moreover, the effect of temperature on a phage may be different from that on the host bacterium. Many years ago, Doerr and Grüninger (1922) reported that a coliphage failed to reproduce at 43° although the uninfected bacterium grew well at this temperature. Interest in the effect of superoptimum temperatures on phage infection has continued. In a study of the effect of elevated temperatures on phage production in *Escherichia coli* K-12, Groman and Suzuki (1962) showed that, at 44°, phage yield was decreased to 2–5% of that at 37°; the host bacterium grew equally well at both temperatures. They concluded that the decreased yield is due primarily to an increased rate of lysis. The effect of suboptimum temperatures on the kinetics of phage production has been studied by Maaløe and his colleagues. Maaløe (1950) observed that *E. coli* infected with phage T-4 and maintained at 36°, began to lyse after 22 minutes, whereas bacteria similarly infected and maintained at 19° began lysing only after 140 minutes, and gave a yield of progeny which was decreased by 40% as compared with that at 36°. The longer that the bacteria were kept at 36°, before being transferred to 19°, the sooner lysis began at the lower temperature. Later, Maaløe in collaboration with his colleagues (Weis Bentzon *et al.*, 1952) established that transfer to a temperature of 19° affected the rate of the lytic process to a smaller extent than it affected the rate of maturation, and that this explained the decreased yield at 19°.

Some of the most interesting experiments on the effects of temperature on phage reproduction have been done with mutant phages, the reproduction of which in the host bacterium is differently affected by temperature as compared with the parent phage. The majority of these temperature-sensitive (*ts*) mutants have been obtained from coliphages (Epstein *et al.*, 1963; Edgar and Lielausis, 1964; Tessman, 1965; Dowell and Sinsheimer, 1966) although similar mutants have been obtained from phage P1 (which infects *Shigella dysenteriae*; Bertani and Nice, 1954), SP3 (with *Bacillus subtilis* as a host; Nishihara and Romig, 1964a, b), phage ϵ^{15} (infective in salmonellae; Uetake *et al.*, 1964), and staphylococcal phages (Beumer-Jochmans, 1951). There are also a few reports of *ts* mutants of RNA phages (Davern, 1964; Pfeifer *et al.*, 1964).

A *ts* mutant may differ in any one of the several ways from the parent, temperature-insensitive strain. For example, Epstein *et al.* (1963) described mutants of coliphage T-4 which form plaques at 25° but not at 42°, as well as mutants which form plaques at 42° but not at 25°;

the wild type for both classes of mutant plaqued at 25° and 42°
Experiments have been done with many of these *ts* mutants to discover
the nature of the temperature-sensitive gene expression. With some *ts*
mutants, the lesion is associated with synthesis of the nucleic acid
(Epstein *et al.*, 1963; Pfeifer *et al.*, 1964); with others, it has been shown
that the mutant phage produces a heat-sensitive lysozyme (e.g.
Streisinger *et al.*, 1961). But the principal reason for this interest in *ts*
phage mutants is that they provide useful tools for mapping the phage
genome. The mapping technique was pioneered by Epstein *et al.* (1963)
and their paper should be perused for details of the technique.

When a temperate, infective phage enters a potential host, one of two
sequences of events can take place. Either the phage multiplies vegetatively and lyses the bacterium; alternatively, the phage establishes a
symbiotic relationship with the host bacterium, when the host bacterium
is described as lysogenic. There is evidence that temperature can
influence the course of events that take place and that, at low temperatures, the lysogenic sequence is favoured. For example, Sussman and
Jacob (1962) showed that a lambda phage would lysogenize in a strain
of *E. coli* at 32° but not at 40°. Lysogenic bacteria, which had been
isolated and maintained at 32°, would lyse and produce phages only
after the temperature was raised to 40° for 1 hour. Similar results were
reported with *Shigella dysenteriae* and phage P1 (Bertani and Nice,
1954), in which the lytic development was prevented at temperatures of
20° and below.

2. *Physiological Bases of Growth Responses*

Micro-organisms, in common with all other living cells, contain
molecular species, including proteins, nucleic acids and lipids, the
properties of which are affected by temperature. Accordingly, microbial
physiologists have studied the effects of temperature on these cell
constituents in the hope that the data obtained would help them to
explain the effects of temperature on the growth of micro-organisms.
The most heat-sensitive cellular constituents, at least over the range of
temperatures in which the majority of micro-organisms grow, are
proteins, and by far the greatest amount of work has been done on the
effects of temperature on the catalytic activities of proteins. It is clear,
however, that the microbiologist is still far from being able to explain the
biochemical bases of the effects of temperature on growth of micro-
organisms. The main reason for this is that, despite the large amount of
work that has been reported on the subject, we are still largely ignorant
of the *basic* factors governing the effect of temperature on biological
molecules. Recent studies in this area (see Chapters 2, 3, 4 and 5) have
shown that solution conditions are extremely important in determining

the effect that temperature has on a biological molecule. Since the solution conditions to which molecules are subjected in the living cell are largely unknown, it is hardly surprising that we are unable to explain the biochemical bases of many of the effects of temperature on microbial growth.

Of necessity, the majority of studies on the effects of temperature on microbial cell constituents are done with cell extracts or, when possible, with purified preparations of the constituent. But it is quite likely that temperature has quite different effects on the molecule *in vitro* as compared with *in vivo*. So far, very few studies have been reported which might throw light on possible differences in the temperature-sensitivity of biological molecules *in vivo* and *in vitro*. It is known, however, that substrates and co-enzymes can protect certain enzymes against heat denaturation (Burton 1951). Also, it has been reported by Boyer and his colleagues (1946, 1947) that short- and medium-chain fatty acids can protect some proteins against heat denaturation. In view of the intimate association between many intracellular enzymes and membrane lipids, it would be interesting to know if this type of protection operates at low and high temperatures. Some of the most compelling evidence showing that the temperature sensitivity of enzymes may be different *in vivo* as compared with *in vitro* has come from Eidlic and Neidhardt (1965). These workers isolated two temperature-sensitive (*ts*) mutants of *Escherichia coli*, which grew normally at 30° but failed to grow at 37°; the parent strains of both mutants grew optimally at 37°. Cultures of the mutants, grown at 30°, were transferred to 37°, and extracts of the bacteria assayed for amino acid-activating enzymes. One of the mutants had a temperature-sensitive valyl-t-RNA synthetase, and the other a temperature-sensitive phenylalanine-t-RNA synthetase. However, the activities of each of these enzymes, in extracts of the bacteria grown at 30° and assayed at 30°, failed to show near-normal activities. It must be concluded that the temperature sensitivities of these synthetases are very different when the enzymes are in the cell from when they are in cell extracts.

a. Optimum temperature for growth. It is presumed that a micro-organism grows most rapidly at that temperature at which the various metabolic processes that contribute to growth operate optimally. In all likelihood, there are certain enzymes that act as "pacemakers" while the majority operate at temperatures that are well below their optima. Experiments with cell extracts of *E. coli* have shown that formate dehydrogenase operates in the growing micro-organism at temperatures below the optimum for activity of the enzyme. Thus Johnson and Lewin (1946) demonstrated maximum activity of this enzyme in cell extracts at 80°, a temperature which is over 40° above the optimum temperature for growth of the bacterium, and indeed some 35° above the maximum for growth of the organism. On the other hand, Upadhyay and Stokes (1963b) reported that the hydrogenase activity of intact cells of another strain of *E. coli* showed optimum activity around 35°, a temperature near to the optimum for growth of the bacterium. But before it is possible to explain why a particular micro-organism grows optimally at a certain temperature, it will be necessary to know far more than we do at present about the effects of temperature on the metabolic activities of micro-organisms, and how these activities are integrated into the growth process.

An appreciable amount of work has, however, been done on thermophilic bacilli with the object of discovering why these bacteria are able to grow well at temperatures far above the maxima for growth of most mesophilic and psychrophilic micro-organisms. Two general types of explanation have been offered. The most obvious possibility is that the cell components of thermophils are relatively more heat-stable than their counterparts in other micro-organisms. A second school of thought, which was proposed in the writings of Gaughran (1947) and Allen (1953), suggested that many of the enzymes in thermophilic bacteria are as sensitive to heat as those in mesophilic and psychrophilic micro-organisms, but that rapid resynthesis of the damaged constituents allows the bacteria to grow at high temperatures. Among the evidence adduced to support this hypothesis was the finding that some facultatively thermophilic bacteria do not indeed have heat-stable enzymes, and the report by Allen (1950) that certain thermophils die rapidly in the absence of nutrients at temperatures which permit growth in nutritionally adequate media. Nevertheless, the "rapid resynthesis" hypothesis has not been well received by workers in the field, and was largely disclaimed by Koffler (1957) in a review of the physiology of thermophils.

The consensus of opinion is that the capacity of thermophilic bacteria to grow and reproduce at high temperatures is due to the greater heat stability of their cell components. As early as 1898, Oprescu reported that the extracellular amylase formed by a thermophilic micro-organism was still active after heating at 85° for 30 minutes. Since then, many other enzymes from thermophilic bacilli have been reported to have exceptional heat stability. Among the enzymes that have been studied, in addition to the extracellular amylases, are malate dehydrogenase (Marsh and Militzer, 1952), inorganic pyrophosphatase (Marsh and Militzer, 1956; Mathemeier and Morita, 1964), ATP-ase (Militzer *et al.*, 1951) and aldolase (Thompson and Thompson, 1962). In addition, Campbell and his colleagues have shown that the hydrogenase (Akagi and Campbell, 1961) and the sulphate adenylyl transferase (Akagi and

Campbell, 1962) in the thermophil, *Clostridium nigrificans*, were more heat-stable than the corresponding enzymes in the mesophil, *Desulphovibrio desulphuricans*.

Almost all of these experiments were done with unfractionated cell extracts, and they do not indicate whether the heat stability is an intrinsic property of the enzymes, or whether it is brought about through the action of protective factors in the cell or cell extract. To obtain information on these possibilities, Manning and Campbell (1961) purified and crystallized the thermostable extracellular α-amylase of *Bacillus stearothermophilus*. The crystalline enzyme was electrophoretically homogeneous and extremely resistant to heat inactivation; it catalysed the hydrolysis of starch optimally between 55° and 70°. With this enzyme, therefore, the heat stability appears to be an intrinsic property of the protein molecule.

It would clearly be a very arduous task to examine each of the hundreds of enzymes in a thermophilic bacterium for heat stability. Koffler and Gale (1957) circumvented this problem by examining the effects of high temperatures on the coagulation of the cytoplasmic proteins in cell extracts of the thermophil, *B. stearothermophilus* and the mesophil *Proteus vulgaris*. The crude mixture of cytoplasmic proteins used accounted for approximately half of the total cellular nitrogen. Over 50% of the protein in the mesophil extract, but hardly any of that in the thermophil extract, coagulated when the extracts were heated at 60° and pH 6 for 8 minutes. This experiment can be criticized on the basis that the conditions used did not resemble those that a protein encounters in an organized cell, and that the heating may have caused alterations in protein structure that did not result in coagulation. Nevertheless, the result strongly suggests that additional heat stability is a property possessed by the bulk of the cytoplasmic proteins in the thermophilic bacillus.

Koffler and his colleagues extended their studies on the effects of high temperatures on protein coagulation to isolated bacterial flagella. These organelles provide excellent material for this type of study. They consist of almost pure protein (flagellin) and can quite easily be obtained in a clean form by shaking a suspension of bacteria. Moreover, flagella are highly organized complexes of flagellin molecules, the organization being similar in some respects to that to which proteins are subjected in intracellular structures. In addition, since the dissociation of flagella into flagellin molecules is accompanied by a decrease in viscosity, the effect of heat on flagella can easily be studied viscometrically. The data in Fig. 7 show that, at 40°, the flagella from the mesophil, *Escherichia coli*, are stable, but that there is a marked decrease in viscosity when the suspension is heated to 50° or 60°. On the other hand, flagella from a thermophilic strain of Bacillus, when subjected to similar heat treatments, showed no evidence of breakdown. Indeed, a temperature of 75° was required before the viscosity of the suspension of thermophil flagella decreased (Koffler et al., 1957). These findings support the observation, made earlier by McCoy (1937), that the H-agglutinogen of the thermophil, Clostridium thermosaccharolyticum, is much more heat-stable than that in the mesophil, Cl. butyricum.

A more detailed examination of these mesophil and thermophil flagella suggested that the relatively greater heat stability of the thermophil organelles is due to intrinsic properties of the protein molecules and probably not to the action of protective materials. Thus, the thermophil flagellin appears to possess more numerous and more strategically located hydrogen and possibly also hydrophobic bonds, as compared

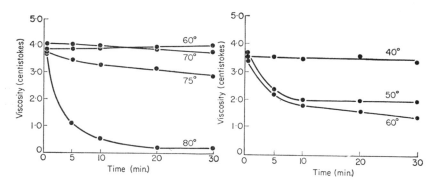

FIG. 7. Effect of different temperatures on the viscosity of suspensions of flagella from (a) a mesophilic strain of *Escherichia coli*, and (b) a thermophilic bacillus (strain 11330). From Koffler (1957).

with the mesophil flagellin. Additional evidence for the view that the comparative stability of the thermophil flagella resides in the protein monomers has been adduced by Abram and Koffler (1965), who demonstrated that reconstitution of the monomers occurred at high temperatures and that the reconstituted polymer was heat-stable.

The heat stability of nucleic acids from thermophilic bacilli has also been investigated. The melting temperature (T_m value) of the DNA from a thermophilic bacillus was shown by Marmur (1960) to be comparable to that of DNAs from mesophilic micro-organisms, and he concluded that there was no apparent relationship between the thermal stability of the DNA and the ability of the thermophil to grow at higher temperatures than the mesophils. However, the ribosomal (r-)RNA of thermophilic bacilli does have a greater heat stability than that in *E. coli* (Teece and Toschi, 1960; Mangiatini et al., 1962; Saunders and Campbell, 1966). Analyses of the ribosomes from the thermophil and the mesophil showed that the differences in overall composition were slight, and would probably not account for the differences in the heat stability of the intact organelles. Saunders and Campbell (1966) suggested that the greater stability of the thermophil ribosomes may be a reflection of differences in the composition and structure of the ribosomal protein. But, since the proteins from the two types of ribosome had very similar amino acid compositions, any differences in the properties of the proteins must be rather subtle. An interesting observation made by Teece and his colleagues (Mangiatini *et al.*, 1962; Teece and Toschi, 1960), was that the RNA from the thermophilic bacillus that they studied had a greater heat stability in the ribosome than in the isolated state.

b. *Superoptimum temperatures.* At temperatures above the optimum, the rate of growth of a micro-organism usually decreases rapidly (see Fig. 1; p. 153). Explanations for this rapid decline in growth rate, and the subsequent cessation of growth, have been sought by a number of workers. Most investigators have done experiments in which cultures grown at, or just below, the optimum temperature are transferred to a temperature a few degrees above the maximum for growth. By examining the biochemical behaviour of organisms transferred in this way, with that of organisms maintained at the optimum temperature, information has been obtained on the biochemical bases for the rapid decline in growth rate at the higher temperatures.

Enzymes have long been known to be the most heat-labile of cell constituents, and several reports have suggested that the decline in the growth rate of micro-organisms at superoptimum temperatures is caused, in part at least, by the heat denaturation of enzymes. Edwards and Rettger (1937) reported good agreement between the maximum temperatures for growth of several bacilli and the minimum temperatures at which certain of their respiratory enzymes (catalase, indophenol oxidase, succinate dehydrogenase) were inactivated. Evison and Rose (1965), in this Laboratory, made a comparative study of the biochemical bases of the effects of supermaximum temperatures on three micro-organisms—strains of Arthrobacter (maximum temperature about 32°), Candida (about 22°) and *Corynebacterium erythrogenes* (about 27°). When cultures which had been grown at or near the optimum temperature were transferred to a temperature 3°–5° above the maximum for growth, there was a decrease in the rate of respiration of exogenous glucose and of endogenous reserves by each of the organisms. Further examination showed that the activities of many of the TCA cycle enzymes in the Arthrobacter and Candida were diminished after the transfer of organisms to the supermaximum temperature. In the Arthrobacter, the isocitrate dehydrogenase activity decreased more

than that of any other TCA cycle enzyme; in the Candida, the pyruvate
dehydrogenase was most sensitive to the temperature shift. The majority
of the TCA cycle enzymes in these organisms were irreversibly inactivated. In *C. erythrogenes*, however, the temperature shift had little if
any effect on the activities the majority of the TCA cycle enzymes.
These results support the findings of Edwards and Rettger (1937)
regarding the heat lability of respiratory enzymes. Further support
came from the report by Hagen and Rose (1961, 1962) that the maximum temperature for growth of a psychrophilic strain of *Cryptococcus*
was caused, in part, by the inactivation of certain TCA cycle enzymes.

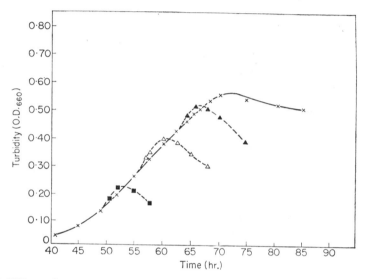

Fɪɢ. 8. Effect of transferring cultures of a psychrophilic strain of *Serratia* from
5° (×), which is the optimum temperature for growth, to a supermaximum temperature of 19·5° after different periods of incubation. From Hagen *et al.* (1964).

A quite different explanation for the behaviour of a micro-organism
at temperatures above the optimum for growth was revealed by Hagen
et al. (1964). These workers used a psychrophilic strain of *Serratia* which
had been isolated by K. Eimhjellen from flounder eggs, and which has a
maximum temperature for growth of around 18°. When cultures of this
bacterium, that had been grown at 5°, were transferred to 19·5°, the
bacteria rapidly lysed (Fig. 8). After examining the kinetics of lysis, and
the nature of the products released from the bacterium during lysis,
Hagen and his colleagues concluded that there had been a breakdown of
certain cytoplasmic membrane constituents, but only after the onset of
lysis. The temperature shift was thought to have caused the activation

of one or more autolytic enzymes in the bacterium, and the activity of these enzymes led to the breakdown of the cytoplasmic membrane.

Another type of lesion which may contribute to the rapid decline in the rate of growth of a micro-organism is the breakdown of RNA. Califano (1952) showed that exposure of buffered suspensions of bacteria to supermaximum temperatures led to a leakage of RNA from the bacteria, and that the temperature at which the process was initiated varied with the species of bacterium but was related to the maximum temperature for growth. This effect was confirmed, using suspensions of *Aerobacter aerogenes* in buffers at 47°, by Strange and Shon (1964) who suggested that the rates of growth (and death) of the bacteria were directly affected by the rapid intracellular accumulation of RNA nucleotides. In their study on the biochemical bases of the effects of supermaximum temperatures on micro-organisms, Evison and Rose (1965) failed to detect any marked intracellular accumulation or excretion of ultraviolet-absorbing compounds by the organisms after exponential-phase cultures had been transferred to the supermaximum temperatures, probably because of the protective effect of medium constituents that had been reported by Strange and Shon (1964). It would seem, therefore, that the heat lability of RNA is not an important factor in the decrease in the rate of growth of micro-organisms at temperatures above the optimum for growth.

c. *Suboptimum temperatures*. At temperatures below the optimum, the rate of growth of micro-organisms declines although not as rapidly as at temperatures above the optimum. The Arrhenius plots (Fig. 1; p. 153) show that, at suboptimum temperatures, the growth rate declines linearly but, near the minimum temperature, there may be an inflection in the curve. Similar curves have been obtained with other micro-organisms. The fundamental question that needs to be answered regarding the behaviour of micro-organisms at suboptimum temperatures was stated quite succinctly by Foter and Rahn as long ago as 1936, when they observed that, since growth and respiration consist of chemical reactions, they should in theory continue, although at a greatly diminished rate, until the medium in which the micro-organisms are suspended freezes solid. This behaviour is found with psychrophils but not with mesophils. In the past ten years, several workers have studied the physiological basis for the decreased growth rate of micro-organisms at suboptimum temperatures, and in particular have attempted to explain the apparently atypical behaviour cf mesophilic micro-organisms at near-zero temperatures. As a result of these studies, two main hypotheses have been forwarded. These hypotheses, as we shall see, are not mutually exclusive, although very much more work is required before either of them can be proved.

To Ingraham (1958) goes the credit for having focused attention on the problem after it had lain fallow for many years. He studied the effect of temperature on the rate of growth of the mesophil, *Escherichia coli* ML 30, and a psychrophilic pseudomonad; his results are shown in Fig. 1 (p. 153). From these data, the temperature characteristic for the mesophil was calculated to be about 14,000 cal./mole and that for the psychrophil, 9,000 cal./mole. Since the psychrophil had a lower temperature characteristic for growth over the linear range as compared with the mesophil, Ingraham and Bailey (1959) examined the effects of temperature on the activities of three enzymes (glucose 6-phosphate-, isocitrate-, and malate dehydrogenase) in cell extracts of the bacteria in order to discover whether the enzymes in the psychrophil had lower activation energies than their counterparts in the mesophil. It was found, however, that the activation energies were similar, if not identical, for the enzymes examined. It was possible that other enzymes in the psychrophil had lower activation energies than the corresponding mesophil enzymes, and that Ingraham and Bailey had, perchance, not chosen to study one of these. Burton and Morita (1965) have since shown that the malate dehydrogenase from the psychrophil, *Vibrio marinus*, has an activation energy only half that of the corresponding enzyme from a mesophilic strain of *E. coli*.

However, Ingraham and Bailey's (1959) paper included further data which directed attention to another possible difference in the physiology of mesophils and psychrophils. They reported that the temperature coefficients (Q_{10} values) for the oxidation of glucose over the range 10°–30°, and of acetate and formate over the range 15°–30°, were less for the psychrophil than for the mesophil, a result similar to that for the effect of temperature on the rates of growth of the organisms over these ranges. On the basis of these data, Ingraham and Bailey (1959) suggested that the differences in the responses of the mesophil and the psychrophil to low temperatures might be due to differences in some aspects of the biochemical organization of the organisms rather than in the properties of individual enzymes.

The first indication of an aspect of cellular organization which might form the basis of the difference in the response to near-zero temperatures came from a report by Baxter and Gibbons (1962). These workers compared the effects of temperature on the respiratory activities of a psychrophilic strain of the yeast *Candida* and a mesophilic strain of *Candida lipolytica*, and found that the psychrophil respired endogenous reserves at a greater rate than the mesophil at all temperatures up to 30° and, while the psychrophil oxidized exogenous glucose at an appreciable rate even at 0°, virtually no exogenous substrate was oxidized by the mesophil at temperatures below 5°. These data suggested that the psychrophil, but not the mesophil, was able to transport sugars into the cell at temperatures below 5°. Baxter and Gibbons then suggested that the main factor determining the minimum temperature for growth of a mesophilic micro-organism is the inactivation of the solute-transport mechanisms. Rose and Evison (1965) in this Laboratory have reported evidence which supports this view. They showed that the

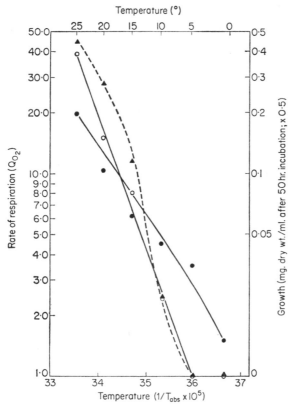

FIG. 9. Effect of temperature on the rate of respiration of endogenous reserves (●) and of exogenous glucose (○) by, and on growth (▲) of, *Candida utilis* NCYC 321. Replotted from data of Rose and Evison (1965).

minimum temperatures for growth of mesophilic strains of Arthrobacter and *Candida utilis* were approximately the same as those at which the organisms ceased to respire exogenous glucose and to accumulate the non-metabolizable sugar glucosamine (Fig. 9).

If psychrophils do in general differ from mesophils in being able to transport solutes into the cell at near-zero temperatures, the problem is to explain how the transport mechanisms differ in the two groups of micro-organisms. There are three main types of physiological lesion that could lead to the failure of mesophils, as distinct from psychrophils, to accumulate solutes at temperatures below 5°–10°, Firstly, there is the possibility that the solute-carrier molecules or permeases—which we shall assume to be proteins, an assumption for which there is much experimental evidence—in the psychrophil membrane differ from those in the mesophil membrane in that they are susceptible to inactivation at near-zero temperatures. A second possible explanation is that the carrier molecules in the two classes of organisms do not necessarily differ in their susceptibility to inactivation at near-zero temperatures but that, in the mesophil membrane but not in the psychrophil membrane, they are prevented from combining with solute molecules as a result of some change in the molecular architecture of the membrane at near-zero temperatures. A third possibility is that, at low temperatures, the provision or expenditure of energy that is necessary for the active uptake of solutes is prevented in mesophils but not in psychrophils.

It is now established that proteins (and presumably therefore permeases) can denature at low temperatures. Brandts, in Chapter 3 of this book, discusses some of the evidence for this; other reports have come from Kavanau (1950) for yeast invertase and other hydrolytic enzymes, Maier et al. (1955) for intestinal phosphatase and turnip peroxidase, Hultin (1955) for yeast invertase, Graves et al. (1965) for pyruvate decarboxylase from rabbit skeletal muscle, Havir et al. (1965) for argininosuccinase from steer liver, Shukuya and Schwert (1960) for glutamate decarboxylase from E. coli, Duodoroff and Shuster (1962) for β-hydroxybutyrate dehydrogenase from Rhodospirillum rubrum, and Dua and Burris (1963) for a "nitrogenase" from Clostridium pasteurianum. In the microbial cytoplasmic membrane, there are probably a score or more different species of permease; one type, for example, transports monosaccharides, while there are others for neutral, basic and acidic amino acids, growth factors and inorganic ions. Since permeases differ in their affinity for solutes, they must differ in structure and possibly therefore in their susceptibility to inactivation following denaturation at near-zero temperatures. It would seem likely, as a result, that the transport of individual classes of solute into a micro-organism could be inactivated at different temperatures. It then follows that the minimum temperature for growth would be that at which an exogenous solute ceases to be accumulated in sufficient quantities, following the inactivation of the permease. The minimum temperature for growth of a mesophil would then depend, to some extent, on the composition of the growth medium, and a micro-organism might appear to be psychrophilic when growing in one medium and, because of the low temperature inactivation of a permease, mesophilic when growing in another medium. To date, there have been no reports of such a type of behaviour. Admittedly, no one appears to have searched for this type of behaviour, but it is not unreasonable to assume that it would have been reported by now. If the inactivation of permeases at low temperatures is to be adduced as a basis for the minimum temperature for growth, much more data will be required on the effects of low temperatures on the uptake of individual solutes. Almost all of the data so far reported are for the uptake of sugars. However, Quetsch and Danforth (1964) have shown that the uptake of uric acid and xanthine by *Candida utilis* is prevented at temperatures below 4°, which is just a few degrees below the minimum temperature for growth of this yeast. Moreover, these workers presented evidence that each of the purines was taken up by a different solute transport system, so that it would seem that two different permeases are similarly inactivated at this temperature.

The notion that permease molecules in the membrane are prevented from combining with the solute at low temperatures as a result of changes in the molecular architecture of the membrane is an extremely difficult hypothesis to test in view of our profound ignorance concerning the structure and function of membranes. Clearly, the functioning of a carrier molecule in the membrane must depend to a great extent on the correct orientation of the permeases in the membrane, a subject about which almost nothing is known. However, since permeases appear to be molecules that easily undergo conformational changes, it is conceivable that their correct orientation in the membrane may be determined in part by lipid molecules which themselves have considerable mobility since they exist in micelles. Possibly, therefore, the lipids in the mesophil membrane can orient the permease molecules correctly only at temperatures above 5°–10°.

Clues as to the ways in which the orienting ability of membrane lipids might change at low temperatures have come from studies on the physics and chemistry of phospholipids. Phospholipids have a liquid–crystalline nature, one result of which is that the fatty acid chains in the molecule can be in a liquid state at a temperature many degrees below the melting point of the phospholipid as determined by conventional chemical means (Byrne and Chapman, 1964). If one assumes that a permease is functioning in a membrane which, according to the views of Luzzati and Husson (1962) and Kavanau (1965) is in the "open" configuration (Fig. 10), then it would appear essential for the fatty acid chains in the phospholipids to be in the liquid state, if the permease is to undergo the conformational changes that are thought to take place during solute transport. Luzzati and Husson (1962) have suggested that the membranes of many cells exist rather critically on the borderline of a transition between the liquid and the solid state of the fatty acid chains.

Conceivably, therefore, at near-zero temperatures, the side chains in the phospholipids of mesophils solidify thereby preventing the permeases from undergoing a conformational change.

Byrne and Chapman (1964) also reported that the presence of unsaturated fatty acid chains in phospholipids decreased the melting temperature of the chains. It has been known for many years that the degree of unsaturation in lipids from poikilotherms increases when the temperature at which the organisms are grown is decreased. Terroine

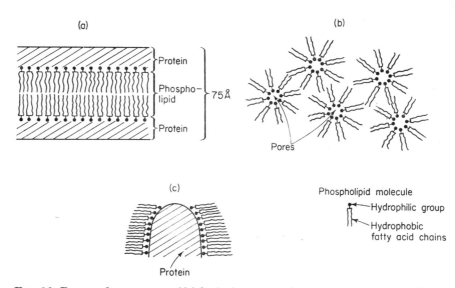

FIG. 10. Proposed structures of biological unit membranes. (a) shows the trilaminar structure as seen in electron micrographs of thin sections of cells. (b) shows a surface view of a structure of the type proposed by Luzzati and Husson (1962), showing phospholipid molecules lining a pore. (c) shows a section through a structure of type (b) with a protein (permease) molecule in the pore.

and his colleagues (1927, 1930) first reported this effect in microorganisms, and more recently it has been confirmed using the very sensitive gas–liquid chromatographic technique for mesophilic and psychrophilic strains of *Candida* by Kates and Baxter (1962) and for *E. coli* ML 30 by Marr and Ingraham (1962). Marr and Ingraham (1962) showed that the proportion of unsaturated fatty acids in lipids extracted from *E. coli* increased as the growth temperature was decreased from 35° to 10° in cultures grown in glucose–minimal medium or in a more complex medium. These workers emphasized, however, that the fatty acid composition of the bacterium grown at any one temperature varied with the chemical composition of the growth medium, and they concluded that this did not indicate a direct relationship between the fatty acid composition and the minimum temperature for growth of the bacterium.

If psychrophilic micro-organisms are able to grow at 0° and below because the phospholipids in their membranes are capable of remaining in the liquid state at these low temperatures, it should be possible to show that the total amounts of unsaturated fatty acids in a psychrophil grown at 0° is greater than the total amounts in a related mesophilic species grown near its minimum temperature for growth in a medium of the same composition, and harvested at a comparable stage of growth. Such data have not as yet been reported. It is also possible that mesophilic micro-organisms are not able to make an adjustment in their fatty acid composition below a certain temperature (the minimum for growth). This hypothesis could be tested experimentally by transferring a culture of a mesophilic organism from the optimum temperature for growth, to temperatures just above and just below the minimum, and following any changes that may occur in the fatty acid composition of the organisms. Shaw and Ingraham (1965) reported that exponential-phase cultures of *E. coli* ML 30, grown in a glucose–salts medium and transferred from 37° to 10°, showed a lag period of about 5 hr. at the lower temperature before growth commenced. During this lag period, the proportion of unsaturated fatty acids in the bacterial lipids increased. But Shaw and Ingraham also varied the composition of the medium to obtain more information on the changes that occurred in the fatty acid composition of the bacterial lipids. In cultures grown at 37°, the availability of glucose was made to limit growth, and glucose was added to the culture that had been transferred to 10° at the end of the lag period. Under these conditions, growth occurred at 10° with bacteria that had a fatty acid composition characteristic of organisms grown at 37°. Shaw and Ingraham concluded that the fatty acid composition of the bacteria does not determine the minimum temperature for growth. It would be interesting to know how these bacteria would have changed in fatty acid composition had they been transferred instead to a subminimum temperature.

No one has yet reported results of experiments designed to show whether ATP production, or expenditure of ATP during the active transport of solutes, is inactivated in mesophils at near-zero temperatures. However, Baxter and Gibbons (1962) and Rose and Evison (1962) showed that the respiration of endogenous reserves by mesophilic yeasts and bacteria proceeded at a measurable rate at 0°, although their data did not indicate whether respiration at these low temperatures was coupled with ATP production. Experiments on the effects of low temperatures on the possible uncoupling of oxidative phosphorylation will need to be done on mitochondria isolated from organisms; so far, this aspect of oxidative phosphorylation does not appear to have been investigated. The possible effect of near-zero temperatures in preventing ATP expenditure during the active transport of solutes into mesophils is extremely difficult to test experimentally. It has been reported, however, that the enzyme ATPase, which may be involved in the utilization of ATP at the membrane, is particularly susceptible to cold inactivation (Penefsky and Warner, 1965).

It is clear from this account that much remains to be done before it will be possible to explain the molecular basis of the effects of near-zero temperatures on solute uptake in mesophilic micro-organisms, or before the physiological importance of this inactivation can be fully evaluated.

Although it was Ingraham's early observations that led to the discovery of permease inactivation to explain the minimum temperature for growth of mesophilic micro-organisms, recent work in his laboratory has been concerned with another aspect of the physiology of micro-organisms at low temperatures. Stated briefly, Ingraham believes that, at temperatures below the optimum for growth of mesophilic micro-organisms, there is a progressively more effective derangement of the biochemical mechanisms that regulate the activity and synthesis of enzymes, and that this derangement leads ultimately to the cessation of growth. In a micro-organism growing in a particular medium, at a specified temperature, there is a complex balance between induction and repression of the synthesis of enzymes that catalyse reactions on metabolic pathways, and in the extent to which the activities of enzymes that have been synthesized are regulated by end-product inhibition. To examine the effect of low temperatures on this dynamic metabolic state, studies have been made on the effect of temperature on the induction of enzyme synthesis. This is a process which has for some time been known to be very sensitive to temperature changes (Knox, 1953; see also Section IID, p. 198). A report by Ng et al. (1962) suggested that growth of E. coli ML 30 at low temperatures damaged the bacteria in such a way that the growth rate was decreased. These workers showed that the glucose repression of β-galactosidase synthesis by this bacterium occurred at a temperature co-incident with that at which the "damage" was observed in the bacteria. Ingraham and his colleagues (Marr et al., 1964) followed up this work by making a more detailed study of the effects of temperature on the kinetics of induction of β-galactosidase synthesis in E. coli ML 30. They studied synthesis of the enzyme during exponential growth in a succinate-minimal medium over the range 10°–43° for a strain with a constitutive ability to synthesize the enzyme, and in an inducible cryptic strain, induced maximally or submaximally with isopropylthio-β-galactoside (which unlike lactose does not lead to the production of glucose). The differential rates of enzyme synthesis were identical for the constitutive strain and for the fully induced strain. The rates were constant from 20° to 43°, and decreased proportionately with a decrease in temperature below 20°. It was concluded therefore, that, in the absence of glucose repression, the ability of *E. coli* to synthesize β-galactosidase decreases at low temperatures. Marr *et al.* (1964) explained this result by postulating that temperature affects the synthesis of the repressor protein. A personal communication from Ingraham has revealed that he would now prefer to explain these data by assuming that the affinity of the inducer for the repressor protein is decreased at low temperatures.

The effect of temperature on the affinity of low molecular weight compounds for allosteric proteins has since been studied in Ingraham's laboratory using other organisms. O'Donovan *et al.* (1965) isolated a number of cold-sensitive (*cs*) mutants of *E. coli* ML 30 which have much higher minimum temperatures for growth (around 20°) as compared with the parent bacterium which is able to grow down to about 8°. In a study of one of these mutants (KII 27), O'Donovan and Ingraham (1965) showed that its requirement for histidine at low temperatures could be attributed to its synthesis of a PR–ATP pyrophosphorylase (the enzyme that catalyses the first reaction on the pathway to histidine synthesis) that is 1000 times more sensitive to feedback inhibition at 37° by histidine than is the same enzyme from the parent. At temperatures below 37°, the affinity for histidine increases with the enzymes from the mutant and the parent, but only with the mutant enzyme is it sufficient to cause a cessation of growth in the absence of exogenous histidine.

Ingraham and his colleagues have therefore established, in elegant fashion, that the affinity of an allosteric protein for a low molecular weight compound can be affected by temperature. It will be interesting to see whether these experiments can be extended to natural psychrophilic and mesophilic micro-organisms and to discover whether this effect contributes to, or even determines, the minimum temperature for growth of micro-organisms. Meanwhile, it is worth noting that the two theories—solute uptake inactivation and allosteric protein modulation—may have a common molecular basis, since permeases appear to have many of the properties of allosteric proteins.

B. VIABILITY

1. *Elevated Temperatures*

Microbiologists have long appreciated that temperatures above the maximum for growth can kill micro-organisms. The application of this phenomenon, in the form of heat sterilization, was instrumental in the development of microbiology as a discipline, and it is mainly because of this economic importance that the literature on the effect of elevated temperatures on micro-organisms has become so voluminous.

a. Factors affecting heat resistance. It is now generally accepted that the effects of elevated temperatures on micro-organisms are very complex indeed, and that the lethal effect is influenced by a large number of factors. It is all the more regrettable, therefore, that so few studies have been done in which all of the known factors (except that which is being studied) have been carefully controlled. This stricture applies particularly to the control of the nutritional environment, for only a handful of experiments have been reported on the effects of elevated temperatures on micro-organisms grown in a chemostat.

The viability of a micro-organism, when subjected to temperatures above the maximum for growth, is conditioned by four main groups of factors. These have been discussed at some length in an article by Wood (1957) and in an excellent review by Hansen and Riemann (1963).

Nature of the organism. One would expect that the heat resistance of micro-organisms would differ from one species or strain to the next, and indeed this seems to be so. Nevertheless, there are very little data in which the heat resistance of individual strains has been compared under carefully controlled conditions. An interesting finding, however, reported by Wood (1957), was that diploid strains of *Saccharomyces cerevisiae* are more heat resistant than haploid strains.

Growth conditions. The environmental conditions under which an organism is grown, and the age of the organisms, can affect their ability to survive at an elevated temperature. Several studies have been carried out on the effect of the temperature of incubation. In general, the heat resistance of bacteria and yeasts increases with an increase in growth temperature (Elliker and Frazier, 1938). This may be the result of a selection of strains with a greater heat resistance. But the heat resistance has also been reported to be greater when organisms are incubated at suboptimum temperatures, as compared with the optimum temperature for growth. Anderson and Meanwell (1936) found this to be true for a species of *Streptococcus*.

Not much has been reported on the effect of the chemical composition of the growth medium. Moreover, when it has been studied, this factor has been found to have relatively little effect on the heat resistance of micro-organisms. For example, Lembke (1937) observed no difference in the heat resistance of a strain of *Escherichia coli* when the organisms were grown on meat extract–peptone–agar as compared with organisms grown on lactose–agar.

In contrast, the effect of the age of the organism has received far more attention and has been shown to be important. Exponentially growing micro-organisms are generally less resistant to heat stress than organisms in the stationary phase of growth. White (1953) made a careful study of the effect of culture age on the resistance of *Streptococcus faecalis* to a temperature of 60° (Fig. 11) for a fixed period of time. The heat resistance of organisms from very young cultures increased rapidly with age, but then dropped precipitously as the culture entered the exponential phase of growth. Thereafter, the organisms gradually acquired a greater resistance to heat stress. Similar results were later reported by Lemcke and White (1959) for a strain of *E. coli*.

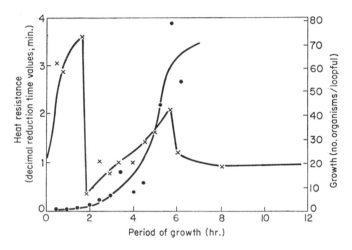

FIG. 11. Effect of the age of the culture on the resistance of *Streptococcus faecalis* strain L 5 to heating at 60° in saline. The bacteria were grown at 37°. Viability was measured by plating dilutions on nutrient agar and incubating at 37°. Crosses indicate heat resistance; circles indicate growth as determined by microscopic counts on a loopful of culture. From White (1953).

Nature and duration of the heat stress. Understandably, perhaps, in view of the commercial importance of heat sterilization, the majority of workers who have studied the effects of heat stress on micro-organisms have used temperatures that are well above the maximum for growth of the organism, temperatures at which the viability of a population of organisms decreases quite rapidly. Some micro-organisms, such as the Arthrobacter and Candida strains studied by Evison and Rose (1965), are killed at temperatures only 3°–5° above the maximum for growth (Fig. 12). However, Evison and Rose (1965) found that cultures of *Corynebacterium erythrogenes*, when transferred from 15°, which is around the optimum temperature for growth, to 30°, a temperature about 3° above the maximum for growth, did not die even after 48 hr. at the supermaximum temperature (Fig. 12).

The first detailed quantitative study of the killing of suspensions of bacteria at elevated temperatures was by Dame Harriette Chick (1910). Her report emphasized the time factor in the inactivation process, and recognized the importance of the *survival curve* which is a plot of the

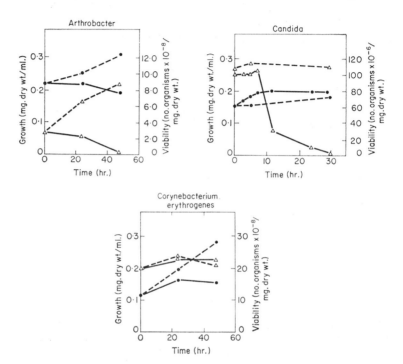

FIG. 12. Effect of change in incubation temperature on growth (○) and viability (△) of strains of Arthrobacter, Candida and *Corynebacterium erythrogenes*. Cultures of the Arthrobacter were transferred from 20° to 37° after 72 hr. incubation; cultures of Candida from 10° to 25° after 120 hr.; and *C. erythrogenes* cultures from 15° to 30° after 120 hr. Continuous lines indicate the activities of organisms at the higher temperatures; dashed lines, the activities at the lower temperatures. From Evison and Rose (1965).

logarithm of the number of survivors in the suspension against the time of heating (Fig. 13). Quite often, the survival curve is exponential (curve A; Fig. 13). An exponential curve suggests that death of the organisms is caused by a monomolecular reaction, and some investigators have read a great deal into this interpretation. There is, however, no reason to believe that the killing is caused by a monomolecular reaction, any more than one should believe that such a reaction is important in the cleaning of clothes, a process which also is described by an exponential curve (Wyss, 1951). An exponential curve simply indicates that a constant fraction of the population is killed per unit of time, and is explained by assuming that the chance of an organism being killed is independent of its previous history of heat exposure.

Quite often, however, non-exponential survivor curves are obtained (curves B and C; Fig. 13), and many workers have attempted to explain this deviation from non-linearity. When an inactivation process is described by a curve of type B, it is assumed that organisms of unequal heat resistance are present in the population (Krishna Jyengar *et al.*, 1957). Curves of type C, on the other hand, are generally attributed to

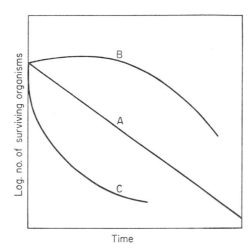

FIG. 13. Different types of survival curves for the death of micro-organisms in a population. See text for explanation.

clumping of the organisms in the population, or to the need for a certain amount of heat damage to take place before individual organisms are killed.

Many attempts to derive a quantitative expression for the killing of micro-organisms in a population at elevated temperatures have been made. The *thermal death point*, which is the lowest temperature at which a suspension of micro-organisms in aqueous medium is completely killed in 10 minutes, was used for many years until the importance of the time factor was realized. It is more usual nowadays to refer to the *thermal death time* (F value) which is the time required to kill a suspension of micro-organisms at any predetermined temperature (Sykes, 1958). An exponential survival curve can be described by the D *value* or *decimal reduction time*, which is the time required to kill 90% of the

7+T.

organisms in a suspension. If the logarithms of the D values are plotted against temperature, a straight line is usually obtained. This is known as the *thermal death time curve*; its slope is referred to as the z value, and is expressed as the increase in temperature required to decrease the D value to one-tenth of its value at the lower temperature. Schelhorn (1960) reported that yeasts often have z values around 3°–5°, non-spore-forming bacteria around 4°–6°, and Aspergillus conidia about 5°.

There are many reports on the influence of the composition of the suspending fluid on the killing of micro-organisms at elevated temperatures. The presence of water greatly decreases the heat resistance of micro-organisms, a fact that was first appreciated by Koch as early as

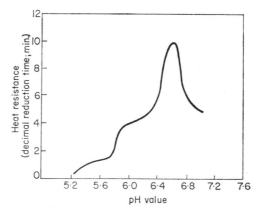

FIG. 14. Effect of pH value on the heat resistance of *Streptococcus faecalis*. The bacteria were grown at 37° and suspended in citrate-phosphate buffers at 60°. From White (1963).

1881 and which is now exploited in commercial and industrial heat sterilization. Even superheated steam acts as dry air and, at 140°–150° it has less killing effect on micro-organisms than water at 100° (Precht *et al.*, 1955). At least part of the explanation of the effect of water is that it affects the susceptibility of proteins to heat denaturation. This, in turn, probably explains why the presence of solutes, especially salts and organic compounds, protects organisms against heat denaturation. The pH value of the suspending fluid has a very marked effect on the heat resistance of micro-organisms. The resistance of bacteria is generally greatest when they are suspended in a solution with a pH value near 7·0 (Fig. 14). Yeasts and moulds behave similarly, although in general they prefer lower pH values for growth. Baumgartner and Hersom (1956) found, however, that the ascospores of *Byssochlamys fulva* were more resistant at pH 3·0 than at pH 7·0.

The density of the suspension also affects the heat resistance of the organisms. Generally, there is an increase in the heat resistance as the density is increased. This may be simply because highly resistant organisms are present in greater numbers per unit volume of suspension as compared with more dilute suspensions. But another factor which is probably important is that some organisms are protected against thermal death by constituents which leak out of cells. Some micro-organisms apparently increase their heat resistance when they are grown in the presence of other micro-organisms. For example, Peppler and Frazier (1941) reported that the heat resistance of lactobacilli was increased when the bacteria were grown in mixed culture containing *Candida krusei*, and that it could be enhanced by adding to the bacterial culture compounds similar to those excreted during the growth of *C. krusei*. But a recent report by Dimmick (1965b) emphasizes how little is yet known about the effects of elevated temperatures on micro-organisms, and describes some complex rhythmic responses of *Serratia marcescens* at high temperatures.

Estimation of survivors. There is no convenient way of counting dead micro-organisms, so that the effect of a heat treatment on the viability of a suspension of organisms can only be assessed accurately by measuring the capacity of the surviving organisms to multiply when incubated in suitable media. Generally this is done by counting the number of colonies that appear on plates of nutrient medium that have been spread with a small volume of a suitably diluted suspension of organisms and incubated at an appropriate temperature. However, the plate culture method has some drawbacks, particularly in that it does not permit an estimate to be made of the number of organisms in a population that are capable of only a limited number of divisions. Postgate *et al.* (1961) have developed a slide culture method which overcomes certain of these disadvantages, but the method has yet to gain wide acceptance. On the whole, rich complex media give higher recovery values than nutritionally simpler media (Nelson, 1943). Also, the best temperatures for incubation of the plates or slides seem to be just below the optimum for growth of the organism (e.g. Williams and Reed, 1942).

b. *Biochemical basis of thermal death.* Microbiologists are almost entirely ignorant of the biochemical basis of viability in micro-organisms, so that one can hardly expect them to be able to explain the killing action of elevated temperatures. It is presumed, meanwhile, that one or more of the temperature-sensitive constituents of the organisms (discussed in Section II.2a) are inactivated, and that this renders the organisms incapable of multiplication. Factors such as the inactivation of nucleic acids, which generally occur at temperatures well above the maximum for growth, will also be involved in addition to more temperature-sensitive processes such as protein denaturation.

2. Low Temperatures

The majority of studies on the viability of bacteria at temperatures below the minimum for growth have been concerned with temperatures at which ice forms in the suspending fluid. Very little indeed has been reported on the viability of mesophilic micro-organisms at temperatures below their minimum for growth but above about $-2°$ at which temperature ice usually forms in the suspending fluid. However, Ryan and Kiritani (1959) reported on the rate of death of *E. coli* in stationary-phase cultures at different temperatures; they showed (Fig. 15) that there was a progressive decline in the viability of the bacterial cultures maintained at temperatures between 37° and 0°, the specific death rate

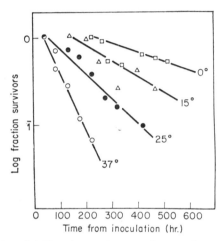

Fig. 15. Decrease in viability in stationary-phase cultures of *Escherichia coli* grown at different temperatures. Cultures maintained at 37°, 25° or 15° in the stationary phase had been grown at the same temperature. Cultures maintained at 0° were grown at 37°. From Ryan and Kiritani (1959).

at 37° being 14.2×10^{-3} and at 0°, 4.6×10^{-3}. The specific death rate, k, was calculated from the equation $N_t = N_0 e^{-kt}$, in which N_t is the number of viable bacteria at time t, and N_0 the number at zero time.

Rather more data have been reported on a phenomenon first described by Sherman and Albus (1923), who found that sudden chilling to 0° of dilute suspension of *E. coli* caused a loss of viability. The phenomenon has come to be known as "cold shock", and has since been reported with other strains of *E. coli* (Hegarty and Weeks, 1940; Meynell, 1958), and with strains of *Pseudomonas aeruginosa* (Gorrill and McNiel, 1960), *Aerobacter aerogenes* (Strange and Dark, 1962), *Salmonella typhimurium* (Gorrill and McNiel, 1960), and *Serratia marcescens* (Strange and Ness, 1963). Gram-positive bacteria are generally thought not to be sensitive to cold shock, although Ring (1965a, b) described a similar phenomenon in *Streptomyces hydrogenans*. Susceptibility to cold shock is usually found only in bacteria from exponential-phase cultures, and is greater with bacteria that have been grown in chemically defined media than with organisms grown in complex media (Strange, 1964). Also, the decline in the viability of a population is greatest when the organisms are suspended in a chemically simple diluent; distilled water is often the most effective. Strange and Dark (1962) showed that subjecting a thick suspension of *A. aerogenes* (containing 2–3 mg. dry wt. equiv./ml.) to a cold shock caused a release from the bacteria of solutes, which included u.v.-absorbing compounds, amino acids and ATP. These results suggest that cold shock affects the cytoplasmic membrane of the bacteria and causes changes in membrane permeability. One of us (J.F.) has recently studied cold shock in a mesophilic and a psychrophilic pseudomonad. In suspensions incubated at − 2°, the loss of viability and the release of endogenous solutes were much smaller with the psychrophil than with the mesophil. It would seem, therefore, that the psychrophil membrane, if such is the site of action of cold shock, is less affected by near-zero temperatures, and one is tempted to surmise that this may be related to its probably greater content of unsaturated fatty acid residues as compared with the mesophil membrane lipids.

a. *Death by freezing.* When the temperature of a suspension of micro-organisms, in buffer or medium, is lowered to a point at which ice forms in the suspension, a proportion of the organisms in the suspension are killed, as judged by their inability to form colonies when plated on nutrient media. This effect has been termed "death by freezing". Repeated freezing and thawing is often used to enhance this killing effect. Numerous studies have been made on the death of micro-organisms by freezing, and it has been shown that the process is influenced by a large number of factors, the principal ones of which are discussed below. The early literature on the subject has been well reviewed by Wood (1957) and Ingraham (1962).

Factors affecting death by freezing. Several claims have been made regarding the relative susceptibility of different species of micro-organisms to death by freezing. But few of these studies have been done under conditions in which all of the factors affecting the process were maintained constant, so that one should treat with caution some of the conclusions drawn from these experiments. Among the generalizations that have been made are that moulds and yeasts are generally more resistant to freezing than vegetative bacteria, and that bacterial spores are more resistant than the corresponding vegetative forms. It has also been claimed that psychrophils, as a class, are no more or less susceptible than mesophils. With regard to bacteria, Haines (1938) claimed that the more resistant forms were to be found among the Gram-positive organisms, a generalization that has been supported by Proom (1951). This conclusion is interesting in view of the finding that cold shock is experienced only by Gram-negative bacteria.

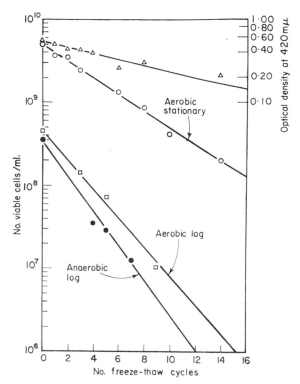

FIG. 16. Effect of the phase of growth, and of aeration of the culture, on the turbidity of, and the viability of the organisms in, a suspension of *Escherichia coli* ML 30 after repeated freezing and thawing. △ indicates turbidity, and ○ the viability of a suspension of aerobically grown, stationary-phase bacteria in 10% spent growth medium. □ indicates viability of aerobically grown, exponential-phase bacteria in 1% spent growth medium. ● indicates the viability of anaerobically grown exponential-phase bacteria in 1% spent growth medium. Statistical analysis showed that the slopes of the lower two curves do not differ significantly. From Packer *et al.* (1965).

The physiological state of the organisms also influences their susceptibility to death by freezing although the amount of data on the subject is meagre. Toyokawa and Hollander (1956) reported that organisms from exponential-phase cultures of *E. coli* were less resistant than those from stationary-phase cultures. A difference in susceptibility between *E. coli* grown in nutrient broth under aerobic and anaerobic conditions was reported by Harrison and Cerroni (1956), but could not be confirmed by Packer et al. (1965) using cultures grown in a glucose–salts medium (Fig. 16).

The effect of the rate of cooling has not been extensively studied. Mazur (1961a) showed, however, that, when Saccharomyces cerevisiae was rapidly cooled to −30° or below, fewer than 0·01% of the population survived; but when the cells were cooled slowly to the same temperature, up to 50% of the yeasts survived. Previous work by Mazur and his colleagues (1957) had shown that this behaviour was not found with Pasteurella pestis, for which the number of surviving bacteria was high regardless of the rate at which the suspensions were cooled to −30°. However, when the suspensions of bacteria were cooled to −45° or below, the amount of killing was much greater. In general, it is thought that the rate of killing declines as the temperature is lowered, and the rate is said to be negligible below about −50°.

Rather more is known about the effect of the composition of the suspending fluid on the killing of micro-organisms by freezing. It is evident from the work of Packer et al. (1965) that very different results are obtained if the bacteria are suspended in a glucose-free salts medium than if they are frozen in nutrient broth. Packer and his colleagues (1965) also reported the existence in filtrates from stationary-phase cultures of E. coli ML 30 of one or more compounds that protected the bacteria against death when they were frozen in glucose-free salts medium. A number of compounds are known to protect organisms against death by freezing, the main ones that have been studied being sugars and glycerol. The incorporation of glycerol into the suspending fluid has been used routinely for preserving suspensions of micro-organisms and animal cells such as erythrocytes. Suspending fluids with low pH values increase the mortality rate, probably because of the concentration of H^+ in the fluid following ice formation.

Apart from the effect of the storage temperature, very little is known of factors that affect the survival of micro-organisms in the frozen state. However, Ashwood-Smith et al. (1965) found that, when a strain of E. coli was suspended in phosphate buffer (pH 7·0) and maintained in the frozen state at different subzero temperatures, there was an appreciable increase in the sensitivity of the bacteria to death by u.v.-radiation between −10° and −79°.

The rate of rewarming does not appear to have a marked effect on the survival of organisms in the suspension, but the nature of the medium used for plating out the suspensions does. In general, the number of survivors scored is greater when dilutions of the population are plated out on a nutritionally complex medium than on glucose–salts media. Those organisms that are capable of growing on the complex medium but not on the simple medium have been described as "metabolically injured" (Straka and Stokes, 1959; Arpai, 1962; Nakamura and Dawson, 1962). Postgate and Hunter (1963) studied this phenomenon in some detail using populations of continuously grown *Aerobacter aerogenes*, and they concluded that the metabolic injury was not due to osmotic sensitivity or to the presence of toxic materials in the agar; nor were they able to find that mutation to nutritional exigence was a contributing factor. As a result of studying metabolic injury in *Aerobacter aerogenes* and *E. coli*, Macleod and his colleagues (1966) concluded that freezing damaged the cytoplasmic membranes in the bacteria, with the result that toxic ions, which are present in trace amounts, can penetrate the bacteria. The enriched media permit growth of the metabolically injured bacteria by providing compounds that chelate the toxic metal ions. Clearly, the phenomenon of metabolic injury deserves closer study which could well reveal some interesting facts regarding the effect of subzero temperatures on microbial metabolism.

Physiological basis of death by freezing. The mechanisms by which freezing kills micro-organisms have been the subject of considerable experimentation and discussion. It was first of all assumed that micro-organisms were killed during freezing as a result of the formation inside the cells of ice, which occupies a greater volume than the water from which it derives and could presumably, therefore, cause death of the cells by crushing. Formation of intracellular ice has been observed microscopically in many types of cells, including yeasts (Nei, 1960). Mazur (1961a) concluded that intracellular ice formation is more extensive in rapidly cooled than in slowly cooled *S. cerevisiae*, and is responsible for the higher mortality found in rapidly cooled suspensions. But the situation is much less clear with bacteria, and Luyet (1962) obtained no evidence for the formation of ice crystals in frozen staphylococci. Keith (1913) first suggested that micro-organisms died during freezing because of the formation of extracellular ice which leads to an enormous increase in the concentration of dissolved solutes in the unfrozen medium and consequently a rapid loss of water from the organisms. A similar process may well occur following the freezing of bacteria, for the relatively large surface area: volume ratio of bacteria as compared with other micro-organisms would cause a correspondingly rapid loss of water following the formation of extracellular ice.

Mazur (1961b; 1965) made further observations on the physiology of frozen *S. cerevisiae*, and concluded that death by freezing is not caused simply by the crushing effect of ice crystals. Rapid cooling of yeast to $-30°$ results in death and in certain morphological alterations including a loss of the central vacuole; it also causes a 50% decrease in volume. The decrease in volume was shown to result from the loss of a solution containing 11–16% solutes. These endogenous solutes were estimated to have a molecular weight less than 600. It was concluded that freezing damaged the cytoplasmic membrane and allowed the escape of low-molecular weight solutes. A similar release of u.v.-absorbing compounds, following freezing of E. coli, was reported by Lindeberg and Lode (1963) which suggests that death by freezing may have a similar physiological basis in bacteria and yeasts.

b. *Freeze-drying.* Freeze-drying has been used for preserving micro-organisms for many years. It is one of the most successful means of preserving large numbers of microbial cultures, and is now used routinely by almost all of the major culture collections (Brady, 1960; Floodgate and Hayes, 1961; Clark, 1962). Freeze-drying of micro-organisms has been well reviewed by Heckly (1961).

The principle of freeze-drying is that the organisms are desiccated while in the frozen state. Below the vapour pressure of ice (which, at 0°, is 4 mm. Hg), water is removed in the gas phase directly from the solid state. Under these conditions, the viability of the organisms is to a large extent preserved. Two main techniques have been used for freeze-drying micro-organisms. The method adopted by Swift (1937) employs dehydration under high vacuum by means of a desiccating agent; the Flosdorf and Mudd (1935) technique is based on the sublimation of water through a manifold into a separate condenser. Other methods which have been described in the past 30 years are essentially embellishments of these basic techniques.

Many factors have been shown to affect the survival of micro-organisms during freeze-drying, and these factors have been discussed in detail in reviews by Fry (1954) and Greaves (1960). The main factors are the nature of the organism and the conditions under which it is grown, the nature of the suspending medium, the density of organisms in the suspension, the degree of vacuum and the drying temperature, and the temperature and moisture and gas contents of the freeze-dried culture. Certain generalizations regarding the effects of these factors have been made, although in many instances on the basis of insufficient data. In general, Gram-positive bacteria survive better than Gram-negative strains (Fry, 1954; Steel and Ross, 1963). The nature of the suspending medium has a marked effect on the survival of freeze-dried micro-organisms. Heller (1941) concluded that the best medium for freeze drying E. coli and Strep. pyogenes was nutrient broth or peptone water; serum gave good results with these bacteria though not as good as nutrient broth. Fry and Greaves (1951) advocated another suspending medium which they called "Mist. desiccans", and which contains 1 vol. nutrient broth + 3 vols. serum, supplemented with 7·5% (w/v) glucose; this suspending medium is now widely used. Glycerol has also been

7*

extensively used in suspending fluids. Conflicting claims have been made regarding the effect of the density of organisms on the survival of freeze-dried micro-organisms. Stamp (1947) opined that low cell concentrations gave higher percentage survival rates, but the results of Steel and Ross (1963) were at variance with this conclusion. It is generally agreed that the presence of moisture and oxygen is deleterious to the survival of freeze-dried micro-organisms. Lion *et al.* (1961) and Dimmick *et al.* (1961) have suggested that the formation of free radicals may cause death of freeze-dried bacteria, and Heckly *et al.* (1965) have evidence that the presence of oxygen and moisture enhances free radical formation.

In recent years, a technique known as *ultradeep freezing* has been increasingly used to preserve micro-organisms. In this technique, a suspension of micro-organisms is rapidly cooled to a temperature of $-196°$ or lower, using liquid nitrogen as the refrigerant; the suspension is then stored at this temperature. Now that apparatus for ultra-deep freezing is available at modest cost, the technique has gained wide acceptance. Hwang (1960) has reported good recoveries of bacteria and fungi stored at these very low temperatures.

C. MICROBIAL GENOME

Temperature is known to affect the properties of the two macromolecular species, namely DNA and protein, that comprise the genome of the living cell. Hardly anything is known of the effect of temperature on the genome proteins. Much more work has been done on the effect of temperature on microbial DNA, mainly with *in vitro* experiments; this work is reviewed in Chapter 3 of this book (p. 25). Suffice to mention at this juncture that the effects that have been studied have been mainly at high temperatures, and probably have little physiological significance in growing micro-organisms.

Mutation rate is a phenomenon which is of paramount importance, and several workers have investigated the effect of temperature on the rate of spontaneous mutation. The majority of the studies have indicated that the rate of mutation/mutable unit/hr. has the same temperature coefficient as the rate of growth, so that the rate of mutation/mutable unit/generation is the same at all temperatures (Witkin, 1953; Ryan and Kiritani, 1959). The temperatures studied have usually been within the growth range for the organisms, although Ryan and Kiritani (1959) also included data on the rate of mutation at $0°$ for a mesophilic strain of *E. coli*. Reports by Zamenhof (1960) and Chiasson and Zamenhof (1966) have described the effects of higher temperatures, around $105°–155°$, on the induction of mutations in spores of *Bacillus subtilis*. The proportion of mutants formed increased as the temperature was increased from 105°–115°, but declined with a further rise in temperature to 155° (Chiasson and Zamenhof, 1966). Of particular interest was their finding that the proportions of auxotrophs formed for individual amino acids showed maxima at different temperatures.

Several reports have appeared concerning the effects of temperature on extrachromosomal genetic elements in micro-organisms. In a study of cytoplasmic mutation to respiration deficiency in *Saccharomyces cerevisiae*, Ycas (1956) observed higher frequencies in organisms grown at 40° than in those grown at 30°. Gutz (1957) obtained similar results with *S. carlsbergensis* grown at 28° and 7°. A more extensive study of this temperature effect was carried out by Ogur *et al.* (1960) using several

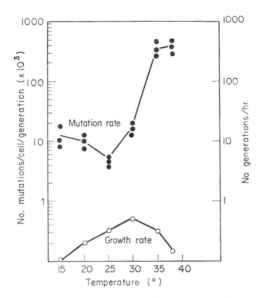

FIG. 17. Effect of temperature on the rate of growth and the rate of mutation of *Saccharomyces cerevisiae* strain 14940. From Ogur *et al.* (1960).

strains of Saccharomyces over the range 15°–38°. Plots of the rate of mutation/cell/generation against temperature gave curves with a marked minimum (Fig. 17). Ogur *et al.* (1960) explained these minima by assuming that unbalanced growth at high and low temperatures in the growth range led to an increase in the probability of an irreversible loss of an organelle that is essential to the biosynthesis of the respiratory system. Unfortunately, little if anything has been reported on the effects of temperature on other extrachromosomal genetic elements in micro-organisms, for these effects are probably of considerable ecological importance.

Another property of the microbial genome which has been shown to be affected by temperature is the frequency of crossing over, the magnitude of the effect depending on the organism and upon the nature of the linkage groups. Using a measure that was probably related to the second division segregation frequency of mating type in *Ustilago hordei*, Hüttig (1931) obtained a U-shaped curve with a minimum at 8° when he plotted the frequency against temperature. Rizet and Engelmann (1949) obtained similar results with *Podospora anserina*, depending upon the mutant pair that was crossed. Using *Neurospora crassa*, Towe and Stadler (1964) reported that the rate of crossing over within linkage group VI was considerably greater at 18° than at 25°, a result that was confirmed by McNelly-Ingle *et al.* (1966) for linkage group I in this mould.

D. SYNTHESIS AND ACTIVITY OF ENZYMES

1. *Total Protein Synthesis*

During the past 20 years, much has been learned about the molecular events that take place during protein synthesis in living cells. More recently, this picture has been embellished by the discovery of the regulatory mechanisms that operate during protein synthesis and also those that control enzyme activity. However, with one or two exceptions, very little has been reported on the effect of temperature on the individual steps in protein synthesis.

Protein synthesis proceeds at a decreased rate as the temperature is decreased, in common with all metabolic processes. Goldstein *et al.* (1964) showed that protein synthesis takes place in *E. coli* at 0°, and that the rate of synthesis of total protein at this temperature was about 350 times slower than at 37°. A few data have been reported on the ways in which the various components of the protein-synthesizing system in micro-organisms are affected by low temperatures. Several workers (e.g. Tempest and Hunter, 1965) have shown that the amount of DNA in each micro-organism, expressed as a percentage of the dry weight, does not alter significantly as the temperature of incubation is lowered. It would seem, however, that the synthesis and activity of the ribosomes is affected, although evidence on this point is meagre. Schaechter *et al.* (1958) examined the macromolecular composition of *Salmonella typhimurium* as affected by temperature, and showed that this composition was not a function of growth rate when this rate was altered by changing the temperature over the range 37°–25°. Tempest and Hunter (1965) examined the effect of temperatures between 25° and 40° on the macromolecular composition of populations of *Aerobacter aerogenes* grown in a chemostat at a fixed rate under different conditions of substrate limitation. They showed that the RNA content of the bacteria increased as the temperature was decreased from 40° to 25°. They assumed that the rate of protein synthesis per unit of ribosome was constant at a particular temperature. Lowering the temperature decreased ribosomal activity so that, in order to maintain a constant growth rate, the bacteria synthesized additional RNA to compensate. Tempest and Hunter (1965) explained the apparent discrepancy between their results and those of Schaechter *et al.* (1958) by assuming that the salmonellae contained their maximum content of ribosomes (a condition which is assumed to be fulfilled in fast-growing organisms in a batch culture), and that a decrease in temperature could not then be compensated for by a further increase in ribosomal content.

Clearly, much remains to be discovered about the effects of temperature on protein synthesis, and in particular it would be instructive to know how the process is affected by much lower temperatures than those that have so far been studied.

2. *Regulation of Enzyme Synthesis*

Rather more is known about the effects of temperature on the regulation of synthesis of individual enzymes than on the synthesis of total protein. Reference has already been made to the earlier reports that certain processes of enzyme induction are particularly sensitive to temperature; see Knox (1953) for a review of the earlier literature on this subject. More recently, Halpern (1961) found that synthesis of glutamate decarboxylase in *E. coli* is inducible at 37° but partly constitutive at 30°. Tryptophan has been shown to induce tryptophanase synthesis in another wild-type strain of *E. coli* at 30° but not at temperatures below 15° (Ng and Gartner, 1963). A number of workers have isolated mutant strains of micro-organisms with temperature-sensitive induction processes, and have used them to study the kinetics of regulation of enzyme synthesis. Thus, Horiuchi and Novick (1961) isolated a mutant strain of *E. coli* which synthesized β-galactosidase constitutively at 43·5° but needed the presence of an inducer to synthesize the enzyme at 14°. The review article by Kjeldgaard (1967) should be consulted for further information on the use of *ts* mutants in studies on the regulation of enzyme synthesis.

Since the discovery of enzyme repression and the relationship of this process to enzyme induction through the Jacob-Monod model, further reports have appeared showing that the repression of enzyme synthesis, like enzyme induction, is often very sensitive to temperature. Gallant and Stapleton (1963) isolated a mutant of *E. coli* B in which the repression of synthesis of alkaline phosphatase by inorganic phosphate decreases as the temperature is increased from 20° to 40°. Repression of synthesis of alkaline phosphatase by inorganic phosphate was not affected by temperature in the parent. Another example has been reported by Udaka and Horiuchi (1965), who isolated a mutant strain of *E. coli* in which repression of the synthesis of certain arginine pathway enzymes (ornithine carbamoyltransferase and argininosuccinase) by arginine decreased as the temperature was raised from 20° to 42°.

Most of the workers who have reported these effects have suggested explanations for their molecular basis. Horiuchi and Novick (1961), Gallant and Stapleton (1963), and Udaka and Horiuchi (1965) postulated that, in the mutant strains, the aporepressor was thermolabile, and so caused a derepression of enzyme synthesis at high temperatures. An alternative explanation (J. L. Ingraham; personal communication) is that the affinity of the aporepressor for the corepressor is decreased at high temperatures much more in the mutant than in the parent.

Reports by Szer and Ochoa (1964) and Friedman and Weinstein (1964) have drawn attention to another mechanism by which temperature may affect the regulation of enzyme synthesis, namely by influencing the fidelity of the translation of m-RNA during protein synthesis. Friedman and Weinstein (1964), using a cell-free amino acid-incorporating system from the thermophil, *Bacillus stearothermophilus*, found that the leucine-phenylalanine ambiguity, which is manifested when poly-U is used as a messenger, is greatly increased at low temperatures in the growth range. They suggested that this ability of temperature to affect the reading of a m-RNA may explain the behaviour of *ts* mutants of phages and bacteria which synthesize enzymes at low but not at high temperatures, since the low temperature, by inducing an ambiguity in the translation, may partially correct the effects of the mutated codon.

3. *Alterations in Metabolic Activity*

There are many other reports which indicate that temperature can alter the metabolic activities of micro-organisms, although the manner in which these modifications in metabolism are brought about are, in most instances, unexplored. These effects of temperature on microbial metabolism may well be important in relation to the activity of micro-organisms in natural environments, and they clearly merit more detailed study.

The metabolism of carbohydrates by certain micro-organisms often seems to be very sensitive to temperature. This may be an inherent property of carbohydrate metabolism, or simply that carbohydrate metabolism has been studied far more extensively than many other areas of metabolism. A differential effect of temperature on carbohydrate metabolism in heterofermentative lactic acid bacteria was reported by

Thiel (1940), who showed that there was an increase in the ratio of the amounts of acetic acid formed to sugar utilized as the temperature of incubation was lowered. A similar effect for gas production by a coliform bacterium was described by Hopton (1958). The fermentation of sugar by a psychrophilic strain of *Aerobacter aerogenes* was shown by Greene and Jezeski (1954) to give rise to acid and gas below 30° but only to acid at temperatures above 30°. Upadhyay and Stokes (1963a, b) observed a similar effect on acid and gas production by an unclassified bacterium (which appeared to be intermediate between an Aeromonas and an enterobacterium) and showed that the effect was explained by the temperature-sensitive nature of the hydrogenase-synthesizing system in the bacterium. Another report of the effect of temperature on carbohydrate metabolism has come from studies on *Saccharomyces carlsbergensis* which synthesizes diacetyl in much greater amounts at 5° than at higher temperatures up to 20° (Denshchikov *et al.*, 1962). This effect is of some commercial importance, since it leads to the development of undesirable organoleptic qualities during the lagering of beer (Farrell and Rose, 1965).

There are indications that, with many micro-organisms, the synthesis of polysaccharides, either capsular or intracellular, is greater at low than at high temperatures in the growth range. Regrettably, however, this effect has not yet been accorded any systematic study despite its potential ecological importance. It has been known for some time that the synthesis of extracellular dextran by many *Leuconostoc* species and lactic acid bacteria is greater at low temperatures; some of these bacteria produce almost no dextran at 37° whereas, at 25°, the culture becomes extremely viscous due to the accumulation of extracellular dextran. This effect has been attributed to the production by these bacteria of a dextransucrase that is very rapidly inactivated at temperatures above 30° (Neely, 1960) and, with a lactobacillus, to the temperature-sensitive nature of the dextransucrase-synthesizing system (Dunican and Seeley, 1963). This temperature effect is not confined to the production of extracellular polysaccharide, for Tempest and Hunter (1965) found that an increase from 3·3% to 8·9% in the dry weight of carbon-limited continuously grown *A. aerogenes*, when the incubation temperature was decreased from 35° to 25°, was accounted for by carbohydrate. Tempest and Hunter did not indicate whether the increase was attributable to the more extensive laying down of polysaccharide reserves or to an increase in the amount of cell-wall polysaccharide. Synthesis of cell-wall polysaccharide in the thermophilic bacilli, *B. stearothermophilus* and *B. coagulans*, was shown by Forrester and Wicken (1966) to be influenced by temperature. In both organisms, there was an increase in the proportion of mucopeptide and a decrease proportion of teichoic acid in the walls from bacteria grown at 55° as compared with the walls of bacteria grown at 37°. In view of the effects of temperature on the cell size of some micro-organisms (see Section II.A.1.d, p. 164), it would seem that this effect merits a more rigorous exploration.

The production of other surface structures, in addition to capsules, has also been shown to be affected by temperature. It has been known for some time that flagella synthesis is markedly affected by temperature in the range in which the organism grows. Frequently, the synthesis of flagella is favoured at low temperatures in the growth range and absent at higher temperatures in the range. Mironescu, as early as 1899, reported that a typhoid-like bacillus produced flagella at 23° but not at 38°. A similar behaviour has since been reported for strains of *E. coli* (Morrison and McCapra, 1961), *Salmonella typhi* (Nicolle and Trenel, 1902; Felix *et al.*, 1934), *Bacillus inconstans* (Braun and Löwenstein, 1923), *Pasteurella pseudotuberculosis* (Arkwright, 1927; Preston and Maitland, 1952), *Salmonella paratyphi* B (Jordon *et al.*, 1934), *Bordetella bronchiseptica* (Lacey, 1953) and certain psychrophilic bacteria (Schubert, 1952; Schubert and Schubert, 1953). The opposite effect, namely the synthesis of flagella at high but not at low temperatures in the growth range, has been reported for other psychrophilic bacteria by Schubert and Schubert (1953), for *Salmonella paratyphi* C by Quadling (1958), and for *Phytophthora infestans* by Ferris (1954). A report by Orr and Taylor (1965) critically discusses the desirability of retaining flagella production as a taxonomic criterion in the classification of Gram-negative bacteria in view of the marked effect of temperature on the synthesis of these organelles.

Roberts and Doetsch (1966) have further examined the effect of temperature on flagella production, and have studied the regeneration of flagella in certain psychrophilic and mesophilic bacteria that had been experimentally deflagellated. The thermophil, *B. stearothermophilus* 11330, resynthesized flagella at 20°, a temperature below the minimum for growth of the bacterium. None of the mesophilic bacteria that were examined could resynthesize their flagella at 45° after being grown at 28°. The psychrophil, *Pseudomonas fragi*, could resynthesize flagella at 4°, but not at 28°, after it had been grown at 4° or 28°.

Temperature has also been shown to affect production of other antigenically active surface structures in a number of micro-organisms. For example, the B antigen in certain strains of *E. coli* was shown by Ørskov (1956) to be synthesized in greater amounts at 18° than at 37°, while Lacey (1960) found that the X antigen of certain *Bordetella* species was synthesized at 37° but not at 25°. The virulence, too, of some organisms is known to be affected by the temperature at which the organisms are grown. Fukui and his colleagues (1959, 1960) showed that *Pasteurella pestis* from cultures grown at 5° showed lower virulence than bacteria from cultures grown at 37°. When organisms from cultures grown at 5° were incubated aerobically for 6 hr. at 37°–41° in a medium containing phosphate, amino acids, an oxidizable sugar and gluconate, virulence was restored; under these conditions, there was no significant growth (Naylor *et al.*, 1961). A similar effect of temperature on the virulence of *Klebsiella pneumoniae* has been reported by Cardinale *et al.* (1965), while the Lippincotts (1965) have studied the effect of temperature on the virulence of the plant pathogen, *Agrobacterium tumefaciens*. An interesting example of the effect of temperature on the properties of a cell-surface component has been discovered in this Laboratory (Stanley and Rose, 1967a). Several strains of *Corynebacterium xerosis*, as well as certain other corynebacteria, form clumps when cultures that have been grown at 30° are rapidly cooled with vigorous aeration to 15°. The clumping appears to be caused by changes in the properties of a cell-surface protein which becomes sticky only at low temperatures.

There are several indications that pigment production by micro-organisms increases when the organisms are incubated at temperatures below the optimum for growth. The most quoted example is the production by *Serratia marcescens* of the red pigment, prodigiosin, which is favoured at temperatures between 20° and 25° although the optimum temperature for growth of the bacterium is nearer 37°. The biochemical basis of this effect has been reported by Williams *et al.* (1965), who showed that the enzyme that catalyses the last step in the biosynthesis, namely the coupling of a monopyrrole with a bipyrrole to give the linear tripyrrole prodigiosin, is abnormally sensitive to temperature. With other examples of temperature-sensitive pigment production, enzyme synthesis and not enzyme action has been shown to be involved. Such an explanation has been proposed to explain the production of a red pigment by the silk-worm pathogen, *Bacillus cereus* var. *alesti*, at 15° but not at 28° (Uffen and Canale-Parola, 1966).

E. DIFFERENTIATION

By far the greatest number of studies on differentiation in unicellular micro-organisms have been concerned with bacterial endospore formation and germination, and the following brief account of the effect of temperature on microbial differentiation will be restricted to the effects on endospore formation and germination in bacilli.

Endospore formation and germination, and vegetative growth, are often differently affected by temperature. Thus, the span between the maximum and minimum temperatures for various stages of the sporulation processes are often greater than that for vegetative growth, although the optimum temperatures are often about the same (Williams et al., 1957; Curran and Pallansch, 1963; Knaysi, 1964). Thermophilic and mesophilic spore-forming bacilli have been known for some time, and Sinclair and Stokes (1964) and Larkin and Stokes (1966) have recently isolated psychrophilic clostridia and *Bacillus* spp. which grow and sporulate at 0°.

The formation of an endospore in a vegetative cell (or sporangium), and the subsequent germination of that spore, involve a complex sequence of events each of which may be differently affected by temperature. The temperature of the sporulation medium influences the rate of spore formation and the number of spores formed. Spore formation is usually most rapid at or near the optimum temperature for growth of the vegetative bacteria (Murrell, 1961; Murrell and Warth, 1965). But, once spore formation has commenced, drastic changes in temperature are required to prevent completion of the process. For example, Hardwick and Foster (1952) found that transfer of a washed suspension of sporulating *Bacillus mycoides* from 30° to 4° for one month did not delay the completion of sporulation when the suspension was returned to 30°. Temperature-sensitive mutants of *B. cereus* var. *lacticola* have been isolated by Lundgren and Beskid (1960). These mutants produce normal spores at 28° but show an abortive sporulation at 37°. A curious effect was reported by Long and Williams (1960), who found that, at 55°, spore formation by, but not vegetative growth of, *B. stearothermophilus* is sensitive to oxygen.

Temperature has also been shown to affect the properties of the bacterial endospore. One of the most striking properties of spores is their heat resistance, and nearly 70 years ago Weil (1899) reported that the heat resistance of *B. stearothermophilus* spores increased as the temperature of the sporulating medium was raised. This observation has since been confirmed with other bacilli and with clostridia (Halvorson, 1962; Murrell, 1961). It is thought that the increased heat resistance is a result of an increase in the content of dipicolinic acid in the spore cortex, and also of a decrease in the ratio of the amounts of Mg^{2+} to Ca^{2+} present (Murrell and Warth, 1965). However, the situation is more complex than would appear from these observations for, when spores with large differences in heat resistance (as much as 10^5) were heated under conditions of controlled water activity (a_w), the difference in heat resistance decreased to less than 10-fold (Murrell and Scott, 1957). Long and Williams (1960) have reported other differences in spore composition as a result of subjecting *B. stearothermophilus* to high temperatures during sporulation, including an increase in the degree of unsaturation in the spore lipids. This finding complements that of Sugiyama (1951), who found that supplementing the sporulation medium with long-chain fatty acids caused an increase in the heat resistance of *Clostridium botulinum* spores.

Before germinating, spores may enter a state of dormancy, which is often induced by heat treatment. Several workers (Curran and Evans, 1937; Nelson, 1943; Knaysi, 1948) have shown that heat-treated spores are more nutritionally exacting than untreated spores. Powell (1950) showed that, after storage, the rate of initiation of germination decreased as the temperature was lowered. Spores stored at $-20°$ for four months by Halvorson and Church (1957) showed an increase in the rate of respiration of endogenous reserves and of glucose as compared with freshly harvested spores.

Some spores require a period of heat activation before they begin to germinate (Murrell, 1961). The Q_{10} of heat activation has been calculated to be about 5, and the lower the temperature of spore formation the greater is the response to heat activation (Curran and Evans, 1945). The amount of heating required for maximum activation varies greatly for different spores, clostridial spores requiring about 25 minutes at 80° (Uehara and Frank, 1965). Very severe heating will kill spores. Thus Edwards *et al.* (1965) found that the inactivation of *B. subtilis* spores was accelerated more by increases in temperature than by increases in exposure time.

The initiation of spore germination, as measured by a loss in heat resistance and in spore refractility, is very susceptible to changes in temperature. In general, the initiation of germination is most rapid at temperatures near the optimum for growth of the vegetative bacteria. Nevertheless, there are instances in which initiation of germination has been observed at temperatures above the maximum, or below the minimum, for growth (Murrell, 1961). Germination of *B. cereus* spores in an amino acid mixture cannot be initiated below 18° (Keynan *et al.*, 1958); but, if the process is initiated at 18°, it can then be continued at 0°. The effect of temperature on the initiation of germination of *B. cereus* spores has also been reported to be influenced by the pH value of the medium (Vas and Proszt, 1957; Keynan *et al.*, 1965). It has also been shown by several workers (Ohye and Scott, 1957; Segner *et al.*, 1966) that spores of *Clostridium botulinum* type E can germinate and grow vegetatively at around 5°. These observations have caused considerable concern to those involved in the processing of foodstuffs, particularly fish (Cann *et al.*, 1965).

III. Economic Importance of the Temperature Relationships of Micro-organisms

The applied microbiologist is mainly concerned with the activities of micro-organisms as they are involved in the cycling of elements in the biosphere, and in industrial and commercial processes. The temperature relationships of micro-organisms are important in many areas of applied microbiology; some of the main temperature effects are discussed briefly in the following pages. In a previous review (Farrell and Rose, 1965), we discussed the applied aspects of low temperature microbiology, and this review should be perused for more detailed treatment of the subject.

A. MICROBIAL ACTIVITY IN NATURAL ENVIRONMENTS

In a few natural environments, such as compost heaps, hot springs, and guysers, the micro-organisms present are growing at or near their optimum temperature for growth. But large areas of the world's surface support microbial populations under conditions in which the temperature rarely rises above 15°–20°. Under these conditions, therefore, the micro-organisms are continually subjected to suboptimum temperatures. Both soil and marine microbiology are still in essentially descriptive stages of development, and it will be many years before the microflora of these habitats are fully described. As such, it is regrettable that many soil and marine microbiologists still attempt to isolate micro-organisms at temperatures that are far higher than those that the micro-organisms have experienced in the soil or the sea, for such practices must inevitably give misleading results.

Approximately four-fifths of the world is covered by water, the temperature of which can range from as low as − 2° to 20° (Sverdrup et al., 1942); however, the main bulk of the ocean rarely exceeds a temperature of 5° (Zobell, 1962). One would therefore expect the majority of marine micro-organisms to be psychrophilic. This is probably true, but as yet very few studies have been reported on the temperature characteristics of marine micro-organisms. The effect of temperature on the activities of marine micro-organisms is discussed further in Chapter 17 of this book (p. 592).

The areas around the poles are the coldest on earth. Nevertheless, micro-organisms occur in these areas, as discussed in Chapter 16 (p. 555). In some respects, more is known about the Antarctic and Arctic microbial flora than the marine microflora. Many of the micro-organisms isolated from the polar regions are extremely well adapted to the low temperatures that prevail in these areas, and they have low minimum as well as low maximum temperatures. The importance of using suitable precautions when isolating micro-organisms from Antarctic lakes was recently demonstrated by our colleague, S. O. Stanley (See Section II.A, p. 159). An examination of the temperature characteristics of the predominant bacteria which he isolated from the Deception Island lakes showed that a third had maximum temperatures for growth of around 20°. Clearly, these micro-organisms would have been lost had the isolation been done in a warm laboratory (Stanley and Rose, 1967b).

Man's recent pre-occupation with the potentialities of space travel has led to a renewed interest in the possible existence of life on other planets. Many of the larger planets are thought to have temperature regimes that are very different from those that prevail on earth, particularly with regard to the extremes of temperature that are experienced, and some biologists have studied the survival of terrestrial micro-organisms in simulated planetary environments. Packer et al. (1963) have compiled a useful review of the temperature relationships of micro-organisms as they might relate to the activities of terrestrial micro-organisms on Mars.

B. EXPLOITATION OF MICROBIAL ACTIVITY

Man has developed a wide range of manufacturing processes in which microbial activity, either in mixed populations or in pure culture, is encouraged and exploited. In many of these processes, the temperature relationships of the micro-organisms are important. For example, after the pulp and beans of cacao have been scooped from the pods, the material is gathered into mounds and, as a result of microbial thermogenesis, the mass of material can reach temperatures of 40°–50° for 4–5 days. This process, which is an integral part of the curing of the cacao beans, frees the beans from the pulp and prevents them from germinating. Most of the thermogenesis is caused by thermophilic bacteria and yeasts, although thermophilic moulds are also thought to participate (Chatt, 1953). Microbial thermogenesis is also important during the curing of tobacco (Garner, 1946).

In most industrial microbiological processes, micro-organisms are grown in pure culture, with the object of producing microbial cell material, such as baker's yeast, or a commercially important chemical, such as antibiotics, or to bring about a chemical transformation in a substrate (Rose, 1961). These industrial processes are usually conducted at or near the optimum temperature for the particular activity that is required of the micro-organism.

C. PREVENTION OF MICROBIAL ACTIVITY

Industry and commerce deal with a wide range of materials that are prone to attack by micro-organisms. Foremost among these perishable commodities are foodstuffs, and one of the main concerns of food microbiologists is to prevent the unwanted growth of micro-organisms in food and food materials. One of the main ways of preventing microbial activity in perishable materials is to subject the materials to temperatures that kill the micro-organisms present; this is heat sterilization.

Alternatively, the material can be stored at a temperature that is below the minimum for growth of potential spoilage micro-organisms. Both heat sterilization, and chilling and freezing, raise microbiological problems that are often peculiar to the individual material and to the conditions used. It is important to stress that, while heat sterilization kills micro-organisms, chilling and freezing usually does not. In the following paragraphs there is an epitome of the principles that underlie the use of heat sterilization and of chilling and freezing.

1. Heat Sterilization

The principles and practice of heat sterilization are familiar to most biologists, and necessarily so to microbiologists since they are indispensable to the practice of microbiology. Sykes's (1958) book should be perused for a detailed account of sterilization by heat. Heat sterilization presents few problems when the material that is to be sterilized can be raised to a sufficiently high temperature to kill all of the micro-organisms present. Problems arise when, because of the nature of the material, the heat treatment that can safely be given is not sufficient to kill all of the organisms present. This situation is common in the food industry, since many foods cannot be subjected to a severe heat treatment often because this leads to a loss of organoleptic qualities. Partial heat sterilization is therefore often practised in the food industry. The main problems that arise as a result of partial heat sterilization are from the growth of vegetative and spore forms of micro-organisms that have a high resistance to heat. Often, these micro-organisms are thermophilic strains of *Bacillus* or *Clostridium*, largely because of the exceptional heat resistance of the spores of these bacteria, which can withstand temperatures well over 110° for 30 minutes. For details of the microbial spoilage of food, the reader cannot do better than consult the book by Frazier (1958).

2. Chilling and Freezing

Low-temperature storage is now widely used to prevent growth of unwanted micro-organisms on a wide range of perishable materials including banked blood and pharmaceuticals such as vaccines. But, as far as the bulk of preserved material is concerned, these applications are relatively minor compared with the use of low temperatures in preserving food and food materials. Communities in the Arctic have, for centuries, preserved perishable foodstuffs by storing them at the low ambient temperatures that obtain in this region, but the practice has only become widespread in the more temperate regions of the world following the introduction of refrigeration and deep-freezing equipment into industry and the home. Goresline (1962) has written a most readable account of the growth of the chilled and frozen-food industry. Some idea of the rate at which the industry has grown is seen from the fact that, between 1949 and 1959, the output of commercial frozen foods in the U.S.A. increased from 1516 million pounds to 6565 million pounds per annum, and there is reason to believe that, since 1959, the expansion has continued at about the same rate.

The literature on the microbiology of chilled and frozen foods is voluminous. Fortunately, there are several review articles which provide valuable digests of the literature, including those by Borgstrom (1955; 1962), Elliott and Michener (1960), Peterson (1962), Michener and Elliott (1965), and Silverman and Goldblith (1965).

The success of chilling and freezing as a means of preserving food and food materials depends to a large extent on the size and nature of the initial microbial population on the material. Some foods always have a high initial count of micro-organisms. Freshly drawn poultry, for example, invariably contains a large population of coliform bacteria, while fish has a markedly psychrophilic flora. Many vegetables, on the other hand, have comparatively low initial counts.

The treatment of the food during the chilling or freezing process very considerably affects its microbial population. Cleanliness in the plant is of paramount importance if the microbial count is to be kept as low as possible. Problems often arise as a result of the defrosting of frozen foods for, during the defrost cycles in a frozen-food cabinet, the temperature can rise above 0° long enough to allow the growth of psychrophilic micro-organisms.

Growth of some spoilage micro-organisms on chilled and frozen foods, such as the growth of yeasts in chilled grape juice (Pederson et al., 1959), does not greatly affect the organoleptic qualities of the food, although it does render it less acceptable for consumption. But the activities of other micro-organisms can be sufficiently extensive to cause the development of off-flavours and changes in the texture of the food. The biochemical changes involved in the spoilage of food are mostly poorly understood. But changes in the physical and organoleptic qualities of chilled and frozen foods are often caused by the activities of microbial proteolytic enzymes. Peterson and Gunderson (1960) isolated a psychrophilic strain of *Pseudomonas fluorescens* from defrosted chicken pies. They found that the development of off-flavours and odours in the defrosted pies occurred in advance of the growth of large numbers of the psychrophilic pseudomonad, and were probably caused by the liberation of intracellular proteolytic enzymes from the bacteria originally present, and by the unusually high activity of these enzymes at low temperatures. Particular attention has been given to the possible production of toxins by pathogenic bacteria in chilled and frozen foods, but there is no reason to believe that this is important or that, at present, it constitutes a hazard to public health. However, the activities of certain micro-organisms need to be scrutinized with great care. Mention has already been made of the ability of *Clostridium botulinum* type E spores to germinate and grow at near-zero temperatures (see p. 205), and, in view of the number of reports during the past few years of aflatoxin production by moulds, it is clear that this too must be watched carefully.

ACKNOWLEDGEMENTS

Work from this laboratory reported in this review was supported by grants from the Science Research Council, and the Nuffield Foundation, for which we express our thanks. One of us (A.H.R.) is grateful to Dr. John L. Ingraham, of the Department of Bacteriology, University of California, Davis, California, U.S.A., for the hospitality afforded him during a stay in his laboratory, and especially for many valuable discussions. We also wish to thank those publishers and authors who have given us permission to reproduce published data.

References

Abram, D. and Koffler, H. (1965). *Bact. Proc.* 30.
Adams, M. H. (1955). *Virology* **1**, 336.
Adant, M. (1928). *Compt. rend. Soc. Biol.* **99**, 1244.
Akagi, J. M. and Campbell, L. L. (1961). *J. Bact.* **82**, 927.
Akagi, J. M. and Campbell, L. L. (1962). *J. Bact.* **84**, 1194.
Allen, M. B. (1950). *J. gen. Physiol.* **33**, 205.
Allen, M. B. (1953). *Bact. Rev.* **17**, 125.
Anderson, E. B. and Meanwell, L. J. (1936). *J. dairy Sci.* **7**, 182.
Arkwright, J. A. (1927). *Lancet* **i**, 13.
Arpai, J. (1962). *Appl. Microbiol.* **10**, 297.
Arrhenius, S. (1889). *Z. phys. Chem.* **4**, 226.
Arrhenius, S. (1908). *Ergeb. Physiol.* **7**, 480.
Ashwood-Smith, M. J., Bridges, B. A. and Munson, R. J. (1965). *Science* **149**, 1103.
Azuma, Y., Newton, S. B. and Witter, L. D. (1962). *J. dairy Sci.* **45**, 1529.
Baumgartner, J. G. and Hersom, A. C. (1956). "Canned Foods; an Introduction to their Microbiology", 4th ed. 291 pp. J. and A. Churchill Ltd., London.
Bausum H. T. and Matney, T. S. (1965). *J. Bact.* **90**, 50.
Baxter, R. M. and Gibbons, N. E. (1962). *Canad. J. Microbiol.* **8**, 511.
Bertani, G. and Nice, S. (1954). *J. Bact.* **67**, 202.
Beumer-Jochmans, M. P. (1951). *Ann. Inst. Pasteur* **80**, 536.
Borgstrom, G. A. (1955). *Advanc. food Res.* **6**, 163.
Borgstrom, G. A. (1962). In "Low Temperature Microbiology", p. 197. Campbell Soup Co., Camden, New Jersey.
Boyer, P. D., Lum, F. G., Ballou, G. A., Luck, J. M. and Rice, R. G. (1946). *J. biol. Chem.* **162**, 181.

Boyer, P. D., Ballou, G. A. and Luck, J. M. (1947). *J. biol. Chem.* **167**, 407.

Brady, B. L. (1960). In "Recent Research in Freezing and Drying", (A. S. Parkes and A. U. Smith, Eds.), p. 243. Blackwells, Oxford.

Braun, H. and Löwenstein, P. (1923). *Z. Bakteriol.* **91**, 1.

Brock, T. D. and Brock, M. L. (1966). *Nature, Lond.* **209**, 733.

Brooks, F. T. and Hansford, C. G. (1923). *Brit. mycol. Soc. Trans.* **8**, 113.

Brown, A. D. and Weidemann, (1958). *J. appl. Bact.* **21**, 11.

Buetow, D. E. (1962). *Exp. Cell Res.* **27**, 137.

Burns, V. W. (1962). *Progr. Biophys.* **12**, 1.

Burton, K. (1951). *Biochem. J.* **48**, 458.

Burton, S. D. and Morita, R. Y. (1965). *Bact. Proc.* 20.

Byrne, P. and Chapman, D. (1964). *Nature, Lond.* **202**, 987.

Califano, L. (1952). *Bull. Wld. Hlth. Org.* **6**, 19.

Cann, D. C., Wilson, B. B., Hobbs, G. and Shewan, J. M. (1965). *J. appl. Bact.* **28**, 431.

Cannefax, G. R. (1962). *J. Bact.* **83**, 708.

Cardinale, M., Hubbard, C. V. and Fukui, G. M. (1965). *Bact. Proc.* 67.

Chatt, E. M. (1953). "Cocoa; Cultivation, Processing, Analysis", 302 pp. Interscience, New York.

Chiasson, L. P. and Zamenhof, S. (1966). *Canad. J. Microbiol.* **12**, 43.

Chick, H. (1910). *J. Hyg., Camb.* **10**, 237.

Clark, W. A. (1962). In "Low Temperature Microbiology", p. 285. Campbell Soup Co., Camden, New Jersey.

Cochrane, V. W. (1958). "Physiology of Fungi", 524 pp. Wiley and Sons, New York.

Cooney, D. G. and Emerson, R. (1964). "Thermophilic Fungi", 188 pp. W. H. Freeman & Sons, San Francisco.

Copeland, J. J. (1936). *Ann. N.Y. Acad. Sci.* **36**, 1.

Curran, H. R. and Evans, F. R. (1937). *J. Bact.* **34**, 179.

Curran, H. R. and Evans, F. R. (1945). *J. Bact.* **49**, 335.

Curran, H. R. and Pallansch, M. J. (1963). *J. Bact.* **86**, 911.

Davern, C. (1964). *Austral. J. Biol. Sci.* **17**, 726.

Davey, C. B., Miller, R. J. and Nelson, L. A. (1966). *J. Bact.* **91**, 1827.

Denshchikov, N. T., Rylkin, S. S. and Zhvirblyanskaya, A. Y. (1962). *Mikrobiologia* **31**, 112.

Dimmick, R. L. (1965a). *Appl. Microbiol.* **13**, 846.

Dimmick, R. L. (1965b). *J. Bact.* **89**, 791.

Dimmick, R. L., Heckley, R. J. and Hollis, D. P. (1961). *Nature, Lond.* **192**, 776.

Doerr, R. and Grüninger, W. (1922). *Z. Hyg.* **97**, 209.

Doudoroff, M. and Shuster, C. W. (1962). *J. biol. Chem.* **237**, 603.

Dowell, C. E. and Sinsheimer, R. L. (1966). *J. molec. Biol.* **16**, 374.

Dua, R. D. and Burris, R. H. (1963). *Proc. nat. Acad. Sci., Wash.* **50**, 169.

Dunican, L. K. and Seeley, H. W. (1963). *J. Bact.* **86**, 1079.

Edgar, R. S. and Lielausis, I. (1964). *Genetics* **49**, 649.

Edwards, O. F. and Rettger, L. F. (1937). *J. Bact.* **34**, 489.

Edwards, J. L., Busta, F. F. and Speck, M. L. (1965). *Appl. Microbiol.* **13**, 851.

Eidlic, L. and Neidhardt, F. C. (1965). *J. Bact.* **89**, 706.

Elliker, P. E. and Frazier, W. C. (1938). *J. Bact.* **36**, 83.

Elliott, R. P. and Heiniger, P. K. (1965). *Appl. Microbiol.* **13**, 73.

Elliott, R. P. and Michener, H. D. (1960). *Conf. Frozen Food Quality, U.S. Dept. Agric., Albany, California*, p. 40.

Epstein, R. H., Bolle, A., Steinberg, C. M., Kellenberger, E., Boy de la Tour, E. Chevalley, R., Edgar, R. S., Susman, M., Denhardt, G. H. and Lielausis, A (1963). *Cold Spr. Harb. Symp. quant. Biol.* **28**, 375.

Erikson, D. (1955). *J. gen. Microbiol.* **13**, 127.

Evison, L. M. (1966). M.Sc. thesis: University of Newcastle upon Tyne.

Evison, L. M. and Rose, A. H. (1965). *J. gen. Microbiol.* **40**, 349.

Farrell, J. and Rose, A. H. (1965). *Advanc. appl. Microbiol.* **7**, 335.

Felix, A., Bhatnagar, S. S. and Pitt, R. M. (1934). *Brit. J. exp. Pathol.* **15**, 346.

Fell, J. W. (1961). *Antonie van Leeuwenhoek* **27**, 27.

Ferris, V. R. (1954). *Science* **120**, 71.

Floodgate, G. D. and Hayes, P. R. (1961). *J. appl. Bact.* **24**, 87.

Flosdorf, E. W. and Mudd, S. (1935). *J. Immunol.* **29**, 389.

Fogg, G. E. (1961). *Bact. Rev.* **20**, 148.

Forrester, I. T. and Wicken, A. J. (1966). *J. gen. Microbiol.* **42**, 147.

Forster, J. (1887). *Z. Bakteriol. Parasitenk.* **2**, 337.

Forster, J. (1892). *Z. Bakteriol. Parasitenk.* **12**, 431.

Foter, M. J. and Rahn, O. (1936). *J. Bact.* **32**, 485.

Frank, H. A. (1962). *J. Bact.* **84**, 68.

Frazier, W. C. (1958). "Food Microbiology", 472 pp. McGraw-Hill, New York.

Friedman, S. M. and Weinstein, I. B. (1964). *Proc. nat. Acad. Sci., Wash.* **52** 988.

Fry, R. M. (1954). In "Biological Applications of Freezing and Drying", (R. J. C Harris, Ed.), p. 215. Academic Press, New York.

Fry, R. M. and Greaves, R. I. N. (1951). *J. Hyg., Camb.* **49**, 220.

Fukui, G. M., Naylor, H. B., Lawton, W. D., Janssen, W. A. and Surgalla, M. J (1959). *Bact. Proc.* 100.

Fukui, G. M., Lawton, W. D., Ham, D. A., Janssen, W. A. and Surgalla, M. J (1960). *Ann. N.Y. Acad. Sci.* **88**, 1146.

Gallant, J. and Stapleton, R. (1963). *Proc. nat. Acad. Sci., Wash.* **50**, 348.

Garner, W. W. (1946). "The Production of Tobacco", 516 pp. Blakiston, Philadelphia.

Gaughran, E. R. L. (1947). *Bact. Rev.* **11**, 189.

Gessner, F. (1955). Hydrobotanik. Band I. Energiehaushalt Deutscher Verlag der Wissenschaften. Berlin, E. Germany.

Goldstein, A., Goldstein, D. B. and Lowney, L. I. (1964). *J. molec. Biol.* **9**, 213.

Goresline, H. E. (1962). In "Low Temperature Microbiology", p. 5. Campbell Soup Co., Camden, New Jersey.

Gorrill, R. H. and McNiel, E. M. (1960). *J. gen. Microbiol.* **22**, 437.

Graves, D. J., Sealock, R. W. and Wang, J. H. (1965). *Biochemistry* **4**, 290.

Greaves, R. I. N. (1960). In "Recent Research in Freezing and Drying", (A. S. Parkes and A. U. Smith, Eds.), p. 203. Blackwells, Oxford.

Greene, V. W. and Jezeski, J. J. (1954). *Appl. Microbiol.* **2**, 110.

Groman, W. B. and Suzuki, G. (1962). *J. Bact.* **84**, 431.

Gutz, H. (1957). *Naturwiss.* **44**, 545.

Hagen, P-O. and Rose, A. H. (1961). *Canad. J. Microbiol.* **7**, 287.

Hagen, P-O. and Rose, A. H. (1962). *J. gen. Microbiol.* **27**, 89.

Hagen, P-O., Kushner, D. J. and Gibbons, N. E. (1964). *Canad. J. Microbiol.* **10**, 813.

Haines, R. B. (1931). *J. exp. Biol.* **9**, 45.

Haines, R. B. (1938). *Proc. Roy. Soc. B* **124**, 451.

Halldal, P. and French, C. S. (1958). *Plant physiol.* **33**, 249.

Halpern, Y. S. (1961). *Biochem. Biophys. res. Commun.* **6**, 33.

Halvorson, H. (1962). In "The Bacteria", (I. C. Gunsalus and R. Y. Stanier, Eds.), vol. 4, p. 223. Academic Press, New York.
Halvorson, H. and Church, B. D. (1957). J. appl. Bact. 20, 359.
Hansen, N-H. and Riemann, H. (1963). J. appl. Bact. 26, 314.
Hardwick, W. A. and Foster, J. W. (1952). J. gen. Physiol. 35, 907.
Harrison, A. P. and Cerroni, R. E. (1956). Proc. Soc. exp. Biol. N.Y. 91, 577.
Heckly, R. J. (1961). Advanc. appl. Microbiol. 3, 1.
Heckly, R. J., Dimmick, R. L. and Campbell, J. E. (1965). Bact. Proc. 34.
Hegarty, C. P. and Weeks, O. B. (1940). J. Bact. 39, 475.
Heller, G. (1941). J. Bact. 41, 109.
Hess, E. (1934). Contrib. Canad. Biol. Fisheries, Ser. C. 8, 489.
Hoffman, H. and Frank, M. E. (1963). J. Bact. 85, 1221.
Hopton, J. W. (1958). J. gen. Microbiol. 19, 507.
Horiuchi, T. and Novick, A. (1961). Cold Spr. Harb. Symp. quant. Biol. 26, 247.
Hotchkiss, R. D. (1954). Proc. nat. Acad. Sci., Wash. 40, 49.
Hulett, J. R. (1964). Quart. Rev. chem. Soc. 18, 227.
Hultin, E. (1955). Acta Chem. Scand. 9, 1700.
Hüttig, W. (1931). Z. Bot. 24, 529.
Hwang, S. W. (1960). Mycologia 52, 527.
Ingraham, J. L. (1958). J. Bact. 76, 75.
Ingraham, J. L. (1962). In "The Bacteria", (I. C. Gunsalus and R. Y. Stanier, Eds.), vol. 4, p. 265. Academic Press, New York.
Ingraham, J. L. and Bailey, G. F. (1959). J. Bact. 77, 609.
Ingraham, J. L. and Stokes, J. L. (1959). Bact. Rev. 23, 97.
Tennison, M. W. (1935). J. Bact. 30, 603.
Johnson, B. F. and James, T. W. (1960). Exp. Cell Res. 20, 66.
Johnson, F. H. and Lewin, I. (1946). J. cell. comp. Physiol. 28, 1.
Johnson, F. W., Eyring, H. and Polissar, M. J. (1954). "Kinetic Basis of Molecular Biology", 874 pp. Wiley and Sons, New York.
Jordon, E. O., Caldwell, M. E. and Reiter, D. (1934). J. Bact. 27, 165.
Kates, M. and Baxter, R. M. (1962). Canad. J. Biochem. Physiol. 40, 1213.
Kates, M. and Hagen, P-O. (1964). Canad. J. Biochem. Physiol. 42, 481.
Kavanau, J. L. (1950). J. gen. Physiol. 34, 193.
Kavanau, J. L. (1965). "Structure and Function of Biological Membranes", vols. I and II, 760 pp. Holden-Day, Inc., San Francisco.
Keith, S. C. (1913). Science 37, 877.
Kempner, E. S. (1963). Science 142, 1318.
Keynan, A., Issahary-Brand, G. and Evenchik, Z. (1965). In "Spores", (L. L. Campbell and H. O. Halvorson, Eds.), vol. 3, p. 180. Amer. Soc. Microbiol., Ann Arbor, Michigan.
Keynan, A., Halman, M. and Avi-Dor, Y. (1958). Abstr. Proc. 7th. Int. Congr. Microbiol. 37.
Kjeldgaard, N. O. (1967). Advanc. microbial Physiol. 1, 39.
Kluyver, A. J. and Baars, J. K. (1932). Proc. Koninkl. Akad. Wetenschap. Amsterdam 35, 370.
Knaysi, G. (1948). Bact. Rev. 12, 19.
Knaysi, G. (1964). J. Bact. 87, 619.
Knox, R. (1953). In "Adaptation in Micro-organisms; Symp. Soc. gen. Microbiol." (R. Davies and E. F. Gale, Eds.), p. 184. University Press, Cambridge.
Koffler, H. (1957). Bact. Rev. 21, 227.

Koffler, H. and Gale, G. O. (1957). *Arch. Biochem. Biophys.* **67**, 249.

Koffler, H., Mallett, G. E. and Adye, J. (1957). *Proc. nat. Acad. Sci., Wash.* **43**, 464.

Koser, S. A. (1926). *Proc. Soc. exp. Biol. N.Y.* **24**, 109.

Krishna Jyengar, M. K., Laxminarayana, H. and Iya, K. K. (1957). *Ind. J. dairy Sci.* **10**, 90.

Lacey, B. W. (1953). *J. gen. Microbiol.* **8**, iii.

Lacey, B. W. (1960). *J. Hyg., Camb.* **58**, 57.

Landman, O. E., Bausum, H. T. and Matney, T. S. (1962). *J. Bact.* **83**, 463.

Langridge, J. (1963). *Annu. Rev. plant Physiol.* **14**, 441.

Larkin, J. M. and Stokes, J. L. (1966). *J. Bact.* **91**, 1667.

Lawrence, N. L., Wilson, D. C. and Pederson, C. S. (1959). *Appl. Microbiol.* **7**, 7.

Lembke, A. (1937). *Z. Bakteriol. Abt.* **2**, **96**, 92.

Lemcke, R. M. and White, H. R. (1959). *J. appl. Bact.* **22**, 193.

Lewis, W. C. McC. (1918). *J. chem. Soc.* **131**, 471.

Lichstein, H. C. and Begue, W. J. (1959). *Proc. Soc. exp. Biol. N.Y.* **105**, 500.

Lindeberg, G. and Lode, A. (1963). *Canad. J. Microbiol.* **9**, 523.

Lindt, W. (1886). *Arch. exp. Pathol. Pharmakol.* **21**, 269.

Lion, M. B., Kirby-Smith, J. S. and Randolph, M. L. (1961). *Nature, Lond.* **192**, 34.

Lippincott, J. A. and Lippincott, B. B. (1965). *Bact. Proc.* 16.

Lochhead, A. G. (1926). *Soil Sci.* **21**, 225.

Long, S. K. and Williams, O. B. (1960). *J. Bact.* **79**, 629.

Lundgren, D. G. and Beskid, G. (1960). *Canad. J. Microbiol.* **6**, 135.

Luyet, B. (1962). In "Low Temperature Microbiology", p. 63. Campbell Soup Co., Camden, New Jersey.

Luzzati, V. and Husson, F. (1962). *J. cell Biol.* **12**, 207.

Maaløe, O. (1950). *Acta Pathol. Microbiol. Scand.* **27**, 680.

Maaløe, O. (1962). In "The Bacteria", (I.C. Gunsalus and R. Y. Stanier, Eds.), vol. 4, p. 1. Academic Press, New York.

Maaløe, O. and Lark, K. G. (1954). In "Recent Developments in Cell Physiology", (J. A. Kitching, Ed.), p. 159. Academic Press, New York.

Maas, W. K. and Davis, B. D. (1952). *Proc. nat. Acad. Sci., Wash.* **38**, 785.

Maclean, F. I. and Munson, R. J. (1961). *J. gen. Microbiol.* **25**, 17.

McCoy, E. (1937). *J. Bact.* **34**, 321.

McDonald, W. C. and Matney, T. S. (1963). *J. Bact.* **85**, 218.

MacLeod, R. A., Smith, L. D. H. and Gelinas, R. (1966). *Canad. J. Microbiol.* **12**, 61.

McNelly-Ingle, C. A., Lamb, B. C. and Frost, L. C. (1966). *Genet. Res., Camb.* **7**, 169.

Maier, V. P., Tappel, A. L. and Volman, D. H. (1955). *J. Amer. chem. Soc.* **77**, 1278.

Mangiatini, M. T., Teece, G. and Toschi, G. (1962). *Nuovo Cimento Suppl.* **25**, 45.

Manning, G. B. and Campbell, L. L. (1961). *J. Amer. chem. Soc.* **236**, 2952.

Marmur, J. (1960). *Biochim. biophys. Acta* **38**, 342.

Marr, A. G. and Ingraham, J. L. (1962). *J. Bact.* **84**, 1260.

Marr, A. G., Ingraham, J. L. and Squires, C. L. (1964). *J. Bact.* **87**, 356.

Marrè, E. (1962). In "Physiology and Biochemistry of Algae", (R. A. Lewin, Ed.), p. 541. Academic Press, New York.

Marsh, C. and Militzer, W. (1952). *Arch. Biochem. Biophys.* **36**, 269.

Marsh, C. and Militzer, W. (1956). *Arch. Biochem. Biophys.* **60**, 439.

Mathemeier, P. F. and Morita, R. Y. (1964). *J. Bact.* **88**, 1661.

Mazur, P. (1961a). *J. Bact.* **82**, 662.
Mazur, P. (1961b). *J. Bact.* **82**, 673.
Mazur, P. (1965). *Ann. N.Y. Acad. Sci.* **125**, 658.
Mazur, P., Rhian, M. A. and Mahlandt, B. G. (1957). *Arch. Biochem. Biophys.* **71**, 31.
Mefferd, R. B. and Campbell, L. L. (1952). *Texas Rep. Biol. Med.* **10**, 419.
Meynell, G. G. (1958). *J. gen. Microbiol.* **19**, 380.
Michener, H. D. and Elliott, R. P. (1965). *Advanc. food Res.* **15**, 349.
Militzer, W. E., Tuttle, L. C. and Georgi, C. E. (1951). *Arch. Biochem. Biophys.* **31**, 416.
Mironescu, T. G. (1899). *Hyg. Rdsch.* **9**, 961.
Mitchell, H. K. and Houlahan, M. B. (1946). *Amer. J. Bot.* **33**, 31.
Morrison, R. B. and McCapra, J. (1961). *Nature, Lond.* **192**, 774.
Mučibabić, S. (1956). *J. exp. Biol.* **33**, 627.
Murrell, W. G. In "Microbial Reaction to Environment; Symp. Soc. gen. Microbiol." (G. G. Meynell and H. Gooder, Eds.), p. 100. University Press, Cambridge.
Murrell, W. G. and Scott, W. J. (1957). *Nature, Lond.* **179**, 481.
Murrell, W. G. and Warth, A. D. (1965). In "Spores", (L. L. Campbell and H. O. Halvorson, Eds.), vol. 3, p. 1. Amer. Soc. Microbiol., Ann Arbor, Michigan.
Nakae, T. (1966). *J. Bact.* **91**, 1730.
Nakamura, M. and Dawson, D. A. (1962). *Appl. Microbiol.* **10**, 40.
Naylor, H. B., Fukui, G. M. and McDuff, C. R. (1961). *J. Bact.* **81**, 649.
Neely, W. B. (1960). *Advanc. carb. Chem.* **15**, 341.
Nei, T. (1960). In "Recent Research in Freezing and Drying", (A. S. Parkes and A. U. Smith, Eds.), p. 78. Blackwells, Oxford.
Nelson, F. E. (1943). *J. Bact.* **45**, 395.
Ng, H. (1965). *Bact. Proc.* 20.
Ng, H. and Gartner, T. K. (1963). *J. Bact.* **85**, 245.
Ng, H., Ingraham, J. L. and Marr, A. G. (1962). *J. Bact.* **84**, 331.
Nicolle, E. and Trenel, M. (1902). *Ann. Inst. Pasteur* **16**, 562.
Nishihara, M. and Romig, W. R. (1964a). *J. Bact.* **88**, 1220.
Nishihara, M. and Romig, W. R. (1964b). *J. Bact.* **88**, 1230.
O'Donovan, G. A. and Ingraham, J. L. (1965). *Proc. nat. Acad. Sci., Wash.* **54**, 451.
O'Donovan, G. A., Kearney, C. L. and Ingraham, J. L. (1965). *J. Bact.* **90**, 611.
Ogur, M., Ogur, S. and St. John, R. (1960). *Genetics* **45**, 189.
Ohye, D. F. and Scott, W. J. (1957). *Austral. J. biol. Sci.* **10**, 85.
Oppenheimer, C. H. and Drost-Hansen, W. (1960). *J. Bact.* **80**, 21.
Oprescu, V. (1898). *Arch. Hyg.* **33**, 164.
Orr, D. A. and Taylor, M. M. (1965). *Nature, Lond.* **208**, 1017.
Ørskov, F. (1956). *Acta Pathol. microbiol, Scand.* **39**, 147.
Packer, E. L., Scher, S. and Sagan, C. (1963). *Icarus*, **2**, 293.
Packer, E. L., Ingraham, J. L. and Scher, S. (1965). *J. Bact.* **89**, 718.
Pederson, C. A., Albury, M. N., Wilson, D. C. and Lawrence, N. L. (1959). *Appl. Microbiol.* **7**, 1.
Penefsky, H. S. and Warner, R. C. (1965). *J. biol. Chem.* **240**, 4649.
Peppler, H. J. and Frazier, W. C. (1941). *J. Bact.* **43**, 181.
Peterson, A. C. (1962). In "Low Temperature Microbiology", p. 157. Campbell Soup Co., Camden, New Jersey.
Peterson, A. C. and Gunderson, M. F. (1960). *Food Technol.* **14**, 413.
Pfeifer, D., Davis, J. E. and Sinsheimer, R. L. (1964). *J. molec. Biol.* **10**, 412.
Postgate, J. R. and Hunter, J. R. (1963). *J. appl. Bact.* **26**, 415..

Postgate, J. R., Crumpton, J. E. and Hunter, J. R. (1961). *J. gen. Microbiol.* **2**, 15.

Powell, J. F. (1950). *J. gen. Microbiol.* **4**, 330.

Precht, H., Christopherson, J. and Hensel, H. (1955). "Temperature und Leben" 514 pp. Springer-Verlag, Berlin.

Preston, N. W. and Maitland, H. B. (1952). *J. gen. Microbiol.* **7**, 117.

Proom, H. (1951). *Proc. Soc. appl. Bact.* **14**, 261.

Quadling, C. (1958). *J. gen. Microbiol.* **18**, 227.

Quetsch, M. F. and Danforth, W. F. (1964). *J. cell. comp. Physiol.* **64**, 123.

Ring, K. (1965a). *Biochem. biophys. Acta* **94**, 598.

Ring, K. (1965b). *Biochem. biophys. res. Commun.* **19**, 576.

Rizet, G. and Engelmann, C. (1949). *Rev. Cytol. Biol. Veg.* **11**, 201.

Roberts, F. F. and Doetsch, R. N. (1966). *J. Bact.* **91**, 414.

Rose, A. H. (1961). "Industrial Microbiology", 286 pp. Butterworths, London.

Rose, A. H. and Evison, L. M. (1965). *J. gen. Microbiol.* **38**, 131.

Ryan, F. J. and Kiritani, K. (1959). *J. gen. Microbiol.* **20**, 644.

Saunders, G. F. and Campbell, L. L. (1966). *J. Bact.* **91**, 332.

Schaechter, M., Maaløe, O. and Kjeldgaard, N. O. (1958). *J. gen. Microbiol.* **19**, 592.

Schelhorn, M. L. von. (1960). *Z. Lebensmitteluntersuch* **112**, 383.

Scherbaum, O. H. (1960). *Annu. Rev. Microbiol.* **14**, 282.

Scherr, G. H. and Weaver, R. H. (1953). *Bact. Rev.* **17**, 51.

Schmidt-Nielsen, S. (1902). *Z. Bakteriol. Parasitenk II*, **9**, 145.

Schubert, O. (1952). *Z. Bakt.* **158**, 540.

Schubert, O. and Schubert, R. (1953). *Z. Hyg. Infektkr.* **136**, 639.

Segner, W. P., Schmidt, C. F. and Boltz, J. K. (1966). *Appl. Microbiol.* **14**, 49.

Shafia, F. and Thompson, T. L. (1964a). *J. Bact.* **87**, 999.

Shafia, F. and Thompson, T. L. (1964b). *J. Bact.* **88**, 293.

Shaw, M. K. and Ingraham, J. L. (1965). *J. Bact.* **90**, 141.

Sherman, J. M. and Albus, W. R. (1923). *J. Bact.* **8**, 127.

Shukuya, R. and Schwert, G. W. (1960). *J. biol. Chem.* **235**, 1658.

Sieburth, J. McN. (1964). *Proc. Symp. Exp. Mar. Ecology* 11.

Silverman, G. J. and Goldblith, S. A. (1965). *Advanc. appl. Microbiol.* **7**, 305.

Sinclair, N. A. and Stokes, J. L. (1963). *J. Bact.* **85**, 164.

Sinclair, N. A. and Stokes, J. L. (1964). *J. Bact.* **87**, 562.

Spencer, R. (1963). In "Symposium on Marine Microbiology", (C. H. Oppenheimer Ed.), p. 350. C. C. Thomas, Springfield, Illinois.

Stamp, Lord (1947). *J. gen. Microbiol.* **1**, 251.

Stanley, S. O. and Rose, A. H. (1967a). *J. gen. Microbiol.* in press.

Stanley, S. O. and Rose, A. H. (1967b). *Proc. Roy. Soc. B*, in press.

Steel, K. J. and Ross, H. E. (1963). *J. appl. Bact.* **26**, 370.

Straka, R. P. and Stokes, J. L. (1959). *J. Bact.* **78**, 181.

Strange, R. E. (1964). *Nature, Lond.* **203**, 1304.

Strange, R. E. and Dark, F. A. (1962). *J. gen. Microbiol.* **29**, 719.

Strange, R. E. and Ness, A. G. (1963). *Nature, Lond.* **197**, 819.

Strange, R. E. and Shon, M. (1964). *J. gen. Microbiol.* **34**, 99.

Streisinger, G., Mukai, F., Dreyer, W. J., Miller, B. and Horiuchi, S. (1961). *Cold Spr. Harb. Symp. quant. Biol.* **26**, 25.

Sugiyama, H. (1951). *J. Bact.* **62**, 81.

Sussman, R. and Jacob, F. (1962). *Compt. rend. Acad. Sci.* **254**, 1517.

Sverdrup, H. U., Johnson, M. W. and Fleming, R. H. (1942). "The Oceans", 1087 pp. Prentice-Hall, New Jersey.

wift, H. F. (1937). *J. Bact.* **33**, 411.

ykes, G. (1958). "Disinfection and Sterilization", 396 pp. E. and F. N. Spon Ltd., London.

zer, W. and Ochoa, S. (1964). *J. molec. Biol.* **8**, 823.

eece, G. and Toschi, G. (1960). *Nuovo Cimento Suppl.* **18**, 207.

empest, D. W. and Hunter, J. R. (1965). *J. gen. Microbiol.* **41**, 267.

erroine, E. F., Bonnet, R., Kopp, G. and Vechot, J. (1927). *Bull. Soc. chim. Biol.* **9**, 605.

erroine, E. F., Hatterer, C. and Roehrig, P. (1930). *Bull. Soc. chim. Biol.* **12**, 682.

erry, D. R., Gaffar, A. and Sagers, R. D. (1966). *J. Bact.* **91**, 1625.

essman, E. S. (1965). *Virology*, **25**, 303.

hiel, C. C. (1940). *J. dairy Res.* **11**, 136.

himann, K. V. (1963). "The Life of Bacteria", 2nd. ed., 909 pp. Macmillan, London.

hompson, T. L. and Shafia, F. (1962). *Biochem. Biophys. res. Commun.* **8**, 467.

hompson, P. J. and Thompson, T. L. (1962). *J. Bact.* **84**, 694.

owe, A. M. and Stadler, D. R. (1964). *Genetics* **49**, 577.

oyokawa, K. and Hollander, D. H. (1956). *Proc. Soc. exp. Biol. N.Y.* **92**, 499.

Jdaka, S. and Horiuchi, T. (1965). *Biochem. Biophys. res. Commun.* **19**, 156.

Jehara, M. and Frank, H. A. (1965). In "Spores", (L. L. Campbell and H. Halvorson, Eds.), vol. 3, p. 38, Amer. Soc. Microbiol. Ann Arbor, Michigan.

Jetake, H., Toyama, S. and Hagiwara, S. (1964). *Virology* **22**, 202.

Jffen, R. L. and Canale-Parola, E. (1966). *Canad. J. Microbiol.* **12**, 590.

Jpadhyay, J. and Stokes, J. L. (1963a). *J. Bact.* **85**, 177.

Jpadhyay, J. and Stokes, J. L. (1963b). *J. Bact.* **86**, 992.

Jas, K. and Proszt, G. (1957). *Nature, Lond.* **179**, 1301.

Von Hofsten, A. and Von Hofsten, B. (1958). *Physiol. Plant.* **11**, 106.

Waksman, S. A. and Corke, C. T. (1953). *J. Bact.* **66**, 377.

Weil, R. (1899). *Arch. Hyg.* **35**, 355.

Weis Bentzon, M., Maaløe, O. and Rasch, G. (1952). *Acta Pathol. microbiol. Scand.* **30**, 243.

Welker, N. E. and Campbell, L. L. (1965a). *J. Bact.* **89**, 175.

Welker, N. E. and Campbell, L. L. (1965b). *J. Bact.* **90**, 1129.

White, H. R. (1953). *J. gen. Microbiol.* **8**, 27.

White, H. R. (1963). *J. appl. Bact.* **26**, 91.

White, R., Georgi, C. E. and Militzer, W. E. (1954). *Proc. Soc. exp. Biol. N.Y.* **85**, 137.

White, R., Georgi, C. E. and Militzer, W. E. (1955). *Proc. Soc. exp. Biol. N.Y.* **88**, 373.

Williams, D. J., Clegg, L. F. L. and Wolf, J. (1957). *J. appl. Bact.* **20**, 167.

Williams, O. B. and Reed, J. M. (1942). *J. infect. Dis.* **71**, 225.

Williams, R. P., Goldschmidt. M. E. and Gott, C. L. (1965). *Biochem. Biophys. res. Commun.* **19**, 177.

Williamson, D. H. and Scopes, A. W. (1961). In "Microbial Reaction to Environment; Symp. Soc. gen. Microbiol." (G. G. Meynell and H. Gooder, Eds.), p. 217. University Press, Cambridge.

Witkin, E. M. (1953). *Proc. nat. Acad. Sci., Wash.* **39**, 427.

Witter, L. D. (1961). *J. dairy Sci.* **44**, 983.

Wood, T. H. (1957). *Advanc. biol. med. Phys.* **4**, 119.

Wyss, O. (1951). In "Bacterial Physiology", (C. H. Werkman and P. W. Wilson, Eds.), pp. 179–213. Academic Press, New York.

Ycas, N. (1956). *Exp. Cell Res.* **10**, 746.

Zamenhof, S. (1960). *Proc. nat. Acad. Sci., Wash.* **46**, 101.
Zeuthen, E. (1958). *Advanc. biol. med. Phys.* **6**, 37.
Zeuthen, E. and Scherbaum, O. (1954). In "Recent Developments in Cel̄
    Physiology", (J. A. Kitching, Ed.), p. 141. Academic Press, New York.
Zobell, C. E. (1962). In "Low Temperature Microbiology", p. 107. Campbell Sou▮
    Co., Camden, New Jersey.

Chapter 7

The Effect of Temperature on the Relation between Animal Viruses and their Hosts

K. R. DUMBELL

Department of Virology, The Wright-Fleming Institute of Microbiology, St. Mary's Hospital Medical School, London, W.2, England

I. Introduction

Viruses will multiply only in living cells. The temperatures which can affect the growth of viruses are thus determined by the physiological limits of the supporting host organism or tissue cells. The viruses which will be discussed in this chapter are those which infect warm-blooded animals, whose homeostatic mechanisms ensure that large fluctuations in the ambient temperature are reflected by comparatively small changes in the body temperature. These changes may yet be sufficient to bring about major alterations in the rate of virus growth in the animal. Living animal cells can be grown in tissue culture over a much wider range of temperatures, and much use has been made of cultured cells in an

8+T.

attempt to understand how temperature affects the growth of viruse
inside the cell. Certain organisms respond more readily to changes i
ambient temperature. Among these is the chicken embryo, which is
classical host for virus growth, and one that will be mentioned severa
times in this chapter.

Temperature may also affect the viability of virus particles during th
inactive, seed-like state in which they carry infection from one host t
another. A virus particle in transit is essentially a piece of nucleic aci
encased in a protein coat of varying complexity. Thermal changes ma
bring about the denaturation of any protein molecule or nucleic aci
molecule in the viral structure. The kinetics of the inactivation of viru
suspensions *in vitro* in the region of 50–60° are usually determined b
the inactivation of the most thermolabile among those proteins that ar
essential for the initiation of infection in a new host. Temperature
higher than 60° are necessary to denature nucleic acid chains, and a viru
suspension which has been inactivated at 56° may well have completel
undamaged nucleic acid. Such a virus may be "rescued" in susceptib
cells by superinfection with a related, living virus (Fenner *et al.*, 195
Hanafusa *et al.*, 1959). The rescue may also be made with a superinfectin
virus which is itself unable to multiply because its genome has bee
damaged with nitrogen mustard (Joklik *et al.*, 1960) or because the rescu
attempt is made in cells kept at a temperature above the ceiling tempera
ture for growth of the superinfecting virus (Dumbell and Bedson, 1964
In this latter type of experiment, the re-activated virus must, of cours
be capable of growing at the temperature used in the experiment.

The subject material for the rest of this chapter will be the effect c
temperature on the association between virus and living cells or orgar
isms. This association is normally in a state of flux. Virus may b
spreading from cell to cell and be steadily increasing in amoun
alternatively the total amount of virus present in the host may b
declining towards total elimination. Metastable states are known i
which the amount of virus in a host fluctuates. There is also the poss
bility of virus entering a dormant state in which it is neither active nc
eliminated but from which it may be re-activated. In some circum
stances, the cells of the host may retain portions of the genetic materi
of the virus, but have insufficient information to fulfil a complete cyc
of virus growth. The classical model of a virus invasion is that infectio
is followed by a rapid increase in the amount of virus, leading perhaps t
disease or even death. If death is avoided, virus multiplication eventu
ally slows down and, after a brief equilibrium, the virus declines and
finally eliminated. The dynamic balance between virus and host ma
often be dramatically altered by changes in the environmental tempera
ture. Some examples of this will now be described.

II. Observations on Virus Infections of Experimental Animals

A. COXSACKIE VIRUS INFECTION IN MICE

Boring and his colleagues (Boring et al., 1956; Walker and Boring, 1958) inoculated adult mice with the Conn 5 strain of Coxsackie B virus and then kept them in rooms at 4° or 25°. At 25°, the infection was barely fatal, and produced only a mild pancreatitis; 64 mice survived out of 65 inoculated in their experiments. At 4°, on the other hand, only 2 mice survived out of 61 inoculated. The mice themselves survived the cold environment and their average rectal temperature was lowered a mere 1° by the large change in ambient temperature. It was not possible to say exactly what physiological changes were responsible for the remarkable difference in mortality at the two temperatures. The titre of virus in a 10% suspension of blood two days after infection was approximately $10^4 LD_{50}$ for baby mice in 0·05 ml. of suspension. This was so at both environmental temperatures. By the 4th. day this titre had fallen to less than 10 in the mice at 25° but remained at 10^4 in the mice kept at 4°. This evidence of commencing recovery in the group maintained at 25° was also reflected in the virus content of the pancreas, which remained high in mice kept at 4°. The mice kept at 25° showed a hundred-fold decline between the 2nd. and 4th. day in the amount of virus recovered from the pancreas, even though the average amount on the 2nd. day was greater than that from mice at 4°. Boring and his colleagues also showed that mice inoculated and kept at 4° would recover if they were changed over to a room at 25° two days after infection. Conversely, mice inoculated and kept initially at 25° still suffered a substantial proportion of deaths if changed to 4° as late as four days after inoculation.

B. MYXOMATOSIS IN RABBITS

This is another example of an infection the outcome of which has been shown to be considerably altered by changes in the environmental temperature. Thompson (1938) and Parker and Thompson (1942) had one rabbit survive out of 10 that they inoculated with myxomatosis and kept in a room at 23°; but 28 others which were kept in a warmer room (36°) fared much better, and 23 of them survived. The rabbits at an ambient temperature of 10–23° had a skin temperature of 33–36° and a rectal temperature of 38–39°. The rabbits in the warm room at 36° had a skin temperature of 38–40° and a rectal temperature of 39–40·5°. Under these circumstances, Thompson and his colleague found that inoculations with fibroma virus produced no lesions in the skin when the temperature of this organ was raised to approximately that of the deeper tissues in the body. Inoculation with myxoma virus produced a modified disease in those animals at the high ambient temperature.

Lesions were more sharply demarcated and recovery was the usual outcome. It is worth noting that McKinley and Acree (1937) had failed to modify the course of myxomatosis in rabbits by subjecting them to intermittent fever therapy. They achieved body temperatures of 41–41·5° by induction heating, but the rabbits were given three or four heating periods per day lasting 10 minutes each.

Experiments with myxomatosis were continued by Marshall (1959). He used an attenuated strain of myxoma virus which allowed about 37% of inoculated rabbits to survive after infection. Marshall found that, in a simulated winter environment varying between 20° and − 3°, only 8% of his rabbits survived. In his simulated summer environment (varying between 39° and 26°), 70% of the animals recovered. The clinical course of the disease was more uniform at the altered temperatures, being always mild in the warm room and always severe in the cold room. In the mild room (20–22°) inoculated rabbits had either a mild or a severe infection. Marshall did not find a great difference in the average rectal temperatures of his different groups of rabbits and he was inclined to discount the notion that the effect of temperature on the outcome of infection was simply due to the inhibition of virus growth at the higher temperatures. Nevertheless he found that, on the chorioallantois of the chicken embryo, the growth of myxoma virus was almost completely inhibited at 39°, a temperature at which the yield of rabbit pox virus was not decreased. Marshall also inoculated some rabbits with rabbit pox virus. The mortality among them was not influenced by the ambient temperature, but neither was it if he used a highly virulent strain of myxoma virus.

The rabbits which Marshall kept at low temperatures had high titres of virus in their blood, and the presence of a soluble viral antigen was also demonstrable in the blood. Rabbits in the warm room had a later and more transient viraemia, and soluble antigen was not detected in their blood at any time; specific antibody was detected at least a day earlier on average in this group. Even this finding could not be simply related to the ambient temperature because, in control experiments, rabbits developed haemolysin at the same time at all three temperatures, after they had been injected with washed sheep erythrocytes.

C. OTHER VIRUS INFECTIONS

Coxsackie and myxoma viruses have so far been selected as examples, and others could be cited where the overall effect of temperature on infection is much the same. But this is not invariable. Griffin et al. (1954) found that the mortality among mice that had been infected with vesicular stomatitis virus was indeed altered by environmental temperature, but that the mice kept at 8° survived much better than those maintained at 27° or 35°. They noted that it was necessary for the mice to be introduced to the chosen temperature at least one day before they were infected.

Another example of interest is Newcastle disease of chickens. Sinha *et al.* (1957) found that chickens 6–7 weeks old succumbed more readily to Newcastle disease virus at high environmental temperatures than in a cold environment. At an ambient temperature of 29–32°, the mortality was 100%; at the optimum temperature for the birds (21–24°) the mortality was 95% and it fell to 75% in birds kept at 10–13° and to 55% in birds kept at 0–2°.

The results of experiments in tissue culture will be discussed in a subsequent section, but it seems reasonable to interpolate here some observations of Ruiz-Gomez and Isaacs (1963a). They studied the effect of temperature on the efficiency with which a selected group of viruses would make visible foci of infection (plaques) in monolayer cultures of cells from the chick embryo. The plaquing efficiency of most of the viruses they tested reached a maximum at 35° or 37° and fell sharply at temperatures higher than 37°. But Newcastle disease virus was found to produce more plaques at the highest temperature tested (42°) than at lower temperatures, and it is tempting to think that this observation is relevant to the results of Sinha *et al.* (1957).

III. Experiments with the Chick Embryo

The experiments in animals described in the previous section have given dramatic results in terms of death or recovery when infected animals were kept at different temperatures. However, the interpretation of these results has been clouded by many uncertainties, and several workers have used other types of experiment to help the analysis of the effect of temperature on virus infections in whole animals. One drawback to experiments with animals is their extremely efficient thermostatic mechanisms, so that large changes in ambient temperature have but little effect on the body temperature. This can be partially avoided in experiments with the chicken embryo, which is much more sensitive to changes in ambient temperature. Detailed observation of this point has been recorded by Alexander (1947). Another advantage of the chick embryo is that the situation is not complicated by the development of specific antibody.

A. POX-VIRUS INFECTIONS

Siim (1949) studied the effect of temperature on the outcome of infecting the chick embryo with vaccinia virus. He inoculated 12 day old embryos on the chorioallantoic membrane (CAM) from a stock pool of seed virus. Embryos kept at 32° were all dead by 108 hours after infection. At 34·5°, all were dead by 84 hours and at 37·5° all were dead by 120 hours. At 39·5° some died within the first two days; these were taken as non-specific deaths. After 48 hours, only one more embryo died and 15 embryos survived from the 39 which had been inoculated. Some eggs were inoculated and kept at 35° for 48 hours till the infection was well established and, at this time, were transferred to 39·5°. Controls left at 35° were all dead by 108 hours but, of the 45 transferred to 39·5°, 33 survived. Transfer to 39·5° after 72 hours at 35° did not lead to any survivors among the 18 embryos so treated.

Bedson and Dumbell (1961) extended these observations to other pox viruses from the same serological group as vaccinia. The criterion of infection they used was the production of discrete foci of infection (pocks) on the CAM, and this considerably facilitated quantitative observations. They studied the behaviour of a few strains each of rabbit pox, vaccinia, cowpox, ectomelia, monkey pox, variola major and variola minor viruses. All of these viruses are very closely related but showed differences in the range of temperature which was required to suppress the production of pocks on the CAM. This ranged from variola minor virus, the growth of which was suppressed at 38°, to rabbit pox which was not suppressed at 41° but which failed to grow at 41·5–42°. Bedson and Dumbell (1961) obtained dose-mortality results in the chick embryo for each of the viruses they used, and found that the virulence of the different viruses followed the same order as their ceiling temperatures for growth. All of these mortality experiments were done at 35° but, in other experiments (Dumbell et al., 1961), there was evidence that mortality in chick embryos inoculated with variola virus was markedly diminished if the temperature was raised from 35° to 37°.

The correlation between ceiling temperature and mortality rate in chick embryos was established using only a small number of viruses. This number was subsequently increased (Bedson and Dumbell, 1964) by the inclusion of ten hybrid viruses with a variola/cowpox parentage. With this larger number of viruses, there was no correlation between ceiling temperature for growth and virulence for the chick embryo. The ceiling temperature of the viruses appeared to be a fairly constant parameter over a number of cell systems from different host species (H. S. Bedson and D. McHugh, unpublished observations), but it was clear all along that the virulence ranking would vary from one host species to another. The ceiling temperature for virus growth would appear to be only one of many factors that determine virulence and even in the chick embryo, not one sufficiently important to dominate other determinants involved in the genetic shuffle which produced the hybrids.

Optimum or maximum temperatures for growth of a virus may be very closely correlated with virulence when we consider not a group of different viruses, but a number of strains of the same species of virus. For example, strains of variola major virus have a higher ceiling temperature for growth than strains of variola minor virus (Nizamuddin and Dumbell, 1961). Poliomyelitis is the example which has been studied most intensively, and this will be considered at some length in Section V.A of this chapter. For the moment, it is sufficient to say that the neurovirulence of the different strains of poliomyelitis virus is fairly closely correlated with their maximum temperatures for growth.

Enough has been said about the chick embryo to show that it raises interesting questions about the relation between the maximum growth temperature of a virus and its virulence. This would serve to explain the therapeutic effect of putting infected animals into a warm environment, but it is obviously only a part of the story. Another line of approach is needed. So far temperature has been taken as the main controlled variable in the experimental situations. What happens when viruses are selectively bred to produce variant strains with higher or lower sensitivities to temperature during their growth cycle. This question will be considered in the next section.

IV. Experiments with Viruses Adapted to Grow at Higher or Lower Temperatures

Cell cultures have been the most favoured tool for the selection of virus mutants adapted to growth at higher or lower temperatures as compared with the wild type. In cell cultures, the temperature can be directly and precisely controlled and over a wider range than even the chick embryo will allow. This is especially so for lower temperatures. Cells in culture will survive at 25° or even lower, but life of the chick embryo cannot be maintained for long below 32°. "Cold" variants of viruses have been sought most frequently because these offered the hope of being suitably avirulent for use in prophylactic immunizations. Dubes and his colleagues (Dubes and Chapin, 1956; Dubes and Wenner, 1957; Wenner and Dubes, 1959) made the first deliberate advance in this direction. They passed poliomyelitis virus many times in series at low temperatures. At least one virus strain "passed in tissue culture at 30°" lost its neurovirulence for the monkey. This did not happen in control tissue culture passes at 35–37°. Further adaptation occurred after passes at 23°. These strains had lost the power to infect or immunize by the alimentary route; they did, however, immunize if injected intramuscularly with adjuvants.

Following this lead, Lwoff and Lwoff (1958, 1959) investigated a number of strains of poliomyelitis virus and found a good correlation between their thermosensitivity in KB cells (a line derived from a human carcinoma) and their neurovirulence for the monkey. This was followed by the demonstration (Lwoff and Lwoff, 1960) that revertants could be obtained from virus mutants adapted by passage at low temperatures. Viruses which had been passed at higher temperatures until they had regained their ability to grow at 40° were found to have regained their neurovirulence also. Lwoff and his colleagues (Lwoff *et al.*, 1960) next experimented with strains of poliovirus adapted to different temperatures and injected into mice kept at different ambient temperatures. Mice were injected intracerebrally with 240 plaque-forming units (pfu) of the "hot" variant. Such mice suffered a 100% mortality if kept at 20°, but in a room at 36° only 40% died. The "cold" variant did not produce 100% mortality at 20°; even when 100,000 pfu were injected, the mortality was only 76%, and from 1000 pfu was only 16%. Yet 1000 pfu of this "cold" variant gave a 73% mortality if the mice were kept at 4° instead of 20°.

Perol-Vauchez *et al.* (1961) described a strain of encephalomyocarditis virus which had been adapted by a series of passages at 25°. After nine passes at 25°, the dose of virus required for 50% mortality had increased by a factor of 1500 compared with that of the mild strain. This was for mice kept at 20° where body temperature was 38°. Mice kept at 35° had a body temperature of 39·5° and required twice as much of the cold-adapted strain to show 50% mortality as compared with those kept at 20°. Mice kept in an environment of 4° had a body temperature of 36·5°, and were much more susceptible to the cold-adapted virus, requiring only 1/25th. of the amount of virus needed at 20° to produce 50% mortality.

Prunet (1964) grew the virus of foot and mouth disease on primary explant cultures of calf kidney at 25°, and selected clones of virus which were non-pathogenic to calves and guinea pigs. The cold-adapted viruses produced cytopathic changes in the tissue culture at 25° but lost the power to do this at 37° or 40°.

Kirn and Braunwald (1964) reported that they had selected a "cold" variant of vaccinia virus by passage at low temperature, and that its virulence was also attenuated. Further reference is made to this report in Section V of this chapter.

In 1963, Inoue and Kato described a thermo-efficient mutant of Japanese B encephalitis virus. This mutant was adapted to grow at higher temperatures and had increased virulence for young adult mice

However, not all variants which have been reported have behaved in the manner so far described. H. S. Bedson and K. R. Dumbell (unpublished observations) adapted a strain of variola virus to growth at higher temperatures in the chick embryo, and found that the virulence of this "hot" strain for the chick embryo was much less than that of the parent strain.

V. Effects of Temperature on the Intracellular Growth Cycle of Viruses

A. POLIOVIRUSES

The work now to be described is largely that of Lwoff and his colleagues, and Lwoff (1962) has himself summarized the main findings. In order to characterize the thermosensitivity of a virus in quantitative terms, Lwoff introduced the term "rendement temperature" or, more shortly, "rt". This was that temperature, above the optimum, at which the yield of a single cycle of virus growth was decreased to 10% of the yield at the optimum temperature. Thus a strain of poliovirus with an rt. of 38·3° would have an optimum temperature of 36° and, at 40°, its growth would be almost completely inhibited. At the optimum temperature of 36°, a single cycle of growth takes about 7 hours, beginning with a 3-hour latent phase which is followed by a rapid increase in virus content. If cells are infected with the strain having an rt. value of 38·3°, and maintained for 3 hours at 40°, they can be transferred at this time to 36° and virus will develop normally to the optimum yield. On the other hand, if the cells are infected at 36° and transferred to 40° at different times, the increase in the number of infectious particles continues for about half an hour and then stops. From this it may be concluded that temperatures higher than the optimum do not block events in the first 3 hours of the virus cycle (the latent phase), but that they block some critical event taking place after this time. Carp et al. (1960) found that heavy water (D_2O) partially suppressed the inhibitory effects of high temperature on the development of polio virus. Lwoff and his colleagues investigated this effect in greater detail. At supraoptimum temperatures, D_2O increased the yield of virus but, at the optimum temperature or below, D_2O decreased the yield of infectious virus. A growth cycle experiment showed that the latent phase was prolonged in the presence of D_2O when the temperature was below the optimum. If the D_2O was not added until 4 hours after infection, it had little or no effect. So the replacement of hydrogen in water by deuterium, which increases the strength of some of the hydrogen bonding, has two effects: when increasing the effect of suboptimum temperature it acts during the latent period; when decreasing the effect of supra-optimum temperatures it acts during the secondary phase of the cycle.

It was shown further that urea at about 0·2-M increased the effect of supra-optimum temperatures. But, in view of the present doubt about

8*

the exact mechanism of action of urea, this result does not necessarily imply that urea acted by weakening hydrogen bonds.

Lwoff and his colleagues found that the phase, in the second part of the cycle, which was inhibited by high temperature might be of very short duration. Cells were infected with a strain having an rt. value of 38·5 and kept at 40°. After various intervals, the temperature was lowered to 36° for 5 min. only and then returned to 40°. If this brief lowering of temperature was done between $1\frac{1}{2}$ and $2\frac{1}{2}$ hours after infection, nearly the full yield of virus was obtained. This is a fascinating result but unfortunately it cannot be generalized too far. The rt. value has been used as a marker character for poliovirus strains. A great number of strains have been tested, and it has often been noted that a test might be invalidated by taking a rack of tubes out of the incubator for a brief inspection. But this did not apply to every strain. There are almost certainly many different "heat defects" possible, involving different parts of the virus genome and resulting in different phenotypic effects. Cooper (1964) found that the strain of poliovirus with which he was working contained normally about 1 or 2% of heat-defective mutants. This proportion could be increased to around 10% in the presence of 5-fluorouracil. It is hoped that a collection of heat-defective mutants may make possible a mapping of the poliovirus genome in a manner analagous to that used by Epstein *et al.*, (1963) to map the genome of phage T4 (see Chapter 5, p. 167).

If cells infected with poliovirus were kept for 64–72 hours at 42°, they were apparently "cured" of their infection (Subak–Sharpe, 1962). Subak–Sharpe (1958) had previously shown a similar "curing" of pig kidney cells infected with the virus of foot-and-mouth disease, and incubated at 42·6°. It is not yet known whether such "curing" is due to the selective elimination of infected cells or to the elimination (or permanent inhibition) of the virus in the eclipse phase within the infected cells.

A similar curing has been noted with variola virus infection of the chicken embryo (K. R. Dumbell and H. S. Bedson, unpublished observations). Another factor which needs to be taken into account is the presence of natural inhibitors of virus infections called interferons. Ruiz-Gomez and Isaacs (1963b) have shown that interferon production may increase as the temperature is raised. This may have a bearing on the "curing" of infected cell cultures kept at supra-optimum temperatures.

B. POX VIRUSES

Dumbell and Bedson (1964) have shown that pox viruses retain properties associated with the earlier part of their growth cycle even when production of new, infectious virus is inhibited by high temperature. These viruses may induce non-genetic re-activation of other pox viruses, and the virus genome appears able to take part in genetic interaction. This latter result strongly suggests that the virus genome can replicate at supra-optimum temperatures, but direct evidence of this was produced only recently by Kirn and his colleagues (Scherrer *et al.*, 1965) for a "cold" mutant of vaccinia virus. They showed, by acridine orange staining, that typical intracytoplasmic inclusion bodies appeared at 36° and at 41°; but at 41° no active virus was formed. Kirn *et al.* (1965) had previously shown that supra-optimum temperatures inhibited the secondary phase of development of their "cold" vaccinia mutant, and that the events that occur in the first 3 hours of the cycle in KB cells were not influenced.

In conclusion it seems obvious that small variations in temperature can bring about major alterations in the course of virus infections in cell cultures. Even if the full mechanism has not been elucidated, enough has been learned to make the continued study of this branch of virology an exciting prospect.

References

Alexander, R. A. (1947). Onderstepoort *J. vet. Sci Animal Industry* **22**, 7.
Bedson, H. S. and Dumbell, K. R. (1961). *J. Hyg., Camb.* **59**, 457.
Bedson, H. S. and Dumbell, K. R. (1964). *J. Hyg., Camb.* **62**, 147.
Boring, W. D., ZuRhein, G. M. and Walker, D. L. (1956). *Proc. Soc. exp. Biol. Med. N.Y.* **93**, 273.
Carp, R. I., Kritchevsky, D. and Koprowski, H. (1960). *Virology* **12**, 125.
Cooper, P. D. (1964). *Virology* **22**, 186.
Dubes, G. R. and Chapin, M. (1956). *Science* **124**, 586.
Dubes, G. R. and Wenner, H. A. (1957). *Virology* **4**, 275.
Dumbell, K. R. and Bedson, H. S. (1964). *J. Hyg., Camb.* **62**, 133.
Dumbell, K. R., Bedson, H. S. and Rossier, E. (1961). *Bull. Wld. Hlth. Org.* **25**, 73.
Epstein, R. H., Bolle, A., Steinberg, C. M., Kellenberger, E., Boy de la Tour, E., Chevalley, R., Edgar, R. S., Susman, M., Denhardt, G. H. and Lielausis, A. (1963). *Cold Spr. Harb. Symp. quant. Biol.* **28**, 375.
Fenner, F., Joklik, W. K., Holmes, I. H. and Woodroofe, G. M. (1959). *Nature, Lond.* **183**, 1340.
Griffin, T. P., Hanson, R. P. and Brandly, C. A. (1954). *Proc. AM. Vet. M.A.* 192.
Hanafusa, T., Hanafusa, H. and Kamahora, J. (1959). *Virology* **8**, 525.
Inoue, Y. K. and Kato, H. (1963). *Virology* **21**, 222.
Joklik, W. K., Abel, P. and Holmes, I. H. (1960). *Nature, Lond.* **186**, 992.
Kirn, A. and Braunwald, J. (1964). *Ann. Inst. Pasteur* **106**, 427.
Kirn, A., Braunwald, J. and Scherrer, R. (1965). *Ann. Inst. Pasteur* **108**, 330.
Lwoff, A. (1962). *Cold. Spr. Harb. Symp. quant. Biol.* **27**, 159.
Lwoff, A. and Lwoff, M. (1958). *C.R. Acad. Sci.(Paris)* **246**, 190.
Lwoff, A. and Lwoff, M. (1959). *C.R. Acad. Sci. (Paris)* **248**, 154.
Lwoff, A. and Lwoff, M. (1960). *Ann. Inst. Pasteur* **98**, 173.

Lwoff, A., Tournier, P., Lwoff, M. and Cathala, F. (1960). *C.R. Acad. Sci. (Paris)* **250**, 2644.

McKinley, E. B. and Acree, E. G. (1937). *Proc. Soc. exp. Biol. Med.* **36**, 414.

Marshall, I. D. (1959). *J. Hyg., Camb.* **57**, 484.

Nizamuddin, M. and Dumbell, K. R. (1961). *Lancet* **i**, 68.

Parker, R. F. and Thompson, R. L. (1942). *J. exp. Med.* **75**, 567.

Perol-Vauchez, Y., Tournier, P. and Lwoff, M. (1961). *C.R. Acad. Sci. (Paris)* **253**, 2164.

Prunet, P. (1964). *Ann. Inst. Pasteur* **106**, 18.

Ruiz-Gomez, J. and Isaacs, A. (1963a). *Virology* **19**, 1.

Ruiz-Gomez, J. and Isaacs, A. (1963b). *Virology* **19**, 8.

Scherrer, R., Kirn, A. and Braunwald, J. (1965). *Ann. Inst. Pasteur* **108**, 413.

Siim, J. C. (1949). *Acta med. Scand. Suppl.* **234**, 304.

Sinha, S. K., Hanson, R. P. and Brandly, C. A. (1957). *J. inf. Dis.* **100**, 162.

Subak-Sharpe, H. (1958). *Nature, Lond.* **182**, 1803.

Subak-Sharpe, H. (1962). *Cold Spr. Harb. Symp. quant. Biol.* **27**, 172.

Thompson, R. L. (1938). *J. inf. Dis.* **62**, 307.

Walker, D. L. and Boring, W. D. (1958). *J. Immunol.* **80**, 39.

Wenner, H. A. and Dubes, G. R. (1959). *Amer. J. Hyg.* **70**, 335.

Chapter 8

Heat Responses of Higher Plants

J. LANGRIDGE AND J. R. McWILLIAM

*Division of Plant Industry, Commonwealth Scientific
and Industrial Research Organization,
Canberra, A.C.T., Australia*

This chapter considers most of the known effects of temperature upon flowering plants, and in particular data that seem to lead to the formulation of general principles. The survey commences with the broader aspects of plant-temperature relationships, those dealing with ecology, distribution and genetics. An attempt is then made to interpret these relationships by a progressively more specialized discussion. This includes growth responses to temperature, their physiological bases and, finally, possible mechanisms for their determination at the cellular and molecular level.

I. Heat Ecology

Given adequate reproductive dispersal, the distribution of plants in nature is primarily determined by their response, especially during germination and reproduction, to the major climatic and edaphic factors of the environment. Amongst these major ecological variables, temperature is always prominent, in that it limits not only the distribution of plants but also the diversity of plant forms that can colonize or develop in a particular region.

As a determinant of the geographical range of plants, temperature assumes increasing importance as it deviates from the general biological norm (about 20°). Thus, it is probably least significant under the most favourable thermal conditions such as the tropics where moisture and soil fertility play the dominant role. Here the evolutionary diversity possible under non-limiting temperature conditions is exemplified by the high density and complexity of species characteristic of tropical rain forests.

Temperate regions typically include a more pronounced cyclic variation in temperature and, although they support a less diverse flora, there is clearer evidence of specific adaptation to both soil and air temperature. Seasonal changes in soil temperature have evoked recognition systems on the part of the plants whereby the start of their life cycles entails obligatory low temperature (stratification) requirements for germination. A similar close adaptation by climatic races to prevailing temperatures is reflected in the correlation between growing ability and the temperature of the native habitat. This has been especially examined by Clausen et al. (1948), Hiesey (1953a, b) and Hiesey et al. (1961) in Achillea, Poa and Mimulus, and by Cooper (1964) in Dactylis and Lolium, either under controlled conditions or at contrasting transplant stations. Reproductive behaviour may also become closely associated with the temperature of the environment. Cooper and McWilliam (1965) demonstrated a close correlation, in ecotypes of Phalaris tuberosa, between the requirement for low temperature (vernalization) and the winter temperature of the place of origin (Fig. 1).

With temperate plants, there is reason to believe that their distribution is partly dependent upon the occurrence of favourable night temperatures. Since growth in many species occurs predominantly at night, the duration and period of suitable night temperature provides an effective measure of the growing season. Long exposures to high night temperatures can be very detrimental to many plants, although exposure to the same temperature during the day is not injurious. Went (1957a) has suggested that intolerance to high night temperatures may represent an important limitation to the growth of temperate plants in the tropics.

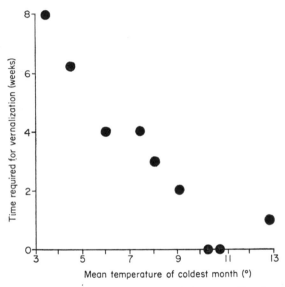

FIG. 1. Relationship between the time required for vernalization and the winter temperature of the place of origin for a range of Mediterranean ecotypes of *Phalaris tuberosa*. From Cooper and McWilliam (1965).

In latitudes beyond the temperate zones and at higher altitudes, temperature plays an increasingly important role and it is often the plant's ability to adjust to low temperatures that determines its survival in these regions. Thus, the main factor influencing the altitude of the tree line in alpine regions is considered to be the mean temperature during the growing season (Zotov, 1938; Wardel, 1965). In Australia, a mean temperature of about 10° for the warmest month is the best single climatic parameter defining this upper level of the tree vegetation (Costin, 1965). Daubenmire (1954) has suggested that the particular altitude demarking this junction between the arboreal and shrub vegetation represents a point on the scale of diminishing heat supply above which thermal energy is not sufficient to support the development of a large stem. At lower elevations, the phenomenon of temperature inversion with the formation of "frost pockets" can also cause a reversal in the usual altitudinal zonation of vegetation (Moore, 1966).

Low winter temperatures can also restrict the distribution of plants by limiting photosynthesis. Saeki and Nomoto (1958) have shown that the natural distribution in Japan of the broad-leaved evergreen tree *Cinnamomum* is determined largely by winter temperatures. In the south, it has an advantage over the deciduous species because of its ability to maintain positive net assimilation during the mild winter months, but in the colder northern environments of Japan, this advantage is lost due to a depression of photosynthetic activity during the winter. This limitation seems to apply generally to broad-leaved evergreen species, as few are adapted to environments with low winter temperatures. Many evergreen coniferous species, on the other hand, are adapted to grow under the most severe winter conditions, and once hardened, show a high degree of low-temperature tolerance (Parker, 1963), enabling them to exploit extreme alpine and subarctic environments.

Although virtually all metabolic activity in plants is restricted to a narrow range of temperatures from 0–50°, plants can survive at temperatures outside this range either by modification of their internal temperatures, or by appropriate escape mechanisms such as dormancy. For example, certain conifers in alpine and subarctic regions can tolerate temperatures down to $-30°$, whereas at the other extreme in continental desert environments, the shrub vegetation and succulents can withstand temperatures up to 60° (Oosting, 1958). Long-term survival in these environments, however, is not possible unless thermal conditions moderate periodically to permit growth and reproduction.

Attempts have been made to explain the distribution of plants with respect to temperature on the basis of the temperature optima of species for growth and reproduction. However, the optimum temperature for growth of plant populations can be only a very general concept, as plants rarely experience prolonged periods under such conditions. Also, in a number of species, ecotypes adapted to different and often contrasting climates, have similar temperature optima when studied under controlled conditions. This suggests that the temperature range, rather than the temperature optimum, is more important in determining plant distribution, as it represents the limits within which the species is best able to maintain its ecological position. Major differences in the temperature range of plants with contrasting distributions have been demonstrated. Evans *et al.* (1964), in a review of the influence of temperature on the growth of grasses, pointed out the marked difference between the Festucoid grasses and the more tropical non-Festucoid species in their response to air and soil temperatures. In addition to the adaptation to lower and higher temperatures that one might expect in these dissimilar groups, there is also a major difference in their response to lower temperatures. The more temperate (Festucoid) species (*Phalaris, Poa, Dactylis, Lolium*) grow actively at temperatures of 15° and below, whereas many of the non-Festucoid species (*Paspalum, Cynodon, Sorghum, Zoysia*) cease growth or are killed by temperatures between 10° and 15°. This intolerance of moderately low (above-freezing) temperatures shown by tropical species appears to be a fairly general phenomenon, and imposes a major temperature limitation on their distribution.

II. Genetic Basis of Temperature Response

Amongst the environmental factors to which plants must develop adaptive characters or responses, temperature is one of the most important. Not only must the genotype be able to produce fixed or adaptable phenotypes to withstand periods of unfavourable temperatures, but it must also develop adaptive systems in which growth and reproduction are geared to cyclic changes in temperature. The genetic ability to resist the injurious effects of extreme temperatures, by systems in which the phenotype remains virtually constant, rests on buffering phenomena known as homeostasis or canalization. Where the genotype adapts to temperature change by an alteration of phenotype, the genetic phenomenon is one of adaptive flexibility. Although most temperature responses include both of these reaction systems, the genetics of temperature adaptation is best treated according to the type of genetic control that is postulated.

A. HOMEOSTASIS AND HETEROSIS

Since any natural temperature regime, even one close to the growth optimum, fluctuates continuously and erratically, provision is needed to ensure that the growth pattern predetermined by the genes is sustained. Such provision is ultimately under genetic control and presumably produces changes in metabolism to buffer, or to compensate for, the influence of shifting temperature. From studies with animals, it has been concluded that the ability of a genotype to buffer the organism against environmental fluctuations is directly dependent on the level of heterozygosity (Lerner, 1954). It is not clear that this is so in plants, for the experiments of Griffing and Langridge (1963) indicated that heterozygosity in *Arabidopsis thaliana* gave significant phenotypic stability only in response to temperatures above the optimum for growth. Thus hybrids were found to possess greater buffering capacities than the homozygous parents to high temperature stress, but not to other environmental stresses (Fig. 2). Such hybrid superiority is better designated as specific high temperature-dependent heterosis. Excluding the effect of heterosis at high temperatures, the contribution of heterozygosity to homeostasis in this plant appears to be very little. Nevertheless, different homozygous ecotypes of *Arabidopsis* showed considerable differences in their homeostatic efficiency with respect to growth temperature over the range 16–31°. Significant high temperature-dependent heterosis also occurs in maize, but in the particular geno-

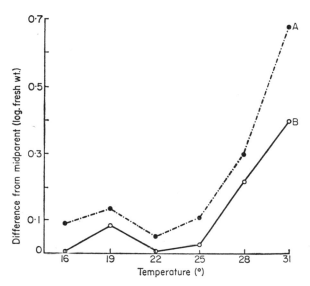

Fig. 2. Relationship between growth temperature and heterosis for growth rate in *Arabidopsis thaliana* (Griffing and Langridge, 1963). A, shows data for F1 minus midparent; B, F2 minus midparent.

types tested there was also heterosis at low temperatures due to non-allelic mutations affecting chloroplast development (McWilliam and Griffing, 1965).

Within a species many genotypes may be found which have taken different evolutionary paths in adapting to environmental fluctuation. In terms of reproductive ability, the optimum genetic strategy appears to be a compromise between resistance and sensitivity to climatic change. This has been particularly well shown by Finlay and Wilkinson (1963), who found that in barley, *Hordeum vulgaris*, varieties with high phenotypic stability all have low mean yields of grain when tested in a range of environments. These genotypes produce such stable phenotypes that they are unable to exploit high-yielding environments. With varieties which are very sensitive to environmental change, mean seed yield was again quite low, for such genotypes fail to reproduce at all under very poor conditions.

The results with *Arabidopsis* suggest that the ability to grow over a range of constant temperatures, up to about the growth optimum, depends principally on the forms and arrangements of homozygous loci. Above this optimum, resistance to temperature inhibition depends upon many of the loci being present in the heterozygous state. The genetic condition that leads to this high temperature-dependent heterosis seems to result from the high frequency with which mutation produces temperature-sensitive alleles; i.e. conditional mutant genes which specify enzymes and other proteins the structures of which are so altered that they are inherently unstable at high temperatures. Therefore, abnormal phenotypes only appear when temperatures above the optimum have denatured these unstable proteins. Since different genotypes can be expected to have different series of temperature-sensitive alleles, hybrids between them will have a higher resistance to heat because of the shielding effect of dominance.

It thus appears that, while developmental homeostasis is a mechanism of resistance to large deviations in environment, additional margins of safety may be required particularly under high temperature conditions. These are provided genetically by diploidy, heterozygosity and the evolution of dominance to the appropriate level, features calculated to provide excesses in the amounts of enzymes formed.

B. ADAPTIVE FLEXIBILITY AND GENETIC ASSIMILATION

When the environmental temperature changes markedly, but not to lethal limits, and these changes occur frequently or for long periods during the plant's life cycle, buffering of the phenotype cannot be maintained. For survival under temperature changes of this nature, the genotype needs to be able to develop adaptive phenotypes. Such changes in phenotype may be transient and reversible if the adaptation is to temporary, especially cyclic, shifts in temperature, or they may be irreversible adaptations to the temperature in which development occurs. However, if the plant is adapted to a habitat where the temperature remains reasonably constant, correspondingly little genetic or phenotypic flexibility will be needed for survival. Such habitats are gained by ephemerals which complete their life cycle during a relatively constant part of the season, and thus escape periodic adjustment of phenotype. On this basis, aquatic plants would be expected to possess less phenotypic stability than terrestrial plants. In this respect, Evans (1963) has noted that modification of the photosynthetic rate to changed temperature conditions appears to be common and extensive in water plants but much more limited in land plants.

In most flowering plants, periodic changes in the environmental temperature, both diurnal and seasonal, are very important in shaping the constitution of the genotype. Adjustment to diurnal change is quite conclusively shown by the frequently demonstrated inability of the genotype to reproduce itself in conditions of very constant temperature. When peas are grown at a constant temperature approaching the optimum, they develop less well than comparable plants growing in diurnally varied temperatures (Highkin, 1958). This deleterious effect becomes progressively more severe in succeeding generations kept at constant temperature until, at the sixth generation, the plants are non-viable. Plants debilitated in this way may be restored to their normal vigorous phenotype only after several generations of growth in diurnally fluctuating temperatures. Similarly, Hillman (1956) has reported that tomato plants lose much of their chlorophyll and become stunted when grown at constant temperatures or with constant illumination. It is possible that the temperature change is required by the tomato to initiate or maintain an endogenous metabolic rhythm, even though such rhythms are themselves independent of temperature. However, Evans (1963) found that only very small shifts in temperature, for example a change in amplitude of 2° about every two minutes, produced significant improvements in the growth of tomato plants.

Apparently, these genotypes, which are dependent upon temperature change for their proper functioning, have shifted from a flexible adaptation when the phenotype altered only in the presence of the stimulus, to phenotypic alterations which automatically occur whether the environmental stimulus is present or not. This alteration from a flexible adaptation to a fixed adaptation to a particular stimulus occurs by a process termed *genetic assimilation* by Waddington (1953).

While the significance of adaptation to diurnal temperature changes is poorly understood, adjustment of the plant to seasonal temperature cycles has obvious survival value. Through adapting to them, plants are able to synchronize their reproductive cycles which is an especially important matter for cross-fertilized plants. Also, the ability to undergo these phenotypic modifications enables them to survive unfavourable portions of the environmental cycle or to utilize efficiently the more favourable times for growth and reproduction. Thus, depending on their genotype, plants may become more or less dormant in mid-summer or winter during periods of temperature and water stress, develop temporary cellular resistance to heat or cold, and utilize temperature change for the initiation of germination and reproduction.

Some of these developmental adaptations to temperature are of the physiological trigger type, probably based on relatively simple genetic systems. In a winter annual strain of *Arabidopsis thaliana*, Napp-Zinn (1962) demonstrated that only four to five genes were involved in determining the plant's cold requirement for vernalization. Although this system requires few genes, it seems to be genetically more complex than those usually found in vernalizable plants.

At the other end of the scale of genetic complexity are hereditary systems controlling such phenomena as winter hardiness. Attempts at genetic analysis have only led to the conclusion that very many polygenes are concerned in their determination. In such cases of adaptive phenotypic modification, it is uncertain whether or not this depends on any special characteristic of the genotype. In outbreeding plants, flexibility of various kinds is believed to be dependent on heterozygosity, so that recombination and segregation will give a high proportion of well balanced genotypes in each generation. This is flexibility due to population diversity and cannot apply to the phenotypic modifications displayed by inbreeding plants.

C. PHENOTYPIC CHANGES AT EXTREME TEMPERATURES

In a stable environment, the genotype is continually re-adjusted each generation to counteract the deleterious consequences of mutation and recombination.

The occurrence of even a single mutation can sensitize the genotype to the environment, and cause the phenotype to fluctuate widely. This uneven expression of a newly arisen mutant implies that any new allele requires a shifting and adjustment in the genetic background to render it stable in phenotype production. This adjustment is most efficient for the most frequently encountered environment since it is the environment itself that selects alleles and combinations of genes. When the environment changes beyond its usual range, conditional alleles, especially temperature-sensitive ones which were previously shielded from selection, show up as climatic lesions. There is usually not a sudden deterioration of a major part of the genome.

If, however, the change to higher or lower temperatures is slow or a progressive gradient exists, the genotype also has an opportunity to change adaptively. Evidence for such adaptive adjustments may be found in the tolerances of plant genotypes that form a temperature cline and in the occurrence of thermophils and psychrophils in continuous extreme temperature environments.

It has very frequently been found that, after prolonged exposure at temperatures only slightly above the optimum for growth of the plant, growth may stop or become abnormal, often because a single reaction becomes limiting. With a further slight increase in the growing temperature, another reaction may fail and it is evident that certain gene products are becoming progressively inactivated as the temperature rises. These heat inactivations do not directly involve the genes because the plant will resume growth when placed at a lower temperature.

Such high-temperature lesions occur very commonly in microorganisms and are probably equally frequent in flowering plants, although more difficult to detect. Langridge and Griffing (1959) studied high temperature-induced growth deficiencies in *Arabidopsis thaliana* grown in aseptic culture. At 31·5°, five races out of 43 possessed very abnormal phenotypes including chlorotic leaves, twisted stalks and suppressed lamina growth. Two of these races failed to respond to supplements, but two others became normal on the addition of biotin to the medium, while the defective growth of a fifth race was partially relieved by cytidine. Appropriate crosses showed that these high-temperature defects were inherited as single genes which are probably controlling thermolabile enzymes. These temperature-sensitive alleles readily accumulate in plants because they occur very frequently as a result of spontaneous mutation, about one-tenth of all forward mutations being of this type. Since they have deleterious effects only at high temperatures, they are relatively resistant to elimination by natural selection. In fact, there may be a selective advantage attached to the possession of the temperature-sensitive biotin alleles under certain conditions (Langridge, 1965). Experiments showed that, although all races of *Arabidopsis* are sterile when grown at 30°, those with the high-temperature biotin requirement cease growth at 30° before going into the reproductive phase and are able to resume growth and reproduce when the temperature falls. Normal plants, which do not undergo a shut-down of growth and development at high temperatures, fail to reproduce and are unable to regenerate at lower temperatures. It is believed that a deficiency in the biosynthesis of biotin, because it is an essential vitamin of especially high activity, leads to a general halt in synthetic reactions, thus avoiding the danger of unbalanced growth.

Temperature lesions similar to the above have been found in cultivated plants by Ketellapper (1963). He demonstrated that retarded growth at high and low temperatures could be accelerated with various organic compounds, including sucrose. However, most of these supplements gave only small and variable increases in growth perhaps because of interference from conditioning or even from carry-over effects from the previous generation (Lang, 1963).

As compared with high temperature-induced defects that can be circumvented by nutritional supplements, low-temperature lesions capable of such repair are quite rare, even in micro-organisms (Langridge, 1963). Three examples have been reported in flowering plants. Ketellapper (1963) obtained an increase in dry weight at low temperatures in *Cosmos sulphureus* by the application of thiamine, and in *Solanum melongena* by a mixture of ribosides. When variety Concurrent of *Linum usitatissimum* (flax) is grown under low-temperature conditions, growth ceases and the leaves become yellow (Millikan, 1945). Since the plants turn green on spraying with ferrous sulphate solution, there is apparently a cold impairment of a specific ion transport system in this plant. Other low-temperature lesions may result from a breakdown in the genetic control mechanism for enzyme production, from a disturbance of interdependent reaction rates, or from cold-produced overbonding of a particularly susceptible enzyme.

III. Temperature and Growth Responses

The effect of temperature on growth is exceedingly complex as virtually all cell processes in the plant are influenced simultaneously, and temperature effects are usually compounded with other environmental influences. Moreover, temperature changes may act directly to modify existing physiological processes, or they may have inductive effects whereby the plant undergoes an altered pattern of development subsequent to the imposition of the temperature change.

The thermal efficiency of plants, usually measured as the amount of heat required to complete a full cycle of development, varies considerably. For crop plants this heat requirement can be measured in units which represent a summation of positive temperatures above a fixed base or "zero point of vital activity". This base temperature has been determined experimentally and represents the lower limit of temperature at which appreciable growth can occur. It varies for different plants from as low as 4° for certain cereals up to 15° for cotton (Wilsie, 1962). A summation of the daily heat demands, usually calculated as day-degrees, gives a total for any specified period, e.g. from planting to maturity. This method of measuring the plant's overall response to temperature has limitations, and a number of modifications have been suggested to include such factors as the duration of photoperiod, altitude, and date of planting. Despite these shortcomings, it has proved useful for characterizing the length of the growing season for crop plants and for predicting harvest dates (Nuttonson, 1956; Fisher, 1962).

A more accurate way of characterizing the plant's response to temperature is to define the cardinal temperature points, the upper and lower limits of tolerance, and also the optimum temperature for growth within this range. The provision of better controlled-environment facilities in recent years has provided a great deal of information of this sort (see reviews by Went, 1953, 1957a, 1961).

These cardinal temperatures for germination and growth vary markedly between major plant groups, but it must be emphasized that, even within a species, they are not absolute, since they vary with age and with the stage of development of the plant. In general there are three major phases of development, namely germination, vegetative growth, and reproduction, when distinct effects of temperature can be recognized. These effects are expressed either directly or indirectly both as changes in developmental rate and in the morphological characters of the plant. Outside these temperature limits for growth the survival of plants is determined by their tolerance to thermal injury.

A. INTERNAL PLANT TEMPERATURES

The temperature of plant tissues is often very different from ambient air temperature, because many plants have mechanisms to maintain a more favourable internal micro-environment when exposed to high or low temperatures. Leaf temperatures in particular are very often above air temperatures during the day, the difference varying according to the radiation load, the air movement, the leaf thickness and the reflecting characteristics of the leaf surface (Billings and Morris, 1951; Ansare and Loomis, 1959; Kuiper, 1961). At night, leaves are usually below air temperature (Tanner, 1963), although the difference is seldom more than 5° (Gates et al., 1964). Wolpert (1962) has calculated that a leaf in daylight in a 10 m.p.h. breeze loses 63% of its absorbed heat by convection, 23% by transpiration and 9% by reradiation. The remaining 5% is used for metabolic activity in the leaves. Leaf hairs improve conductive cooling by increasing the surface area of the leaf, particularly in cacti where they are very numerous. Closure of stomata on the other hand is claimed to decrease transpirational cooling especially under conditions of low air movement (Cook et al., 1964). However, Gale and Poliakoff-Mayber (1965) and Tanner (1963), who treated leaves with anti-transpirants, found that stomatal closure caused only a small increase in leaf temperature.

In a study of the leaf temperatures of *Mimulus* (musk) plants growing along a temperature and altitudinal transect from 400 to 3,200 m., Gates et al. (1964) found that the leaves had a remarkable ability to remain cooler than warm air and warmer than cool air. Over a gradient of temperature from a maximum of 45° at the lowest altitude to 20° at the highest, the leaves maintained a temperature close to 30°. The actual leaf temperature crossed over from below to above air temperature at about 30°, and Gates et al. (1964) claimed that this ability of *Mimulus* to cross over at relatively low temperatures resulted from active transpiration.

Increases in leaf and stem temperatures of alpine plants by as much as 22° above ambient under full insolation have also been reported (Salisbury and Spomer, 1964; Tranquillini, 1964). These temperature differentials are experienced at low air temperatures and are obviously important in assimilation under these unfavourable conditions (Fig. 3).

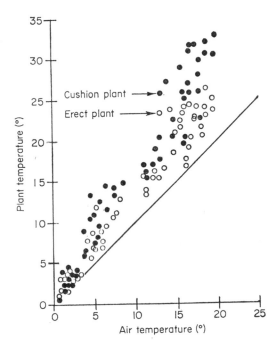

FIG. 3. Relationship between plant temperature and air temperature for cushion plants (●) and erect plants (○). The data were obtained at high elevation (3800 m.) in the Rocky Mountain National Park in Colorado, U.S.A. They are representative of those obtained on three occasions under cloudy and bright conditions. The line indicates equal plant and air temperatures. From Salisbury and Spomer (1964).

In a study of the heat resistance of a group of desert plants in Mauretania, Lange (1959) found plants which maintained their leaf temperatures above and below air temperature. *Citrullus* maintained leaf temperatures at as much as 15° below ambient, whereas in plants such as *Phoenix* (Date), leaf temperatures as high as 53·3° were recorded, an increase of 13° above air temperature. Even higher temperatures, up to 30° above air temperature, have been found in the leaf joints of the desert cactus (*Opuntia*) when the leaves were fully exposed to incident light (Konis, 1948).

The temperature of other plant organs such as stems and fruits can also reach a value above or below air temperature. In some instances, the increase in temperature can be attributed to increased respiration, as in the spadix of *Araceae* (Went, 1961) but usually, as in leaves, there is an increase due to insolation during the day and cooling below ambient temperature at night (Hopp, 1947; Angus, 1962). Some of the highest temperatures, often causing severe "sun scald", have been recorded in bark (Geiger, 1959), and in young plants growing on exposed soil. The roots generally maintain a more even temperature especially in the subsoil, as the soil mass is buffered against temperature fluctuations; large temperature gradients may, however, arise between the shoots and the roots. In high latitudes during sunny periods in the spring when the soil is still frozen, these gradients can result in severe desiccation of the shoots (Voight, 1951), a condition known as "winter drought".

B. GERMINATION

The temperature at which a seed is placed may have significant effects, immediately and eventually, on the plant's development. The simplest action of temperature is its direct effect on germination, and it is well known that seeds will germinate only if the prevailing temperature is suitable. Some seeds require an initial low temperature, or more rarely a high temperature, as a preconditioning to facilitate germination subsequently at a more favourable temperature. Quite frequently, the temperature-induced preconditioning is not for completion of the germination process but, as in vernalization, for sensitization to a following seasonal change in the environment. Finally, the temperature of germination may become reflected in a generalized change in growth pattern which may even be transmitted through subsequent generations.

The optimum temperatures for the germination of most seeds fall between 15° and 30°, although higher optima (35–40°) have been reported for tropical species such as *Paspalum* and *Saccharum* (sugar cane) (Williams and Webb, 1958; Poljakoff-Mayber, 1959), and lower optima for many cold temperate species including conifers (Stearns and Olson, 1958) and rock plants (Schroeder and Barton, 1939).

Correlated with this difference in the optimum temperature is a change in the temperature range for germination. With tropical species, the range is clearly shifted to higher temperatures, with a minimum between 10° and 20°, whereas many temperate species such as wheat, peas and pasture grasses germinate at temperatures down to 0°. The temperature range over which seeds will germinate is often wider than the range for survival of seedlings. *Hyparrhenica hirta*, for example, is a summer-growing perennial grass which will germinate at temperatures down to 4°, but fails to survive as a seedling at temperatures much lower than 15° (J. R. McWilliam, unpublished observations).

The inhibiting effects of high temperatures on the germination of imbibed seed, and the requirement for low temperatures to break dormancy and to satisfy vernalization requirements, are discussed in later sections. In this respect, the particular temperature requirements for germination are largely dependent on the physiological age of the seed. The need for prechilling, for example, declines with the age of the seed, and the temperature optimum for germination often becomes broader and higher.

Experiments indicating that the temperature experienced during the germination of seed can influence the subsequent development of the derived plants, even when grown under optimum conditions, have been reported for the groundsel, *Senecio vulgaris*, by Knapp (1957) and more recently for peas by J. Highkin and A. Lang (unpublished obervations).

Many investigators (see Lang, 1965b) have demonstrated the beneficial effect of diurnal temperature fluctuations on germination. Such treatment, by increasing the ability of seeds to germinate and by accelerating the germination process, decreases the variation in germination time. Toole *et al.* (1955) suggested that this beneficial effect of temperature variation resulted from an alteration in the rates of metabolic reactions, giving a balance of reactants at one temperature favourable for succeeding reaction rates with different temperature coefficients. Another possibility is that diurnal fluctuations relate to the physiological control exercised through an internal endogenous clock. The cycle change in this instance acts as a trigger to "start" the clock or to keep it running (Ruddat, 1960; Lang, 1965b).

C. VEGETATIVE GROWTH

The temperature range over which plants can survive in nature may be as large as 90° (see above). However, the difference in the maximum and minimum temperatures at which most plants cease effective growth is much smaller than this, and for most domesticated plants it is about 30°.

The minimum temperature for the growth of crop plants such as peas, rye, and wheat ranges from −2° to 5°, whereas sorghum and melons require a temperature of from 15° to 18° to make any appreciable growth. A comparable situation is found in a comparison of minimum temperature requirements for the growth of wild plants native to temperate and tropical latitudes. Likewise, the maximum temperature for growth of temperate-zone crops ranges from 35° to 40° with the more thermophilic species such as corn and cotton extending to as high as 45°.

The temperature at which plants achieve optimum growth also varies for different species, although most plants, either temperate or tropical, grow best in the range 25° to 35°. One problem in defining the optimum temperature is the tendency for growth rates to fall with time, especially at more elevated temperatures, so that, in any definition of the optimum temperature, the time factor should be taken into consideration.

A good example of a temperature-growth response study in plants has been presented by Friend et al. (1962a, b; 1964), who studied the effect of temperature on the growth of wheat. Using relative growth rate as a measure of response, they found that the highest growth rates occurred at 30°, but that these growth rates declined with increasing plant age, and that temperatures above 30° accelerated the decline. Over the entire growth period, the weighted mean relative growth rate was greatest at 25°. The final weight of the plants, however, depended both on the rate and duration of growth. A similar pattern of response to temperature has been shown for the growth of cocksfoot seedlings (Davidson and Milthorpe, 1965). When wheat was harvested at the same physiological stage of growth (anthesis), the highest total dry weight was achieved at 10°, because the longer growth period compensated for the slower growth rate. Increasing temperatures in wheat between 10° and 25° also cause progressively higher rates of leaf initiation, emergence and expansion, and result in an increased leaf-area ratio (leaf area/plant weight). The net effect of an increase in temperature on the whole plant thus depends on the difference between the increase in dry matter, resulting from an increase in the active assimilating surface, and the loss of dry weight through increased respiration (Friend et al., 1962a). Thus the concept of optimum temperature for growth is a dynamic one, in that the temperature changes with the stage of development, the age of the plant, the duration of exposure, and the particular growth criterion used to evaluate performance. In addition to these internal factors, the optimum temperature is also obviously influenced by other factors of the environment.

Plant roots, as distinct from the shoots, in general have a lower temperature optimum for growth, presumably because of their adaptation to the cooler soil conditions. Also roots appear to be more sensitive to sudden fluctuations in temperature (Muromtsev, 1963), which have a direct effect on their growth and thus an indirect influence on the aerial parts of the plant. In particular, low root temperatures have a marked effect on the pattern of translocation, and can cause a redistribution of carbohydrate within the shoot. It has also been shown that high or low temperatures retard the uptake of the elements N, P, and K, and also inhibit the absorption of water thereby decreasing shoot growth (Bloodworth, 1960; Korovin et al., 1961; Gukova, 1961; Grobbelaar, 1963). High soil temperatures, in conjunction with long days, are also considered to be the major factor in determining the time of onset of summer dormancy in certain perennial grasses (Laude, 1953; Ketellapper, 1960a).

Another factor which is undoubtedly significant in the plant's response to temperature is the phenomenon of overshoot which has been investigated in tomatoes by Went (1958). He found that, after a period of growth at a night temperature below optimum, transfer to a higher temperature above the optimum resulted in a temporarily increased rate of growth well above the maximum steady rate possible at that new temperature. Similar examples of overshoot following rapid changes in temperature have been found for growth in *Chrysanthemum* (Schwabe, 1957) and for respiration in many plants (Forward, 1960). One suggested explanation for overshoot with temperatures above the optimum is that the excess of sugar accumulated at the suboptimum temperature provides a temporary source of additional energy for the apex on transfer to the higher temperature. In general, the overshoot with rising temperatures is greater than that with falling temperatures and, according to Evans (1963), with the overshoot in the respiration rate of cotton leaves during periodic temperature fluctuations, they do not cancel each other out.

D. REPRODUCTION

During the early stages of floral development, low night temperatures may cause a marked decrease in the number of functional florets as shown for gladioli (Shelo and Halevy, 1963) and for *Elymus junceus* (Clary, 1965). Also, during the later stages of flowering from meiosis through fertilization and fruit set, there is a narrowing of the temperature range for normal development. Night temperature is particularly critical for many plants during this period, and both high and low temperatures have a detrimental effect on fruit set in tomato (Went, 1962). It has further been shown that this response is under genetic control and can be modified by selection (Schaible, 1962; Curme, 1962). A similar effect has been found in certain varieties of rice in which low night temperatures during anthesis can cause a marked decrease in grain fertility (A. A. McDonald, unpublished observations). In other crops, such as grapes and peas, exposure to high night temperatures during the flowering period greatly decreases fruit set (Tukey, 1958; Lambert and Linck, 1958) and in beans, the early development of the seedlings (Kleinert, 1961). Although the nature of the temperature-induced limitation imposed at this critical stage is not fully understood, this reaction to unfavourable night temperatures appears to be widespread among flowering plants. At a later stage, during the ripening of the fruit or grain, although temperature is less critical, high temperatures can decrease total yield, as in cereals, by increasing grain respiration (Asana and Williams, 1965).

E. THERMOPERIODICITY

Many plants are adapted to fluctuating temperatures and develop optimally under such conditions. In the absence of any fluctuation, growth may be abnormal as in tomato plants kept under constant temperature and continuous illumination (Hillman, 1956). Growth of these plants can be restored to normal by resuming diurnal fluctuations of either light or temperature. Highkin (1958) has also shown that, when peas are first grown at constant temperature, no injury occurs but, after several generations under this condition, the ability of the plant to grow is seriously impaired. Went (1957b) has reported the curious finding that peas grown under conditions of constant light and temperature are more variable in phenotype than genetically identical peas grown in a fluctuating environment.

The requirement for a diurnal fluctuation in temperature, although long appreciated by horticulturalists, was first demonstrated by Went (1944a, b). He showed that tomatoes exposed to fluctuating temperatures gave greater stem elongation, dry matter production and fruit set than plants grown at any one constant temperature. The optimum night temperature was about 17° and the optimum day temperature 26°. The night temperature optimum, however, decreased with decreasing light intensity and with increasing plant age. This phenomenon has since been found in other species (Dorland and Went, 1947; Viglierehiv and Went, 1957; Went, 1957a). In many plants such as tomato, tobacco and chili pepper, investigated by Went and his coworkers, night temperature has a more pronounced effect on growth than day temperature, whereas in others such as peas and *Sequoia*, growth is largely determined by day temperature (Went, 1957a; Monselise and Went, 1958; Hellmers and Sundahl, 1959).

The optimum range of day and night temperatures varies for different species as shown in Fig. 4 (Went, 1957a). These various thermoperiods are a reflection of the plant's natural adaptation to differential day and night temperatures. The optimum day–night differential for succulents adapted to dry continental climates, for example, is much higher than for tropical species (Went, 1961).

On the other hand, some plants appear to be insensitive to diurnal thermoperiodicity and the generality of this phenomenon has been questioned. Hussey (1965) has shown that the optimum temperature regime for vegetative growth of young tomato seedlings is close to 25° and, at this age, the effects of day and night temperature on total dry matter production show a considerable degree of independence. The optimum night temperature, however, decreases with age as previously shown by Went (1945). The superiority of constant temperatures over alternating day and night temperatures for the growth of young plants has also been reported for cucumbers (Milthorpe, 1957), french beans (Dale, 1964), and for growth at any age in peanuts (Fortainer, 1957), sugar cane (Glaziou et al., 1965) and wheat (Friend, 1965).

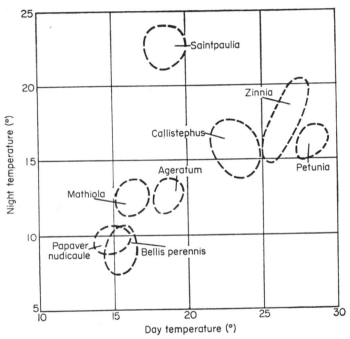

Fig. 4. Relationship between optimum day temperature (abscissa) and optimum night temperature (ordinate) for several annual plants. From Went (1957a).

The nature of thermoperiodic responses in sensitive plants depends upon the amplitude and frequency of the temperature change. Even the continuous momentary fluctuations in the environment sometimes referred to as "climatic noise" are significant in plant growth, and presumably plants may be adapted to them as they are to fluctuations of longer duration (Evans, 1963). Other responses to thermoperiod are either diurnal with a 24-hour cycle, or they represent a seasonal response based on an annual cycle. This seasonal response is characteristic of many bulbous plants, biennials and deciduous trees, and is discussed later in connection with dormancy.

The mechanism underlying thermoperiodicity is not clear, but if different physiological processes occur during night and day, they may respond differently to temperature. In tomatoes during the day, photosynthesis has a high temperature optimum, whereas growth is greater at night and has a lower optimum (Went, 1961). The absence of a thermoperiodic response in young seedlings, in which the tissues are in an active state of growth, is possibly because high night temperatures do not cause excessive respiration which is a feature of older plants under these conditions.

Among the plants that require cyclic fluctuations in the temperature and light environment, some appear to possess an inner cyclic time-measuring device (clock) based on a 24-hour cycle. For the optimum growth of these plants the external periodicity must be synchronized with the periodicity of the internal clock. Went (1957b), Ketellapper (1960b) and Overland (1960) have evidence that the internal clock, although largely independent of temperature, slows down with decreasing temperature and speeds up with increasing temperature, thus losing its synchrony with the external circadian cycle. This is claimed to cause at least part of the decrease in the rate of growth of plants under unfavourable temperature conditions. These authors have shown further that this type of growth retardation can be offset by adjusting the period of the external light–dark cycle so that it is in register with the endogenous clock. Tropical plants such as *Saintpaulia* and *Begonia*, if exposed to 10° on a 24-hour photocycle, cease growth and ultimately die. If the photocycle is lengthened to 32 hours, they develop well and remain healthy (Went, 1957b).

F. MORPHOGENESIS

Because of the widespread effect of temperature on most developmental processes in plants, it is not intended in this survey to do more than sketch in some examples of the more striking direct effects of temperature on the external form of the plant. The altered morphology produced by a changed developmental pattern is usually fixed, but the pattern itself may be reversed by a return to the original temperature. These temperature influences differ from the long-lasting and often permanent inductive effects such as vernalization and dormancy, in that they represent adaptive reponses to the immediate environment. This morphological flexibility enables plants to adapt more successfully to fluctuating environments. The capacity to change applies only to morphogenetic centres such as the growing points which are capable of continued growth. These centres can respond directly to temperature by modifying the rate or pattern of leaf primordia production, or by developing floral organs.

The rate of growth of the plant apex responds only slightly to temperatures between 17° and 27°, but it is markedly decreased by chilling at temperatures as low as 5° (Schwabe, 1963). In cereal rye, following such a low temperature (vernalization) treatment, the growth of the apex is accelerated even although it remains vegetative (Gott et al., 1955). This response has also been shown for the rate of initiation of leaf primordia, which responds to temperature in much the same way as the apex. The subsequent step, the rate of leaf growth or appearance, is more directly influenced by temperature as in Chrysanthemum (Schwabe, 1963) and in grasses. The average rate of leaf appearance in the grass Phalaris increased from 0·08 per day at a day/night temperature of 9°/4° to 0·19 per day at 24°/19° (Cooper and McWilliam, 1965). During this phase of leaf growth, cell expansion is more important than cell division, and it is possible that temperature exerts a greater influence on expansion than on the earlier stages of cell division. This effect may be mediated through a change in the supply of carbohydrate as suggested by Schwabe (1963).

During the initiation and expansion of leaves, temperature may profoundly influence their eventual size and shape, characteristics which are determined at an early age presumably through some control exercised at the time of cell division and cell expansion. In wheat, Friend (1965) has shown that an increase in temperature over the range 10° to 30° results in narrower and thinner leaves. This effect of temperature on leaf length and width was brought about primarily by an increase in cell length; the number of cells along the lamina showed little variation. Schwabe (1957) has also demonstrated that the size and shape of Chrysanthemum leaves reflect the temperature conditions under which they were developed. Leaves initiated at 17° or lower, and subsequently transferred to higher temperatures, are smaller, with a higher degree of dissection than leaves developed throughout at the higher temperature. Similar effects have been produced in other species (Fisher, 1954; Milthorpe, 1956; Njoku, 1957). The decrease in length of the first few leaves of winter cereals following seed vernalization has been regarded as a measure of the degree of vernalization. Recently, however, Hurd (1964) has shown that low temperature is not essential, and that the decrease in length is due to an inhibition during restricted germination of the earliest phases of leaf extension growth.

An interesting morphogenetic response, although not strictly within the scope of the present discussion, is that of tuberization. This process is a typical inductive effect, as the initiation of tubers occurs subsequent to the appropriate treatment. In a tuber-forming plant such as potato,

9 + T.

although there are interactions between temperature and photoperiod
night temperature is the most important limiting factor in tuber initia
tion and development. Low night temperatures between 10° and 17
are optimum for both processes but, under conditions of high nigh
temperatures near 25°, tuberization is inhibited irrespective of the day
temperature and the duration of the photoperiod (Gregory, 1965).

At the descriptive level, a good deal is now known about the effect o
environmental factors such as temperature on development, but vir
tually nothing is known of the mechanisms whereby these factor
modify the phenotype. Possible mechanisms include effects on meta
bolic rates controlling the availability of substrate particularly carbo
hydrate for growth, and changes in the regulation of the endogenou
levels of hormones in the tissues (Booth et al., 1962; Ballard and Wild
man, 1964, Hurd, 1964). Ultimately, at the level of the differentiating
organ, the visible alterations in form are brought about by changes in
the rate or plane of cell division.

G. THERMAL INJURY

As the temperature extends either above or below the extreme limits
for growth, thermal injury increases until finally the plant dies due to
metabolic failure. Resistance to extremes of heat or cold is a function o
the genotype as expressed in the properties of the protoplasm and in
the ability of the cells to repair damage to proteins or to the protein
synthesizing system. Another major factor in the survival of plants at
temperature extremes is the ability to undergo hardening, which is a
temporary adaptation which conveys enhanced resistance to either heat
or cold.

The type of thermal injury suffered by plants varies according to the
temperature of exposure. At freezing temperatures, dehydration and
structural damage to protoplasm and plasma membranes, due to the
formation of ice crystals within the plant, are a major cause of injury and
death, particularly in plants not adapted to low temperatures. Frozen
soil can also cause injury through heaving, a lifting of the soil due to
ice formation, which causes gross structural damage and desiccation of
the roots. At temperatures between 0° and 15°, many tropical plants
are unable to grow and may be severely damaged by long exposure to
these conditions. A common symptom of damage by such non-freezing
temperatures is retarded growth and chlorosis especially in seedlings
germinated or grown at these temperatures. In a low temperature-
sensitive line of maize reported by McWilliam and Griffing (1965), the
plants are unable to make chlorophyll at temperatures below 16°, and
the same effect has been reported in other thermophilic plants after chilling treatment (Klages, 1942). As discussed below, these low tempera-

ture lesions may be caused by the derangement of cellular control systems. Exposure, usually of long duration, to non-lethal high temperatures severely inhibits growth; metabolism becomes disrupted, toxic products accumulate and there is a depletion of essential metabolites. A good example is the critical temperature-dependence of chlorophyll formation in Marquis wheat (Friend et al., 1962a). A rise of about 0·5° at a temperature of 34·0° changes the pattern of normal chlorophyll accumulation and growth, to one of inhibition of chlorophyll formation and early death. Finally, at yet higher temperatures, injury and death are thought to result from the denaturation of proteins with irreversible coagulation of protoplasm. These damaging effects of high and low temperatures on plants have been the subject of a number of comprehensive reviews (Levitt, 1951; Joslyn and Diehl, 1952; Went, 1953; Levitt, 1956; Petinov and Molotkovsky, 1961; Langridge, 1963; Parker, 1963; Alexandrov, 1964).

The nature of heat- and cold-resistance in plants, and the molecular theories of hardening, are discussed in Section VI (p. 280). Resistance to heat and cold is thought to be closely associated with the colloidal-chemical properties of the protoplasm. These include the capacity for hydration of protoplasmic colloids and the degree of protoplasmic viscosity. For example, succulents especially cacti which are highly heat-resistant, are known to contain large amounts of bound water and to have high protoplasmic viscosity (Lange and Schwemmle, 1960; Henckel, 1964). Heat-resistant plants have also been shown to possess protective mechanisms based on respiration (Petinov and Molotkovsky, 1957). Under the influence of heat there is a fall in the respiratory quotient. This results in the accumulation of organic acids as intermediates in respiration, and these acids function as a source of protein and also as a substrate for the detoxification of endogenous ammonia which builds up at high temperatures. Foliar sprays of $ZnSO_4$ are believed to increase heat resistance in the same way, by lowering the respiratory quotient and causing an accumulation of organic acids (Petinov et al., 1964). The protective actions of sugars against injury caused by high temperatures have been reported by Molotkovsky and Zhestkova (1964), and their role is thought to be in stabilizing respiration and protecting the active surface of mitochondria against heat damage. Sugars are also important in cold resistance, and it has been observed by Sakai (1965) that, the greater the effectiveness of cold-hardening treatment, the greater is the rate of conversion of starch into sugar. Sakai (1962) has also demonstrated the protective action of sugar at low temperatures with cabbage leaf tissue. Sections in a hypotonic solution were able to survive freezing at temperatures down to − 70°.

The age of the tissue can also be important in frost tolerance. Hudson and Brustkern (1965) have shown that the freezing process and frost tolerance of young leaves of moss plants differ from those of mature leaves. The difference appears to lie in the ability of the cells of mature leaves to lose their water more rapidly and thus avoid the damaging effects of intercellular ice formation which occurs in younger leaves. The process of hardening is usually accompanied by a general decrease in growth which explains the terms "summer and winter dormancy" that are used to describe the condition of evergreen perennial or biennial plants during extremes of heat or cold. Apart from growth changes, there are few if any definitive morphological characteristics which can be used to identify cold- or heat-resistant plants.

During the process of cold-hardening, which is generally effective below about 6°, the degree of hardiness acquired is a reflection of the hardening temperature. In hardy species, the effective prefreezing temperature depends on the degree of cold hardiness and the duration of the hardening treatment. Dormant willow twigs, for example, can withstand the temperature of liquid nitrogen after appropriate hardening, but the hardening temperature required is lower for twigs collected during early spring than during winter (Sakai, 1965). The reversibility of cold-hardening is also shown by the rapidity with which plants, such as winter wheat, lose their resistance to cold once exposed to warm conditions, and the lack of resistance in cold-tolerant plants during the summer.

The acquisition of cold tolerance by chemical means has recently been reported. Kuiper (1964) has shown that the cold resistance of young bean plants can be markedly enhanced by the feeding of decenyl-succinic acid through the roots. The presence of this unsaturated fatty acid causes an increase in the permeability of cells when it penetrates the lipid membrane, and enables normally frost-susceptible bean seedlings to resist a frost of $-5°$. A similar protective effect was achieved when decenylsuccinic acid was sprayed on flowers of certain fruit trees before exposure to freezing temperatures.

The tolerance of plants to heat often increases with increasing age and, as with cold resistance, it is developed by prior exposure to high temperatures or moisture stress (Laude and Changule, 1953). In fact, heat resistance and drought resistance have much in common as have been shown by Henckel (1964). In this process of heat-hardening, the intensity as well as the duration of heat treatment is important. It is generally accepted that the exposure time for heat damage decreases logarithmically as the temperature rises, and this relationship appears to hold equally well for heat-hardening. Brief exposures, for as little as 30 seconds at 50°, have been effective in increasing the heat tolerance of many cultivated plants (Yarwood, 1961a). However, the lag period between heat-hardening and the test exposure to heat must be sufficient to allow heat adaptation to occur (Yarwood, 1964). In more extreme cases, where brief exposure of a leaf to high temperatures causes severe damage, the heat injury can be translocated and cause injury in an adjacent untreated leaf (Yarwood, 1961b). Nothing is known of the nature of the translocated stimulus responsible for this effect, which resembles a similar phenomenon in animals. Heat shocks have been shown to increase the overall thermostability of proteins, and also the stability of the bond between chlorophyll and protein in the chloroplast which renders the chloroplast more stable to heat (Lyutova, 1963). Heat-hardening is also effective with plant tissues *in vitro* (Schroeder, 1963) which suggests that the processes involved are localized and probably occur at the level of the individual cell.

IV. Physiological Basis of Temperature Response

A. PHOTOSYNTHESIS

Photosynthesis combines a sequence of photochemical, physical, and biochemical processes, of which one or more may be limiting at any given time depending on the external conditions. Although the direct effect of temperature on photosynthesis concerns only the biochemical aspects, it is indirectly involved in all three processes through their mutual interaction. Under natural conditions, photosynthesis occurs over a wide range of temperatures, the actual limits being set by the genotype of the species and the level of such external factors as light intensity and CO_2 concentration. For most mesophilic plants, photosynthesis occurs at an appreciable rate from 10° to 35°.

One factor which complicates any analysis of the effect of temperature on photosynthesis is the possibility of internal leaf temperatures being either higher or lower than the ambient air temperature (see Section III.A, p. 242). The needles of conifers, for example, on a sunny day in winter may have an internal temperature 20° higher than the air temperature (Tranquillini, 1964). An increase of this magnitude could have a profound influence on the photosynthetic activity of evergreens in winter, as the temperature difference is usually greatest when air temperatures are low. Some alpine plants similarly have leaf temperatures well above the ambient temperature (Salisbury and Spomer, 1964) while, at high air temperatures, cooling or heating of leaves can occur (Lange, 1959). The adaptive significance of such modifications of the internal temperatures of leaves has been demonstrated by Gates et al. (1964) in altitudinal races of *Mimulus*. The optimum temperature for photosynthesis in all races was close to 30°, despite the fact that the temperatures from the lowest to the highest altitude decreased from

40° to 20°. The reason for the apparent lack of photosynthetic adapta‐
tion to these temperatures became clear when it was found that the leaf
temperatures at all sites remained close to 30°.

Changes in the rates of photosynthesis with temperature are com‐
plex. In general, at normal concentrations of CO_2 (about 300 p.p.m.) and
saturating light intensities, the increase in the rate of fixation of CO_2
with increasing temperature is greatest at temperatures just above 0°.
The relatively high Q_{10} values reported for photosynthesis at these low
temperatures reflect the limitations imposed by biochemical processes
(Murata and Iyama, 1963; Stålfelt, 1960). Over a wide range of median
temperatures, photosynthesis is little affected by changes in tempera‐
ture because, under these conditions, the diffusion of CO_2, which is only
slightly affected by temperature, becomes the limiting factor. Finally,
at high temperatures, photosynthesis decreases rapidly to zero due to
thermal impairment of the photosynthetic apparatus. The rapid decline
in apparent photosynthesis (total photosynthesis minus respiration)
with increasing temperatures above the optimum is also caused by the
increase in respiration although, as shown by Decker (1944), as the
limits of temperature tolerance are approached the decline in apparent
photosynthesis is too great to be explained by increasing respiration
alone.

When plants are grown under saturating light intensity and CO_2
concentration, that is when the main photochemical and physical
limitations to photosynthesis are removed, there is a marked response
of photosynthesis to temperature (Gaastra, 1963; Fig. 5). Under these
conditions the photosynthetic process has a Q_{10} value of about 2 which
is typical for enzyme-controlled reactions. Although this represents a
highly artificial situation, the principle of increased assimilation at high
temperatures and CO_2 concentrations has been successfully applied to
the growing of glasshouse crops. Also some of the highest values ever
recorded for photosynthetic efficiency and net assimilation rate have
been obtained in Australia with millet, *Pennisetum*, and Jerusalem
artichoke, *Helianthus*, grown under natural conditions of high light
intensity and temperature (Begg, 1965; A. A. Warren-Wilson, personal
communication). Moss *et al.* (1961) also found that they were able to
increase significantly the net assimilation rate of corn by increasing the
temperature in the field.

Although temperature coefficients and activation energies for photo‐
synthesis are of about the same magnitude for most plants, it is well
known that different species have different temperature optima and
temperature ranges for photosynthesis. Psychrophilic plants from al‐
pine and arctic environments are capable of photosynthesis at tempera‐
tures below 0°, and often show maximum rates of true photosynthesis at

temperatures below 10°. Also certain coniferous species show positive net assimilation rates at temperatures as low as −7° (Pisek and Rehner, 1958; Stålfelt, 1960). At the other extreme, many thermophilic plants do not attain their maximum rate of photosynthesis below 40°, and are capable of photosynthesis at 50° (Rabinowitch, 1956). In this category, certain desert succulents show extraordinary adapta-

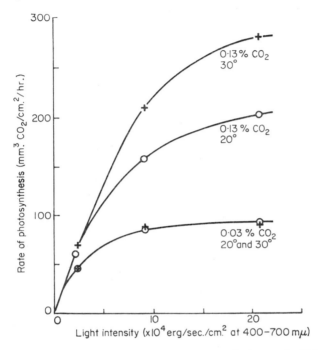

FIG. 5. Rate of photosynthesis of a cucumber leaf in relation to the light intensity at two different temperatures and in the presence of a limiting concentration (0·03%, v/v) or a saturating concentration (0·13%, v/v) of carbon dioxide. From Gaastra (1963).

tion to high temperatures. MacDougal and Working (1921) showed that the cactus, *Opuntia*, grows and presumably photosynthesizes without thermal injury at 58°. Also Wood (1932) found that *Atriplex* continued photosynthesis at leaf temperatures up to 55° under semi-arid conditions in Australia. Possibly the most remarkable adaptation to extreme temperatures in the plant kingdom is provided by the algae. On the bare rocks of the polar region the encrusting algae survive at surface temperatures which can change from −60° to 10° or higher within a few hours, whereas other species of blue-green algae that grow in hot thermal springs carry out photosynthesis at temperatures between 50° and 73° (Inman, 1940; Marrè, 1962; Kempner, 1963).

This thermal adaptation of the photosynthetic process is also apparent in latitudinal races of many native plants. In these plants, the temperature for optimum net photosynthesis in the different populations is well correlated with the temperature of the natural environment (Miller, 1960; Bjorkman et al., 1960; Mooney and Billings, 1961; Klekoff, 1965). Similar relationships have been found for contrasting crop and pasture species (El-Sharkawy and Hesketh, 1964; Murata and Iyama, 1963).

Temperature adaptation of photosynthesis may also be achieved by developmental flexibility, thereby permitting plants in a given habitat to adjust to seasonal changes in the environment. Long exposure to low or high temperatures, provided they are not injurious, induces a reversible shift in the optimum temperature for photosynthesis in the direction of the imposed temperature. Such shifts, if too extreme, can result in a prolonged suppression of photosynthesis. The capacity for such adaptation varies considerably with different species (Stålfelt, 1960; Semikhatova, 1960), and may well be an important factor in the natural distribution of plants (Mooney and West, 1964).

At both extremes of temperature (relative to the tolerance of the particular species), a decreased rate and ultimately cessation of photosynthesis are brought about by a temporary or permanent impairment of the photosynthetic system. At low temperatures, when injury does not directly result from mechanical damage to the protoplasm due to freezing and thawing, cessation of photosynthesis may have several causes. Low temperatures, especially below 10°, may cause a rapid increase in viscosity, and a decrease in the permeability of membranes thereby impeding the diffusion of CO_2 and the translocation of photosynthetic products (Rabinowitch, 1956); or as Langridge (1963) has suggested, the temperatures may be too low for activation of one or more of the enzymes involved in photosynthesis. Similarly at high temperatures, thermal inactivation of enzymes, as discussed in Section VI (p. 279) appears to be the main reason for the progressive decline and ultimate cessation of photosynthesis.

B. RESPIRATION

Physiologically active cells of most plants cease respiration at a little below 0°, but when plants are hardened to low temperatures or when seeds are dried to prevent freezing damage, respiration is possible at lower temperatures. For example, Zeller (1951) was able to detect respiration in cold-hardened winter cereals at −7°. The upper temperature limit for respiration is determined by the thermostability of the cytoplasmic proteins and, with the exception of thermophilic species, most plants die between 45° and 55°. Dehydrated organs such as seeds

and spores can survive at higher temperatures (Ben-Zeev and Zamenhof, 1962). At these extreme temperatures, and even at moderately
high temperatures, there is a marked depression in the rate of respiration with time, due presumably to the progressive inactivation of
enzymes. This time-shift effect makes it difficult to define optimum temperatures for respiration, although they are usually taken as the
temperature at which a maximum steady rate of respiration can be
maintained.

Temperature also influences the age-dependent decline in respiratory
and mitochondrial activity in plant leaves. High temperatures accelerate, and low temperatures decelerate, this decline, which occurs
normally even at optimum temperatures (Geronimo and Beevers, 1964).
These changes in respiratory activity in the dark, due to temperature
and time–age relationships, when computed on a whole plant basis are
largely responsible for the variation in net assimilation rate under different environmental conditions. Japanese workers in particular have
analysed changes in dry matter accumulation in terms of net gain from
the excess of photosynthesis over respiration (Takeda, 1961; Hiroi and
Monsi, 1963). In general, the decreased growth rate with increasing
temperature above the optimum is mainly caused by increased respiratory losses during the dark period; the ratio of photosynthesis to
respiration is inversely related to temperature (Friend, 1965). The net
assimilation, calculated on a leaf area basis, also declines with time
even under constant conditions, and especially under conditions of
rapid growth and self-shading of leaves (Thorne, 1961).

Information on the temperature coefficients and activation energies
for respiration have been reviewed by Forward (1960). In general,
activation energies and Q_{10} values for the aerial parts of plants decline
steadily as the temperature rises and, over the range 10°–30°, the Q_{10}
value is usually between 2 and 2·5. The corresponding Q_{10} values for
respiration in roots follow the same pattern, although in tomato the
existence of especially low Q_{10} values at higher temperatures suggests
that the rate of gas diffusion also may limit respiration (Jensen, 1960).

The rates of respiration of plants from different environments have
been compared to obtain evidence for the specific thermal adaptation
of the respiratory process. Most comparisons have involved plants
from widely different species ranging from arctic to tropical environments. Although in some instances few or no differences were found,
there does appear to be some respiratory compensation for temperature,
with northern populations having higher respiration rates especially
at lower temperatures (Stocker, 1935; Wager, 1941; Scholander and
Kanwisher, 1959; Mooney and Billings, 1961). Those arctic species
which show higher rates of respiration often have higher concentrations

9*

of sugar in their underground organs as compared with plants from more moderate climates. Low temperature-induced hydrolysis of starch to sucrose would provide the necessary substrate for active respiration early in the season in addition to its role in increasing cold resistance (Mooney and Billings, 1960).

C. TRANSLOCATION OF MATERIALS

There is no doubt that temperature influences the translocation of organic compounds within the plant, and most studies indicate a general increase in the rate of translocation with increasing temperature with an optimum between 25° and 30° and a Q_{10} value greater than unity (Hewitt and Curtis, 1948; Swanson and Bohning, 1951; Swanson, 1959; Whittle, 1964). However, Went and Hull (1949) have claimed that the rate of translocation increases with decreasing temperature in decapitated stems of tomato and, more recently, several workers have demonstrated a temperature independence for the primary process of translocation (Hsia et al., 1963; Swanson and Geiger, 1965).

In searching for principles governing the relationship between temperature and translocation, it must be appreciated that translocation is a complex phenomenon, and is made up of a series of sequential processes which are all influenced to a greater or lesser degree by temperature. These include the availability of materials in the leaves and their movement into the translocating pathway from the assimilating organ (source), both of which processes depend on metabolic activity. Also included is the radial translocation of materials from the conducting elements into the surrounding tissue, and finally their removal at sites of high metabolic activity.

It is not surprising therefore that raising or lowering the temperature of the whole plant, or of particular parts of the plant such as the roots or the leaves, influences the general pattern of movement of organic materials (mostly sugars) from the sources to the sites of metabolic activity. For example, lowering the temperature around the roots, which are important sites of metabolic activity in plants, alters the translocation of assimilates from the leaves. Sekioka (1963a, b) found that the accumulation of labelled material from the leaves of sweet potatoes was greater when the roots were maintained at 30°, and decreased at higher and lower temperatures. A similar effect of low temperatures in decreasing the rate of translocation in sugar cane has been demonstrated by Burr et al. (1958) and Hartt (1965). The chilling of roots in both sets of experiments caused a greater decrease in the movement of materials than cooling the tops of the plants, suggesting that the main effect of temperature in these plants was on the metabolism of the roots. Fujiwara and Suzuki (1961) have also stressed the importance of top and root temperatures. They reported that the rate of translocation in barley reached its maximum when the tops of the plants were maintained at the optimum temperature for photosynthesis and the roots maintained at the optimum temperature for respiration.

The majority of recent studies support the view that the translocation of sugars is retarded when the plant is subjected to low temperatures. In soybean, translocation from the leaves is inhibited when either the entire plant or the petioles are chilled to a temperature of 1–3°. This low-temperature inhibition is readily reversed by increasing the temperature (Thrower, 1965). Several hypotheses have been offered to explain this effect of low temperatures on translocation, including an increased viscosity of protoplasm, and an effect on the respiratory reactions responsible for energizing the translocation process (Esau et al., 1957). Less specific, but undoubtedly of major importance, is the effect of low temperatures on the centres of growth which constitute the main sites for metabolism of substances moving in the plant. The importance of such sites of metabolic activity in determining the velocity of movement of materials is well established (Nelson, 1962; Thrower, 1965), and it is becoming clear that the regulation of their activity by temperature is a major factor controlling the pattern of translocation over the entire plant.

In addition to studies involving the whole plant, attempts have also been made to investigate the effect of temperature on the primary processes of translocation by controlling the temperature around short sections of leaf petiole. The rate of movement of ^{14}C-labelled compounds through sugar beet and soybean petioles chilled to temperatures close to 0° has been studied by Mortimer (1961) and Thrower (1965). They showed that chilling prevents the movement of materials for periods of up to four hours, but that the low-temperature inhibition is reversible with a return to normal temperatures. Hsia et al. (1963), however, did not find this temperature dependence in wheat. The movement of ^{14}C-labelled compounds out of the supplying organ (leaf), and their movement into the receiving organ (ear), could be decreased by lowering the temperature to 5–8° around either organ, but decreasing the temperature around the translocating pathway, the internode between the source and the site of metabolic activity, had no effect on translocation. This has recently been confirmed by Swanson and Geiger (1965) working with a simplified translocating system. They showed that the major decrease in the rate of translocation caused by chilling the petiole is reversible with time, and in fact, petioles chilled well in advance of labelling showed no decrease in the rate of translocation of materials out of the leaf. This decrease in low-temperature inhibition with time has also been reported in bean leaf petioles by Swanson and Bohning (1951).

These results, and also the finding that HCN applied to the petiole moves into the leaf and blocks the entry of sucrose into the conducting tissue (Mortimer, 1961), indicate that localized applications of cold may inhibit metabolic processes in the leaf and not the translocating mechanism itself. The available information thus suggests that the movement of materials along the translocating pathway in the conducting tissue of the petiole or stem, is largely independent of temperature, but that the movement into and out of the pathway is temperature-dependent because it is linked to metabolic processes.

D. FLOWERING

The two environmental factors which dominate the control of flowering in plants are the duration of the photoperiod and temperature. In the following discussion emphasis will be given to the effect of temperature, including the direct effects which have an immediate influence on the flowering process, and certain indirect effects which are expressed subsequent to the temperature experience.

1. *Direct Effects*

Some of the best known studies of the direct effects of temperature on flowering are those of Blaaw and his coworkers with bulbs, which have characteristic temperature requirements for the initiation and development of flowers. This work has been reviewed recently by Hartsema (1961). Although flower formation in bulbous and tuberous plants is generally favoured by higher temperatures, there are some species with much lower temperature optima. Wedgwood iris, for example, remains vegetative indefinitely when stored at 25°, but rapidly initiates the formation of flowers when the temperature is lowered to 13°. Low temperatures (13°) promote flower initiation by favouring the export of gibberellin-like substances from the young leaves and scales to the apex whereas, at higher temperatures (25°), no such flower-inducing compounds are produced (Rodrigues Pereira, 1961, 1962, 1965). Exogenous gibberellin applied to the apex, however, does not initiate flower formation in Wedgwood iris although it accelerates subsequent flowering (Halevy and Shoub, 1964). In addition to their action on bulbous and tuberous plants, low temperatures are required to promote the flowering of plants such as cabbage and brussels sprouts (Zeevaart, 1963), and are known to cause rapid and synchronous flowering in several tropical orchids when given as a brief treatment (Went, 1961).

Once the apex has received the floral stimulus, its subsequent development is strongly influenced by temperature, as in wheat and certain long-day grasses. Increased temperatures accelerate the development of the inflorescence, resulting in a shortening of the interval between initiation and anthesis (Evans, 1960a; Friend *et al.*, 1963).

Temperature also interacts with day-length in controlling flowering. As a general rule, the flowering in long-day plants is inhibited by high temperatures, whereas the opposite response pertains in short-day plants. The pattern of response of long- and short-day plants to temperature during flowering may explain the preponderance of short-day plants under conditions of high night temperatures in the tropics, where appropriate photoperiods for either long- or short-day plants occur (Evans, 1964). For an intermediate-day plant, such as sugar cane, favourable photoperiods occur either in the autumn or in the spring but, with few exceptions, flower initiation occurs only in the autumn. Burr *et al.* (1957) claim that this is the result of low temperatures limiting flowering in the spring, rather than decreasing day-length favouring flowering in the autumn.

Temperature and the duration of the photoperiod are also known to influence sex expression in flowers of monoecious and dioecious species. In general, male sex expression is favoured by high temperatures and short days, and the female expression by short days and low temperatures (Heslop–Harrison, 1957; Nitsch, 1965). However, temperature appears to be more critical than day-length, and the temperature of the dark period to be more important than that of the light period. This has been demonstrated by Saito (1961), who showed that Japanese cucumber produced female flowers at temperatures below 17° even under continuous light.

2. *Indirect Effects (Vernalization)*

One of the most important indirect effects of temperature on flowering is the action of low temperatures in potentiating plants to respond fully to inductive conditions. This process, which is known as vernalization, was once restricted to the low temperature treatment of seeds, but is now used generally for cold treatment at all stages of plant growth. This subject has been the topic of a number of recent detailed reviews (Chouard, 1960; Purvis, 1961; Napp-Zinn, 1961; Zeevaart, 1963; Salisbury, 1963; Lang, 1965a).

The ability to respond to vernalization is not universal, and where responses occur, these may be either obligate or facultative. Vernalization is a feature of many temperate perennial forage grasses and winter cereals and of biennials such as *Hyoscyamus niger* (henbane). Plants which respond to vernalization as seedlings, usually have a subsequent long-day requirement.

The role of vernalization in controlling flowering in plants is thought to be associated with the promotion of flowering in the spring. However, in most temperate environments, perennial plants are fully vernalized long before the end of winter, and in these plants, the more important role of vernalization might be to prevent flowering in the autumn. In perennial grasses, such as *Lolium* and *Phalaris*, the duration of the vernalization requirement increases with increasing perenniality and shows adaptive variation in response to climate (Evans, 1960b; Cooper and McWilliam, 1965).

As with many other climatic responses that have been investigated, vernalization requirements have proved to be under polygenic control (Davern *et al.*, 1957; Cooper, 1960). In some plants, a simpler mode of inheritance has been revealed by partitioning the response. Thus Pugsley (1963) demonstrated a single gene difference governing the vernalization response in two Australian spring wheats. Similarly in *Hyoscyamus niger*, a single gene is responsible for the difference between the annual and biennial forms (Abegg, 1936).

In cereals with no absolute cold requirement, vernalization has proved effective in hastening flowering at every stage from fertilization to floral initiation (Purvis, 1961). In other plants, the ability to vernalize germinating seed varies due to the existence of a so-called juvenile phase, when the seedling is unable to respond to cold treatment (Sarkar, 1958). The existence of a juvenile phase suggests that some prerequisite for vernalization, such as the presence of a specific precursor or substrate reserves, may be limiting during this period.

The importance of reserve materials for vernalization has been demonstrated by Kruzhilin and Shvedskaya (1960). In the imbibed seed, these reserves are supplied by the endosperm, and in the plant by reserve organs (bulbs and tubers) or from materials photosynthesized in the leaves. As a rule, the velocity coefficients for the rate of vernalization are higher in well-developed seedlings than in seeds (Evans, 1960b; McCown and Peterson, 1964).

The operative temperature for vernalization lies between the extreme limits of $-4°$ and $12–14°$, but the most effective temperature is between $1°$ and $7°$ if applied for sufficient time and in the presence of oxygen. The site of perception of the low temperature stimulus during vernalization is considered to be the primary meristem of the bud or stem, and it has been claimed by Wellensiek (1962) that the process can only proceed in dividing cells. The possibility of vernalizing seeds at temperatures below $0°$, however, suggests that, provided the genes are being expressed, mitosis itself may not be essential.

The progress of vernalization treatment, as measured subsequently by the flowering response under inductive conditions, follows a typically sigmoid curve, suggesting that some form of autocatalytic reaction is involved. In this sense it differs from photo-induction which is much closer to an all-or-none reaction.

The application of discontinuous low temperature produces less response than continuous treatment with the same total exposure to cold. Also, high temperatures (30–35°), given immediately after vernalization treatments, cause devernalization or an annulment of the effect. The occurrence of devernalization may have detrimental effects on seed yields under field conditions (Lindsey and Peterson, 1962). The vernalization process is progressively stabilized to heat with increasing vernalization treatment, and this stability can be further enhanced by maintaining the material at 12–15° for several days immediately after the completion of the vernalization treatment (Purvis and Gregory, 1952).

One further interesting aspect of vernalization is that the vernalized state can be conserved in plants held in non-inductive conditions for long periods (Sarker, 1958). It is also self-perpetuating, as evidenced by its transmission through several cell divisions, to buds arising from those previously vernalized.

Attempts to extract a specific substance or product of vernalization (vernalin) have been partially successful. Diffusates obtained from vernalized seeds have evoked a small response when applied to unvernalized seed, but the relatively weak stimulation obtained suggests that, if a specific substance is concerned, it is very difficult to extract in a stable form (Highkin, 1955). Tomita (1964) has obtained extracts from vernalized plants, such as winter rye and radish, which promote flowering in unvernalized plants. The uridylic acid-like fraction was especially effective in flower promotion, and Tomita suggests that, in cold-requiring plants, this flowering substance might be related to a nucleic acid component such as uridylic acid or uridine diphosphate. Possibly the best evidence for the existence of vernalin is still the transmission of the vernalized state by grafting (Melchers, 1937).

A number of mechanisms have been proposed for the overall vernalization reaction, and these have been reviewed by Purvis (1961). All of the proposed mechanisms embody the concept of a thermolabile intermediate formed from a precursor at low temperatures. The completion of vernalization then depends on the further conversion of this intermediate product at an appropriate temperature to the final thermolabile substance, vernalin.

The ability of gibberellins to replace, or partly substitute for, the vernalization requirement in many plants, has been reviewed by Lang (1965a). Also it is known (Chailakhyan et al., 1964) that the amounts of endogenous gibberellins in many plants increase following vernalization. The relationship between gibberellin and vernalization is however, still obscure, and it is doubtful if gibberellin and vernalin are the same. Gibberellin appears more likely to be a precursor or cofactor which acts in a similar fashion to vernalin, i.e. it potentiates the apex to respond to the inductive photoperiod.

Very little is known of the biochemistry of the vernalization response, and it is difficult to think of a unifying principle underlying all of the various responses. The activity of a specific RNA during vernalization has been postulated (Hess, 1961) but rigorous evidence for its existence, or for differences in protein synthesis following vernalization, have not been forthcoming.

E. DORMANCY

The development of true dormancy in the seeds, buds, and underground organs of plants prevents germination and growth under optimum conditions of temperature, light and nutrition. Recent reviews of this subject have been presented by Vegis (1964, 1965), Stokes (1965), Barton (1965), and Evenari (1965). The nature and degree of dormancy vary considerably within and between species, and are undoubtedly of major importance in the adaptation of plants to recurrent adverse environmental conditions.

Smith and Kefford (1964) have recognized three major phases in the winter dormancy reaction of buds, and these stages apply equally well to other types of dormant organs. The stages are (1) dormancy development, (2) release from dormancy leading to the non-dormant state, and (3) the initiation and resumption of active growth. During the first stage of dormancy development in buds, the duration of the photoperiod is clearly the important environmental factor, although it is primarily the temperature that determines the rate of response to the photoperiod. In seeds and in many underground organs, temperature is the major influence. When dormancy is complete, plant organs, especially buds and seeds, acquire increased resistance to extremes of climate including frost and heat. Also, in many deciduous woody plants, the onset of dormancy is the essential first step in the development of winter hardiness (Tumanov et al., 1964). For the release from dormancy, many woody plants and seeds have a requirement for low temperatures (chilling) which, when satisfied, potentiates the organ to respond to increasing temperatures which initiate the resumption of growth.

Vegis (1963, 1964, 1965) in detailed reviews of dormancy in higher plants has emphasized the importance of temperature in the induction, maintenance, and breaking of dormancy and has drawn attention to the temperature response in buds and seeds during the various phases of dormancy. For most species, there is a narrowing of the temperature range for seed germination and bud break with the onset of dormancy, and a widening of the range again during the post-dormancy phase.

In climates characterized by hot dry summers, the seeds and underground organs of many perennial plants lose their ability to germinate or develop at high temperatures. This is a condition known as *relative dormancy*, as these seeds or plants retain their ability to develop at low temperatures. This has been shown for seeds of Mediterranean pasture plants (Ballard, 1961; Cooper and McWilliam, 1965), for several perennial grasses (Laude, 1953) and also for many bulb species (Hartsema, 1961). Under these conditions, true dormancy would be of little advantage, as the survival of these plants is ensured by their inability to develop at elevated temperatures.

A narrowing of the temperature range due to an increase in the minimum temperature required for germination and bud break is less common. Rees (1961) has demonstrated this effect in the seeds of the tropical oil palm which have a high temperature requirement for germination which resembles the phenomenon known as stratification in the seeds of temperate plants (see below). Also the buds of a number of deciduous trees will break dormancy under favourable photoperiods at high temperatures, but not at low (Wareing, 1956; Vegis, 1964). Similarly, it has been shown that potato tubers immediately after harvest are able to sprout only within a narrow temperature range above 30°, which presumably protects them from premature sprouting in the autumn (Vegis, 1964).

Many seeds which experience true dormancy, along with the dormant buds on many woody species, require a period of after-ripening low temperature treatment known as *stratification* to break dormancy. In seeds, this treatment is effective only if they are imbibed and aerated. During this after-ripening low temperature treatment, *Fraxinus* (ash) seeds produce a growth-promoting substance which apparently counteracts the effect of the endogenous inhibitor responsible for the dormancy (Villiers and Wareing, 1965). There is a marked similarity in the mode of action and in the kinetics of low temperature in the breaking of dormancy and in vernalization although, unlike vernalization, stratification can be replaced in many species by long periods of dry storage at room temperature. This tends to be the rule with those species that are capable of some germination without stratification, such as the cereals and grasses (Crocker and Barton, 1953).

Exposure to high temperatures has been used to break dormancy in seeds of *Malva verticillata* (Ruge, 1955). However, more commonly this treatment induces a condition known as *secondary dormancy*, particularly in seeds that have completed ripening. This effect can occur in seeds that normally show little dormancy reaction, and the effect is more pronounced if the moisture content of the seed is high (Pisarev and Zhilkina, 1951).

The dwarf habit of seedlings grown from unchilled embryos is common in Rosaceous species, and can persist for long periods. Peach seedlings, grown without experiencing low temperatures, have remained in this physiologically dwarfed condition for up to 10 years (Flemion, 1959). Normal growth occurs following exposure to low temperatures and also following certain photoperiodic and hormone treatments (Flemion, 1959; Stokes, 1965). Also the dwarfing response is quantitative; it decreases with increasing stratification, and is limited in its effect to the primary shoot, the secondary shoots and roots being unaffected.

Little is known of the mechanisms which control the narrowing and widening of the temperature ranges for germination and bud break during the onset and recovery from dormancy. There is evidence that the amounts of endogenous gibberellin-like substances in dormant organs are increased by chilling, both in seeds (Frankland and Wareing, 1962) and in woody perennials (Chailakhyan et al., 1964). Further, applications of gibberellin can substitute for stratification, shorten the rest period, break the dormancy of buds and generally widen the temperature range for growth in many dormant organs (see the reviews by Lang, 1965b; Vegis, 1964 and Smith and Kefford, 1964). This suggests an important role for gibberellins in the regulation of dormancy release.

The action of exogenously supplied gibberellin in replacing the cold requirement may be through its role as a general mobilizing hormone that stimulates the release of sugars and proteins as suggested by Paleg (1961), or it may function as a derepressor of the genes controlling the synthesis of α-amylase (Varner and Chandra, 1964) or other essential enzymes (Tuan and Bonner, 1964).

V. Cellular Aspects of Temperature Response

A. BIOPHYSICAL RESPONSES

The principal effect of temperature upon the protoplasm of plant cells is believed to be brought about through its influence on the water of the cells. Changes in temperature can alter drastically the amount of intracellular water, as well as inducing important modifications in water structure and water binding (see Chapter 2, p. 5). The water content of the cell fluctuates considerably with changes in temperature, and is usually higher in the cold (Bělehrádek, 1963) when it increases the hydration of proteins. Genetic factors, which change the normal hydration–temperature response, may help in conferring hardiness on the cell.

With a decrease in temperature, the protoplasmic gel tends to solate reversibly and stabilizes the cellular membranes in the open and expanded configuration, thus altering their permeability (Kavanau, 1965). Also, hydration shells around uncharged polar groups of organic molecules increase in size. An increase in temperature within physiological limits has the opposite effect; it promotes gelation and stabilizes the closed configuration of membranes.

In addition to the changes involving water, gas solubilities alter considerably with temperature change, and the solubility of carbon dioxide and oxygen in the cytoplasm increases as the temperature is lowered. These solubility changes can cause profound alterations in cellular metabolism especially in those processes which involve the exchange of CO_2. For example, the low temperature-induced rise in dissolved CO_2 in the cell, due to increased solubility and slower diffusion out of the cell, will tend to depress decarboxylation because of mass action effects, and favour CO_2 fixation (Leopold, 1964). At the same time, oxygen saturation of the respiratory system will be achieved at lower partial pressures, so causing an increase in energy production from respiration and a depression of terminal CO_2 production. Temperature alterations also induce morphological changes in protoplasm, but the significance of such changes is not clear. It would be anticipated that the viscosity of protoplasm would decrease as the temperature rises, since water, and solutions of proteins, are affected in this way by a rise in temperature. However, both increases and decreases in protoplasmic viscosity with increased temperature have been reported, and some plants show a viscosity maximum either with temperature change or with time at a given temperature. Frey-Wyssling (1952) has concluded that there is probably a cellular control mechanism influencing protoplasmic viscosity.

Another activity of protoplasm which shows readily discernible temperature effects is protoplasmic streaming, higher temperatures giving accelerated streaming. In the alga *Nitella*, the rate–temperature curve for streaming is logarithmic between 7° and 20° with a Q_{10} of 1·8 (Frey-Wyssling, 1952). Above 25°, the streaming rate decreases and, in most plants, it ceases reversibly between 30° and 40°. Belikov *et al.* (1963) have noted that, in barley coleoptiles first grown at 17° and then placed at 44°, the rate of protoplasmic streaming is first accelerated but soon slows down and ceases altogether after 4–5 hours at this temperature. The cessation of streaming is frequently used as an index of cellular heat injury, especially by the Russian workers. Streaming also stops at low temperatures above freezing, and plants sensitive or insensitive to temperature may be differentiated on the basis of their ability to continue streaming in the cold (Lewis, 1956). In chill-sensitive plants, protoplasmic streaming stops suddenly when the temperature of the tissue is dropped below 10°, although streaming continues in cells from chill-resistant plants almost to 0°. Lyons *et al.* (1963) have suggested that the capacity for protoplasmic streaming in resistant cells at these low temperatures is determined by the greater resilience or flexibility of their membranes. They measured the permeability of the membrane system of plant cells and also analysed the membranes for fatty acid residues. This approach was used to test the generality of the findings of Richardson and Tappel (1962), who reported differences in the flexibility of mitochondrial membranes from warm- and cold-blooded animals. These changes in flexibility were correlated with differences in the degree of saturation of the fatty acid residues in the membrane lipids. In the plants studied, those that survived low non-freezing temperatures had markedly greater mitochondrial membrane permeability and a noticeably higher proportion of unsaturated fatty acid residues than had mitochondrial membranes from species sensitive to cold. Lyons *et al.* (1963) therefore proposed that, as the temperature is lowered below about 10°, cellular membranes with a high content of saturated fatty acid residues become increasingly rigid, whereas membranes relatively rich in unsaturated fatty acid residues remain flexible down to 0°. If membranes become unduly rigid, it is supposed that oxidative phosphorylation, which is associated with mitochondrial membranes, is inhibited and ATP production is consequently decreased.

The permeability of the cell to water and to solutes also shows marked changes with temperature. The temperature coefficient for permeability to water has been reported as being between 1·3 and 1·6 in some plants, and 2 to 3 in others (Kramer, 1955). The first of these temperature coefficient values corresponds to that expected for the free diffusion of molecules across a membrane in response to a concentration gradient. However, the more usual temperature coefficients of 2–3 are too high for a simple diffusion process and suggest that the passage of ions and molecules across membranes is an energy-linked activity. The process of ion absorption may, in fact, have both a temperature-sensitive and a temperature-insensitive component. However, it has proved difficult to separate temperature effects on the structural integrity of semipermeable membranes from those on metabolically-dependent active transport. At high temperatures, there is a large increase in the excretion of water-soluble substances from the cell. This excretion begins abruptly at a certain temperature suggesting that the cellular membranes have become disorganized rather than that energy has become unavailable for the retention of solutes. However, with a decrease in the temperatures of the root systems of temperate plants such as the tomato, there is a progressive slowing down of mineral uptake (Shakov and Golubkova, 1960). This suggests an energy deficit due to sluggish metabolism or possibly an excessive viscosity of the protoplasm.

B. CELL DIVISION AND CELL ENLARGEMENT

Both cell division and cell enlargement have temperature coefficients between 2 and 3, and occasionally higher (Mazia, 1961). In the mitotic division of plant cells, the duration of the entire division cycle and the individual stages of this process are differently affected by temperature. Within certain temperature limits, a straight line is given when the logarithm of the velocity of cell division is plotted against the reciprocal of the temperature, and it is evident that the division process relies heavily upon metabolic energy. Meiosis shows temperature responses similar to those of mitosis although there is greater evidence of chromosomal irregularities at high temperatures. These follow temperature disturbance of the complex processes of chromosome pairing and chiasma formation. Crossing-over generally increases in frequency with increased temperature.

Heat shocks arrest the course of mitosis and also cause reversion of premetaphase chromosomes to the resting stage. When the temperature is slowly decreased, dividing nuclei complete their division but no new mitoses begin. A rapid drop in temperature causes a complete stoppage of cell division and mitosis ceases whatever the stage. Since the initiation of nuclear division is more sensitive to high or low temperature shock than the actual division process, temperature treatment is often used to synchronize cell division. A series of temperature shocks, if not too prolonged, will result in the gradual accumulation of all cells in the predivision stage.

It is not known how extreme temperatures suppress the onset of cell division, but some of their effects on nuclear division are suspected to result from an interference in spindle formation and function (Mazia, 1961). The spindle, which is composed mostly of protein, is believed to depend upon a sol-to-gel transformation (Marsland, 1957), and its formation is therefore very sensitive to temperature. Alternatively, high and low temperatures may prevent nuclear divisions from proceeding beyond the metaphase because of an impairment in ATP generation. The sea urchin egg requires about three times as much energy for cell division as is available from respiration (Scholander et al., 1958) and there is good evidence from other systems that the processes of phosphorylation are readily damaged by temperature extremes.

As with cell division, the enlargement of cells has temperature coefficients which indicate that chemical reactions are governing the process, and that temperature is not simply changing the tensile properties of the cell wall. Chao and Loomis (1947) found that the stems of the dandelion, *Taraxacum*, and the hypocotyls of the bean, *Phaseolus*, which were not undergoing cell division, had temperature coefficients usually between 2 and 3 within the interval 0–30°, with a maximum rate of elongation at 30°. Although the rate of elongation increased with increasing temperature, the duration of elongation decreased. The final length therefore depends upon the balance between the two processes, but high temperatures result in decreased cell lengths. The measurements of Burström (1956) indicate that, with increasing temperatures, the cell wall plasticity which is believed to be the plasticity of the pectin matrix, disappears but that the elasticity remains. He assumed that there were two phases of elongation involving plasticity and elasticity, and that these were differently sensitive to changes in temperature. Furthermore, he deduced that active cell wall synthesis should have a higher temperature coefficient than passive stretching. As a result of this work, Burström (1956) proposed that an increase in temperature causes primarily an increased concentration of native auxin, which in turn leads to more rapid cell wall synthesis but a shortened duration of elongation and a decreased cell length. In support of this, Gustafson (1946) has reported that plants usually contain a lower concentration of auxin at lower temperatures. However, the precise relationships existing between temperatures, especially low temperatures, auxin and cell growth are still unclear. Preston and Hepton (1960) found that, although auxin usually has a pronounced effect upon the extensibility of the cell walls of *Avena* coleoptiles, it is quite without effect at 0°. It seems more probable that the suppression of cell elongation at low temperatures may result, not from an insufficiency of auxin, but from a breakdown in the metabolic systems through which auxin exerts its effect.

C. CELLULAR METABOLISM

Many of the effects of temperature upon the metabolism of plant cells arise from changes in the rates of individual reactions. A rise in temperature, for example, accelerates the rates of reactions according to their activation energies, displaces equilibria in the endothermic direction, and causes both reversible and irreversible denaturation depending on the duration and severity of the heat treatment. Thus the effects of temperature changes on cell metabolism depend primarily on the inherent properties of the cell's enzymes, especially their activation energies and resistance to heat- and cold-inactivation.

If a particular reaction has a high activation energy, or if the activation energy changes to a higher value at low temperatures, the rate of this reaction may become a limiting factor as the temperature decreases. This appears to happen in bacteria, for those bacteria that are capable of growth at low temperatures are relatively resistant to rate limitation because their enzymic reactions have low activation energies (Ingraham, 1958). However, there is as yet no evidence that this type of adaptation occurs in flowering plants. The activation energies for photosynthesis and respiration are much the same in both arctic and tropical plants (Rabinowitch, 1956; Forward, 1960).

More frequently, cellular metabolism alters when a branched or coupled reaction system, catalysed by enzymes with different activation energies, suffers a change in temperature. If, for example, there are two enzymes of very different activation energies each modifying the same substrate to initiate separate metabolic pathways, a rise in temperature stimulates one reaction pathway much more than the other. This results in an accumulation of one end-product, which may perhaps be inhibitory in excess, and a deficiency of the other end-product. This must be a common metabolic effect of a change in temperature, although verified instances of it in plants are rare. Growth inhibitions in flowering plants at extreme temperatures have been attributed to an imbalance in metabolism causing the accumulation of toxic products (Joslyn, 1949) or leading to metabolic derangement (Kushnirenko, 1961).

In theory, temperature changes can also affect metabolic rates by causing a displacement of equilibrium conditions. An increase in temperature would be expected to suppress an exothermic reversible reaction and favour an endothermic one. Such a mechanism has been considered by Oota *et al.* (1960) as an explanation of effects of temperature on the lipid $\rightleftharpoons$ hexose $\rightleftharpoons$ sucrose equilibria in cotyledons. The lipid $\rightleftharpoons$ hexose reaction, being exothermic, may shift to the left with a rise in temperature, while the endothermic hexose $\rightleftharpoons$ sucrose conversion may be hastened. Similarly, James (1953) has interpreted the sweetening of potatoes at low temperatures as due to a temperature-induced shift in the starch $\rightleftharpoons$ sucrose equilibrium. The heat of reaction for conversion of starch to sucrose is about 3.7 kcal./mole, so that high temperatures would favour starch formation and low temperatures the formation of sugar. On the other hand, Arreguin-Lozano and Bonner (1949) believe that the low-temperature sweetening of potatoes results from quantitative changes in enzymes converting starch to sucrose. It is probable that thermal shifts in equilibria establish apparent temperature optima of certain reactions but do not cause marked changes in the concentrations of metabolic intermediates.

As the temperature is lowered, there is an increase in the solubility of

CO_2 and oxygen, and alterations may therefore occur in the enzymic reactions which involve CO_2 exchange. In particular, low temperatures can induce a diversion of CO_2 to organic acid formation as has been demonstrated in *Bryophyllum* (Pucher *et al.*, 1948) and in grapes (Kliewer, 1964). This shift in metabolism may also be aided by the fact that, being an exothermic reaction, the oxidation of sugars to organic acids would be favoured by a lowered temperature. Thomas and Ranson (1954) have shown that, during acid production in the dark in plants possessing a crassulacean acid metabolism, the fixation of CO_2 and the accumulation of organic acids are inversely related to temperature between 12° and 32°. This increased CO_2 and bicarbonate content of the cell sap, as well as the accumulation of organic acids, leads to a decrease in pH value and consequently to changes in enzyme activity. In addition to acids, sugars particularly sucrose, increase in amount in plants kept at low temperatures for reasons not well understood, although causes such as depressed metabolism, breakdown of control systems, and changes in equilibria have been advanced.

It is evident that an alteration in temperature will result in extensive changes in the amounts and types of available substrates in the cell with consequent changes in respiration patterns. A temperature-induced change of respiratory substrate from sugar to organic acids or lipids would therefore be expected to cause a drift in the respiratory quotient (R.Q.). A lowered R.Q. value would indicate that there is a conversion of lipid to sugar or of sugar to organic acids accompanying respiration, since the products are more highly oxidized than the substrates. Potato tubers, for example, exhibit a low R.Q. value at 0° with an associated accumulation of citric and malic acids (Forward, 1960). The reverse effect of high temperatures is exhibited by *Vigna sesquipedalis* (Oota *et al.*, 1960). In this plant, high R.Q. values and alcohol production were a feature of the metabolism at higher temperatures.

At temperatures at which severe damage occurs, disturbances due to changes in metabolic rate in plant cells are over-shadowed by various types of irreversible derangements. It is frequently observed that photosynthetic ability seems to be especially sensitive to heat, whereas respiration, even if its energy yield is decreased, is much less sensitive. As a result of this disproportionate inactivation at relatively high temperatures, an excessive proportion of the photosynthetic products may be respired, and plants may become stunted and retarded in growth. Apart from protein denaturation and mechanical effects on cells, much of this thermal damage may stem from the inactivation of electron-transport systems. Cellular oxidation and reduction systems may be expected to be particularly sensitive to extreme temperatures. These oxido-reductions involve complex enzyme-coenzyme catalysts; they depend upon the integrity of mitochondrial membranes and are readily subject to a separation of electron transfer from energy transfer by a wide range of compounds. This last type of inhibition might frequently follow from the production of intracellular uncoupling agents as a result of a temperature-induced rate imbalance. Thus Semikhatova and Bushuyeva (1963) found that mitochondrial preparations from pea seedlings became progressively weaker in their ability to esterify phosphate above 20–25°; there was no phosphorylation at 35°. They suggested that thermal damage, which often occurs in peas under field conditions, is the result of an uncoupling of oxidation and phosphorylation. Similarly, the experiments of Belikov et al. (1963) on barley coleoptiles suggested that the main cause of heat death was the destruction of the electron-transport system.

Electron-transfer mechanisms seem to be very sensitive to cold damage also. In this respect, Heber and Santarius (1964) have demonstrated a correlation between freezing injury and ATP destruction. Of a number of individual enzymes tested for inactivation by freezing in vivo and in vitro, only those concerned with photosynthetic and oxidative phosphorylation proved to be sensitive. They considered that dehydration of the protoplasm by freezing was responsible for the inactivation of phosphorylation systems leading to an inability of the cell to produce sufficient amounts of ATP to maintain metabolism. Since the addition of sugars prevented the uncoupling or destruction of ATP synthesis in photosynthesis or respiration, they proposed that a relationship existed between sugar content and frost hardiness (see Section VI, p. 280).

VI. Molecular Aspects of Temperature Response

The effects of temperature on plants are primarily exerted through the influence of heat on the synthesis, stability and activity of controlling molecules such as enzymes (Fig. 6) and on molecular complexes such as occur in membranes, which in turn produce changes in cellular metabolism. As macromolecular biochemistry advances, the interpretation of the influence of heat at this level of complexity becomes easier to visualize. It is only recently that this perspective of the action of heat has reached a reasonably firm basis mainly through studies with microorganisms. The purpose of this section is to extrapolate this molecular aspect of heat response to the higher level of organization presented by flowering plants. The validity of such an extrapolation rests on the now generally accepted view that the genetic code is a universal one and that only minor differences exist between organisms in the transcription and translation of genetic information. However, this aspect of the temperature response of plants can only be presented in a conjectural fashion at present, for the molecular bases of the very important processes of development and differentiation are still practically unknown.

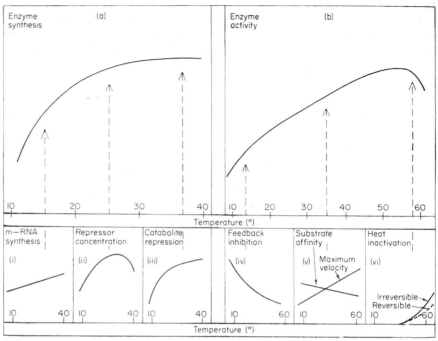

FIG. 6. Graphs showing the general types of relationship between temperature and enzyme synthesis and activity.

Curve (a) shows the effect of temperature on the synthesis of the inducible enzyme β-galactosidase by *Escherichia coli* (Marr *et al.*, 1964). The smaller graphs below curve (a) refer to parts of this curve and show the effect of temperature on (i) the postulated rate of m-RNA synthesis by RNA polymerase from *E. coli* (Mehrotra and Khorana, 1965), (ii) the relative amounts of repression produced by the regulator gene that controls expression of the lactose operon in *E. coli* (Marr *et al.*, 1964), (iii) the repression by glucose (catabolite repression) of the synthesis of β-galactosidase by *E. coli* (Ng *et al.*, 1962).

Curve (b) is an idealized curve showing the effect of temperature on enzyme activity. The smaller graphs below curve (b) show the effect of temperature on (iv) the feedback inhibition of the first enzyme (PR-ATP pyrophosphorylase) on the pathway to histidine biosynthesis in a mutant strain of *E. coli* (O'Donovan and Ingraham, 1965), (v) maximum velocity and substrate affinity of β-galactosidase from *E. coli* (Wallenfels and Malhotra, 1961), (vi) the reversible and irreversible inactivation of a typical enzyme; these are idealized curves.

A. REPRESSION AND DEREPRESSION OF GENES

Heat, within physiological limits, has little effect on the integrity of genes themselves, for the heat resistance of DNA is determined by the proportion of guanine-cytosine base pairs, a property which is not a reflection of the ecological temperature. Thus Evreinova *et al.* (1961) showed that the blue-green alga, *Mastigocladus laminosus*, which has a high temperature optimum for growth, had DNA with a melting temperature (a property which is taken as a measure of its thermal stability; see p. 80) similar to related organisms with a lower optimum temperature for growth.

However, where the action of genes is subject to control systems, these controlling elements may be more sensitive to temperature than either the genetic material or the primary gene products; in fact, temperature often serves as an inducer, as in vernalization, or a repressor as in secondary dormancy, of gene action. In the flowering plants, evidence is accumulating that the lack of cellular activity in dormant embryos and buds is due to their genes being in a repressed state; i.e. the DNA of the nucleus is unable to direct specific protein synthesis. It has long been known that the onset of germination and the breakage of dormancy are associated with an increase in RNA formation (Oota, 1964). Recently, Tuan and Bonner (1964) have shown that, in dormant potato buds, this RNA formation appears to be DNA-dependent in that it is inhibited by actinomycin D, which is known to decrease specifically the production of m-RNA. Moreover, the chromatin (a DNA-protein complex) isolated from dormant potato buds is very inefficient in carrying out the DNA-dependent synthesis of RNA, whereas the chromatin of buds treated with the dormancy-breaking chemical, ethylene chlorhydrin, is highly active. On the basis of this work, the well-known effects of temperature in producing germination and bud-break (Vegis, 1963) may soon be capable of explanation in molecular terms.

At the level of gene repression, temperature, in addition to its effect on major physiological processes such as growth initiation and flower induction, is likely to be an important factor wherever induced enzyme formation occurs. Where the properties of inducible enzymes have been studied in micro-organisms, it has very frequently been found that the temperature range for production of the enzyme is much narrower than the temperature range for its catalytic activity. Thus a temperature-induced impairment of the control system for a particular enzyme may lie behind a temperature-sensitive failure in a metabolic activity. In an inducible enzyme system, temperature can influence enzyme synthesis by changing the effective concentration of the specific repressor. There are a number of examples of temperature-dependent repressions of enzyme synthesis in bacteria, the general trend being towards increased repression with decreasing temperature. This effect is not necessarily due to an increase in the actual concentration of repressor molecules, but may be a consequence of a progressive loss in the response of the control system to the inducer. For example, wild type

Escherichia coli, which is inducible for tryptophanase at 30°, cannot be induced to form this enzyme below 15° (Ng and Gartner, 1963).

It has been suggested by Marr *et al.* (1964) that the various reports of increased nutritional requirements by bacteria at low temperatures may be interpretable on the basis of a cold-induced repression. This proposal is the more acceptable since no convincing reason in terms of enzyme structure and function has yet been offered for low temperature-induced biochemical deficiencies. An explanation of this sort may hold for low temperature chlorosis in flowering plants. According to Sachs (1865), there is a threshold temperature below which plant species will not make chlorophyll (or functional chloroplasts), and that this threshold temperature varies with the species.

One of the best examples of a temperature-dependent control system in flowering plants is that for invertase in the sugar cane (Sacher *et al.*, 1963). The amounts of invertase in this plant decrease four-fold between 18° and 34°, the decrease being almost linear with increasing growth temperature. The repressor of invertase synthesis, most probably glucose, seemed to prevent the DNA-dependent synthesis of invertase rather than the activity or stability of the enzyme. As with the bacterial control systems, temperature appeared to be affecting the concentration or activity of the repressor.

B. PROTEIN SYNTHESIS

The details of the processes whereby DNA directs the synthesis of specific proteins are now reasonably well understood. Protein synthesis goes through many stages involving quite unstable templates and intermediates, and the overall process may be expected to be profoundly sensitive to temperature changes. Nevertheless, the temperature factor has been little studied as yet. When an organism is grown at different temperatures, it is usual to find that the activity of a particular enzyme in the organism varies strongly with the growth temperature. However, these data often confuse enzyme synthesis with enzyme denaturation.

At the level of protein synthesis, there are several steps where temperature is likely to be particularly important. At low temperatures, the release of newly-formed m-RNA from the DNA template may become the limiting step in protein formation (Mehrotra and Khorana, 1965). This step is therefore rendered more difficult at low temperatures, and this may account for the slowing down in protein formation observed in cold-treated plants. Once released from the template, m-RNA is broken down at a rate varying with the temperature, for the presence of the 2′-OH group on the sugar residue of RNA renders the phosphodiester bonds much more sensitive to hydrolysis than those of DNA (Ginoza *et al.*, 1964). This breakdown results in striking changes in the proportions of different proteins synthesized when these are coded from the one m-RNA (Nishi and Zabin, 1963). It appears that the aminoacyl-s RNA synthetases, besides serving as amino-acid adaptor molecules in protein assembly, when charged with amino acids act also as repressors of amino acid biosynthesis (Eidlic and Neidhardt, 1965). The extent of regulation of the biosynthetic enzymes varies with temperature, and where there is restricted growth at high temperatures as occurs with a heat-induced metabolic deficiency, there would be a general increase in the levels of repressors for various enzymes. This may explain in part the changes in levels of metabolites such as amino acids, sugars and organic acids so often observed in tissues of plants that have been exposed to unfavourable temperatures.

With respect to the adaptation of the organism to temperature, rates of protein synthesis have been implicated by the studies of Allen (1950) on thermophilic bacteria. These bacteria were found to be resistant to death at 55° only so long as protein formation could continue. This led to the conclusion that thermophils have enzymes with the usual thermosensitivity, but are able to survive because a more heat stable protein-forming system allows them to replace the proteins lost by heat denaturation. This proposal has received some direct experimental support from the work of Hancock (1957) who examined the rates of glycine incorporation in a soil bacillus that would grow at 55°, but not at 37°. He concluded that this bacterium possessed a more heat-resistant protein-synthesizing system than ordinary bacteria, enabling it to balance thermal inactivation at 55° with the synthesis of new protein. Some plant physiologists similarly believe that heat-resistant plants respond to high temperatures with accelerated protein synthesis either to avoid serious damage to the cells (Henckel, 1964) or to eliminate the injury caused by heating (Alexandrov, 1963). Kinetin (6-aminofurfuryl purine) is considered to increase the heat resistance of *Nicotiana rustica* leaves by stimulating the accumulation of amino acids, thereby favouring higher rates of protein synthesis (Englebrecht and Mothes, 1960). However, processes other than accelerated protein synthesis must be important in heat resistance, for Lark and Adams (1953) have shown that organisms such as isolated T5 bacteriophages, in which no resynthesis of components is possible, may vary by as much as 5,000-fold in high-temperature stability. Also, thermophilic bacteria derive much of their ability to survive at high temperatures because of the especially stable structure of their proteins (Koffler, 1957).

C. PROTEIN STABILITY

In thermophilic bacteria, many individual enzymes, as well as the total bulk of cytoplasmic protein, have been found to be inherently more stable to heat than the corresponding proteins of mesophilic forms (Langridge, 1963). This enhanced stability appears to result from an increase in the number or strength of the hydrogen and hydrophobic bonds which are important in maintaining the tertiary structures of proteins (Koffler, 1957; Campbell and Cleveland, 1961). Little will be said here of this aspect of heat resistance because practically nothing is known of the stability of plant proteins to heat. However, there is good evidence that many poikilothermic animals, which face problems of heat adaptation similar to those of plants, have proteins with a heat stability that is correlated with the environmental temperature. Such correlations have been shown for collagens (Gustavson, 1956), myosins (Connell, 1961), adenosine triphosphatase (Vinogradova, 1963) and other enzymes (Kusakina, 1963). Moreover heat stability may be genetically induced in a protein by a single amino acid substitution as has been shown in tryptophan synthase (Henning and Yanofsky, 1962) and tobacco mosaic virus (Aach, 1960).

It might be expected, therefore, that the proteins of desert plants would be of the heat-resistant type because the tissues of these plants often reach very high temperatures. No study of this matter appears to have been made, although the enzymes of cacti have been reported to have high temperature optima (Sanwal and Krishnan, 1961a, b). They found that neither the aldolase nor the phosphatase of *Nopalea dejecta* reached its maximum velocity of reaction after 15 minutes of incubation at 60°.

Other ways in which proteins may be protected from inactivation include the binding of enzymes into membranes or cell particles. This mechanism has been found to operate for several enzymes in bacilli (Militzer and Burns, 1954) and for pectinesterase in plant tissues (McDonnell *et al.*, 1945).

Stability may also be conferred on proteins by the elaboration of heat-protective substances by the plant. Thus Wood (1932) concluded that the ability of the desert plant, *Atriplex vesicarium*, to withstand heat depended upon the stabilizing effect of the high salt content of the leaves. This plant has a temperature optimum for photosynthesis between 40° and 50° and a content of KCl and NaCl varying between 8 and 30% of the leaf dry weight. More generally, protective substances seem to be formed as a phenotypic response to unusual or seasonal temperature extremes, the plant reverting to the more sensitive state when the stringent temperature conditions pass. This is part of the phenomenon of hardening which will be considered in the following paragraphs.

D. MOLECULAR ASPECTS OF HARDENING

The various known types of cellular hardening are to some extent related phenomena, since cold-hardening also increases heat- and drought-hardiness, while drought-hardening increases heat- and frost-resistance. However, it is doubtful if heat hardening gives much resistance to cold, and heat-resistant species are not always drought-resistant.

The curve of cell heat resistance shows, in many plants, a change towards a steeper slope at about the temperature at which protoplasmic streaming ceases (Alexandrov, 1964). The flatter slope below this point is believed to result from metabolic disturbances with a consequent accumulation of toxins, or from starvation resulting from the differential thermal coefficients for photosynthesis and respiration. The steeper slope above the transition point is believed to be more the result of protoplasmic protein denaturation.

The evidence for protein denaturation by heat comes mainly from the facts that the temperatures that induce heat injury are in the same range as those that cause denaturation. Moreover, the temperature coefficients are very high for both phenomena, and the process of hardening appears to increase the stability of plant proteins. It has been convincingly shown by Alexandrov and Fel'dman (1958), and confirmed by other workers, that heat hardening results in a stabilization of the cell proteins. They demonstrated that the degree of heat-hardiness obtained by exposing tissues of *Tradescantia fluminensis* to different temperatures was closely paralleled by the resistance of the tissues to protein denaturants such as ethanol and acetic acid. Hardening did not, however, change the responses of the proteins to the action of inhibitors of catalytic activity.

Assuming then that hardening results from the developed resistance of cellular proteins to unfavourable temperatures, there are three conceivable classes of molecular mechanism for this hardening.

The first is that hardened cells have their proteins protected from temperature inactivation by an increased concentration of antidenaturants. Substances reported to have such a protective effect include sugars, organic acids, vitamin C, B^{2+}, Ca^{2+} and other ions. Such compounds, particularly sugars, almost certainly increase resistance to heat damage and are probably especially important in lessening low temperature injury. Heber and Santarius (1964) have shown that, whereas most individual enzymes are not appreciably inactivated by freezing, the enzyme systems of electron transport in plant photosynthesis are very frost-sensitive. This breakdown in ATP synthesis, interpreted as an uncoupling of oxidative phosphorylation, is prevented by the accumulation of sugars in the protoplasm. More generally, protectants are believed to help maintain the structural integrity of the cytoplasm by changing viscosity, increasing hydrophily and altering permeability (Meyer *et al.*, 1960), but the details are still unclear. It is possible that, at high temperatures, these protectants do not prevent the initial damage to proteins, but create conditions in which repair or restoration of activity is facilitated.

A second possible explanation for the hardened condition is that it results from changes in the structure of protein molecules which increase their temperature stability. Since hardening is temporary, this hypothesis implies that reversible changes in non-covalent bonding leading to a more stable protein tertiary structure are induced by extreme temperatures. It is uncertain whether this more stable structure is impressed upon existing proteins as a consequence of high temperature, or whether only proteins synthesized at the higher temperatures are capable of adopting a "resistant" configuration. Various hypotheses exist in favour of the interpretation that it is existing proteins that are modified, the older ideas assuming that resistance depends on the degree of hydration of the protoplasmic proteins. Thus some workers believe that decreased hydration leads to increased heat resistance (e.g. Sapper, 1935), while others find that an increased water content in the cell increases resistance to heat (e.g. Henckel, 1964). There are undoubtedly changes in colloidally- and osmotically-bound water in plant cells during hardening, but temperature effects on transpiration, water uptake and metabolism obscure their significance.

On the assumption that frost injury is due to a denaturation of the structural proteins of the protoplasm, Levitt (1962) has presented a closely reasoned hypothesis of cold hardening based on resistance towards sulphydryl group oxidation. The injury is thought to result from a combination of the removal of intermolecular water to form ice, and a compression of the dehydrated protein molecules favouring disulphide bond formation between them. Structural proteins might then undergo partial unfolding or there might be damage to semipermeable membranes especially with thawing because of these sulphydryl-disulphide interchanges. On this hypothesis of frost injury, the primary effect of hardening would be to increase the resistance of proteins to the formation of new disulphide bonds. As experimental support for this mechanism of frost hardening, Levitt and his coworkers have shown that, with hardening, there is an increase in the number of sulphydryl groups in the protoplasmic proteins (or a relative decrease in the number of disulphide bonds formed) as compared with plants incapable of hardening. Also, a series of wheat varieties, differing in their relative hardiness to low temperatures, had contents of sulphydryl groups which were proportional to their hardiness, but only after hardening had taken place. Levitt believes that heat injury may have a similar molecular basis, in that the heat, by increasing molecular movement and removing bound water, allows the proteins to approach close enough together for intermolecular disulphide bond formation to take place. Frost resistance would then also confer heat resistance by maintaining the "sulphydryl state". So far, the sulphydryl-disulphide theory of frost injury and hardiness has received little experimental support. Heber and Santarius (1964) found that no oxidation of protein sulphydryl groups occurred during the inactivation of photophosphorylation in wheat and spinach by freezing. This inactivation, they believe, resulted from the dehydration of the system by ice formation. They concluded that the oxidation of sulphydryl groups is a secondary event in frost injury and has little to do with the primary action of frost.

A third explanation for hardening is based on the proposal that hardening occurs in plants that are capable of accelerating their rate of protein synthesis at extreme temperatures. This hypothesis, originally due to Lepeschkin (1935), and elaborated for thermophilic bacteria by Allen (1950), cannot apply to low-temperature hardening where metabolic rates generally are greatly depressed. The meagre evidence bearing on this hypothesis has been discussed above.

VII. Conclusions

A plant growing under the most favourable temperature conditions for its particular developmental stage is usually adversely affected by a temperature change. However, the magnitude of the change required to produce depression depends upon the genotype of the plant. Few plants are visibly affected by small temperature changes, for all of them have genetic mechanisms based on homeostasis and heterosis which buffer them against environmental fluctuations. Larger temperature changes may induce phenotypic alterations in certain plants but these are gene-controlled adaptive modifications and not pathological ones. In other plant species, similar changes in temperature, away from the apparent optimum, have favourable effects on some processes but overriding depressing effects on more numerous or more important ones. The favourable action of increased temperatures is primarily kinetic, while that of decreased temperatures is due mainly to increased gas solubility. The depressing action is exerted firstly at the level of gene action, by inhibiting protein synthesis, secondly upon enzymic products causing rate limitation or rate imbalance, and thirdly upon substrate availability by decreasing intracellular gas concentrations and changing permeability, transport efficiency and organelle function. Temperature influences of the first type, which affect the function and timing of gene action, may be much more important in plants than in micro-organisms, because it is probable that complex systems of gene regulation underly morphogenetic processes. No firm evidence for this view is yet available

10+T.

for plants although there are suggestions that genes are in their repres
sed states during seed and bud dormancy, and their triggered releas
may be mediated by heat or cold. Data showing temperature effect
upon plant proteins, other than the expected influence on the velocit
of enzyme action, are at present restricted to demonstrable changes i
protein stability following cold- or heat-hardening. Much better know
is the action of temperature change in producing effects upon substrat
concentration leading to shifts in metabolism. Among these are th
promotion of organic acid-type metabolism, and accelerated hydrolysi
of starch, with consequent changes in ion adsorption, translocation o
photosynthetic products and possibly electron-transport system
through membrane impairment.

Extreme temperature deviations cause the deaths of cells and even o
whole plants. At high temperatures, these effects are suspected, but no
proved, to result from enzyme inactivation and eventually bulk protei
coagulation. At temperatures below freezing, dehydration, membran
rupture and perhaps cell wall damage are the primary causes of injury

The ecological distribution of plants is reflected in their density an
variety by the facility with which they can evolve means of toleratin
or mitigating the unfavourable influences of temperature. Plants ar
most numerous and diverse where temperature does not limit growt
and reproduction while, in more thermally harsh environments, th
frequency of species and the number of individual plants steadily de
clines. Adaptation towards one temperature extreme seems usually t
be accompanied by a correspondingly increased sensitivity towards th
other extreme; i.e. the survival range is moved on the temperatur
scale and not merely extended.

In many instances, the temperature distribution of a species i
limited by its special thermal requirements for the initiation of
development phase such as germination, flowering and bud-break. Th
lack of convincing explanations for temperature action on these develop
mental processes is perhaps the largest gap in our knowledge of plant
temperature relations. To explain how a vernalized meristem retains it
temperature stimulus for very long periods, and how it transmits thi
state to non-vernalized meristems derived from it, requires cellular an
molecular systems which at present are difficult even to visualize.

References

Aach, H. G. (1960). Z. Vererbungslehre. **91**, 312.

Abegg, F. A. (1936). J. agric. Res. **53**, 493.

Alexandrov, V. Ya. (1963). Abstracts, Internat. Symp. on Cytoecology, Leningra
pp. 5–6.

Alexandrov, V. Ya. (1964). Quart. Rev. Biol. **39**, 35.

Alexandrov, V. Ya. and Fel'dman, N. L. (1958). *Botan. Z.* **43**, 194.

Allen, M. B. (1950), *J. gen. Physiol.* **33**, 205.

Angus, D. E. (1962), *CSIRO, Div. Meteorol. Phys. Tech. Paper.* **12**, p. 1.

Ansare, A. Q. and Loomis, W. E. (1959), *Amer. J. Bot.* **46**, 713.

Arreguin-Lozano, B. and Bonner, J. (1949). *Plant Physiol.* **24**, 720.

Asana, R. D. and Williams, R. F. (1965). *Austral. J. agric. Res.* **16**, 1.

Ballard, L. A. T. (1961). *Austral. J. biol. Sci.* **14**, 173.

Ballard, L. A. T. and Wildman, S. G. (1964). *Austral. J. biol. Sci.* **17**, 36.

Barton, L. V. (1965). *In* "Handbuch der Pflanzenphysiologie", (W. Rutland, Ed.), Vol. xv/11, p. 699. Springer, Berlin.

Begg, J. E. (1965). *Nature, Lond.* **205**, 1025.

Bělehrádek, J. (1963). Abstracts, Internat. Symp. on Cytoecology, Leningrad, pp. 16–17.

Belikov, P. S., Dmitrieva, M. I. and Kirillova, T. V. (1963). Abstracts, Internat. Symp. on Cytoecology, Leningrad, pp. 17–18.

Ben-Zeev, N. and Zamenhof, S. (1962). *Plant Physiol.* **37**, 696.

Billings, W. D. and Morris, R. J. (1951). *Amer. J. Bot.* **38**, 327.

Bjorkman, O., Florell, C. and Holmgren, P. (1960). *Kungl. Lantbrukshogskolans. Annaler. Uppsala.* **26**, 1.

Bloodworth, M. E. (1960). *Trans. 7th Int. Congr. Soil. Sci.* **1**, 153–163.

Booth, A., Moorby, J., Davies, C. R., Jones, H. and Wareing, P. F. (1962). *Nature, Lond.* **194**, 204.

Burr, G. O., Hartt, C. E., Brodie, H. W., Tanimoto, T., Kortshak, H. P., Takahashi, D., Ashton, F. M. and Colemna, R. E. (1957). *Annu. Rev. plant Physiol.* **8**, 275.

Burr, G. O., Hartt, C. E., Tanimoto, T., Takahashi, D. and Brodie, H. W. (1958). *Radioisotopis Sci. Research, Proc. Intern. Conf. Paris*, 1957, **4**, 351.

Burström, H. (1956). *Plant Physiol.* **9**, 682.

Campbell, L. L. and Cleveland, P. D. (1961). *J. biol. Chem.* **236**, 2966.

Chailakhyan, M. K., Nerrasova, T. V., Khlopenkova, L. P. and Lozhnikova, U. N. (1964). *Plant Physiol.* (U.S.S.R.) (Engl. Transl.) **10**, 389.

Chao, M. D. and Loomis, W. E. (1947), *Bot. Gaz.* **109**, 225.

Chouard, P. (1960). *Annu. Rev. plant. Physiol.* **11**, 191.

Clary, W. P. (1965). *Agron. J.* **57**, 4.

Clausen, J., Keck, D. D. and Hiesey, W. M. (1948). Carnegie Inst. Wash. Publ. No. 581, pp. 129.

Connell, J. J. (1961). *Biochem. J.* **80**, 503.

Cook, G. D., Dixon, J. R. and Leopold, A. C. (1964). *Science* **144**, 546.

Cooper, J. P. (1960). *Ann. Bot.* **24**, 232.

Cooper, J. P. (1964). *J. appl. Ecol.* **1**, 45.

Cooper, J. P. and McWilliam, J. R. (1965). *J. appl. Ecol.* **3**, 191.

Costin, A. B. (1965). Proceedings VII Inqua Congress, Boulder, Col., U.S.A.

Crocker, W. and Barton, L. V. (1953). "Physiology of Seeds", p. 130. Chronica. Bot. Waltham, Mass.

Curme, J. H. (1962). *In* "Plant Science Symposium", p. 99. Campbell Soup Co., Camden, New Jersey.

Dale, J. E. (1964). *Ann. Bot.* **28**, 127.

Daubenmire, R. F. (1954). Butler Univ. Bot. Studies. **11**, 119.

Davern, C. I., Peak, J. W. and Morley, F. H. W. (1957). *Austral. J. agric. Res.* **8**, 121.

Davidson, J. L. and Milthorpe, F. L. (1965). *Ann. Bot.* **29**, 407.

Decker, J. P. (1944). *Plant Physiol.* **19**, 679.

Dorland, R. E. and Went, F. W. (1947). *Amer. J. Bot.* **34**, 393.

Eidlic, L. and Neidhardt, F. C. (1965). *Proc. nat. Acad. Sci.*, Wash. **53**, 539.

El-Sharkawy, M. A. and Hesketh, J. D. (1964). *Crop. Sci.* **4**, 514.

Engelbrecht, L. and Mothes, K. (1960). *Ber. deut. Botan. Ges.* **73**, 246.

Esau, K., Currier, H. B. and Cheadle, V. I. (1957). *Annu. Rev. plant Physiol.* **8** 349.

Evans, L. T. (1960a). *New Phytol.* **59**, 163.

Evans, L. T. (1960b). *J. agric. Sci.* **54**, 410.

Evans, L. T. (1963). *In* "Environmental Control of Plant Growth", (L. T Evans, Ed.), p. 421. Academic Press, New York.

Evans, L. T. (1964). *In* "Grasses and Grasslands", (C. Barnard, Ed.), p. 126 Macmillan, London.

Evans, L. T., Wardlaw, I. F. and Williams, C. N. (1964). *In* "Grasses and Grass lands", (C. Barnard, Ed.), p. 102. Macmillan, London.

Evenari, M. (1965). *In* "Handbuch der Pflanzenphysiologie", (W. Rutland, Ed.) Vol. xv/11, p. 804. Springer, Berlin.

Evreinova, T. N., Davydova, I. M., Sukover, A. P. and Goriunov, S. V. (1961) *Dokl. Akad. Nauk. S.S.S.R.* **137**, 213.

Finlay, K. W. and Wilkinson, G. N. (1963). *Austral. J. agric. Res.* **14**, 742.

Fisher, D. V. (1962). *Proc. Amer. Soc. hort. Sci.* **80**, 114.

Fisher, F. J. F. (1954). *Nature, Lond.* **173**, 406.

Flemion, F. (1959). *Con. Boyce Thompson Inst.* **20**, 57.

Fortainer, E. J. (1957). Mededel Landbouwhogeschool Wageningen. **57**, 1.

Forward, D. F. (1960) *In* "Handbuch der Pflanzenphysiologie", (W. Rutland Ed.), Vol. xii–2, p. 234. Springer, Berlin.

Frankland, B. and Wareing, P. F. (1962). *Nature, Lond.* **194**, 313.

Frey-Wyssling, A. (1952). "Deformation and Flow in Biological Systems" pp. 552. North Holland Publishing Co., Amsterdam.

Friend, D. J. C. (1965). *In* "The Growth of Cereals and Grasses", (F. L. Milthorpe and J. D. Ivins, Eds.). Butterworths, London.

Friend, D. J. C., Helson, V. A. and Fisher, J. E. (1962a). *Canad. J. Bot.* **40**, 939

Friend, D. J. C., Helson, V. A. and Fisher, J. E. (1962b). *Canad. J. Bot.* **40** 1299.

Friend, D. J. C., Fisher, J. E. and Helson, V. A. (1963). *Canad. J. Bot.* **41**, 1663– 1674.

Friend, D. J. C., Helson, V. A. and Fisher, J. E. (1964). *Canad. J. Bot.* **43**, 15.

Fujiwara, A. and Suzuki, M. (1961). *Tohoku. J. Agric. Res.* **12**, 363.

Gaastra, P. (1963). *In* "Environmental Control of Plant Growth", (L. T. Evans Ed.), p. 113. Academic Press, New York.

Gale, J. and Poljakoff-Mayber, A. (1965). *Plant Cell Physiol.* **6**, 111.

Gates, D. M., Hiesey, W. M., Milner, H. W. and Nobs, M. A. (1964). Carnegie Inst. Wash. Year Book. **63**, 418.

Geiger, R. (1959). "The Climate Near the Ground", (Transl. by M. N. Stewart) pp. 494. Harvard Univ. Press, Cambridge, Mass.

Geronimo, J. and Beevers, H. (1964). *Plant Physiol.* **39**, 786.

Ginoza, W., Hoelle, C. J., Vessey, K. B. and Carmack, C. (1964). *Nature, Lond* **203**, 606.

Glaziou, K. T., Bull, T. A., Hatch, M. D. and Whiteman, P. C. (1965). *Austral. J biol. Sci.* **18**, 53.

Gott, M. B., Gregory, F. G. and Purvis, O. N. (1955). *Ann. Bot.* **21**, 87.

Gregory, L. E. (1965). *In* "Handbuch der Pflanzenphysiologie", (W. Rutland, Ed.), Vol. xv/1, p. 1328. Springer, Berlin.

Griffing, B. and Langridge, J. (1963). *In* "Symposium on Statistical Genetics and Plant Breeding", pp. 368–390. Raleigh, North Carolina.

Grobbelaar, W. P. (1963). Mededel. Landbouwhogeschool Wageningen, **63**, 1.

Gukova, M. M. (1961). *Dokl. Akad. Nauk.* **139**, 1055.

Gustafson, F. G. (1946). *Plant Physiol.* 21, 49.

Gustavson, K. H. (1956). "The Chemistry and Reactivity of Collagen", p. 342. Academic Press, New York.

Halevy, A. H. and Shoub, J. (1964), *J. hort. Sci.* **39**, 120.

Hancock, R. (1957). *J. gen. Microbiol.* **17**, 480.

Hartsema, A. M. (1961). *In* "Handbuch der Pflanzenphysiologie", (W. Rutland, Ed.), Vol. XVI, p. 132. Springer, Berlin.

Hartt, C. E. (1965). *Plant Physiol.* **40**, 74.

Heber, U. W. and Santarius, K. A. (1964). *Plant Physiol.* **39**, 712.

Hellmers, H. and Sundahl, W. P. (1959). *Nature, Lond.* **184**, 1247.

Henckel, P. A. (1964). *Annu. Rev. plant Physiol.* **15**, 363.

Henning, U. and Yanofsky, C. (1962). *Proc. nat. Acad. Sci. Wash.* **48**, 183.

Heslop-Harrison, J. (1957). *Biol. Rev.* **32**, 38.

Hess, D. (1961). *Planta.* **57**, 13.

Hewitt, S. P. and Curtis, D. F. (1948). *Amer. J. Bot.* **35**, 746.

Hiesey, W. M. (1953a). *Evolution* 7, 297.

Hiesey, W. M. (1953b). *Amer. J. Bot.* **40**, 205.

Hiesey, W. M., Nobs, M. A. and Milner, H. W. (1961). Carnegie Inst. of Wash. Year Book. **60**, 381.

Highkin, H. (1955). *Plant Physiol.* **30**, 390.

Highkin, H. R. (1958). *Amer. J. Bot.* **45**, 626.

Hillman, W. S. (1956). *Amer. J. Bot.* **43**, 89.

Hiroi, T. and Monsi, M. (1963). *Bot. Mag.* Tokyo. **76**, 121.

Hopp, R. (1947). *Proc. Amer. Soc. hort. Sci.* **50**, 103.

Hsia, C. A., Wan, H. S. and Wang, P. T. (1963). *Acta. Bot. Sinica.* **11**, 338.

Hudson, M. A. and Brustkern, P. (1965). *Planta* **66**, 135.

Hurd, R. G. (1964), *J. exp. Bot.* **15**, 381.

Hussey, G. (1965). *J. exp. Bot.* **16**, 373.

Inman, O. (1940). *J. gen. Physiol.* **23**, 661.

Ingraham, J. L. (1958). *J. Bact.* **76**, 75.

James, W. O. (1953). "Plant Respiration", p. 282. Clarendon Press, Oxford.

Jensen, G. (1960). *Physiol. Plant.* **13**, 822.

Joslyn, M. A. (1949). *Advanc. Enzymol.* **9**, 613.

Joslyn, M. A. and Diehl, H. C. (1952). *Annu. Rev. plant Physiol.* **3**, 149.

Kavanau, J. L. (1965). "Structure and Function in Biological Membranes", Vol. 2, p. 555. Holden-Day, San Francisco.

Ketellapper, H. J. (1960a). *Physiol. Plant.* **13**, 641.

Ketellapper, H. J. (1960b). *Plant Physiol.* **35**, 238.

Ketellapper, H. J. (1963). *Plant Physiol.* **38**, 175.

Kempner, E. S. (1963). *Science* 142, 1318.

Klages, H. K. W. (1942). "Ecological Crop Geography", p. 615. Macmillan, New York.

Kleinert, E. C. (1961). *Z. Bot.* **49**, 345.

Klekoff, L. G. (1965). *Ecology* 46, 516.

Kliewer, W. M. (1964). *Plant Physiol.* **39**, 869.

Knapp, R. (1957). *Z. Naturforsch.* **12**B, 564.

Konis, E. (1948). *Palest. J. Bot. Jerus. Ser.* 5, 46.

Koffler, H. (1957). *Bact. Rev.* **21**, 227.

Korovin, A. I., Sycheva, Z. F. and Bystrova, Z. A. (1961). *Dokl. Akad. Nauk.* (*Bot. Sci.*) (Engl. Transl.), **137**, 78.

Kramer, P. J. (1955). *In* "Handbuch der Pflanzenphysiologie", (W. Rutland, Ed.), Vol. 1, p. 194. Springer, Berlin.

Kruzhilin, A. S. and Shvedskaya, Z. M. (1960). *Plant Physiol.* U.S.S.R. (Engl. Transl.) **7**, 237.

Kuiper, P. J. C. (1961). Mededel, Landbouwhogeschool, Wageningen, **61**, (7) 1.

Kuiper, P. J. C. (1964). *Science* **146**, 544.

Kusakina, A. A. (1963). Abstracts, Internat. Symp. on Cytoecology, Leningrad, pp. 35–36.

Kushnirenko, S. (1961). *Fiziol. Rast.* **8**, 345.

Lambert, R. G. and Linck, A. J. (1958). *Plant Physiol.* **33**, 347.

Lang, A. (1963). *In* "Environmental Control of Plant Growth", (L. T. Evans, Ed.), p. 405. Academic Press, New York.

Lang, A. (1965a). *In* "Handbuch der Pflanzenphysiologie", (W. Rutland, Ed.), Vol. xv/1, p. 1380. Springer, Berlin.

Lang, A. (1965b). *In* "Handbuch der Pflanzenphysiologie", (W. Rutland, Ed.), Vol. xv/11, p. 848. Springer, Berlin.

Lange, O. L. (1959). *Flora* (*Jena*) **147**, 595.

Lange, O. L. and Schwemmle, B. (1960). *Planta* **55**, 208.

Langridge, J. (1963) *Annu. Rev. plant Physiol.* **14**, 441.

Langridge, J. (1965). *Austral. J. biol. Sci.* **18**, 311.

Langridge, J. and Griffing, B. (1959). *Austral. J. biol. Sci.* **12**, 117.

Lark, K. G. and Adams, M. H. (1953). *Cold Spr. Harb. Symp. quant. Biol.* **18**, 171

Laude, H. M. (1953). *Bot. Gaz.* **114**, 284.

Laude, H. M. and Changule, B. A. J. (1953). *J. range Mangt.* **6**, 320.

Leopold, A. C. (1964). "Plant Growth and Development", p. 466. McGraw-Hill, New York.

Lepeschkin, W. W. (1935). *Protoplasma* **23**, 349.

Lerner, I. M. (1954). "Genetic Homoestasis", p. 134. Oliver and Boyd, Edinburgh

Levitt, J. (1951). *Annu. Rev. plant. Physiol.* **2**, 245.

Levitt, J. (1956). "The Hardiness of Plants", p. 278. Academic Press, New York

Levitt, J. (1962). *J. theoret. Biol.* **3**, 355.

Lewis, D. A. (1956). *Science* **124**, 75.

Lindsey, K. E. and Peterson, M. L. (1962). *Crop Sci.* **2**, 71.

Lyons, J. M., Wheaton, T. A. and Pratt, H. K. (1963). *Plant Physiol.* **39**, 262.

Lyutova, M. I. (1963). *Dokl. Akad. Nauk, Biol. Sci. Sec.* **149**, 532.

MacDougal, D. T. and Working, E. B. (1921). Carnegie Inst. Wash. Year Book **20**, 47.

McCown, R. L. and Peterson, M. L. (1964). *Crop Sci.* **4**, 388.

McDonnell, L. R., Jansen, E. F. and Lineweaver, H. (1945). *Arch. Biochem* **6**, 389.

McWilliam, J. R. and Griffing, B. (1965). *Austral. J. biol. Sci.* **18**, 569.

Marr, A. G., Ingraham, J. L. and Squires, C. L. (1964). *J. Bact.* **87**, 356.

Marrè, E. (1962) *In* "Physiology and Biochemistry of Algae", (R. A. Lewin, Ed.) p. 541. Academic Press, New York.

Marsland, D. (1957). *In* "Influence of Temperature on Biological Systems" (F. H. Johnson, Ed.), pp. 111–126. Amer. Physiol. Soc. Washington.

Mazia, D. (1961). *In* "The Cell", (J. Brachet and A. E. Mirsky, Eds.), Vol. **3** p. 77. Academic Press, New York.

Mehrotra, B. D. and Khorana, H. G. (1965). *J. biol. Chem.* **240**, 1750.

Melchers, G. (1937). *Biol. Zbl.* **57**, 568.

Meyer, B. S., Anderson, D. B. and Böhning, R. H. (1960). "Introduction to Plant Physiology", 541 pp. D. van Nostrand Co., Princeton, New Jersey.

Militzer, W. and Burns, L. (1954). *Arch. Biochem. Biophys.* **52**, 66.

Miller, V. J. (1960). *Proc. Amer. Soc. hort. Sci.* **75**, 700.

Millikan, C. R. (1945). *J. Dept. Agr., Victoria.* **43**, 133.

Milthorpe, F. L. (1956). *In* "The Growth of Leaves", (F. L. Milthorpe, Ed.). Butterworths, London.

Milthorpe, F. L. (1957). *In* "Control of the Plant Environment", (J. P. Hudson, Ed.), p. 140. Butterworths, London.

Molotkovsky, Yu. G. and Zhestkova, I. M. (1964). *Plant Physiol. U.S.S.R.* **11**, 254.

Monselise, S. P. and Went, F. W. (1958). *Plant Physiol.* **33**, 372.

Mooney, H. A. and Billings, W. D. (1960). *Amer. J. Bot.* **47**, 594.

Mooney, H. A. and Billings, W. D. (1961). *Ecol. Monographs* **31**, 1.

Mooney, H. A. and West, M. (1964), *Amer. J. Bot.* **51**, 825.

Moore, R. M. (1966). Australia—UNESCO Symposium on Arid Zone Climatology with special Reference to Microclimatology, Canberra Paper No. 20.

Mortimer, D. C. (1961). *Plant Physiol.* **36** (suppl.), xxxiv.

Moss, D. N., Musgrave, R. B. and Lemon, E. R. (1961). *Crop Sci.* **1**, 83.

Murata, Y. and Iyama, J. (1963). *Proc. crop Soc. Japan* **31**, 315.

Muromtsev, I. A. (1963). *Plant Physiol. (U.S.S.R.)* (Engl. Transl.), **9**, 334.

Napp-Zinn, K. (1961). *In* "Handbuch der Pflanzenphysiologie", (W. Rutland, Ed.), Vol. xvi, p. 76. Springer, Berlin.

Napp-Zinn, K. (1962). *Z. Vererbungslehre* **93**, 154.

Nelson, C. D. (1962). *Canad. J. Bot.* **40**, 757.

Ng. H., Ingraham, J. L. and Marr, A. G. (1962). *J. Bact.* **84**, 331.

Ng. H. and Gartner, T. K. (1963). *J. Bact.* **85**, 245.

Nishi, A. and Zabin, I. (1963). *Biochem. Biophys. res. Commun.* **13**, 320.

Nitsch. J. P. (1965) *In* "Handbuch der Pflanzenphysiologie", (W. Rutland, Ed.), Vol. xv/1, p. 1537. Springer, Berlin.

Njoku, E. (1957). *New Phytologist* **56**, 154.

Nuttonson, M. Y. (1956). *Amer. Inst. Crop. Ecol.* Study 18, Washington, D.C.

O'Donovan, G. A. and Ingraham, J. L. (1965). *Proc. nat. Acad. Sci. Wash.* **54**, 451.

Oosting, H. J. (1958). "The Study of Plant Communities", p. 389. Freeman and Co., San Francisco.

Oota, Y. (1964). *Annu. Rev. plant Physiol.* **15**, 17.

Oota, Y., Fuju, R. and Sunobe, Y. (1960). *Physiol. Plant.* **9**, 38.

Overland, L. (1960). *Amer. J. Bot.* **47**, 378.

Paleg, L. G. (1961). *Plant Physiol.* **36**, 829.

Parker, J. (1963). *Bot. Rev.* **29**, 124.

Petinov, N. S. and Molotkovsky, Yu, G. (1957). *Plant Physiol. U.S.S.R.* (Engl. Transl.), **4**, 221–227.

Petinov, N. S. and Molotkovsky, Yu. G. (1961). *In* "Arid Zone Research xvi. Plant-Water Relationships in Arid and Semi-arid Conditions", Symposium UNESCO, p. 275. Columbia Univ. Press, New York.

Petinov, N. S., Molotkovsky, Yu. G. and Fedorov, P. S. (1964). *Dokl. Akad. Nauk Biol. Sci. Sec.* **153**, 1649.

Pisarev, V. E. and Zhilkina, M. D. (1951) *Agrobiologiya* **5**, 61.

Pisek, A. and Rehner, G. (1958). *Ber. Dtsch. Bot. Ges.* 71.

Poljakoff-Mayber, A. (1959). *Bull. Res. Counc.* Israel, **7D**, 93.

Preston, R. D. and Hepton, J. (1960). *J. exp. Bot.* **11**, 13.

Pucher, G. W., Leavenworth, C. S., Ginter, W. D. and Vickery, H. B. (1948). *Plant Physiol.* **23**, 123.

Pugsley, A. T. (1963). *Austral. J. agric. Res.* **14**, 622.

Purvis, O. (1961). *In* "Handbuch der Pflanzenphysiologie", (W. Rutland, Ed.), Vol. xvi, p. 76. Springer, Berlin.

Purvis, O. N. and Gregory, F. G. (1952). *Ann. Bot.* **16**, 1.

Rabinowitch, E. I. (1956). "Photosynthesis and Related Processes", **2**, pt. 2, 1211 and 1236. Interscience, New York.

Rees, A. R. (1961). *Nature, Lond.* **189**, 74.

Richardson, T. and Tappell, A. L. (1962). *J. cell Biol.* **13**, 43.

Rodrigues Pereira, A. S. (1961). *Science* **134**, 2044.

Rodrigues Pereira, A. S. (1962). *Acta. Botanica Neerlandica* **11**, 97.

Rodrigues Pereira, A. S. (1965). *J. exp. Bot.* **16**, 405.

Ruddat, M. (1960). *Z. Bot.* **49**, 23.

Ruge, U. (1955). *Beitr. Biol. Pflanz.* **31**, 409.

Sacher, J. A., Hatch, M. D. and Glasziou, K. T. (1963). *Plant Physiol.* **16**, 836.

Sachs, J. (1865). "Handbuch der Experimental Physiologie der Pflanzen", pp. 10–11, W. Engelmann, Leipzig.

Saeki, T. and Nomoto, N. (1958). *Bot. Mag. Tokyo*, **71**, 235.

Saito, T. (1961). *J. Jap. Soc. Hort.* **30**, 1.

Sakai, A. (1962). *Nature, Lond.* **193**, 89.

Sakai, A. (1965). *Nature, Lond.* **206**, 1064.

Salisbury, F. B. (1963). "The Flowering Process", 234 p. Pergamon Press, New York.

Salisbury, F. B. and Spomer, G. G. (1964). *Planta* **60**, 497.

Sanwal, G. G. and Krishnan, P. S. (1961a). *Enzymologia* **23**, 85.

Sanwal, G. G. and Krishman, P. S. (1961b). *Enzymologia* **23**, 249.

Sapper, J. (1935). *Planta* **23**, 518.

Sarkar, S. (1958). *Biol. Zbl.* **77**, 1.

Schaible, L. W. (1962). *In* "Plant Science Symposium", p. 89. Campbell Soup Co., Camden, New Jersey.

Scholander, P. F., Leivestad, H. and Sundnes, G. (1958). *Exp. cell Res.* **15**, 505.

Scholander, S. I. and Kanwisher, J. T. (1959). *Plant Physiol.* **34**, 574.

Schroeder, C. A. (1963). *Nature, Lond.* **200**, 1301.

Schroeder, F. M. and Barton, L. V. (1939). Contr. Boyce Thompson Inst. **10**, 235.

Schwabe, W. W. (1957). *In* "Control of the Plant Environment", (J. P. Hudson, Ed.), p. 16. Butterworths, London.

Schwabe, W. W. (1963). *In* "Environmental Control of Plant Growth", (L. T. Evans, Ed.), p. 311. Academic Press, New York.

Sekioka, H. (1963a). *Sci. Bull. Fac. Agr. Kyushu. Univ.* **20**, 107.

Sekioka, H. (1963b). *Sci. Bull. Fac. Agr. Kyushu Univ.* **20**, 119.

Semikhatova, O. A. (1960). *Bot. Zhur.* **45**, 1488.

Semikhatova, O. A. and Bushuyeva, T. M. (1963). Abstracts, Internat. Symp. on Cytoecology, Leningrad, p. 60.

Shakov, A. A. and Golubkova, B. M. (1960). *Dokl. Akad. Nauk. S.S.S.R.* **135**, 486.

Shelo, R. and Halevy, A. H. (1963). *Israel J. agric. Res.* **13**, 141.

Smith, H. and Kefford, N. P. (1964). *Amer. J. Bot.* **51**, 1002.

Stålfelt, M. G. (1960). *In* "Handbuch der Pflanzenphysiologie", (W. Rutland, Ed.), Vol. v, p. 100. Springer, Berlin.

Stearns, F. and Olson, J. (1958). *Amer. J. Bot.* **45**, 53.

Stocker, O. (1935). *Planta* **34**, 402.

Stokes, P. (1965). In "Handbuch der Pflanzenphysiologie", (W. Rutland, Ed.), Vol. xv/11, p. 746, Springer, Berlin.

Swanson, C. A. (1959). In "Plant Physiology—A Treatise", (F. C. Steward, Ed.), Vol. 2, p. 481. Academic Press, New York.

Swanson, C. A. and Bohning, R. H. (1951). Plant Physiol. 26, 557.

Swanson, C. A. and Geiger, D. R. (1965). Plant Physiol. 40 (Suppl.), x/vii–x/viii.

Takeda, T. (1961). Japan. J. Bot. 17, 403.

Tanner, C. B. (1963). Agron. J. 55, 210.

Thomas, M. and Ranson, S. L. (1954). New Phytol. 53, 1.

Thorne, G. N. (1961). Ann. Bot. 23, 366.

Thrower, S. L. (1965). Austral. J. biol. Sci. 18, 449.

Toole, E. H., Toole, V. K., Borthwick, H. A. and Hendricks, S. B. (1955). Plant Physiol. 30, 473.

Tomita, T. (1964). In "Régulateurs Naturels de la Croissance Végétale", No. 123, p. 635. Colloq. Intern. C.N.R.S. Paris.

Tranquillini, W. (1964). Annu. Rev. plant Physiol. 15, 345.

Tuan, D. Y. H. and Bonner, J. (1964). Plant Physiol. 39, 768.

Tukey, L. D. (1958). Proc. Amer. Soc. hort. Sci. 71, 157.

Tumanov, N. N., Kuzina, G. V. and Karnikova, L. D. (1964). Plant Physiol. U.S.S.R. (Eng. Transl.), 11, 592.

Varner, J. E. and Chandra, G. Ram. (1964). Proc. nat. Acad. Sci. Wash. 52, 100.

Vegis, A. (1963). In "Environmental Control of Plant Growth", (L. T. Evans, Ed.), p. 265. Academic Press, New York.

Vegis, A. (1964). Annu. Rev. plant Physiol. 15, 185.

Vegis, A. (1965). In "Handbuch der Pflanzenphysiologie", (W. Rutland, Ed.), Vol. xv/11, p. 534. Springer, Berlin.

Viglierehiv, D. R. and Went, F. W. (1957). Amer. J. Bot. 44, 449.

Villiers, T. A. and Wareing, P. F. (1965). J. exp. Bot. 16, 519.

Vinogradova, A. N. (1963). Abstracts, Internat. Symp. on Cytoecology, Leningrad, pp. 78–79.

Voigt, G. K. (1951). Wis. Acad. Sci. Lett. Trans. 40, 241.

Waddington, C. H. (1953). Evolution 7, 118.

Wager, H. G. (1941). New Phytol. 40, 1.

Wallenfels, K. and Malhotra, O. P. (1961). Advanc. carb. Chem. 16, 239.

Wardel, P. (1965). N.Z. J. Bot. 3, 113.

Wareing, P. F. (1956). Annu. Rev. plant Physiol. 5, 183.

Wellensiek, S. J. (1962). Nature, Lond. 195, 307.

Went, F. W. (1944a) Amer. J. Bot. 31, 135.

Went, F. W. (1944b) Amer. J. Bot. 31, 597.

Went, F. W. (1945). Amer. J. Bot. 32, 469.

Went, F. W. (1953). Annu. Rev. plant Physiol. 4, 347.

Went, F. W. (1957a). "The Experimental Control of Plant Growth", pp. 343. Chronica Botanica, Waltham, Mass.

Went, F. W. (1957b). In "Influences of Temperature on Biological Systems", (F. H. Johnson, Ed.), p. 163. Amer. Physiol. Soc. Washington, D.C.

Went, F. W. (1958). In "Physiological Adaptation", (C. L. Prosser, Ed.), p. 126. Amer. Physiol. Soc. Washington, D.C.

Went, F. W. (1961). In "Handbuch der Pflanzenphysiologie", (W. Rutland, Ed.), Vol. xvi, p. 1, Springer, Berlin.

Went, F. W. (1962). In "Plant Science Symposium", p. 149. Campbell Soup Co., New Jersey.

Went, F. W. and Hull, H. M. (1949). Plant Physiol. 24, 505.

Whittle, C. M. (1964). *Ann. Bot.* **28**, 339.

Williams, R. C. and Webb, B. C. (1958). *Agron. J.* **50**, 235.

Wilsie, C. P. (1962). "Crop Adaptation and Distribution", p. 448. W. H. Freeman, San Francisco.

Wood, J. G. (1932). *Austral. J. exp. biol. med. Sci.* **10**, 89.

Wolpert, A. (1962). *Plant Physiol.* **37**, 113.

Yarwood, C. E. (1961a). *Science* **134**, 941.

Yarwood, C. E. (1961b). *Nature, Lond.* **192**, 887.

Yarwood, C. E. (1964). *Phytopathol.* **54**, 936.

Zeevaart, J. A. D. (1963). *In* "Environmental Control of Plant Growth", (L. T. Evans, Ed.), p. 289. Academic Press, New York.

Zeller, O. (1951). *Planta* **39**, 500.

Zotov, V. (1938). *N.Z. J. Sci. Tech.* **19**, 474.

Chapter 9

Insects and Temperature

KENNETH U. CLARKE

*Department of Zoology, University of Nottingham,
Nottingham, England*

I. Introduction

Much of the information that has been gained about insects comes from the work of scientists who have approached these animals from the viewpoint of geneticists, biochemists, physiologists or ecologists. Their choice of material underlines the fact that the basic processes of insects are similar to those of other animals, and the responses they make to environmental temperature are similar to those of any other poikilothermous animal. This chapter includes a survey of the effects of temperature, so far as they are known, on all aspects of insect life, and shows how these basic responses are influenced by the type of animal organization which is characteristic of insects.

The class Insecta comprises a group of terrestrial Arthropoda in which are recognized a number of Orders the origins of which can be traced back to Carboniferous times. The diversity of organization shown by these Orders is relatively small, the greatest changes being associated with the origin of wings, the development of a pupal stage in the life cycle, and modifications of mouthparts arising from the exploitation of diverse food resources. Throughout the Class, the pattern of organization of cells into tissues, tissues into organs, and the disposition of organs throughout the body are surprisingly constant. Contrasting with this uniformity is the presence of a wealth of different kinds of insects, as shown by the fact that more than one million living species have been recorded. Structural differences between insect species tend to be small, but biological differences, particularly those required by the temperature and humidity regimes of climate and habitat, are pronounced.

The data which have accumulated about the effects of temperature upon insects can be arranged in a number of ways. The approach adopted here considers the properties of the insect type of organization as a system that first, must obey the laws and concepts of thermodynamics; second, has constants that are dictated by the information content of the zygote and are dynamically maintained throughout life; third, is co-ordinated within itself and with the environment; fourthly, can be altered in response to environmental changes. The chapter concludes with a tentative suggestion of a mechanism of response which can embrace most if not all of the observed changes. I believe that the advantages of this approach are that it permits an orderly account of the effects of temperature at all levels of any type of animal organization, particularly with regard to the comparisons it makes possible, and the basis it provides for theoretical and practical investigations.

II. Application of Thermodynamic Principles to Insect Systems

It is now generally agreed that the application of thermodynamic principles to living organisms is conditioned by certain concepts additional to the classical laws of the discipline. Thus, many of the chemical reactions which take place in living cells are irreversible. Moreover, these reactions are held by various constraints in steady states widely different from those they would assume if governed by simple chemical equilibria (Hill, 1931). The materials and energy to accomplish this flow through the system, thus permitting a decrease in entropy (increase in organization) in the animal without violating the classical laws of thermodynamics. Burton (1939), Reiner and Spiegelman (1945), Denbigh *et al.* (1948) and Bertalanffy (1964) have shown that the properties of open systems parallel the properties of living organisms. Most of the confirmatory work has been with micro-organisms and little has been done to consider the problems that arise when the increased complexity of body organization of multicellular organisms has to be dealt with. In the following pages, an attempt is made to orientate what is known about the energy requirements of insects and the manner in which they conform to these ideas.

A. INSECTS AS NON-ISOLATED SYSTEMS

The first condition for applying thermodynamic principles to insects is to demonstrate that no insect exists as an isolated system. As far as energy is concerned, this is self-evident since energy in the form of heat is exchanged with the environment under all known conditions. Non-isolated systems are those through which there is a flow of energy but not of matter, or those through which there is a flow of both energy and matter. The former are called closed systems, the latter, open systems.

In strict application of these definitions, all insects should be regarded as open systems since they respire, as shown by a flow of oxygen into, and of carbon dioxide out of, the animals, under all normal environments. Some insects can survive periods at a very low temperature ($-196°$), but it is not known if gas exchange takes place at these temperatures. Gas exchange has been observed in larvae of *Chironomus* at $-15°$ when the insect was partially frozen (Scholander *et al.*, 1953). Some insects (Cynipidae) can be active at temperatures as low as $-20°$ (Kinsey, 1942) and presumably respire normally at these temperatures (Fig. 1). In view of distinctions to be made later, it is more useful to regard respiration as a "non-isolating" phenomenon along with heat exchange, and to reserve the term "open system" for the flow of food and water, and "closed system" to denote the lack of flow of these substances through the insect.

1. *Energy Exchange*

The conditions for the exchange of heat energy with the environment are set whenever the body temperature of the insect is different from that of its surroundings. Heat may be lost or gained by conduction, convection, and/or radiation.

In many insects, heat exchange by conduction can be ignored since only very small areas of the tarsi are normally in contact with the substratum (Parry, 1951), and perfectly still air is a good heat insulator (Gunn, 1942). This cannot be true for aquatic insects, for those living in stored products such as flour, or for wood-boring insects However, there appears to be no information about heat exchange by conduction under these circumstances.

Heat exchange by convection is very important in insects. In the desert locust, *Schistocerca gregaria*, Church (1960) has estimated that 60–80% of the heat produced in flight is lost in this way. Heat loss by convection from a naked insect is similar to that from a smooth cylinder, the rate of heat loss being related to the wind speed, surface temperature

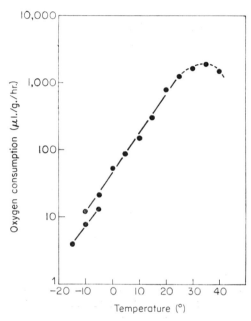

Fig. 1. Oxygen consumption of the larvae of *Anagasta kuhniella* (Zell) over a wide range of temperatures. The upper curve is for the respiration of mature larvae before spinning; the lower curve for prepupal larvae in cocoons. From Salt (1958).

excess and body size (Parry, 1951; Digby, 1955; Shepherd, 1958; Church, 1960). Natural convection must result in some small heat loss from the insect but, as pointed out by Parry (1951), conditions under which this occurs in nature are rare. Forced convection, that is, air moving over the animal due to forces generated outside the system, results in considerable exchanges of heat. Digby (1955) has shown that quite small variations in microclimatic wind speed may cause considerable differences in body temperature. The wind speed over the surface of the animal can be modified by the presence of a more or less thick coat, hairs (as with bumble bees), or scales (in the case of hawk moths).

The presence of these coats greatly diminishes heat loss due to convection (Church, 1960; Fig. 2).

Air sacs between the flight muscles and the body wall can act as heat insulators and diminish heat loss by keeping the surface temperature lower than it otherwise would be (Church, 1960). The subelytral air spaces of beetles may act in the same way (Franz, 1930). Buxton (1924) has shown that, in the beetle *Adesmia*, the temperature of the subelytral air space was within 1° of the body temperature and varied with it.

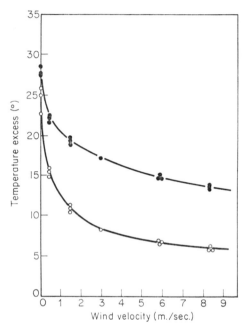

Fig. 2. The effects of wind velocity in normal and denuded *Sphinx ligustri*, artificially heated. Black circles show the effects with hair and legs intact; open circles show the effects with hair and legs removed. Redrawn from Church (1960).

Between species, there appears to be little relationship between body size and the temperature of the insect environment. Within a species, those individuals reared at temperatures towards the lower part of the tolerance range tend to be larger than those reared at the higher temperatures. Within a season, Mer (1936) has observed that the mosquitoes (*Anopheles sacharovi*) that appear at the end of the summer and at higher temperatures tend to be smaller than those appearing in spring at lower temperatures.

Radiant heat falling upon an insect will increase its body temperature above that of the surroundings. Shepherd (1958) found that, in the larvae of the sawfly, *Choristoneura fumiferana*, the increase in body

temperature varied directly with the radiation intensity. Under fixed
conditions, namely a wind speed of 50 cm./sec. and an air temperature
of 20°, Digby (1955) showed that, for radiation intensities from 0–2·0
cal./cm.²/min., body temperature excess had a linear relationship with
radiation intensity. The speed with which the maximum temperature
excess is reached, and also the final temperature attained, vary with the
size of the insect. Under a radiation intensity of 1·5 cal./cm.²/min.,

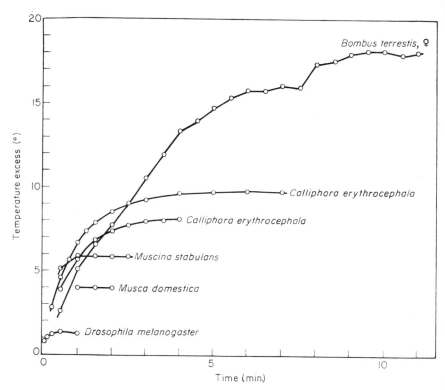

Fig. 3. Increase in temperature excess in different species of insects following
exposure to a radiation intensity of 1·5 cal./cm.²/min., at a wind speed of 50
cm./sec. From Digby (1955).

Drosophila melanogaster reaches its maximum temperature excess of 1°
in less than 1 min.; *Calliphora erythrocephala* (blowfly) that of 9° in 4
min.; and *Bombus terrestris* (bumble bee) that of 17° in 6 min., followed
by a further increase to 18° in 9 min. (Fig. 3).

The degree of absorption or reflection of radiant heat falling on the
body surface varies widely in different insects. Data given by Rucker
(1933), quoted in Parry (1951), for 21 species of insects, mostly beetles,
gave values from 10–74% reflection of radiant heat from the body

surface. Absorption of radiation may be different for different parts of the body surface. In the butterfly, *Parnassius apollo*, 95% of the radiation falling on the prominent black spots of the wings is absorbed, compared with 93% of that falling on the red spots and only 67% of that falling on the creamy outer margin of the wing (Brangham, 1962).

The body colour also is important in influencing the amount of radiation absorbed. Hill and Taylor (1933) showed that black locusts had a body temperature 3–3·5° higher than did the green form of the same animal when both were exposed to sunlight. In the grasshopper, *Calliptamus* (*Kripa*) *coelesyriensis*, which is dimorphic in colour, chocolate-coloured individuals had a body temperature 4–5° higher than the normal pink and buff form when both were exposed under the same conditions (Buxton, 1924).

The absorption of radiant heat, and the consequent body temperature excess, is influenced by the surface area of the insect exposed to the sunlight. Chapman (1959) has shown that hoppers of the red locust, *Nomadacris septemfasciata*, have body temperatures differing by 0–1·5° depending upon their orientation in the sunlight.

Heat loss from the body by long-wave radiation must occur whenever the body temperature is in excess of that of the environment (Shepherd, 1958). Some 10–15% of heat loss from flying locusts is by this means (Church, 1960).

2. Gas Exchange

The consumption of oxygen and the excretion of carbon dioxide are manifestations of the respiratory activity of the insect and continue throughout its existence. Except in one or two aquatic forms, air reaches the cells of the body without the aid of a respiratory pigment, and the oxygen-carrying capacity of the blood is limited by the solubility of oxygen in this body fluid. Insects show considerable independence of oxygen tension in their respiratory rates. For example, the rate is independent of tension over the range 7·5–100% oxygen in *Calliphora erythrocephala* larvae (Fraenkel and Herford, 1938). High oxygen tension does not have a harmful effect until it is at a pressure of several atmospheres (Keister and Buck, 1964), when it can be extremely harmful at certain stages in development (Goldsmith and Schneiderman, 1960).

In the majority of insects, the greater part of the gas exchange takes place through the tracheal system. Simple diffusion is adequate to supply the demands of insects less than 0·1 g. in weight, but heavier insects must supplement diffusion with ventilatory movements. A comparison between the demands for oxygen imposed upon the insect by its normal activity, and those imposed by temperature changes over the viable range, suggests that the tracheal system is not a limiting factor in the effects of temperature upon the respiration of the insect. Polacek and Kubista (1960) showed that, in *Periplaneta americana* at 20°, the oxygen consumption at rest was 0·36 mm.^{3}/mg./hr. and this could increase to 36 mm.^{3}/mg./hr. when the insect vibrated its wings. Richards (1963a) found that, for this insect, oxygen consumption ranged from 0·05 mm.^{3}/mg./hr. at 3° to 0·91 mm.^{3}/mg./hr. at 35°. In the adult fly, *Phromina regina*, oxygen consumption increases from 0·09 μl./mg./hr. at 0° to 5·03 μl./mg./hr. at 45° (Keister and Buck, 1961), while for the butterfly, *Thais cassandra*, at an air temperature of 20–25° the resting oxygen consumption of 4 mm.^{3}/mg./hr. was raised by a nicotine-induced "buzz" to 216 mm.^{3}/mg./hr. (Raffy and Portier, 1931). These last figures show that the tracheal system can easily handle a flow of oxygen to the cells greatly in excess of that induced by a temperature increase. Even if the demands of temperature are added to those of flight, the increase is not great and the variable demands of flight (10–30 mm.^{3}/mg./hr. in *Schistocerca gregaria*; Krogh and Weis-Fogh, 1951) show that this could easily be accommodated by the tracheal system. In aquatic insects, there is some evidence that temperature may influence the mechanisms of gas exchange to the extent of being a limiting factor. Popham (1964) found that the physical gills of *Notonecta glauca* failed to function at 15°, those of *Corixa punctata* at 28°, and those of *Naucoris cimicoides* at 35–40°.

B. OPEN AND CLOSED SYSTEMS IN INSECT ORGANIZATION

A further distinction is made in non-isolated systems between "closed" and "open" systems. By considering gas exchange along with energy exchange as "non-isolating" phenomena, we can distinguish in insects stages in the life history when they approximate to closed systems and stages when they are open systems. A further discussion of the application of these terms will follow after dealing with the flow of water and food through the insect body.

1. *Flow of Water Through the Insect Body*

Water is taken into the insect body by drinking, with the food (Mellanby and French, 1958) or by absorption through the cuticle (Beament, 1964). The intake of water with the food is the most important source in desert-dwelling insects where the hygroscopic food materials retain the dew that condenses from the atmosphere at night, thereby making it available for diurnal species (Buxton, 1924).

The active uptake of water through the cuticle may occur in actively feeding forms (Beament, 1964) but, in non-feeding stages such as eggs and pupae, it is the only way of absorbing water. The eggs of insects, almost without exception, absorb water through the cuticle from their environment; during the course of embryonic development, the amount absorbed may be equal to the weight of the egg. This uptake of water is affected by temperature, and curves for the uptake show differences related to the temperature of rearing (Browning, 1953; Fig. 4).

The water content of the insect body ranges from 50–90% of the total body weight (Wigglesworth, 1950). It is likely to vary in amount in any one insect at different times. In nymphs of the migratory locust, *Locusta migratoria*, the tissues are bathed in a considerable volume of haemocoelic fluid, but in older adults hardly any fluid can be found in the haemocoele (Hoyle, 1954). A decrease in the amount of body water is always associated with an increased resistance of the insect to cold. This

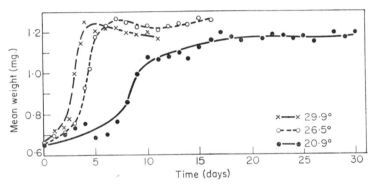

FIG. 4. Changes in the mean weight of eggs of *Gryllulus commodus* during incubation at three different temperatures. The increase in weight is mainly due to the absorption of water from the environment. From Browning (1953).

is partially due to depression of the freezing point of the haemocoelic fluid and partially due to the increased concentration of solutes in it. However, for this to have any appreciable effect on the cold tolerance of the insect, concentrations harmful to the organism would have to be attained (Salt, 1961; Edney, 1957).

Extreme dehydration, when the body water content decreases to 8% or less, occurs in some insects and these animals are very resistant to temperature extremes. The larvae of the fly, *Polypedilum vanderplanki*, in this condition, can be exposed to temperatures down to −270° and up to 106° and show signs of life upon return to normal conditions (Hinton, 1960).

The sites of water loss from the body are the tracheal system, the cuticle, and the gut. As Mellanby (1934) showed in the beetle, *Tenebrio molitor*, under normal conditions the main site of water loss is from the tracheal system. The cuticle is very impermeable over the normal

temperature range of the animal, but there is an upper temperature
above which the permeability of the cuticle rapidly increases until water
loss approaches that of a free water surface (Ramsay, 1935). The
temperature at which this occurs varies for different species of insects
and is related to the requirements of their habitats (Beament, 1945;
Fig. 5). This increased permeability is due to the loss of orientation of
the wax molecules in the thin film of cuticular wax upon which the

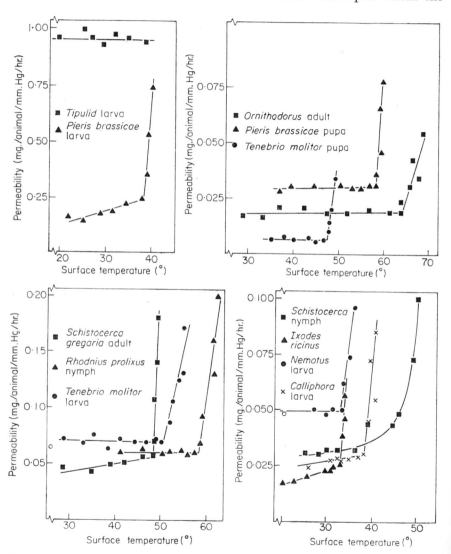

FIG. 5. Changes in the permeability to water of a number of arthropods at various
cuticular temperatures. From Beament (1959).

waterproofing of the cuticle depends (Beament, 1964). In the Orthoptera there may be special areas of the cuticle from which water is lost (Makings, 1964). The rate of evaporation of water is not related to the amount of water present in the body or to the concentration of solutes in the haemocoelic fluid, but is related to the concentration of water vapour in the air around the insect (Beament, 1964).

Other factors being equal, the rate of evaporation from the insect body is proportional to the saturation deficiency of the air; the greater the deficiency, the greater the rate of evaporation (Johnson, 1942). Due to the high latent heat of evaporation of water, this will have a cooling effect upon the insect body. The loss of 1% of the body weight of water by evaporation in an animal weighing 1 g. can lower the body temperature by 5–6°. It is generally estimated that an insect can lose 20–40% of its body weight in the form of water before it dies from desiccation. The cooling effect that can be achieved, although relatively short lived, may nevertheless have survival value for insects in certain habitats (Mellanby, 1932; Buxton, 1930). If there is a flow of water into the animal to compensate for this loss, then it is possible for the insect to become independent of the saturation deficiency of the air, at least over quite a large range. In those individuals of the bug, *Dysdercus fasciatus*, having access to drinking water which the animal can take through a pinhole opening, relative humidities of 20–90% have little effect on the growth of the animal (Clarke and Sardesai, 1959). There appears to be only one estimate of the rate of turnover of water in the insect body. Govaerts and Leclercq (1946), using D_2O, estimated that the body water was completely exchanged in 5–13 days.

Some absorption of water may take place through the insect cuticle. When this happens, the amount of water in the air is more conveniently expressed by the relative humidity than by the saturation deficiency (Beament, 1964).

2. *Flow of Food through the Insect Body*

While in general there is a flow of water into and out of the insect at all stages of its life history, the flow of food into, and excretory products out of, the insect are more restricted. No flow of material occurs through the egg or the pupae, and in species scattered through all the orders of insects there are adults which do not feed, but depend upon reserves laid down in the larvae or nymphal stages. In the feeding stages, the intake of food is not a continuous process, but is shown as a period of "alimentation indispensable" and "alimentation facultative" during an instar (Bounhiol, 1938), and as shorter periods of feeding and non-feeding in the course of its daily activity. In a few species, such as the tsetse fly (Buxton, 1955), there are longer, well-defined cycles of food intake, and egg maturation. The flow of materials through the animal then is intermittent, an important deviation from the conditions assumed in much open-system theory where it is supposedly continuous.

During a feeding stage, the desire to take in food depends upon the internal nutritional demands which are related to general metabolic regulation (Dadd, 1963). The amount passed through the system per day is very variable. Davey (1954) showed that, in the laboratory, nymphs and adults of *Schistocerca gregaria* would consume half their own weight of food per day. Weis-Fogh (1952) confirmed this for adults, and calculated from the energy requirements of flying locusts that, in the field, the insect must eat from $1\frac{1}{2}$–3 times its body weight per day. The total amount of food eaten over any period varies with the temperature at which the insects are kept. In the grasshopper, *Melanoplus atlantus*, for the first 20 days of adult life, food consumption was, in dry weights, 4·8 g. at 27°, 8·9 g. at 32°, and 11·5 g. at 37°; but in the nymphs the total amount consumed was the same at all three temperatures. At alternating temperatures, the amount of food consumed was less than would be expected in terms of weighted means based on requirements at constant temperatures (Parker, 1930). Under unfavourable temperatures, more food may be required to accomplish certain physiological processes than is necessary at favourable ones. In *Anopheles maculipennis messeae*, the amount of food required during the maturation of the eggs is greater at extremes than at normal temperatures (Shlenova, 1938). The sawfly, *Neodiprion sertifer*, uses only 80–85% of its fat reserves to produce eggs at 10°, while at 20° the fat reserves are completely exhausted (Campbell and Sullivan, 1963). Heavy feeding may affect the resistance of the animal to unfavourable temperatures. In the beetles, *Chrysomela gemina* and *C. hyperici*, heavy feeding in the autumn may lead to a decreased frost resistance in the animal (Harris, 1962).

The rates at which food passes through the gut, is digested, and absorbed are also a function of temperature. Schreiner (1952) observed that the passage of fluid through the gut of the honey bee was more rapid when the energy demands were greater, and that the passage of pollen was faster at 37° than at room temperature. In the mosquito, *Aedes aegypti*, the rate of digestion of serum proteins has an average Q_{10} value of 2 between 15° and 35° (Williams, quoted in Clements, 1963), and the digestion of sucrose in *Oxycarenus hyalinipennis*, and the absorption of sugars from the gut, are slower at 19° than at 35° (Bhatnagar, 1963). Frass drop studies can be used as an indication of the rate of feeding, and are a direct measure of the loss of matter from the insect. In larvae of *Neodiprion americanus* and *N. lecontei*, material is passed through the system at temperatures between 6° and 36°, and the rate is greatly influenced by temperature (Green and de Freitas, 1955).

The effects of temperature on the nutritional requirements of insects are hard to judge. Dietary requirements tend to be different at different stages of the life history (House, quoted in Rockstein, 1965) and in many instances are determined by the genetic constitution of the insect (Hinton, 1955; Hinton and Dunlap, 1958). The beetle, *Tribolium castaneum*, kept in an atmosphere with a relative humidity of 70% and fed on ground nuts, takes 45·5 days to complete total development at 35°, 64 days at 30°, and 93·4 days at 25°; corresponding values when fed on wheatfeed are 20·3, 27·2 and 44·6 days respectively (Howe, 1956). Temperature effects on nutrition are also manifest when the insect has become dependent upon some micro-organism for an essential nutrient, and the temperature ranges of the insect and the micro-organism do not coincide. In the cockroach, *Blatella germanica*, the micro-organisms (bacteriods) can effectively be removed from the tissues by exposing the animal to 37–39°. In adults the asymbiotic forms so produced show impaired reproductive abilities. The high temperature prevents the transovarian inheritance of the bacteriods so that the offspring of these animals are also asymbiotic. These nymphs show a greatly diminished growth rate which can be improved by including massive doses of yeast in their diet (Brooks and Richards, 1955). A similar failure to grow after the removal of micro-organisms by exposure to high temperatures has been observed in termites (Cleveland, 1924), and the cockroach, *Periplaneta americana* (Glaser, 1946). Asymbiotic strains of *Sitophilus granarius* have been found in the tropics, and it is suggested that this is the result of the naturally high environmental temperature (Schneider, 1954). In general, however, it seems likely that the diet of an insect normally contains enough nutrients to offset any additional demands that temperature extremes may thrust on the animal.

3. *Insects as Open and Closed Systems*

By strict definition, all insects must be regarded as open systems under all naturally occurring conditions since gas exchange is an exchange of mass with the environment. It is, however, convenient to disregard this, and to determine whether an insect is an "open" or "closed" system on the basis of the flow of food and water into the animal. Of these two criteria, food flow shows the better correlation with other features of insect organization, so that it is useful to regard non-feeding insects as closed systems and feeding insects as open systems. As has been pointed out, eggs, pupae, and some adults do not feed, and should therefore be regarded as closed systems. While this is true of the system as a whole, the actively metabolizing tissues within an egg, pupa or adult are not closed systems, since material flows through them from the reserves of the yolk and fat body. This supply is, however, limited and thus imposes a restriction not necessarily operative in open systems. Thus, in the eggs of the bug *Oncopeltis fasciatus* at subthreshold temperatures, the rate of development is too slow to be completed before the energy reserves are used up, though at higher temperatures the reserves are adequate for development to be completed (Richards, 1958).

C. STEADY AND UNSTEADY STATES IN INSECTS

Throughout the Class Insecta, examples may be found which indicate that it is possible for every stage of the life history (egg, larva, nymph, pupa, and adult) to exist in one of two states; a normal active state, or an inactive state known as diapause. The change from one state to another may be an integral part of the development of the animal or it may occur only in certain environmental circumstances. With few exceptions, mostly insects from high mountain environments, an individual goes into diapause only once during its life history.

The energy requirements of the two states are very different. Taylor and Crescitelli (1937) have shown a close relationship between the heat output and oxygen consumption in the pupae of the moth *Galleria mellonella* (Fig. 6). The relationship is not a very rigid one but close enough to relate oxygen requirements to energy production. In the moth *Platysamia cecropia* at 25°, the oxygen consumption of the prediapause pupae is 0·15 mm.^{3}/ mg./hr., and in the diapausing pupae it is 0·016 mm.^{3}/mg./hr.; the respiratory quotient (0·78) is the same in both states (Schneiderman and Williams, 1953).

The rate of turnover of specific metabolites is also greater in the active than in the diapause state. In protein synthesis the rate of [1-^{14}C] valine incorporation is increased by a factor of two for the midgut, and of 200 for the blood following a change from the diapause to the active state (Skinner, 1960). An increase in the rate of incorporation of [1-^{14}C] glycine into protein has been observed in pupae of the moth *Platysamia cecropia* (Telfer and Williams, 1960) and in *Sphinx ligustri* (Bricteux-Gregoire *et al.*, 1957), and for [^{35}S] methionine incorporation in *Antheraea peryni* (Demjanowski *et al.*, 1952) following a change from the diapause to the active state. Associated with this, there is a low level of incorporation of labelled inorganic phosphate into RNA in diapause pupae which increases with the onset of development (Wyatt, 1959). The ratio of RNA to DNA, which is 5:6 in diapause, becomes 7:4 with the change to the active state (Wyatt, 1959).

In addition to the different level of activity there is evidence that, in diapause, the insect is in, or very close to, a true steady state. Telfer and Williams (1960) observed that the protein content of the blood does not

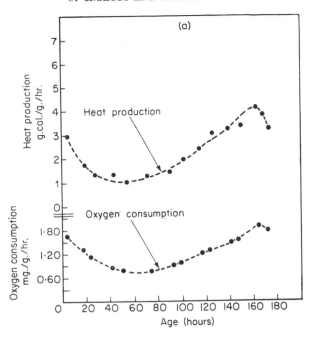

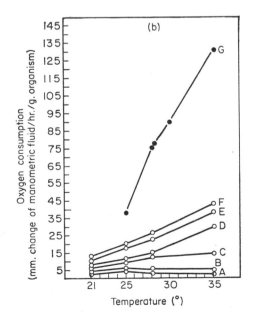

FIG. 6

(a) The relationship between heat production and oxygen consumption in a male pupa of *Galleria mellonella* during development at 30°. From Taylor and Crescitelli (1937).

(b) The effects of temperature on the oxygen consumption of diapausing and non-diapausing *Sceliphron caementarium*. Curve A, animal at beginning of diapause; B, at the middle of diapause; C, at the end of diapause; D, animal coming out of diapause; E, entering pupal stage; F, pupal stage; G, animal ready to emerge. From Bodine and Evans (1932).

change during diapause though some incorporation of amino acids into blood protein could be demonstrated. Protein must therefore be degraded at a rate equal to its formation. From these data they concluded that diapause is a true steady state in which the system is being maintained at a low energy level, possibly by the maintenance of permeability barriers and/or the activation of hydrolytic enzymes. In many insects it has been observed that the diapause state can last for several years and may be regarded as approaching a time-independent state. Whether an organism ever conforms rigidly with the definition of a steady state, in which the rates of change of *all* of the variables vanish (Burton, 1939), is still an unsolved problem. Certainly, as compared

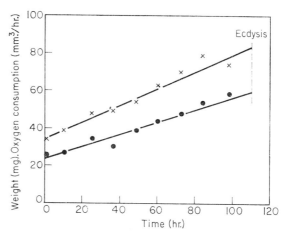

FIG. 7. Fluctuations in weight and oxygen consumption throughout the 4th. instar of *Locusta migratoria*. X denotes weight; O, oxygen consumption. Trend lines were fitted by the method of least squares. From Clarke (1957).

with the active state, the diapause state in insects approaches this condition.

The active state might be called the "unsteady" state and this indeed describes one of its principal features. Heat output is very variable over short intervals of time. In *Periplaneta americana*, with a background heat output of the order of 0·5 cal./g./hr. at 25°, there occur paroxysms of heat output of the order of 5–6 cal./g./hr. occurring every few minutes. The ratio of the maximum to the minimum heat output varies from 2–6 within the temperature range 24°–37° (Calvet and Prat, 1963). Considerable variation in oxygen consumption, associated with the intermittent nature of food intake, is to be found in nymphs of *Locusta migratoria* (Clarke, 1957; Fig. 7). Considerable changes can occur in the amounts of substrates and enzymes present in connection with the normal hazards the insect is likely to encounter. The level of labelled α-glycerophosphate in the thorax of the housefly, *Musca domestica*, which under light cyclopropane anaesthesia is 20·9% of total soluble ^{32}P recovered from the head and thorax, may be decreased to 12·7% by non-flying activity and a little further by flight. Starvation has little effect until the prostration stage is reached when it falls to 11%. The level of ATP in the head of the housefly can be decreased from 35·9 to 14·8% by starvation, an effect that is reversed by feeding glucose to the insect (Winteringham, 1960).

The long-term time-dependent changes that occur in the unsteady state are the growth and development of the insect from the zygote stage to the reproductive stage in the adult instar. These processes tend to be cyclical, the period of each cycle lasting considerably longer than the short-term changes of starvation and activity described above. Practically the whole of the unsteady state duration is occupied by these changes. When any long period of developmental stasis occurs, the insect switches to the steady diapause state. Exceptions may occur in the bug *Rhodnius prolixus* when, prior to a blood meal in each instar, development does not occur but the creature remains active; or in adults such as *Nomadacris septemfasciata* which can remain for a long period in a prereproductive state in the adult instar. Experience shows that, in starved insects, steady states of long enough duration for a basal metabolic rate to be determined do not occur.

The general effect of temperature on growth is to increase the rate of growth with an increase in temperature over the viable range of the species, the response curve being sigmoid in form. The final size reached by the insect varies with temperature, a larger body size usually being attained when they are reared at the lower temperatures of their viable range as shown for *Drosophila melanogaster* by Anders *et al.* (1964). However, little difference was found in the adult weights of *Dysdercus fasciatus* reared at different temperatures (Clarke and Sardesai, 1959). *Locusta migratoria*, when subjected to fluctuating temperatures, are heavier than those held at a mean constant temperature, but do not vary by more than 10% from values founded on weights of individuals grown at the extremes of the range (K. U. Clarke, unpublished observations). The effect of size influences the reproductive rate of the female (Waloff and Richards, 1958), while Huot and Leclercq (1958) have shown that small individuals are more likely to be affected by dietary deficiencies than are large ones. Care should therefore be taken to consider whether the effects of temperature on survival and reproduction are not secondary to the main effect of temperature on adult size.

From this general account of the application of thermodynamic principles to insects, the following basic points emerge. During its life history, an insect is at different stages a closed or an open system. The closed stages (egg, pupa, and non-feeding adult) draw on reserves within the system so that the actively metabolizing tissues within them act as open systems but, since they have limited resources to draw on, can exhaust these reserves under certain circumstances. In the open condition, the flow of material through the system is not constant but intermittent. The rate and amount flowing through varies with temperature, but there is some evidence that the total amount that must flow through to allow the insect to reach a certain stage in development is the same at all temperatures at which the insect remains viable.

Regardless of whether the system is closed or open, it can exist in a steady or an unsteady state. Usually the steady state is a closed system, but the unsteady state occurs regularly in both open and closed systems. The steady state is so, only relative to the unsteady state of the insect. It may be truly steady and time-independent, but is always a low-energy state. The unsteady state is a high-energy state, constantly changing in time both in response to the fluctuations of the environment and to the developmental instructions within the insect's genetic system.

III. Information Content and Constants of the Insect System

One of the characteristics of an open system is that its properties are set by the constants that control it (Bertalanffy, 1950). These constants, in the present theory, are reaction rates and diffusion rates. Their occurrence and their character in the insect must, as in any other animal, depend upon the presence of information which dictates the kinds and amounts of molecules that the insect can synthesize. The bulk of this information is contained within the genetic system, although some is derived from cytoplasmic sources and is passed from parent to offspring in the maternal line (Saunders, 1964; Clarke et al., 1960). By mutation of the genes, crossing over of the chromosomes at meiosis, and alterations in the chromosome number, changes occur in the information passed from the parent to the offspring. These processes, and hence the stability of the genetic information, are influenced by environmental temperature.

A. THE STABILITY OF THE GENOME

The rate of formation of lethal mutants in a population of *Drosophila melanogaster* that had been cleared of them through four generations, and had been tested for the presence of lethal mutants through three generations for the 1st. chromosome and four generations for the 2nd. chromosome, showed an increased mutation rate at high temperatures

(Plough, 1941). Ives (quoted in Plough, 1941) pointed out that the effects of temperature on the formation of lethal and "visible" mutations may not be the same. A few genes which are very unstable under normal conditions occur in *Drosophila virilis*. Their mutation rate is unaffected by many environmental conditions, including a 10° rise in temperature (Demerec, 1932). These studies relate to insects that have been exposed to the appropriate constant temperatures for long periods of time. Brief exposures to temperatures near the lethal limit (temperature shock) can also induce mutations (Plough, 1941). Low temperatures as well as high are effective. Larvae of *Drosophila* exposed to − 6° for 25–40 min. showed a tripling of the rate of production of lethal mutants on the X and 2nd. chromosomes (Birkina, 1938). An inverse relationship between temperature and mutation rate has been observed in *Drosophila* (Gowen and Gay, 1933). The mutation rate at constant temperatures has a Q_{10} value of 2–3 (Plough, 1941).

Zimmering (1963) found that the frequency with which the Y chromosome was lost in male *Drosophila* was significantly higher at 26° than at 18°. In *Talaeporia*, the prevalence of high temperatures during oogenesis favours the appearance of the X chromosome in the female pronucleus, while low temperatures favour its inclusion in the polar body (Davey, 1965). The effect of temperature on the cross-over frequency in *Drosophila* is complex, there being two maxima, one at 14° and the other at 31° (Plough, 1917). White (1934) found that the frequency of chiasma formation did not increase between 0° and 42° in *Locusta migratoria*, between 2° and 45° in *Schistocerca gregaria*, and between 2° and 37° in the grasshopper, *Stenobothrus parallelus*. In addition there was some terminalization of the chiasma in these temperature ranges. This was also observed in *Schistocerca gregaria* at high temperatures by Henderson (1963), who observed a diminution in chiasma frequency in males kept at 40°. All levels of univalence have been observed, depending upon the duration of the temperature treatment and the sensitivity of the individual insect. In *Melanoplus*, Lima-de-Faria (1961) has noted that chiasma formation occurs most frequently at the sites of DNA replication. In general, there is no increase in the frequency of mutations due to changes in temperature that occur while the animal is exposed to the source of radiation (Sollunn and Strömnaes, 1964). The mutational response pattern which results from this is related to the phase of the spermatogenic cycle in the irradiated insect. Recovery from radiation by rejoining of the broken ends of the chromosomes is adversely affected by increasing temperatures (Ives, 1962).

Temperatures towards the extremes of the animal's tolerance range may bring about inactivation of the nuclei. When the egg of the honey bee, *Apis mellifica*, is chilled to 4–6° for 1–4 hr., adult gyandromorphs appear in the population. From 7,000 chilled eggs, 79 of the 3,194 survivors showed the presence of both male and female tissues; none appeared in the controls. The cold inactivates the female pronucleus but allows further development of the male (Drescher and Rothenbuhler, 1963). Similar results have been obtained by exposing the eggs of the silk moth, *Bombyx mori*, to high temperatures. In this insect, the maximum sensitivity to the heat treatment occurs at the anaphase of the first, and at the metaphase of the second, meiotic divisions when the cell is inactivated (Ostryakova-Varshaver, 1958, 1960).

Changes may occur in the ratio of nuclear:cytoplasmic material with changes in temperature. Frankhauser (1942) recorded that, if the unfertilized eggs of *Bombyx mori* are immersed in water at 46° for 18 min., parthenogenesis is induced and, in 25% of the eggs, fusion of the diploid nuclei occur during the early cleavage stages, resulting in tetraploid or partially tetraploid individuals. Henderson (1963) has found that, in *Schistocerca gregaria*, treatment at high and low temperatures can result in the formation of some tetraploid spermatocytes. In the weevil (*Otiorrhynchus dubius*) in addition to the normal bi-sexual diploid race there occurs a tetraploid parthenogenic race which has a 2° lower temperature tolerance (Lindroth, 1954). The ratio of nuclear DNA to cytoplasmic RNA may also change as a result of the different responses of cell growth and cell division to temperature. Bodenstein (quoted in Roeder, 1953) recorded that, in the stick insect, *Dixippus*, at temperatures above 20°, the cell number decreases while cell size begins to increase. These two processes do not compensate for each other, and the overall size of the animal decreases. Li and Yu-lin (1936) found that, in vestigial wings in *Drosophila melanogaster*, the increase in size due to a rise in temperature was brought about by an increase in the number rather than the size of the cells. Richards (1951) also found that, in *Drosophila*, high temperatures promoted cell division and resulted in the formation of smaller cells, at least in the epidermis.

B. TRANSCRIPTION AND TRANSLATION OF THE GENETIC INFORMATION

The genetic system contains information that is decoded in the synthesis of specific proteins and enzymes, which will in turn constitute the system and set its constants. It is here assumed that, in insects, the translation of the code into proteins follows the model given by Jacob and Monod (1961) for micro-organisms, and modified by Goodwin (1963) for multicellular organisms.

There is evidence that temperature may have an important effect on the processes of transcribing and translating the genetic information in insects. Primarily the effect is on the formation of substances at the gene locus. Changes in the quantity of DNA probably do not occur since Evans (1956) found that cold treatment was without effect on the amount of DNA in the grasshopper, *Chortophaga viridifasciata*. In *Chironomus*, larvae which have been kept at 5° for at least 1 hr. and then transferred to 20° show, after $1\frac{1}{2}$–$2\frac{1}{2}$ hr., an accumulation of droplets that appear regularly at certain loci in the chromosomes. These droplets vanish 8 hr. after the transfer. Their formation is attributed to a temporary shift in the balance between reaction and diffusion rates (Beerman, 1959). Stich (1959) observed in the midge, *Chironomus*, that, over a period of 2 days, the nucleolus at the end of the "small" chromosome decreased in size and vanished, while that at the other end increased in size when the insect was transferred from 4° to 20°.

In further discussion on the effects of temperature on the formation of the insect system constants, it is convenient to distinguish between those primarily concerned with energy and maintenance, and those involved with the development of the insect. The former must function throughout the life of the insect; their responses to temperature will not therefore be time-dependent. The processes related to them can continue for long periods under conditions which will restrict RNA formation (Laufer *et al.*, 1964). Developmental effects of temperature, on the other hand, are very largely time-dependent. The occurrence of specific proteins of transient existence has been shown in the pupal development of *Platysamia cecropia, Samia cynthia* and *Phromina regina* (Laufer, 1963), and in *Chironomus thummi* their development may be regulated by the sequence of gene expression and gene repression. The short duration of protein production necessitates the continuous and unrestricted formation of the homologous m-RNA (Laufer *et al.*, 1964).

C. ENERGY AND MAINTENANCE CONSTANTS OF THE SYSTEM

In insects, as in other animals, ATP is the common currency in energy production within the cell. In muscle, the release of energy from ATP is accomplished through the action of the enzyme ATP-ase which splits off the terminal phosphate group of the molecule. The activity of this enzyme in relation to temperature has been extensively studied in insect muscle, and the enzyme has been prepared from the thoracic and femoral muscles of *Locusta migratoria* and *Gastrimargus musicus*. In tests of 5 min. duration, maximum activity of the enzyme occurred at 42° above which temperature it decreased. The response of this enzyme to temperature is not linear over its full range. Between 5° and 20°, the reaction velocity gives a straight line relationship on a log. V versus $1/T$ plot; above 20°, the rate of increase in activity falls off (Gilmour and Calaby, 1952). The enzyme has an extremely high activation energy. Values reported include 21,000 cal./mole (Chin, 1951), 29,600 cal./mole

(Gilmour and Calaby, 1952); for the *Periplaneta americana* enzyme, Davison and Richards (1954) reported a value of 20,000 cal./mole. The enzyme is sensitive to Mg^{2+} and Mn^{2+} ions, and the difference in values may be attributed to differences in the ion content of reaction mixtures used by these investigators. The Q_{10} values for this enzyme are also high. Gilmour and Calaby (1952) found a Q_{10} value of 4 for the enzyme from *Locusta migratoria*, and Davison and Richards (1954) a value of 3·5–4 for the enzyme from *Periplaneta americana*. The former authors considered that the temperature properties of this enzyme offer, at the biochemical level, an explanation for the high degree of dependence of muscular activity in insects upon environmental temperature.

The monosaccharides in insect blood represent only a small proportion of the total carbohydrates present. Variations in the amounts of glucose present have been induced in *Apis mellifica* by extreme heat (Lensky, 1964). Abnormalities in the absorption and utilization of glucose have also been shown to occur in honey bees at low temperatures (Martignoni, 1964). The common sugar of the insect blood is the oligosaccharide, trehalose (Wyatt and Kalf, 1957). The amount present in the blood is influenced by the hormones of the corpora allata (Steele, 1961). The amount of trehalose in the blood of *Calliphora erythrocephala* increases when the insect is exposed to 4° for a period of 12 days (Dutrieu, 1961). Trehalose is hydrolysed by the enzyme trehalase. This enzyme has been purified from insect tissues and shows a maximum rate of hydrolysis at 45°, above which it is rapidly inactivated. It is apparently tolerant to cold since it can be stored at −12° for 2 months without loss of activity (Chefurka, 1965). Trehalase activity has been observed to be specifically decreased in actinomycin D-treated *Drosophila* salivary glands (Laufer et al., 1964), and it was concluded that the antibiotic affected synthesis of the enzyme.

Transglycosidation in some insects, such as the pea aphid, may be dependent on, or vary with, temperature since oligosaccharides have been found in the honey dew of aphids at 20° but not at 15° (Dehn, quoted by Auclair, 1963).

One of the major changes associated with a decrease in temperature is the production of sorbitol and glycerol from glycogen which occurs in some insects (Chino, 1958). Glycerol, which may occur in insect blood in concentrations as high as 5 M, plays an important part in the cold hardiness of many insects (Salt, 1959).

Most insects can probably synthesize all of the fatty acids they require, although a few need dietary sources of some unsaturated fatty acids (Dadd, 1960). House et al. (1958) have found that, by feeding *Calliphora erythrocephala* larvae on a diet of highly saturated lipid, it was possible to increase their heat resistance. The degree of saturation of fatty acids in insects has been observed to vary with the season (Timon-David, 1930), with the diet, and with the stage in the life history (Yuill and Craig, 1937). Little change has been found, at least in the depot fats, in the lipid composition with changes in temperature. Rainey (1938) found only a slight and insignificant difference in the iodine numbers of the lipids from larvae of the fly *Lucilia* reared at 15°, 25° and 35°. Ditman and Weiland (1938) again found only a small tempera-

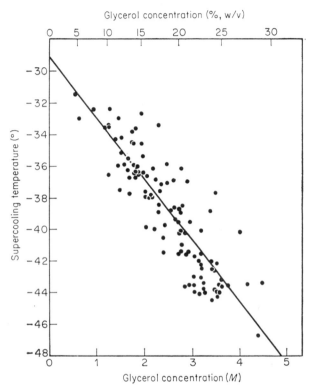

FIG. 8. Relationship between supercooling temperatures and glycerol concentrations in 109 *Bracon cephi* larvae of variable cold hardiness. From Salt (1959).

ture effect on the iodine numbers of lipids in *Heliothus*. Recently Niemierko (1959) has summed up the situation by stating that, while there is good agreement between temperature and the degree of fatty acid saturation in vegetable fats, in insects this relationship does not hold.

The property of some insect lipids to remain liquid at temperatures at which others are solid is related to some property other than the degree of saturation. Of two wood-boring beetles, *Ergates faber* and *Oryctes nasicornis*, the former has liquid and the latter solid lipids at

11+T.

room temperature (Timon-David, 1927). In the aphid, *Rhopalosiphum prunifolia*, the temperature at which the lipid solidifies increased with increased rearing temperature (Ackerman, 1926). In *Melanoplus differentialis*, the lipid globules are liquid, while in *Chortophaga viridifasciata* they are solid at room temperature. Both lipids have the same iodine number; the lower melting point of the former is attributed to the short-chain fatty acids present (Slifer, 1930, 1932).

Temperature-dependent changes in the respiratory rate may be taken as evidence of the different energy requirements of the insect with change in temperature. Such studies should include measurements of

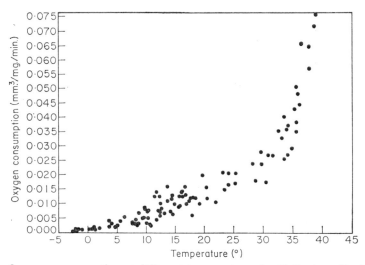

FIG. 9. Oxygen consumption at different temperatures by *Pollenia rudis* showing a plateau in the curve between 20° and 30°. From Argo (1939).

oxygen consumption, carbon dioxide output, and calculations of the respiratory quotients. The majority of studies, however, are of oxygen consumption alone and, as Keister and Buck (1964) have pointed out, the increased oxygen consumption with an increase of temperature is perhaps the most over-confirmed fact in insect physiology. Usually oxygen consumption is low at low temperatures and increases rapidly with rising temperature, the increase terminating abruptly and the consumption falling rapidly as the temperature approaches the upper lethal limit.

Perhaps the most interesting feature shown in the oxygen consumption curves of some insects is the occurrence of a plateau where an increase in temperature is not accompanied by an increase in oxygen consumption. This is shown by adults of the fly *Pollenia rudis* in which no increase occurs between 20° and 30° (Argo, 1939; Fig. 9) and

Phromia larvae where the plateau occurs between 10° and 15° (Keister and Buck, 1961). A similar phenomenon may be found with carbon dioxide excretion, and Slowtzoff (1909) found no increase in the carbon dioxide output of the beetle *Geotrupes stercoralis* between 12° and 24°.

There is some evidence from gas exchange experiments of a shift towards lipid utilization at low temperatures. In hibernating nymphs of *Chortophaga*, the respiratory quotient falls from 0·83 to 0·62 when the temperature drops from 27° to 15° (Kleinman, 1934).

D. TIME-DEPENDENT CONSTANTS OF THE SYSTEM

The duration of insect development at constant temperature decreases as the temperature increases until a temperature is reached near the upper thermal tolerance of the insect, when the duration again increases until this limit is reached. The rate of development also increases as the temperature is raised, and decreases rapidly as the upper thermal limit is approached (Uvarov, 1931). A comparison of the times taken for the successive stages of embryonic development to be reached at 20° and 27° in *Schistocerca gregaria* indicated that all stages were evenly accelerated by an increase in temperature (Fig. 10; Shulov and Penner, 1963). Bates (1947) found that, at high temperatures, the metamorphosis of mosquitoes of the genus *Haemagogus* proceeded at such a rate that the capacity of the species to form tissues was not fully realized. In *Anopheles gambiae*, the number of teeth on the maxillae increases with increasing temperature (Gillies and Shute, 1954), and this may indicate small changes in the relative rates of tissue formation at different temperatures.

The temperature range over which the information contained in a gene can express itself may not correspond with the temperature range for viability of an insect. A strain of the moth, *Panaxia dominula*, has been reported which produces normal colour forms when reared at temperatures above 22°. Below 21°, a new recessive and an intermediate colour form separate out in the ratio of 1:2:1, indicating that the recessive gene could not express itself at temperatures above 22° (Kettlewell, 1944). In *Aedes* subgenus *Ochlerotatus* there are 11 subarctic species in which males develop normally below 23°, but, with increasing temperatures, the male characteristics are progressively repressed and do not appear at all above 28·4° (Horsfall and Anderson, 1964). In *Aedes aegypti* Craig (1965) has shown that sex reversal at high temperatures is dependent upon the presence of an autosomal recessive gene sex-linked in expression. Its presence is not revealed at low temperatures.

Hartung (1947) studied the effects of temperature upon the occurrence of spontaneous tumours in *Drosophila melanogaster*, the susceptibility

to which is inherited. Five strains were studied at five different temperatures between 20° and 30°. Three of the strains showed highest incidence
at low temperatures; in one, temperature had little influence on the
frequency of occurrence, and in the fifth, the incidence was highest at
23–28° and less at temperatures above and below these values. Gardner

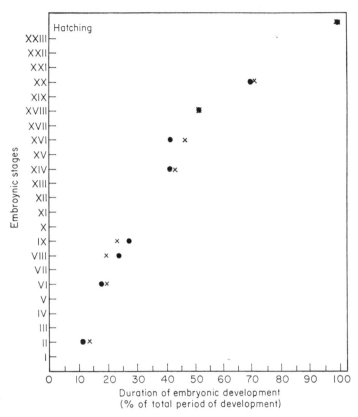

FIG. 10. The duration of the period of embryonic development, from oviposition
to various embryo stages, at 20° (crosses) and 27° (dots) in *Schistocerca gregaria*,
expressed as percentages of the total period of development. From Shulov and
Penner (1963).

and Woolf (1950) found that the expression of the tumorous head increased with increasing temperature, and had a frequency of 93% at
30°. The most favourable temperature regime for the expression and
penetrance of the tumorous head was that of high temperatures in the
embryonic stages and low temperatures in the pupal stages (Hillman,
1962). Akita and Nakayama (1954) found that the expression and
penetrance of vg^{nr} mutant genes in *Drosophila* were kept to a minimum

by subjecting the insect to high temperatures in early development and low temperatures in later stages.

Many observations suggest that the temperature responses of insect heterozygotes and homozygotes are different. In *Drosophila pseudo-obscura*, the longevities of the homozygotes WT/WT and KL/KL at 15° are 166 and 165 days respectively, while that of the heterozygote is 174 days. In some species, the longevity of the heterozygote is intermediate between that of the homozygotes at high temperatures but superior to either at low temperatures (da Cunha, 1960). An examination of F2 individuals of *D. pseudo-obscura* maintained at 19° and 23° showed that the appearance of heterozygotes was favoured; but, if a change of temperature occurred during development, an excess of homozygotes appeared in the population indicating that under these conditions they were superior (Hartmann-Goldstein and Sperlich, 1963).

In order that an insect can develop from one stage of its life history to another, there must be an orderly production in definite sequence of a number of different proteins. The sequence is thought to be ensured by processes of gene repression and derepression (Jacob and Monod, 1961; Goodwin, 1963). The period in which any one protein is produced, when compared with the duration of development of an insect, is relatively short. Goodwin (1963) estimated that some 5 min. may be necessary for the production of a protein molecule, and that, following a transient stimulus that induces synthesis of a particular protein, the system takes from $1\frac{1}{2}$–4 hr. to return to its original state. Production of m-RNA at the gene can be very rapid. Arnold (1965) found that, when the salivary glands of *Drosophila hydei* were immersed in solutions of uridine, which is incorporated into RNA, localization occurred within the nucleolus within 15 sec., and labelled RNA appeared in the cytoplasm within 60 sec. at 17–18°. Against this background it is clear that the effects of a change in temperature will depend very much on when, in the development of the insect, the change occurs.

Most of the information on this aspect of temperature effects comes from subjecting the animal to a temperature shock, that is by exposing it for a brief period to temperatures which would be lethal if the exposure was of longer duration (Goldschmidt, 1938).

Temperature-induced sex reversal in *Aedes aegypti* results only if the shocks are given 2–4 days after ecdysis during the second and third instars; the first and fourth instars are insensitive (Craig, 1965). Tumorous head can be induced in *Drosophila* larvae by temperature shocks, the sensitive period being 20–24 hr. after the egg has been laid (Gardner *et al.*, 1960). If pupae of the moth *Ephestia kuehniella* that have been kept at 18° are exposed to 45°, 40–60 hr. after pupation, there is a narrowing of the central band of the wing pattern (Kuehn and

Henke, 1936). It is not necessary for the duration of the temperature shock to be of the same duration as the sensitive period. With the induction of tumorous head in *Drosophila*, a 4-hr. exposure between 8 and 12 hr. is as effective as a 24-hr. exposure (Gardner *et al.*, 1960) and, in *Ephestia*, the effect can be produced by a temperature shock lasting only 45 min. in a 12-hr. sensitive period.

In many instances the temperature-sensitive period coincides with the beginning of the formation of the affected organ or tissue. Stanley (1935) found that the temperature-sensitive period for the vg allelomorphs in *Drosophila* occurred at that time in the third instar when the wing buds were beginning to form. In tumorous head, however, the temperature-sensitive period was in the embryo stage but the affected organ did not develop until the pupal stage, indicating that considerable lag can occur between the sensitive period and the first visible appearance of its effects.

While the intensity of the temperature shock needs always to be near maximum, the direction of the temperature change is, or can be, important. If the pupae of the butterfly, *Vanessa urticae*, are exposed to a severe high temperature shock, the wing pattern of the adult is altered towards that found in *V. ischnusa* from Sardinia, while extreme low temperatures alter it towards that found in *V. polaris* from Lapland (Goldschmidt, 1938).

In many insects, the effects of a temperature shock are similar to those that result from some known gene mutation occurring within the species. Goldschmidt (1938) has suggested that the common basis for this is an alteration in the rates of gene action or of changes in the balance between rates of action produced by temperature or by mutation. It should be noted that temperature is not the only factor that can produce phenocopies of mutations. Sub-lethal doses of cyanide, Ag^+, quinones and their derivatives, given in larval media, can all produce non-inherited modifications strikingly similar to those caused by mutations and by temperature shocks.

The basic materials for protein synthesis are the amino acids that arise from the digestion and absorption of food or by the activities of micro-organisms. Florkin and Jeuniaux (1964) pointed out that the blood of insects is characterized by a high amino-acidemia which is more pronounced in the *Endopterygota* than the *Exopterygota*. After studying the amino acid compositions of proteins in the fly *Phromina regina*, Henry and Cook (1963) concluded that they were relatively constant throughout development.

The amounts of free amino acids in the larvae and pupae of *Drosophila melanogaster*, with the exception of glutamic acid, vary inversely with temperature; however, the amounts of glutamic acid vary directly with temperature. Additional feeding of glutamic acid at low temperatures led to an increase in the amounts of most other free amino acids in the insect (Anders et al., 1964). Transaminase activity in insects, as in other animals, may be greater at lower than at higher temperatures. McAllan and Chefurka (1961) have observed that the transaminases catalysing the inverconversion of glutamate and aspartate are rapidly inactivated at temperatures above 48°.

In the majority of insects, phenylalanine is an essential dietary requirement. It can be oxidized to tyrosine which is involved in the darkening and hardening of the cuticle following an ecdysis. The first step is the conversion of tyrosine to 3,4-dihydroxyphenylalanine (DOPA), a reaction catalysed by the enzyme tyrosinase (phenolase). This reaction is greatly influenced by temperature. The sigmoid curve which results from the oxidation of monohydroxyphenols by phenolase is thought to be an autocatalytic process due to the release of a protein-aceous activator. With increasing temperatures above 0°, there is a shortening of the lag period and an increase in the rate of activity, but a decrease in maximum activity. This loss of activity results from the release of a heat-stable inhibitor which can be dialysed and, when added to a fully active phenolase preparation, inhibits the enzyme activity (Lewis, 1960). No tyrosinase activity has been noted in *Musca* above 40° (Ohnishi, 1959), or above 25° in *Drosophila* (Lewis, 1960). On the other hand, Bodine and Allen (1938) and Bodine et al. (1944) found that exposure to high temperatures activated the protyrosinase of the diapausing eggs of *Melanoplus*.

The further metabolism of DOPA can occur through one of two path-ways. One leads to the formation of N-acetyl dopamine which functions in the tanning of the proteins and the hardening of the cuticle (Karlson and Sekeris, 1962); the other leads to the formation of melanin (Chefurka, 1965). There are many observations that, at low tempera-tures, the amount of black pigmentation of the cuticle increases as shown by *Melanoplus* (Parker, 1930). Goodwin (1952) has reported that, in the nymphs of locusts, this darkening is entirely due to melanin formation, but in the adult another pigment, insectorubin, is mainly responsible.

IV. Co-ordination of the System Constants

The individual insect starts life as a zygote in which is encoded the information that constitutes the "nature" of the creature. The tran-scription and translation of this information in the insect, as in other multicellular animals, requires the co-ordination and integration of the activities of spatially separated cells. This is brought about, except in the early embryonic stages, by the actions of the nervous and endocrine systems. The control exercised by these systems on cellular processes must not be thought to be rigid and absolute. It is quite possible for the cell to be influenced by the direct action of any properties of the environment without reference to its nervous and endocrine responses. Nevertheless, these systems play a most important part in co-ordinating the selection of encoded information, the integration of cellular processes, and the adjustment of physiological responses and the behaviour pattern exhibited with the internal body needs and the external environmental requirements.

A. TEMPERATURE AND THE NERVOUS SYSTEM

The functions of the nervous system in the regulation of the insect's responses to temperature are: (a) the perception of environmental temperature; (b) the integration of this information with that derived from other sources; and (c) adjustments in the patterns of its own activity which will in their turn influence the activities of the endocrine glands and the patterns of muscular activity of the body.

1. *Temperature Perception*

Temperature has a considerable effect on the information entering the nervous system of the insect through its sensillae, including those that appear to be primarily temperature receptors and those for the perception of other environmental properties.

Studies on the grasshoppers, *Melanoplus femur-rubrum* and *Dissosteira carolina*, have shown that the entire body surface is slightly sensitive to heat. The antennae were very sensitive, the pulvilli and tarsi of the fore and hind legs less so, the ventral and dorsal side of the abdomen still less, while the middle tarsi were only slightly more sensitive than the general body surface (Geist, 1928). In the cricket, *Lyogryllus campestris*, the labial palps were most sensitive, the antennae, fore legs, cerci, ovipositor, middle leg, hind leg, wings, abdomen, prothorax and head showing progressively decreasing sensitivity to temperature stimuli (Herter, 1924). The temperature sensitivity of insects varies widely in different species, blood-sucking insects being especially sensitive (Dethier, 1957), though Wigglesworth (1941) found that a temperature change of $\pm 4°$ around 29–30° was necessary to influence the behaviour of the louse, *Pediculus humanis corporis*. *Aedes aegypti* is sensitive to air temperature changes of 0·5–1·0° (Roth, 1951), *Blatta orientalis* to $\pm 1·0°$, and the ant, *Formica rufa*, to 0·25° (Herter, 1924).

Temperature reception through the antennae has been shown in many insects including the bug, *Pyrrhocoris apterus* (Herter, 1924), the stick insect, *Menexenus semiarmatus* (Cappe de Baillon, 1932), and the beetle, *Dorcus parallelpipedus* (Gebhardt, 1951). Makings (1964) found that the entire antennae were sensitive to heat in *Locusta migratoria*; in *Dorcus parallelpipedus* it is the last three distal segments (Gebhardt, 1951) and the terminal segment only in *Pyrrhocoris apterus* (Herter, 1924). In *M. semiarmatus*, the heat receptor has been identified as a small organ of the 12th. antennal segment (Cappe de Baillon, 1932) while, in the related Phasmid *Carassius morosus*, it is on the 14th. segment (Herter, 1939). In *Rhodnius prolixus*, Wigglesworth and Gillett (1934) showed the long hairs at the tip of the antennae to be sensitive to heat. In general, the identification of the precise temperature receptor sensillium is uncertain. However, a sensillium consisting of a relatively thick-walled, fixed,

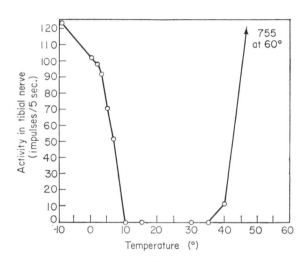

Fig. 11. Effect of temperature on tarsal receptors in *Periplaneta americana*. The preparation was acclimatized to 22° and then subjected to various temperature changes. Impulses were recorded from the tibial nerve. From Kerkut and Taylor (1957).

sharp-pointed hair about 40–50 μ long, curved and lying parallel to the cuticle, has been provisionally implicated in *Rhodnius* and *Pyrrhocoris* (Murray, 1962). Temperature receptors have also been demonstrated on other parts of the body including the maxillary palps of *D. parallelpipedus* (Gebhardt, 1951) and the labial palps of the cockroach *Blabera fusca* and *Lyogrillos campestris* (Herter, 1924).

Temperature receptors occurring on the arolium and pulvilli of the legs of *Periplaneta americana* have been studied by Kerkut and Taylor (1957; Fig. 11). These structures have the characteristics of cold receptors. Electrophysiological studies show that, at temperatures below 13°, the preparation becomes more active, and that changes of 1° magnitude below this temperature cause an increase in activity. Over

11*

the range 0–28°, a 5° increase in temperature produces a transient increase in activity. Prolonged electrical activity is manifest over 30°. On substrata above this temperature, the insect raises its tarsi above the ground.

Some insects have receptors especially adapted for the reception of infrared radiation. In *Melanophila acuminata*, receptors are present on the metathorax and these are sensitive to energy fluxes of 0.6×10^{-4} W./cm.^{2} for radiation of 4 μ wavelength. These beetles deposit their eggs in fresh fire-killed conifers. They can perceive and orientate on a 50 acre area of glowing wood from 6 km. As they approach the glowing wood, the antennae temperature receptors are used for orientation(Evans,1964).

The labellar chemoreceptors of the flies *Phromia regina* and *Sarcophaga bullata* are sensitive to temperature changes, the frequency of discharge changing significantly with temperature changes of as little as 0·1° (Hodgson and Roeder, 1956). These changes in frequency were recorded in response to changes in the temperature of the entire preparation (Hodgson, 1956). When, in *P. regina*, the contact receptors of the tarsus and the labellar hairs were tested with sucrose solutions, it was found that, when the preparation was held at a constant temperature and only the temperature of the stimulating solution altered, there was no change in the threshold value of response over the range 0–37° (Dethier and Arab, 1958). *S. bullata* showed different thresholds of response when tested at different temperatures. The thresholds for sucrose were at 19–20°, 0·14 *M*; at 27–29°, 0·06 *M*; and at 37–39°, 0·17 *M* (Frings and Cox, 1954). Hodgson (1958) found that the salt response of the butterflies *Epargyreus* and *Limenitis* were increased by a 1·2° rise in temperature. *Ceuthophilus gracilipes*, while giving positive responses to chemical stimulation, showed no increase in response following a change from 20 to 30°.

In *Phromia regina*, the tarsal chemoreceptors are coupled with thermoreceptors, but these are not found in association with the labellar chemoreceptors. Data suggest that the responses to hot and cold stimuli by the thermoreceptors counteract the effects of temperature upon the chemoreceptors, and that the response that the animal makes depends upon the total sensory output reaching the central nervous system by these two independent routes (Dethier, 1963). The temperature receptor shows two types of single fibre discharge, a large peak of 0·2–0·5 mV and a small amplitude discharge of 0·05–0·1 mV. The large amplitude spikes are decreased in size by a temperature rise; the small spikes are unaffected. When the temperature drops, the large spikes reappear, and occur at a greater frequency before returning to the normal rate. Some preparations show another fibre stimulated by a temperature rise to fire at a very fast rate (Dethier and Arab, 1958).

Temperature has a considerable effect upon the electrical responses shown by the dark-adapted eye of the grasshopper, *Melanoplus differentialis*, to brief exposures of bright light (Crescitelli and Jahn, 1939). Temperatures down to 0° diminish the magnitude of the response as compared with that given at room temperature (18–22°) and also its rate of development and decline, and lengthen the latent period. These changes are reversible, and the response is the same for any given temperature regardless of whether the temperature is approached by warming up or by cooling down, or whether it is a momentary exposure or one lasting up to 1½ hr. High temperatures (43–56°) produce very varied responses from different individuals. The magnitude of the potential increases up to approximately 36° and then decreases; the optimum temperature varies greatly. With increasing temperature, the discharges become increasingly spike-like and rapid; the "c" wave which is prominent at lower temperatures is depressed. At 34·5° a rhythmic after-discharge appears with a frequency of 13/sec. and persists for 0·5 sec. At 38·5°, the frequency is 15/sec. and it persists for 0·9 sec.; at 40·8°, it is 19/sec., and persists for 1·0 sec. At higher temperatures, the frequency increases, the persistence time is unchanged and its prominence decreases. The pattern is reversible so long as the temperature does not exceed 46–53°. Repetitive stimulation shows no oscillatory discharge at 23·6°, but one appears at 27·3° and increases in prominence up to 42°. An oscillatory discharge does not appear if the light stimulus is of too long a duration, or if the eye is thoroughly light-adapted. These observations indicate that the quality and quantity of information passed to the nervous system from the sense organs varies with temperature, and suggest that the insect may perceive a very different world from its normal one at the extremities of its temperature tolerances.

2. *The Central Nervous System*

The central nervous system will be subject to temperature changes along with the rest of the insect body and these changes are known to produce definite physiological responses.

Electrophysiological studies of the isolated nerve cord of *Periplaneta americana* have shown that there exist in the nerve cord units which respond differently to different temperatures. These units may be grouped into four classes: (a) those that show an increase in frequency of impulses with an increase in temperature; (b) those that show transient changes in frequency with changes in temperature, and soon resume their original level of activity; (c) those that show activity over a restricted part of the temperature range. One unit shows a decrease of activity as the temperature falls from 17·5° to 11°, below which temperature activity again increases; some show activity only at 7° and below, some only at 1°; (d) one unit appears to be relatively unaffected by temperature at least between 10° and 20°. The isolated nerve cord shows a symmetrical response in impulse frequency about a temperature optimum. In insects kept for 4 weeks at 22°, the optimum is 22°; for those kept at 31° it is 31° (Kerkut and Taylor, 1957; Fig. 12).

The transmission of impulses from one neuron to another is influenced by temperature as shown in studies on the sixth abdominal ganglion of *Blabera craniifer*. At low temperatures, a larger potential must be produced in the cercal nerve, as compared with high temperatures, to produce a post-synaptic response (Bernard *et al.*, 1965). The role of acetylcholine and of cholinesterases is the same in the synaptic transmission of nerve impulses in insects as it is in other animals. The amount of acetylcholine in the ventral nerve cord of *Periplaneta americana* increases with increasing temperature between 15° and 35°; at 9°, however, the amount is slightly greater than at 15° or 25° (Colhoun, 1958). Acetylcholine also has been shown to accumulate in the brain of diapausing *Platysamia cecropia* pupae at a faster rate at low temperatures than at high (van der Kloot, 1955). Something is known about the rate at which these changes take place. In *Periplaneta americana* held at 35° for 20 hr. and then transferred to 15°, the concentration of acetylcholine fell from 97·8 µg./g. wet weight of thoracic cord to 84·6 µg./g. in 2 hr., and to the normal value for 15° (72·1 µg./g.) in 20 hr. (Colhoun, 1958).

Cholinesterase has been prepared from the housefly and the rate of activity of the enzyme has been shown to be proportional to temperature up to 30°, with a Q_{10} of 1·3–1·5. There is an irreversible loss of activity above 35° although maximum activity for a 20–30 min. measurement occurs at 40°. Cholinesterase from other sources was less sensitive to temperature (Chadwick, 1957). The acetylcholinesterase activity in the brain of *Platysamia cecropia* decreased just before pupation. Prolonged exposure at 6° did not restore it, but was necessary for its re-appearance when the insect was returned to 25°. At this temperature, enzyme activity re-appeared in 4–5 days. Unchilled brains cannot synthesize acetylcholinesterase. These changes occur only in the brain; the ventral nerve cord does not show changes in acetylcholinesterase activity with diapause (van der Kloot, 1955).

3. *The Motor Neurons*

Studies on the motor units of the nervous system concerned with wing movements have shown that a unit may generate one or two impulses per wing beat. The interval between this pair of impulses has been shown to be strongly dependent upon temperature, a modal value of

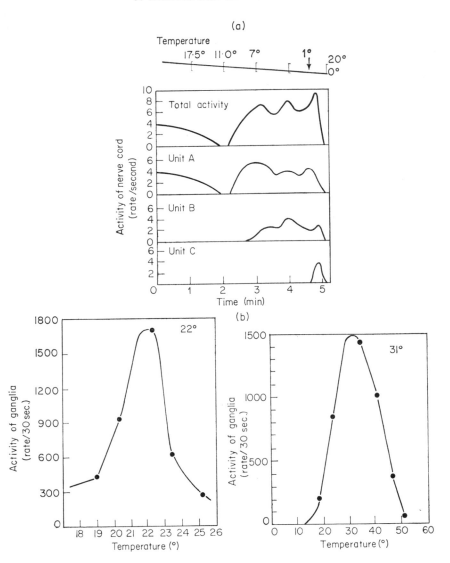

FIG. 12

(a) Effect of a temperature decrease upon the activity of the cockroach (*Periplaneta americana*) nerve cord. The top curve shows the total activity of the nerve cord which is due to three units A, B, and C. The activities of these units are plotted below. (b) Curves showing the effect of temperature on the activity of isolated ganglia from *P. americana*. The insects were kept at 22° and 31° respectively for 4 weeks prior to the observation. From Kerkut and Taylor (1958).

10 msec. at 26° is decreased to 6 msec. at 32°, although the wing beat interval changed only slightly as a result of this temperature change. This temperature response suggests that the pair of impulses were generated by a refractory oscillation during a single long synaptic potential or other state of continued excitation (Wilson, 1965). In dragonflies, the motor impulses to the closure muscle of the spiracle have a frequency which shows temperature dependence and a Q_{10} of 2·7 between 15° and 25° (Miller, 1965).

B. THE ENDOCRINE SYSTEM

There are relatively few observations on the effects of temperature on the endocrine system of the insect. The medial neurosecretory cells of the protocerebrum show no histological evidence of impairment of neurosecretion in 6 day-old adult *Locusta migratoria* kept at temperatures of 15°, 30° and 45°, or for 4-hr. period fluctuations of 30 ± 0·25°, 30 ± 10°, and 30 ± 15° over a 16-day interval (Clarke, 1966). In the brain of the pupae of *Platysamia cecropia*, the secretion ceases to be formed at the beginning of diapause (Williams, 1947), and there is a gradual restoration of neurosecretory activity which takes place spontaneously, but is greatly accelerated by cold (Danilevski, 1965). Temperature may affect the amount of material present in the corpora cardiaca. In a 6 day-old adult *L. migratoria*, the amount of neurosecretory "A" material present in the anterior lobes was less at 15°, than at 30° or 45°. In 16 day-old adults at 30 ± 15° (4-hr. cycle), the corpora cardiaca was completely depleted of neurosecretory material whereas, under the other fluctuations, normal amounts were present (Clarke, 1966).

In the hibernating larvae of *Mormoniella*, the physiological effect of chilling the larvae for 7 days at 5° is almost entirely reversed by subsequent exposure to 25° for 2 days and is completely reversed in 7 days. It is thought that low temperature permits the accumulation of hormone by slowing down its anaerobic breakdown, while high temperatures favour its destruction (Schneiderman and Horowitz, 1958).

Variations with temperature have been observed in the rate at which the prothoracic gland responds to the brain hormone. In the 2nd., 3rd. and 4th. nymphs of *Locusta migratoria*, the peak of mitotic response coincides with the moment of ecdysis at 28° and 43° but, at 25°, the peak does not occur until after 20% of the instar duration has elapsed (Clarke and Langley, 1963a; Fig. 13). In *Rhodnius*, the prothoracic gland shows no histological signs of activity at 36° (Wigglesworth, 1959).

The corpora allata show histological changes associated with the temperatures at which the animals were kept. Six day-old *L. migratoria* have normal corpora allata at 30° but, at 15°, the allatum is shrunken, and the nuclei are irregular in shape, closely packed, and exhibit different staining reactions to methyl green/pyronin stain. At 45° the allatum is smaller than at 30°, and the nuclei stained with methyl green/pyronin show no trace of RNA, a condition that contrasts strongly with the reactions at all other temperatures studied. In insects subjected to

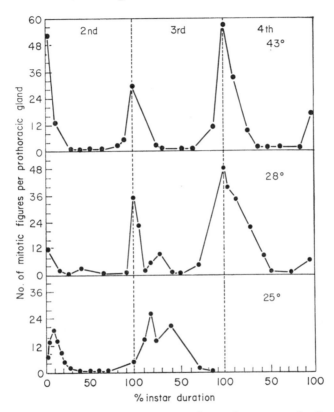

FIG. 13. The time of occurrence of the maximum frequency of mitoses in the prothoracic gland of *Locusta migratoria* at three different temperatures. Vertical dotted lines indicate the moment of ecdysis between the 2nd., 3rd. and 4th. instars. From Clarke and Langley (1963a).

fluctuating temperatures, the allati show increasing signs of hyperactivity and exhaustion as the amplitude of the temperature fluctuation is increased (Clarke, 1966).

There is clear evidence that nervous stimuli of many kinds may influence the secretion of hormones. The release of neurosecretory material is caused by nervous stimulation arising from stretching the abdomen in *Rhodnius* (Wigglesworth, 1934), by the stimulation of stretch receptors in the pharynx of *L. migratoria* (Clarke and Langley, 1963b), by the stimulation of chemoreceptors in *Periplaneta americana* (Davey, 1961), and by hyperactivity of *Blabera craniifera* (Hodgson and Geldiay, 1959). Nervous control of the corpora allata was inferred for *Rhodnius* by Wigglesworth (1936), and demonstrated for the cockroach, *Leucophaea*, by Luscher and Engelmann (1955, 1960) where it has an inhibitory effect.

C. TEMPERATURE AND THE NEURO-ENDOCRINE CONTROL OF THE SYSTEM CONSTANTS

The changes which occur in an insect in response to a change in temperature indicate that, for any given temperature, the insect is in a definite state with regard to the rates of its metabolic reactions, the concentrations of metabolic products and intermediates, and the amount of genetic information in use. It has been pointed out (Clarke, 1960) that this state is that which requires the least consumption of energy to maintain itself; any other state at that temperature would call for a greater expenditure of energy. The achievement of this state, and its maintenance, is the poikilotherm equivalent to the work that homeotherms have to do to maintain constant body temperatures.

Control in response to temperature in a poikilotherm therefore means the maintenance of this state in the face of other environmental changes; the assumption of this state as quickly as possible following a temperature change; and the assumption of the necessary state in anticipation of a temperature change. The mechanisms involved in this control are the neural and endocrine systems of the body, and they achieve it by influencing the reactions that occur at all levels of body organization. It can be demonstrated that those processes that have been described as temperature-dependent are also influenced by these systems.

1. *Control of Cellular Processes*

Many of the intracellular processes of insects can be influenced by insect hormones. The action of these hormones on gene activity has been well documented in the last few years (Clever and Karlson, 1960; Clever, 1962; Becker, 1962; Kroeger, 1963; Sekeris and Karlson, 1964). Hormonal action has also been demonstrated on the microsomal fraction of the cell (Karlson *et al.*, 1964), on the mitochondrion (Clarke and Baldwin, 1960) and on the cytochrome system (Williams, 1947).

Undoubtedly one of the most important constraints to metabolism is the impermeability of the cell wall and of the membranes within the cell. Particles may be separated from the muscle cells of *Locusta migratoria*, reared at 35°, which are capable of completely oxidizing butyrate, but not the higher fatty acids. From locusts reared at 45°, the muscle particles showed differences in the spectrum of fatty acids that could be oxidized, and required coenzyme A for the oxidation of saturated fatty acids of chain length C_8–C_{18}. It is thought that the differences between these particles reside in differences in their permeability which increases with increasing temperature (Meyer et al., 1960). In *Calliphora erythrocephala* and *Phromia terranovae*, there is a direct relationship between the degree of saturation of the fatty acid residues in the phospholipids and the temperature at which the animals were reared. Those reared at the higher temperatures and having the more saturated phospholipid had only a 1° greater temperature tolerance than those reared at lower temperatures. When both were bred at 27°, *C. erythrocephala* was killed at 39° and *P. terra-novae* at 45°. The iodine number of the lipids extracted from both insects reared at their maximum temperature was nearly identical at 75 (Fraenkel and Hopf, 1940). In insects, there is little direct evidence of permeability changes in the cell membrane or in intracellular particles due to changes in hormonal milieu. By analogy with vertebrates, however, such a relationship might be expected.

2. *Control of Physiological Processes*

The complexity of the interactions of endocrine, and neural activity, with temperature in influencing a physiological process can be seen in the factors that affect heart beat frequency in *Periplaneta americana*. Changes in the frequency of heart beat have been observed due to fasting in adults (Jones, 1964), upon feeding (Davey, 1961), and with changes in temperature when the increase gives a linear plot against temperature over the range 12–40° (Richards, 1963b). Endocrine control was demonstrated by Cameron (1953), who showed that the rate of heart beat could be accelerated by a substance, possibly an orthodiphenol, secreted from the corpora cardiaca. Davey (1961) found that this hormone did not act directly upon the heart but on the pericardial cells, and it was from these cells that the accelerating substance was released. The corpora allata also have an effect since the increase following food intake does not occur if the corpora allata are extirpated (Davey, 1962).

The basis of neural control is the presence of an innervation arising from the lateral and segmental nerves (McIndoo, 1945). The entire dorsal vessel is said to be capable of initiating a contraction (Clark, 1927). In the semi-intact heart in cold-adapted cockroaches, the heart stops beating at temperatures slightly above those that induce cold stupor but, in the intact animal, the heart continues beating at temperatures at which the animal is rigid with cold. At these lower temperatures

(9–12°), the plot of heart beat rate against temperature is nonlinear. It is thought that, within this range, the heart is being driven from the nervous system (Richards, 1963b).

Within the insect body there are many processes and reactions proceeding simultaneously, each with its own temperature response curve. Richards (1963b) has stressed the impossibility of correlating the temperature responses of all of these activities, some of which give straight line plots with temperature and others curvilinear plots. Nevertheless, in a poikilotherm, all of these activities must be interrelated and coordinated under diverse temperature conditions. The joint effects of hormonal and nervous influences, as illustrated by the heart beat frequency data already reported, can allow adjustment of these rates so that a harmonious response to temperature change can result. It is possible that the temperature tolerance of the insect is limited by the ability of its control systems to maintain the rates of change of these various processes in their correct relationships with each other.

In this connection Orgel (1964) has noted that the replacement of a partially inactivated enzyme is most speedily achieved by relaxation of the repressor of gene expression visualized in the Jacob and Monod hypothesis. Clarke (1966) observed exhaustion of the neurosecretory material under conditions of extreme temperature stress in *Locusta migratoria* and related this to the need for a maximum rate of enzyme synthesis under these conditions. If the control systems fail, the imbalance that results is harmful to the animal, but it will take time for the effects to reach a lethal level. Such a situation agrees with the temperature and time responses observed near the insect's tolerance limits.

V. Adaptability of the System

From the evidence given in the preceding pages, it will be seen that the insect has a characteristic state for each temperature value within its viable range. However, the temperature tolerances of each state are not identical. In the cockroach, *Blattella germanica*, individuals kept at 35° died sooner than those kept at 25° and these sooner than those kept at 15° when all were exposed to 7°. Similarly, the chill coma temperature is lower with increasingly low temperature of rearing, although cockroaches reared at 15° and 10° showed nearly identical chill coma temperatures. The causes of immobility and death at low temperatures are not known, but irreversible disturbances occur in the nervous systems of cold-immobilized cockroaches (Colhoun, 1954). Death can also result from immobilization at room temperatures where a factor from the corpora cardiaca is involved (Beament, 1958). An increase in the upper lethal temperature from 42° to 44° has been observed in *Aedes aegypti* following a change in rearing temperature from 30° to 37° (Mellanby, 1954). But, in *Anopheles minimus*, a change in the rearing temperature from 30° to 35° had no effect on the upper lethal limit (Muirhead-Thomson, 1940). Mellanby (1954) pointed out that, while treatment with lower temperatures within the viable range conferred some degree of cold tolerance upon the insect, progressively increasing temperature treatments did not confer heat tolerance until they were within 3–4° of the heat coma temperature. The extension of cold tolerance was always greater than the extension of heat tolerance. Cold tolerance can amount to as much as 7·5° below that of an insect from the warm part of its range, and heat tolerance as much as 3–4° above that of an insect from the cool end of its range. In *Tribolium confusum*, animals reared at 30° and then exposed for long periods to 18° showed an increase in their heat and cold tolerances (Edwards, 1958). Various criteria have been used in estimating the temperature limits to which the insect could be subjected (Belěhrádek, 1935). The temperature limits are different for each parameter examined but the pattern of response is similar to that given above.

A. RESPONSES OF THE SYSTEM TO TEMPERATURE CHANGES

Many experiments have been done in which insects have been kept at one temperature and then transferred to another, and observations made on the effects of the transfer on behaviour and metabolic activity. The changes from one temperature to another have been either quickly or slowly accomplished. No terms to describe these changes appear to be in general use in biology but, in engineering, the term "step function" is used when the change from one temperature to another is made as rapidly as possible, and "ramp function" when a slower rate of change occurs. These terms, so descriptive of the type of change, will be employed here.

There are a number of estimates on how long the insect may take to reach its new equilibrium state following a step-function transfer. When insects are exposed for a time exceeding 3 days to a temperature within their viable range and the chill coma temperature then determined (Bělehrádek, 1935), it was found to be lower in insects kept at the lower end than in those from the upper end of their temperature range. If, now, insects are transferred from one temperature to another, and the chill coma temperatures measured at known intervals of time following the transfer, some estimate of the speed of the change can be made. In *Calliphora erythrocephala*, the tsetse fly, *Glossina palpalis*, and the bed bug, *Cimex lenticularis*, no change could be detected after 5 min.; some change occurred after 2 hr., partial acclimatization occurred after 12 hr., and the full chill coma temperature of the system reached after 20 hr. In

Blatta orientalis, a step-function transfer of 30° to 15° required 2–3 day
for the full change to occur (Mellanby, 1939).

In the parasitic wasp, *Dahlbominus fuscipennis,* a step transfer from
23° to 43° is immediately followed by a burst of intense activity. Thi
lasts for 60 min. if the transfer temperature is 42°, and 15 min. if it i
46°. Activity then decreases until many of the animals become immobil
due to heat stupor. In the majority of the population, this occurs 3 hr
after the transfer and is followed by recovery, which is complete withi

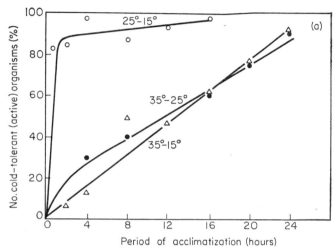

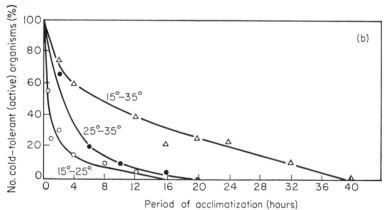

Fɪɢ. 14

(a) Rate of gain of cold tolerance following a step transfer of *Blattella germanic*
from a high to a low temperature. (b) Rate of loss of cold tolerance following a
step transfer from a low to a high temperature in *Blattella germanica.* From
Colhoun (1960).

0 hr. (Baldwin, 1954). In *Tenebrio molitor*, the heat coma point is modified following a transfer to 37° over a period of 20–24 hr. (Mellanby, 954).

Contrary to what might be expected, it appears that the times taken to change from one temperature state to another are not very different at high or low temperatures. If, however, the step function involves transfer to a temperature which will produce cold anaesthesia in the insect, acclimatization cannot occur. In *C. lenticularis*, transfer from 30° to 9·5° allows adaptation to occur but, if the transfer is to 5°, no adaptation occurs (Mellanby, 1939). *Aedes aegypti* shows a similar response (Mellanby, 1960), and Colhoun (1960) found no further acclimatization in *Blattella* below 15° (Fig. 14).

Changes in respiratory activity following a step-function transfer from 30° to 18° have been observed in *Tribolium confusum* where the full change was accomplished within 24 hr. (Fig. 15). When transferred from 30° to 38°, the increase in respiratory activity in the male lasted for 2 days and in the female for 3 days. In the males, the final level of oxygen consumption was higher than that immediately following an exposure to 38°; in the females it returned to this level (Edwards, 1958). Richards and Suanraksa (1962) found that, following a transfer of *Oncopeltis fasciatus* eggs from 25° to 15°, the oxygen consumption decreased within a few hours, but remained some 20% above the final level for some hours; after a transfer from 15° to 25°, there was an overshoot in oxygen consumption lasting 1 hr.

When the transfer of the insect from one temperature to another takes the form of a ramp function, two additional aspects may be learnt about the animal's response. The form of the response curve of the animal may reveal something of the mechanisms involved, and indicate whether the tolerance limits of the animal are wider in response to a ramp than to a step function.

The body temperature reached with both step and ramp functions will depend upon conditions other than the nature of the function. Step-function transfers do not reveal anything of the change since the response will be controlled by the conditions. In ramp-function transfers, however, measurements of the body temperature under carefully controlled conditions can give some indication of metabolic changes that occur in response to the temperature change, and is indeed the only parameter which can be easily followed (Clarke, 1964). In *Locusta migratoria*, when the air temperature is slowly increased from 20° to 40°, the body temperature lags behind the air temperature over most of the period of observation, but approaches the air temperature while the latter is still increasing, and eventually overtakes it to give a body temperature 0·5–1·0° above that of the air. The body temperature is

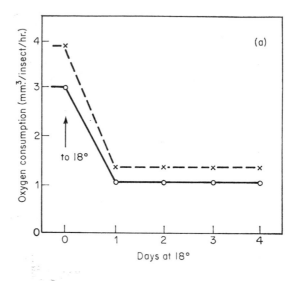

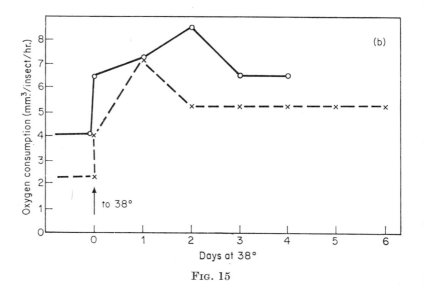

FIG. 15

(a) Changes in oxygen consumption following a step-function transfer of *Tribolium confusum* from 30° to 18°. The broken line indicates the average response of 10 males, and the solid line the response of 10 females. (b) Changes in oxygen consumption following a step transfer of *T. confusum* from 30° to 38°. The broken line indicates the average response of 10 males, and the solid line the response of 10 females. Note the well-defined overshoot following an increase in temperature and its absence following a decrease in temperature. From Edwards (1958).

ield for some time but, due to other factors, details of the return to a ower temperature which takes place within 12 hr. have not been observed. The form of the response curve can be altered by use of sub-lethal doses of cyanide, by surgical interference with the sense organs of the animal, and by starvation (Clarke, 1960; Fig. 16).

Changes in body composition associated with ramp function temperature changes have been observed in the accumulation of glycerol in the tissues of the ant *Campanotus pennsilvanicus pennsilvanicus*. Ants at

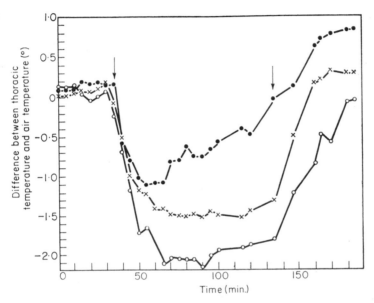

FIG. 16. Differences between the air temperature and the thoracic temperature in adult *Locusta migratoria* during a ramp change of air temperature from 20° to 45°. Vertical arrows indicate the beginning and the end of the temperature change. Dots represent the responses in an insect injected with 2,4-dinitrophenol at the commencement of the experiment; circles, of insects treated with KCN; and crosses, of insects injected with distilled water. From Clarke (1960).

20–25° have no trace of glycerol in their tissues but, when slowly cooled to 0–5° over a period of 6 days, glycerol to a concentration of 10% (live weight) accumulates in the tissues. Warming slowly brings about the disappearance of glycerol from the tissues (Dubach *et al.*, 1959).

Salt (1961) has pointed out that, at a fairly rapid rate of cooling of a few degrees per minute, the undercooling point that can be reached in cold-adapted tissues is not influenced by the rate of cooling. At slower rates, when cooling is extended over hours or days, higher supercooling points may result. This is probably because the temperature of freezing in a supercooled state depends upon a particular molecular event the frequency of occurrence of which increases with time. The time spent in a supercooled state before freezing is clearly longer if cooling is gradual than if it is fast; hence higher cooling points result.

B. ANTICIPATION OF TEMPERATURE CHANGES

As has been pointed out, the insect can exist in one of two states, a high energy, open unsteady state and a low energy, closed, steady state. The latter state is that in which the insect survives adverse conditions of long duration including high and low temperatures which would be lethal or semilethal in the active state. The change from the active to the diapause state cannot apparently be accomplished very quickly. Danilevski (1965) observed in the sawfly, *Dendrolimus pini*, that preparation for the change was most speedily achieved at temperatures which were most favourable to the active state; the process required 30 days at 23° but 60 days at 10–12°. Development may continue at the appropriate rate for the temperature prevailing during this time. Diapause thus appears at the end of the 2nd. and beginning of the 3rd. instar at optimum active state temperatures, but not until the 4th., 5th. and even 6th. instars at suboptimum temperatures. It has already been noted that, if the active state is exposed to temperatures that induce cold anaesthesia, then adaptive changes do not occur (Mellanby, 1939, 1960). There is therefore a basis for the insect to anticipate coming adverse changes in the environment and to assume the resistant phase whilst the conditions are favourable for an active change of state. The intimate relationships between the nervous, endocrine and genetic systems allow for a controlled change in the system constants in response to stimuli which signal the advent of harsh environmental conditions.

Depending upon the ecological requirements of the insect, almost any factor in the environment can act as a signal for the switch from the active to the diapause state. Moderate temperature changes themselves may be sufficient as in the moth, *Telea polyphaemus* (Dawson, 1931), in which a drop in temperature initiates diapause, or in *Spilsoma menthastria* where temperature changes to below 20° or above 27° induce this state (Danilevski, 1965). More often it is a pattern of photoperiod and temperature stimuli which initiates the change. The pattern may be a simple one, as for example with long days and high temperatures maintaining the active state, and short days and low temperatures inducing the diapause state. Alternatively, it may be a complex one as in *Acronycta rumicis* in which rhythmic illumination and cooling will cause all pupae to assume the diapause state; rhythmic cooling of 3 hr. to 0° daily from 26–27° in constant light results in the maintenance of the active stage, and heating to 38° for 3 hr. will cancel the effect of a short day, again leading to the maintenance of the active state (Danilevski, 1965).

The temperature at which diapause is induced will influence its duration. In *Dendrolimus pini*, diapause induced at 30° lasts for 2 days, whereas that induced at 12° lasts for $1\frac{1}{2}$ months. Pupae of the cotton boll worm induced to diapause at 29° required on the average 80·5 days, and those at 19–16°, 41 days, to elapse before resuming the active state (Komarova, 1959).

C. SELECTION OF THE GENOTYPE

Previous sections have included discussions on the state of the insect at any given temperature, its response to temperature changes, and the control of these responses. The system constants which set the tolerances of the individual and condition its responses within these limits are derived from information contained within the genetic system, the content of which is related to the gene pool of the population from which the specimen has been taken. As a natural selective agency, temperature may influence this gene pool directly, and there may be, and often is, a rather exact adaptation of the gene pool to the temperature requirements of the insect's habitat (Muller, 1942). It may also act indirectly by influencing the ability of the population to compete with other populations, and by favouring synchronization of individual responses to environmental requirements.

A direct action is shown in *Drosophila funebris* in which there exist many morphologically indistinguishable races, each characterized by a different temperature tolerance related to the temperatures of their environments (Timofeeff-Ressovsky, 1940). In *Drosophila melanogaster* and *D. simulans*, Tantawy and Mallah (1961) have noted that populations from the Lebanon thrive under a lower and wider temperature range than do those from Uganda which require a higher and narrower range.

The genotype selected will be related to the actual temperatures experienced by the insect. In one habitat these may be very different in insects with different behaviour patterns. Chapman *et al.* (1926) observed the behavioural and temperature tolerances of two species of wasps inhabiting a sand dune area in Minnesota. One, *Bembex* sp., digs into the sand to make deep burrows in which the larvae live. The adult wasp is inactive at temperatures below 25° and is rapidly killed by temperatures above 42°. This wasp is able to work on the sand surface which, on a bright summer's day, may reach 52°, by breaking off its digging activities for frequent flights into the cooler air layer 1–2 ft. above the desert surface. The other species of wasp, a member of the genus *Dasymutilla*, is wingless and cannot escape from the high temperatures of the sand and the surrounding sparse vegetation. These temperatures it has to tolerate; the insect is not killed below 52°.

There are many observations on the distribution of temperatures in different habitats which may be summed up as follows. Widely different temperatures can occur, each over a sufficient area to shelter a number of insects and close enough together to allow the insect to move readily from one to the other. This, coupled with appropriate behavioural patterns, allows the insect to exist in a temperature regime very different from that suggested by climatic and/or single microhabitat records.

These patterns of behaviour may serve to minimize changes in body temperature as indicated by the behaviour of *Locusta migratoria* in a temperature gradient. In such a gradient, the insect will choose the temperature close to that to which it had been exposed prior to being placed in the gradient (Chapman, 1955). The ant, *Formica rufa*, by blocking up the entrance holes to its nest at night, keeps the temperature as much as 10° above that of the surrounding soil. On the other hand, diversity may be deliberately sought. In the larvae of *Tribolium castaneum*, reared in a temperature-choice apparatus, the larvae spends most of its time in the neighbourhood of 29° but pays a short visit to 35° just before pupation, which occurs at 30–31° (Graham, 1964). In many ants, the workers control the rate of development of larvae and pupae by placing them in the warmer or cooler parts of the nest according to the needs of the colony.

The outcome of competition between populations can be different under different temperature regimes. In the warmer parts of Australia, there occurs a subspecies of *Dacus tryoni* designated *neohumeralis*. This subspecies is superior in survival to the type under crowded conditions at 25° but inferior to it at 20° (Andrewartha and Birch, 1960). There are many similar observations in *Drosophila* in which the outcome of competition between mutants has been reversed with a change in temperature.

The ability of a population to recover from some catastrophe, or to survive in competition with some other population within their temperature tolerance ranges, is closely related to its intrinsic rate of increase. Howe (1953) has shown that, in 9 species of beetles of the family *Ptinidae*, differences in intrinsic rates of increase are adequate to account for the frequent occurrence of some species and rarity of others under identical environmental conditions. In *Rhizopertha dominica*, maximum rates of increase occur at 32–35°, and in *Calandra oryzae* at 28–31° (Birch, 1953). The latter insect is a pest in stored grain over the whole of Australia, but the former can only reach high population levels in the warmer parts and is absent altogether in cooler regions such as Tasmania (Andrewartha and Birch, 1954).

The intrinsic rate of increase of a population is a composite factor depending upon the reproductive capacity of the adults, the mortality rate of the population, and the duration of the generation interval.

Howe (1957) found that the total number of eggs laid by the cigarette beetle, *Lasioderma serricorne*, was little affected by temperature over the range 25–37·5° but was low at 20°. In *Haemogogous* mosquitoes, Bates (1947) found that the number of eggs laid at a constant temperature of 25° was the same as under conditions in which the temperature fluctuated between 25° and 35°. In the parasitic wasp, *Collyria puncticeps*, only a small number of eggs are laid at 23–25° but the number can be increased by supplementary feeding with carbohydrates (Boiko, 1962). The daily oviposition rate is increased with a rise in temperature of 20–25° in *L. serricorne* (Howe, 1957), and of 12° in the beetle *Phytodecta* (Waloff and Richards, 1958). In insects which lay their eggs at intervals in batches, temperature affects the numbers produced by influencing the precopulation, pre-oviposition and interoviposition periods. In *Anopheles funestus*, the period from feeding to oviposition takes 2 days at 25·5° and 3 days at 24·7° (Gillies, 1953). Hayward (1962) reported that the number of egg batches of *Dysdercus intermedius* falls at low temperatures; the female produced 7 batches at 28° and only 2 batches at 17·5°, although the number of eggs in each batch was identical.

In *Glossina palpalis*, reproduction does not occur at all in 1–10 day-old flies at 29–30°. Dissection showed that all the females were fertilized, but that abnormalities in the ovary prevented development of the larvae even when the adults were returned to lower temperatures (Mellanby, 1937). The females of *Glossina* have been observed to carry heavier larvae at low than at high temperatures. This is thought to be due to the longer gestation period required at low temperature, which gives the female a better opportunity of obtaining a large blood meal at the appropriate time (Buxton, 1955).

The curve expressing the age at death of individual insects in a population varies with temperature. In *Dysdercus fasciatus*, at low temperatures, the distribution of deaths indicated a fairly constant death rate over the duration of post-embryonic development. At optimum temperatures, most of the population survived to the adult stage, although the population died out over a fairly short interval of adult life. At high temperatures, the mortality rate tended to be high in the 5th. instar, though some adults can live as long or longer at these temperatures than at lower temperatures (Clarke and Sardesai, 1959). The generation interval decreased with increasing temperature, and is one of the main factors responsible for the rise in the intrinsic rate of increase which occurs with rising temperatures (Birch, 1948; Howe 1953). Clarke and Sardesai (1959) also found this factor to be important in *D. fasciatus*, between 20° and 30°, for the generation interval decreased by 4·6 days for each 1° rise in temperature.

Temperature may act as a signal to synchronize the responses of individuals in a population. The times of eclosion from the egg and pupae of the bee, *Megachile rotundata*, occur at random when the insects are kept at constant temperatures of 26°, 29°, 32°, and 35°. If the temperature is alternated between 32° and 22° or between 29° and 22° eclosion follows in the first 6 hr. following a return to the higher temperature (Stephen, 1964). Scott (1936) found that, in *Ephestia kuehniella*, the maximum numbers of adults emerging from the pupae coincided with a fall in temperature, and in *Drosophila* a rhythm of emergence could be initiated in an unphased culture by exposure to a temperature rise of 10° for 4 hr. The period of the rhythm was 24·5 hr at 16° and 24 hr. at 26° (Pittendrigh, 1954).

VI. Conclusions

The final consideration in any discussion on the effects of temperature upon a group of animals is to single out those aspects of their organization which appear to play a leading role in shaping the temperature responses of individual animals. One of the characteristics of insects is the relatively high proportion of their life span spent in growing and developing, and the relatively short period spent as a stable mature adult. In many insects, the period of growth and development occupies from two-thirds to three-quarters of the life span. In some, it is of much greater duration. The mayfly's often-quoted short life of 2 to 3 days applies only to the adult, and the immature stages last, in different species, from several months to 3 years. Exceptions do occur, notably in the long duration of the adult life of the queen in social insects, in which a period of development of a few weeks or months is succeeded by an adult life span of many years. These are specializations which occur in relatively advanced orders of insects.

The significance of this long period of development is that an individual insect must maintain the correct sequence of gene expression and repression and the correct balance in the amounts of gene products in the face of environmentally induced changes in body temperature of considerable amplitude and frequency. How is this done?

It is now widely accepted that, within a cell, m-RNA is synthesized at a gene locus. This m-RNA passes into the cytoplasm where, at a ibosome, it leads to the formation of a specific protein. These reactions are irreversible. Control is exercised by certain of the products that are formed by metabolic pathways being passed back to the gene locus where, after combining with a repressor protein, they repress further formation of m-RNA and hence further production of particular protein species. Within a cell, this system provides a basis for the regulation of developmental instructions that would show considerable temperature tolerance. It will be noted that this scheme for the regulation of protein synthesis can only operate if the system is open, that is, under all conditions some protein synthesis is occurring.

During the development of a multicellular animal such as an insect, the activation and inactivation of genes in different cells have to be co-ordinated in space and in time. This is not merely a matter of organizing the times and places of action of the same gene in different cells, but that of different genes producing different proteins the catalytic activities of which within the cell may be very diverse. From what is known of the temperature response curves of insects, it is very unlikely that un-controlled harmony would prevail except within a very narrow temperature range. Within an insect body, temperature differences of 2–3° between different parts are common; in flying insects, temperature differences of over 10° can occur. These differences in temperature do not appear to form a regular pattern, and are of sufficient magnitude to alter appreciably the rates of processes occuring within the body. The abrupt and frequent changes in temperature to which the insect is subject are also likely to cause chaos in gene expression unless some controlling influence is present.

The molecular messengers of this controlling and co-ordinating system are the hormones, all of which have been shown to influence protein metabolism in one way or another, some at the gene level. With regard to temperature, the functions of hormones, either individually or through joint action, may be considered under two headings; control of the rate at which the system can function, and the selection of specific gene actions.

Changes in the rates of protein formation, directed by different genes, can be accomplished by varying degrees of repressor feedback control. When a protein species is not in "use", this feedback mechanism is sufficient to decrease synthesis of that protein to the minimum rate necessary to maintain the mechanism. A hormone could, by regulating the activity of the repressor, control protein synthesis in the insect. A single hormone, with allosteric properties, would be superior to a number of other substances whose different diffusion rates may well lead to disharmony of action. In the absence of such a hormone, protein synthesis would be decreased to a low level. This gives a basis for the two energy states observed in insects; the low energy and relatively time-independent state corresponding to unsuppressed feedback; the high energy, time-dependent state corresponding to varying degrees of feedback repression.

Such a system has a number of advantages, and its effect may be seen in some of the responses that insects make to temperature. The system allows some autonomy of cell response to its environment. The amount of feedback is related to the use of the molecules produced; if this use increases, feedback will be decreased and protein synthesis increased. This is clearly seen in diapause when tissues can "escape" from their steady state condition and become active in response to wounding. By increasing the amount of hormone present, the growth and development of the animal can be stimulated; by decreasing the amount, it can be slowed down. Such a mechanism can therefore account for the observed increase of growth rates at low, and their decrease at high, temperatures. It also gives a basis for the anticipation of adverse temperature conditions shown by some insect species. The low-energy state may be assumed in response to a hormonal instruction given regardless of prevailing environmental conditions. Changes from one temperature-dependent state to another can also be accelerated by release of this hormone. Studies on the endocrine systems of insects from these varied conditions suggest that neuro-secretion is the source of the hormone involved in this overall genetic control of protein production.

The action of ecdysone in stimulating the expression of specific genes has been observed, but in connection with the pattern of development of the insect rather than as an environmental requirement. Nevertheless changes in the pattern of gene expression have been observed in response to a temperature change. Similarly, the action of the juvenile hormone is associated with developmental rather than environmental requirements, though the exhausted state seen in the corpora allata under conditions of temperature-induced stress suggest that it plays some part in the insect's temperature responses. It must not be supposed that the only sites of action of insect hormones are on the genes, or that this is the only response that temperature changes bring forth in the animal. Control through changes in metabolic constraints, such as the permeability of cells and intracellular organelles, are undoubtedly important, but knowledge of these in the Insecta is more limited and perhaps not so characteristic of the Class.

The release of the hormones from their endocrine glands is to some extent under the control of the nervous system. The patterns of nervous activity which lead to this are conditioned by the information fed into the nervous system from numerous sources, such as information about conditions within the animal's own body, and information about the environment gained by its direct action on the nervous system and by perception of it through the sense organs. Some of these sense organs perceive temperature; others are chemoreceptors and light receptors and are influenced by temperature. To this extent the information that is fed into the nervous system from these receptors is temperature-dependent. That the complex interplay of this sensory information influences the responses of the animal to temperature is indicated by the interaction of environmental signals that stimulate the animal to assume a diapause state prior to the appearance of the conditions it is intended to withstand.

Each individual insect will have its own set of genetic information on which it can draw during development. The tolerance that it can show to temperature is probably limited by the ability of the control system to hold the numerous reactions occurring in the body in some sort of harmony. Limits of the individual's tolerance are reached when the rates of important reactions are so far out of balance that there occurs a disruption of gene expression. The point at which this happens will vary, depending upon the stage of development of the animal at the time of its exposure to the temperature extreme, and will give the well-known relationships between temperature and time of exposure in producing a lethal effect.

At different temperatures, the state of the insect is not just that of an identical system working faster or slower under one set of conditions than under another. Changes occur in the state constants which need information to effect and time to accomplish. The widely different temperature tolerances of different species indicate that the Class contains the genetic information that allows the existence of its organization under a very wide range of environmental temperatures. An individual insect can increase its range of possible state constants by the presence of "silent" genes which act only under certain temperature conditions. These silent genes may be alleles at a locus, as indicated by changes in dominance observed at different temperatures and by the wider temperature tolerances shown by some heterozygotes, or they may occupy different loci in the chromosome. The rate at which protein synthesis can be initiated and maintained will depend upon the number of gene loci concerned in its production. It should be noted that, in many insects, endopolyploidy can lead to a great increase in the number of loci available. Furthermore, polyploid races may have a greater temperature tolerance than their diploid types; also in the Cynipidae that are active at low temperatures, it is the diploid female that has this tolerance, while the haploid male is absent from the winter generation.

Nevertheless the degree to which an individual can increase its temperature tolerance is limited, and new kinds of information for the establishment of new constants must arise, presumably by gene mutation, if very different temperature limits are to be produced. The selection of genotypes under different environmental temperature regimes has been noted.

Thus the Class Insecta has the anatomical and physiological organization which permits its members to survive under a wide range of environmental temperatures. Their ability to do so is manifest in three types of response. The insect may enter a resistant stage, accompanied by extreme dehydration in which all of the metabolic processes are halted or brought to a very low level. In this state, the insect may be exposed to temperatures as low as $-260°$ or as high as $102°$ and recover when returned to its normal temperature range.

In many species, the temperature tolerance of the individual may be increased by its ability to exist in either a high energy and relatively time-dependent state or in a low energy, relatively time-independent, closed steady state. The temperature tolerances of these two states may partially overlap, supplement one another, or be widely different. The low energy state is the resistant state and mechanisms have been developed which allow its assumption prior to the actual occurrence of the stress conditions that have to be endured.

These are mechanisms for increasing the temperature tolerance of the life of an individual insect. The third type of response does not do this, but shifts the temperature scale so that the insect is fully active at temperatures which evoke the formation of the resistant stages in other species. This is associated with the production of new state constants derived from new information produced by mutation and natural selection.

It is thought that the dominant features of the response of the insect type of organization to temperature arise from the chain of reactions that connect environmental changes with the genetic information contained within the animal.

References

Ackerman, L. (1926). *J. exp. Zool.* **44**, 1.
Akita, Y. and Nakayama, T. (1954). *Jap. J. Zool.* **11**, 297.
Anders, F., Drawert, F., Ander, A. and Reother, K. (1964). *Z. Naturforsch.* **19b**, 495.
Andrewartha, H. G. and Birch, L. C. (1954). "The Distribution and Abundance of Animals", University Press, Chicago.
Andrewartha, H. G. and Birch, L. C. (1960). *Annu. Rev. Entomol.* **5**, 219.
Argo, V. N. (1939). *Ann. entomol. Soc. Amer.* **32**, 147.
Arnold, G. (1965). *J. Morph.* **116**, 65.
Auclair, J. L. (1963). *Annu. Rev. Entomol.* **8**, 439.
Baldwin, W. F. (1954). *Canad. J. Zool.* **32**, 157.

Bates, M. (1947). *Ann. entomol. Soc. Amer.* **40**, 1.

Beament, J. W. L. (1945). *J. exp. Biol.* **21**, 115.

Beament, J. W. L. (1958). *J. insect Physiol.* **2**, 199.

Beament, J. W. L. (1959). *J. exp. Biol.* **36**, 391.

Beament, J. W. L. (1964). *Advanc. insect Physiol.* **2**, 67.

Becker, H. J. (1962). *Chromosomia* **13**, 341.

Beerman, W. (1959). *In* "Developmental Cytology", (D. Rudnick, Ed.), pp. 83–103. Ronald Press Co., New York.

Bělehrádek, J. (1935). "Temperature and Living Matter", *Protoplasma Monographien* **8**, 1.

Bernard, J., Gahery, Y. and Boistel, J. (1965). *In* "The Physiology of the Insect Central Nervous System", (J. E. Treherne and J. W. L. Beament, Eds.), Academic Press, London.

Bertalanffy, L. (1950). *Science* **111**, 23.

Bertalanffy, L. (1964). *Helgol. Wiss. Meeresunters.* **9**, 1.

Bhatnagar, P. L. (1963). *Naturwissenschaften* **50**, 445.

Birch, L. C. (1948). *J. animal Ecol.* **17**, 15.

Birch, L. C. (1953). *Evolution, N.Y.* **7**, 136.

Birkina, B. N. (1938). *Biol. Zhurn.* **7**, 653.

Bodine, J. H. and Allen, T. H. (1938). *J. cell. comp. Physiol.* **12**, 71.

Bodine, J. H. and Evans, T. C. (1932). *Biol. Bull.* **63**, 235.

Bodine, J. H., Tahmisian, T. N. and Hill, D. L. (1944). *Arch. Biochem.* **4**, 403.

Boiko, N. L. (1962). *Voprosy ekologii. Kievsk. Univ. Kiev.* **8**, 10.

Bounhiol, J. J. (1938). *Bull. Biol., Paris.* Suppl. 24, 1.

Brangham, A. N. (1962). "The Naturalist's Riviera", 339 pp., Phoenix House Limited, London.

Bricteux-Gregoire, S., Verly, W. G. and Florkin, M. (1957). *Nature, Lond.* **179**, 678.

Brooks, M. A. and Richards, A. G. (1955). *Biol. Bull.* **109**, 22.

Browning, T. O. (1953). *J. exp. Biol.* **30**, 104.

Burton, A. C. (1939). *J. cell. comp. Physiol.* **14**, 327.

Buxton, P. A. (1924). *Proc. Roy. Soc. B* **96**, 123.

Buxton, P. A. (1930). *Proc. Roy. Soc. B* **106**, 560.

Buxton, P. A. (1955). "The natural history of tsetse flies", London School of Hygiene and Tropical Medicine Memoir No. 10.

Calvet, E. and Prat, H. (1963). "Recent Progress in Microcalorimetry", 177 pp. Pergamon Press, London.

Cameron, M. L. (1953). *Nature, Lond.* **172**, 349.

Campbell, I. M. and Sullivan, C. R. (1963). *Proc. Internatl. Congr. Zool.* **16**, 62.

Cappe de Baillon, P. (1932). *Compt. rend. Acad. Sci., Paris* **195**, 557.

Chadwick, L. H. (1957). *In* "Influence of Temperature on Biological Systems", pp. 45–59. American Physiological Society.

Chapman, R. F. (1955). *J. exp. Biol.* **32**, 126.

Chapman, R. F. (1959). *Anti-Locust Bull.*, 33.

Chapman, R. N., Mickel, C. E., Parker, J. R., Miller, G. E. and Kelley, E. G. (1926). *Ecology* **7**, 416.

Chefurka, W. (1965). *In* "The Physiology of Insecta", (M. Rockstein, Ed.), Vol. II. Academic Press, New York.

Chin, C. T. (1951). *Arch. Biochem. Biophys.* **31**, 333.

Chino, H. (1958). *J. insect Physiol.* **2**, 1.

Church, N. S. (1960). *J. exp. Biol.* **37**, 186.

Clark, A. J. (1927). "Comparative Physiology of the Heart", 157 pp. University Press, Cambridge.

Clarke, J. M., Smith, J. M. and Travers, P. (1960). *Genet. Res., Cambridge* 1, 375.

Clarke, K. U. (1957). *J. exp. Biol.* 34, 29.

Clarke, K. U. (1960). *J. insect Physiol.* 5, 23.

Clarke, K. U. (1964). *Helgol. Wiss. Meeresunters.* 9, No. 1–4, 133–140.

Clarke, K. U. (1966). *J. insect. Physiol.* 12, 163.

Clarke, K. U. and Baldwin, R. W. (1960). *J. insect Physiol.* 5, 37.

Clarke, K. U. and Langley, P. A. (1963a). *J. insect Physiol.* 9, 287.

Clarke, K. U. and Langley, P. A. (1963b). *J. insect Physiol.* 9, 411.

Clarke, K. U. and Sardesai, J. B. (1959). *Bull. entomol. Res. Lond.* 50, 387.

Clements, A. N. (1963). "The Physiology of Mosquitoes", 393 pp. Pergamon Press, London.

Cleveland, L. R. (1924). *Biol. Bull.* 46, 177.

Clever, L. (1962). *Gen. Comp. Endocrinol.* 2, 604.

Clever, U. and Karlson, P. (1960). *Exp. Cell Res.* 20, 623.

Colhoun, E. H. (1954). *Nature, Lond.* 173, 582.

Colhoun, E. H. (1958). *J. insect Physiol.* 2, 108.

Colhoun, E. H. (1960). *Entomol. exp. appl.* 3, 27.

Craig, G. B. (1965). *Proc. XII Int. Congr. Entomol.* 263.

Crescitelli, F. and Jahn, T. L. (1939). *J. cell. comp. Physiol.* 14, 13.

da Cunha, A. B. (1960). *Annu. Rev. Entomol.* 5, 85.

Dadd, R. H. (1960). *J. insect Physiol.* 4, 319.

Dadd, R. H. (1963). *Advanc. insect Physiol.* 1, 47.

Danilevski, A. S. (1965). "Photoperiodism and Seasonal Development of Insects", 282 pp. Oliver and Boyd, Edinburgh.

Davey, K. G. (1961). *Gen. comp. Endocrinol.* 1, 24.

Davey, K. G. (1962). *J. insect Physiol.* 8, 579.

Davey, K. G. (1965). "Reproduction in Insects", 96 pp. Oliver and Boyd, Edinburgh.

Davey, P. M. (1954). *Bull. entomol. Res.* 45, 539.

Davison, J. A. and Richards, A. G. (1954). *Arch. Biochem. Biophys.* 48, 485.

Dawson, R. W. (1931). *J. exp. Zool.* 59, 87.

Demerec, M. (1932a). *Proc. nat. Acad. Sci. Wash.* 18, 430.

Demjanowski, S. Y., Vasilyeva, N. V. and Konikova, A. S. (1952). *Biochemistry U.S.S.R.* 17, 529.

Denbigh, K. G., Hicks, M. and Page, F. M. (1948). *Trans. Faraday Soc.* 44, 479.

Dethier, V. G. (1957). *Exp. Parasitol.* 6, 68.

Dethier, V. G. (1963). "The Physiology of Insect Senses", 266 pp. Methuen & Co. Ltd., London.

Dethier, V. G. and Arab, Y. M. (1958). *J. insect Physiol.* 2, 153.

Digby, P. S. B. (1955). *J. exp. Biol.* 32, 279.

Ditman, L. P. and Weiland, G. S. (1938). *Ann. entomol. Soc. Amer.* 31, 578.

Drescher, W. and Rothenbuhler, W. C. (1963). *J. Hered.* 54, 195.

Dubach, P., Smith, F., Pratt, D. and Stewart, C. M. (1959). *Nature, Lond.* 184, 288.

Dutrieu, J. (1961). *Compt. rend. Acad. Sci.* 252, 347.

Edney, E. B. (1957). "The Water Relations of Terrestrial Arthropods", 93 pp. Cambridge Monographs in Experimental Biology No. 5. University Press, Cambridge.

Edwards, D. K. (1958). *Canad. J. Zool.* 36, 363.

Evans, W. G. (1964). *Proc. XII Int. Cong. Entomol.* 286.

Evans, W. L. (1956). *Cytologia* **21**, 417.
Florkin, M. and Jeuniaux, C. (1964). *In* "The Physiology of Insecta", (M. Rockstein ed.), Vol. III, pp. 109–188. Academic Press, New York.
Fraenkel, G. and Herford, G. V. B. (1938). *J. exp. Biol.* **15**, 266.
Fraenkel, G. and Hopf, H. S. (1940). *Biochem. J.* **34**, 1085.
Frankhauser, G. (1942). *Biological Symposia* VI, 21.
Franz, H. (1930). *Biol. Zbl.* **50**, 158.
Frings, H. and Cox, B. L. (1954). *Biol. Bull.* **107**, 360.
Gardner, E. J., Turner, J. H. and Berseth, W. D. (1960). *Genetics* **45**, 905.
Gardner, E. J. and Woolf, C. M. (1950). *Genetics* **35**, 44.
Gebhardt, H. (1951). *Experientia* **7**, 302.
Geist, R. M. (1928). *Ann. entomol. Soc. Amer.* **21**, 614.
Gillies, M. T. (1953). *East African Med. J.* **30**, 129.
Gillies, M. T. and Shute, G. T. (1954). *Nature, Lond.* **173**, 409.
Gilmour, D. and Calaby, J. H. (1952). *Arch. Biochem. Biophys.* **41**, 83.
Glaser, R. W. (1946). *J. Parasitol.* **32**, 483.
Goldschmidt, R. (1938). "Physiological Genetics", 375 pp. McGraw-Hill Book Co. Inc., New York.
Goldsmith, M. H. M. and Schneiderman, H. A. (1960). *Biol. Bull.* **118**, 269.
Goodwin, B. C. (1963). "Temporal Organization in Cells", Academic Press, London.
Goodwin, T. W. (1952). *Biol. Rev.* **27**, 439.
Govaerts, J. and Leclercq, J. (1946). *Nature, Lond.* **157**, 483.
Gowen, J. W. and Gay, E. H. (1933). *Science* **77**, 312.
Graham, W. W. (1964). *Proc. XII Int. Cong. Entomol.* 345.
Green, G. W. and de Freitas, A. S. (1955). *Canadian Ent.* **87**, 427.
Gunn, D. L. (1942). *Biol. Rev.* **17**, 293.
Harris, P. (1962). *Canadian Ent.* **94**, 774.
Hartmann-Goldstein, I. and Sperlich, D. (1963). *Genetics* **48**, 863.
Hartung, E. W. (1947). *J. exp. Zool.* **106**, 223.
Hayward, J. A. (1962). M.Sc. Thesis: University of Nottingham.
Henderson, S. A. (1963). *Heredity* **18**, 77.
Henry, S. M. and Cook, T. W. (1963). *Contrib. Boyce Thompson Inst.* **22**, 133.
Herter, K. (1924). *Z. vergl. Physiol.* **1**, 221.
Herter, K. (1939). *Proc. VII Int. Cong. Entomol.* 740.
Hill, A. V. (1931). "Adventures in Biophysics", p. 55 University of Pennsylvania Press, Philadelphia.
Hill, L. and Taylor, H. J. (1933). *Nature, Lond.* **132**, 276.
Hillman, R. (1962). *Genetics* **47**, 11.
Hinton, H. E. (1960). *Nature, Lond.* **188**, 336.
Hinton, T. (1955). *Genetics* **40**, 224.
Hinton, T. and Dunlap, A. (1958). *Proc. X Int. Cong. Entomol.* **2**, 123.
Hodgson, E. S. (1956). *Anat. Rec.* **125**, 560.
Hodgson, E. S. (1958). *Biol. Bull.* **115**, 114.
Hodgson, E. S. and Geldiay, S. (1959). *Biol. Bull.* **117**, 275.
Hodgson, E. S. and Roeder, K. D. (1956). *J. cell. comp. Physiol.* **48**, 51.
Horsfall, W. R. and Anderson, J. F. (1964). *J. exp. Zool.* **156**, 61.
House, H. L., Riordan, D. F. and Barlow, J. S. (1958). *Canad. J. Zool.* **36**, 629.
Howe, R. W. (1953). *Ann. appl. Biol.* **40**, 121.
Howe, R. W. (1956). *Ann. appl. Biol.* **44**, 356.
Howe, R. W. (1957). *Bull. entomol. Res.* **48**, 9.
Hoyle, G. (1954). *J. exp. Biol.* **31**, 260.

350   KENNETH U. CLARKE

Huot, L. and Leclercq, J. (1958). *Arch. intern. Physiol. Biochem.* **66**, 270.
Ives, P. T. (1962). *Amer. Zoologist* **2**, 417.
Jacob, F. and Monod, J. (1961). *J. molec. Biol.* **3**, 318.
Johnson, C. G. (1942). *Biol. Rev.* **17**, 151.
Jones, J. C. (1964). In "The Physiology of Insecta", (M. Rockstein, ed.), Vol. III pp. 1–107. Academic Press, New York.
Karlson, P. and Sekeris, C. E. (1962). *Nature, Lond.* **195**, 183.
Karlson, P., Sekeris, E. and Maurer, R. (1964). *Z. physiol. Chem.* **336**, 100.
Keister, M. and Buck, J. (1961). *J. insect Physiol.* **7**, 51.
Keister, M. and Buck, J. (1964). In "The Physiology of Insecta", (M. Rockstein, Ed.), Vol. III, pp. 617–658. Academic Press, New York.
Kerkut, G. A. and Taylor, B. J. R. (1957). *J. exp. Biol.* **34**, 486.
Kettlewell, H. B. D. (1944). *Proc. and Trans. South London entomol. and nat. hist. Soc.* **79**.
Kinsey, A. C. (1942). *Biological Symposia VI* 167.
Kleinman, L. W. (1934). *J. cell. comp. Physiol.* **4**, 221.
Komarova, O. S. (1959). *Ent. Obozr.* **38**, 318.
Kroeger, H. (1963). *J. cell. comp. Physiol.* **62**, Suppl. 1, 45.
Krogh, A. and Weis-Fogh, T. (1951). *J. exp. Biol.* **28**, 344.
Kuehn, A. and Henke, K. (1936). *Abh. Ges. Wiss. Göttingen Berlin (N.F.)* **15**, 221.
Laufer, H. (1963). *Ann. N.Y. Acad. Sci.* **103**, 1137.
Laufer, H., Yasukiyo, N. and Vanderberg, J. (1964). *Develop. Biol.* **9**, 367.
Lensky, Y. (1964). *J. insect Physiol.* **10**, 279.
Lewis, H. W. (1960). *Genetics* **45**, 1217.
Li, Ju-Chi and Yu-lin Tsui (1936). *Genetics* **21**, 248.
Lima-De-Faria, A. (1961). *Hereditas* **47**, 674.
Lindroth, C. H. (1954). *Entomol. Tidskr. Stockholm* **75**, 111.
Lüscher, M. and Engelmann, F. (1955). *Rev. suisse Zool.* **62**, 649.
Lüscher, M. and Engelmann, F. (1960). *J. insect Physiol.* **5**, 240.
Makings, P. (1964). *J. exp. Biol.* **41**, 473.
Martignoni, M. E. (1964). *Annu. Rev. Entomol.* **9**, 179.
McAllan, J. W. and Chefurka, W. (1961). *Comp. Biochem. Physiol.* **3**, 1.
McIndoo, N. E. (1945). *J. comp. Neurol.* **83**, 141.
Mellanby, H. (1937). *Parasitology* **29**, 131.
Mellanby, K. (1932). *J. exp. Biol.* **9**, 222.
Mellanby, K. (1934). *Proc. Roy. Soc. B*, **116**, 139.
Mellanby, K. (1939). *Proc. Roy. Soc. B*, **127**, 473.
Mellanby, K. (1954). *Nature, Lond.* **173**, 582.
Mellanby, K. (1960). *Bull. entomol. Res.* **50**, 821.
Mellanby, K. and French, R. A. (1958). *Entomol. exp. appl.* **1**, 116.
Mer, G. (1936). *Bull. Soc. Path. exot. Paris* **30**, 38.
Meyer, H., Preiss, B. and Bauer, Sh. (1960). *Biochem. J.* **76**, 27.
Miller, P. L. (1965). In "The Physiology of the Insect Central Nervous System", (J. E. Treherne and J. W. L. Beament, Eds.), pp. 141–155. Academic Press, London.
Muirhead-Thomson, R. C. (1940). *J. malar. Inst. India.* **3**, 323.
Muller, J. H. (1942). *Biological Symposia VI*, 71.
Murray, R. W. (1962). *Advanc. comp. Physiol. Biochem.* **1**, 117.
Niemierko, W. (1959). In "Biochemistry of Insects", (L. Levenbook, Ed.). *Proc. Fourth International Conference of Biochemistry*, Vol. XII, pp. 185–200. Pergamon Press, London.
Ohnishi, E. (1959). *J. insect Physiol.* **3**, 219.

Orgel, L. E. (1964). *J. molec. Biol.* **9**, 208.
Ostryakova-Varshaver, V. P. (1958). *Tr. Inst. Morfol. Zhivotnykh Akad. Nauk SSSR.* **21**, 81.
Ostryakova-Varshaver, V. P. (1960). *Referat. Zhur. Biol.* No. 45751 (Translation).
Parker, J. R. (1930). *Montana agric. exp. Sta. Bull.* **223**, 132.
Parry, D. A. (1951). *J. exp. Biol.* **28**, 445.
Pittendrigh, C. S. (1954). *Proc. nat. Acad. Sci. Wash.* **40**, 1018.
Plough, H. H. (1917). *J. exp. Zool.* **24**, 148.
Plough, H. H. (1941). *Cold Spr. Harb. Symp. quant. Biol.* **9**, 127.
Polacek, I. and Kubista, V. (1960). *Physiol. Bohemosl.* **9**, 228.
Popham, E. J. (1964). *Proc. XII Int. Cong. Entomol.* 324.
Raffy, A. and Portier, P. (1931). *Compt. rend. Soc. Biol. Paris* **108**, 1062.
Rainey, R. C. (1938). *Ann. appl. Biol.* **25**, 822.
Ramsay, J. A. (1935). *J. exp. Biol.* **12**, 373.
Reiner, J. M. and Spiegelman, S. (1945). *J. phys. Chem.* **49**, 81.
Richards, A. G. (1951). "The Integument of Arthropods", 411 pp. University of Minnesota Press, Minneapolis.
Richards, A. G. (1958). *Proc. X Int. Cong. Entomol.* Vol. 2, pp. 67–72.
Richards, A. G. (1963a). *Ann. entomol. Soc. America* **56**, 355.
Richards, A. G. (1963b). *J. insect Physiol.* **9**, 597.
Richards, A. G. and Suanraksa, S. (1962). *Entomol. Exptl. Appl.* **5**, 167.
Rockstein, M. (1965). "The Physiology of Insecta", Vol. II, 905 pp. Academic Press, New York.
Roeder, K. D. Ed. (1953). "Insect Physiology", 1100 pp. John Wiley & Sons Inc. New York.
Roth, L. M. (1951). *Ann. entomol. Soc. Amer.* **44**, 59.
Salt, R. W. (1958). *Canad. J. Zool.* **36**, 265.
Salt, R. W. (1959). *Canad. J. Zool.* **37**, 59.
Salt, R. W. (1961). *Annu. Rev. Entomol.* **6**, 55.
Saunders, D. S. (1964). *Proc. XII Int. Cong. Entomol.*, 182.
Schneider, H. (1954). *Naturwissenschaften* **41**, 147.
Schneiderman, H. A. and Horowitz, J. (1958). *J. exptl. Biol.* **35**, 520.
Schneiderman, H. A. and Williams, C. M. (1953). *Biol. Bull.* **105**, 320.
Scholander, P. F., Flagg, W., Hock, R. J. and Irving, L. (1953). *J. cell. comp. Physiol.* **42**, Suppl. 1, 1.
Schreiner, T. (1952). *Z. Vergleich. Physiol. Berlin,* **34**, 278.
Scott, W. N. (1936). *Trans. R. ent. Soc. Lond.* **85**, 303.
Sekeris, C. E. and Karlson, P. (1964). *Arch. Biochem. Biophys.* **105**, 483.
Shepherd, R. F. (1958). *Canad. J. Zool.* **36**, 779.
Shlenova, M. F. (1938). *Med. Parasit. Moscow* **7**, 716.
Shulov, A. and Penner, M. P. (1963). *Anti-Locust Bull.* **41**.
Skinner, D. M. (1960). *Anat. Record* **138**, 383.
Slifer, E. H. (1930). *Physiol. Zool.* **3**, 503.
Slifer, E. H. (1932). *Physiol. Zool.* **5**, 448.
Slowtzoff, B. (1909). *Biochem. Z.* **19**, 497.
Sollunn, F.-J. and Strömnaes, O. (1964). *Hereditas* **51**, 1.
Stanley, W. F. (1935). *J. exp. Zool.* **69**, 459.
Steele, J. E. (1961). *Nature, Lond.* **192**, 680.
Stephen, W. P. (1964). *Proc. XII Int. Cong. Entomol.* 350.
Stich, H. F. (1959). *16th. Symp. Soc. for the Study of Development and Growth,* 105.

Tantawy, A. O. and Mallah, G. S. (1961). *Evolution* **15**, 1.

Taylor, I. R. and Crescitelli, F. (1937). *J. cell. comp. Physiol.* **10**, 93.

Telfer, W. H. and Williams, C. M. (1960). *J. insect Physiol.* **5**, 61.

Timofeeff-Ressovsky, N. W. (1940). *In* "The New Systematics", (J.Huxley, Ed.), pp. 73–136. University Press, Oxford.

Timon-David, J. (1927). *Compt. Rend. Soc. Biol. Paris* **96**, 1225.

Timon-David, J. (1930). *Ann. Fac. Sci. Marseille* **4**, 29.

Uvarov, B. P. (1931). *Trans. Entomol. Soc. Lond.* 79.

van der Kloot, W. G. (1955). *Biol. Bull.* **109**, 276.

Waloff, N. and Richards, O. W. (1958). *Trans. R. entomol. Soc. Lond.* **110**, 99.

Weis-Fogh, T. (1952). *Phil. Trans. Roy. Soc. B*, **237**, 1.

White, M. J. D. (1934). *J. Genet.* **29**, 203.

Wigglesworth, V. B. (1934). *Quart. J. micr. Sci.* **77**, 191.

Wigglesworth, V. B. (1936). *Quart. J. micr. Sci.* **79**, 91.

Wigglesworth, V. B. (1941). *Parasitology* **33**, 67.

Wigglesworth, V. B. (1950). "The Principles of Insect Physiology", 544 pp. Methuen & Co. Ltd., London.

Wigglesworth, V. B. (1959). "The Control of Growth and Form: A Study of the Epidermal Cell in an Insect", 136 pp. Cornell University Press, Ithaca.

Wigglesworth, V. B. and Gillett, J. D. (1934). *J. exp. Biol.* **11**, 120.

Williams, C. M. (1947). *Anat. Rec.* **99**, 591.

Wilson, D. M. (1965). *In* "The Physiology of the Insect Central Nervous System", (J. E. Treherne and J. W. L. Beament, Eds.), pp. 125–140. Academic Press, London.

Winteringham, F. P. W. (1960). *Biochem. J.* **75**, 38.

Wyatt, G. R. (1959). *In* "Biochemistry of Insects", (L. Levenbook, Ed.), pp. 161–178. Pergamon Press, London.

Wyatt, G. R. and Kalf, G. F. (1957). *J. gen. Physiol.* **40**, 833.

Yuill, J. S. and Craig, R. (1937). *J. exp. Zool.* **75**, 169.

Zimmerging, S. (1963). *Genetics* **48**, 133.

Chapter 10

The Heat Responses of Invertebrates (Exclusive of Insects)

M. A. McWhinnie

Department of Biological Sciences
De Paul University
Chicago, Illinois, U.S.A.

I. Introduction

Living organisms maintain a state of dynamic balance in their constantly varying environments by the delicate interaction of numerous metabolic reactions. An organism adapted to an environment has the capacity to modulate the rates of various reactions which are sensitive to the flux of the environment. In this manner, a homeostatic equilibrium is efficiently maintained. At the cellular level, these responses are rooted in enzymic systems which respond to environmental signals by quantitative or qualitative biochemical modifications. At this point no reference is made to enzyme concentration or to enzyme activity. The maximum ability of an organism to adjust within the wide range of a variable reflects the genetic capacity of a species. However, within the total scope of genetic competence, there are physiological adjustments which are based on compensatory metabolic responses to environmental variables. Successful adjustment within a gradient marked by an upper and lower limit, under some circumstance, does not represent a fixed zone defining the full adaptational capacity of a species. Apparent physiological limits are influenced by past environmental histories; by many physical quantities; multiple biological variables including age, size, nutritional state; and the abruptness with which the organism meets the change, among others. Thus, the genetic limits become more clearly defined when adaptation limits are experimentally tested and the total range of tolerance and survival is determined.

Through many years, there has been increasing interest in the physiological basis of adaptation to various environments, and in these studies the effects of temperature have been of central importance. Review articles have focused upon special aspects of this factor (Vernberg, 1962; Prosser, 1958; Bullock, 1955; Scholander et al., 1953), and more recently a comprehensive treatise of temperature influences, among other environmental parameters, has been presented (Dill et al., 1964).

Approaches to understanding the mechanisms of adaptation or survival at the extremes of temperature found across the wide spectrum encountered at various latitudes and in different habitats have been through two general types of study. The first of these is found in an extensive literature in which respiration of animals that had been subjected to various temperatures was reported. Comparisons of organisms of the same and different genera at many latitudes have been made, and responses have been measured using adults as well as developmental stages. In addition, experimentally acclimated animals have been studied with respect to their change in respiratory response at a variety of temperatures. Coinciding influences which modify the temperature response have been established through experimental modifications of salinity, light intensity, and available oxygen supply.

In studies of whole organism respiratory response to changes in environmental temperatures, five categories of response patterns have been identified by Precht (1958) and Prosser (1958). The changes include a displacement of response–temperature curves as a consequence of increased or decreased metabolism after acclimation to lower temperatures. In this type of response, there is no change in the ratio of reaction rates when lower and higher temperatures are used in the measurement (e.g. no change in Q_{10} value). This pattern is described as translation and demonstrates no physiological compensation. Metabolic alterations to changed environmental conditions may also be characterized by an increase (or decrease) in the response at one end of a gradient of the environmental variable, but with no proportionate increase corresponding to increments of the variable. These responses, when superimposed upon those measured in animals taken from their normal environmental temperatures, show rotation of the rate–temperature curve. The response after acclimation leads to a decrease in the ratio of rates at two different temperatures which is expressed by a decrease in the temperature coefficient (Q_{10}) for the reaction. This pattern of response confers a degree of physiological (= metabolic) independence upon the acclimated organism, since fluxes in environmental temperature do not elicit corresponding rate changes. This pattern of acclimation change is a consequence of physiological compensation, and the organism responses are no longer a proportionate reflection of temperature variations within a range of relative neutrality. The distinct differences between the two types of responses outlined must find their explanation at the level of biochemical reactions influenced through the environmental stress either quantitatively or qualitatively. Prosser (1958, 1964) has pointed out that these two types of response most probably represent increases in enzyme level or quantitative changes in metabolic pathways. Recent studies provide evidence in support of these interpretations and will be discussed below.

The second general approach to an elucidation of the fundamental mechanisms of adaptation to variations and extremes of temperature has been through a study of biochemical modifications, consequent upon the establishment of acclimation. This approach has been more extensively pursued in homeothermic vertebrates (Smith and Hoijer, 1962) but has some representation in invertebrate studies. Clearly, it is this approach which will provide the molecular basis for the thermogenesis essential to account for activity and syntheses at suboptimum temperatures, as well as survival and cellular homeostasis at superoptimum temperatures.

The first approach has been a fruitful one and has provided the physiological framework within which molecular changes can now be assigned with meaning. It is the second approach which is presently gaining in interest and, correspondingly, yielding a new understanding concerning the molecular mechanisms which underlie behavioural and whole organism physiology in both poikilothermic and homeothermic animals.

II. Temperature Influences at the Organismic Level

A. ACCLIMATION HISTORY

1. *Species and Latitudinal Differences*

It has been noted that a reduction in the Q_{10} value provides a degree of metabolic independence wherein the organism responds less to temperature variation, though across a low-temperature range it may support a higher metabolic rate. This has been shown for the terrestrial isopods *Porcellio laevis* and *Armadillidium vulgare* (Edney, 1964) where animals

12*

acclimated to 10° for 14 days showed increased oxygen consumption at 10°, with no increase when measured at 20° and a decline at 30°. Exposed to the same acclimation temperatures, *P. laevis* showed greater O_2 uptake than *A. vulgare*, verifying species differences. Aquatic species of amphipods show similar responses (Wautier and Troiani, 1960). *Gammarus pulex* showed a 25% greater O_2 consumption than did a *Niphargus* sp. when both were acclimated to 10°; however, both showed little variation in their responses to temperatures between 10° and 20°, but an increase in Q_{10} from 20° to 30°. The lethal temperatures were species-specific and the *Niphargus* sp. exhibited higher heat resistance, dying at 28–29° while the upper limit for *Gammarus* was closer to 20°.

The extent of acclimation which is achieved by organisms maintained at temperatures reflects their past temperature histories. Based upon latitudinal distribution and therefore environmental temperature gradients, studies of the crustacean decapod *Uca* sp. have confirmed that temperate species show higher oxygen consumption at elevated temperatures than do tropical species when both have been acclimated at 15° (Vernberg, 1959). Similarly, temperate-acclimated species consumed more O_2 at 36° than did the tropical species. Alternately, tropical species showed higher lethal temperatures than those from temperate regions until both were acclimated to 15°; inter-specific differences with respect to a high lethal temperature were lost while cold lethal temperatures remained lower for temperate species after acclimation (Vernberg and Tashian, 1959). This same type of latitudinal and therefore temperature effect has been studied further (Vernberg and Vernberg, 1966) using *Uca rapax* and *U. uruguayensis* from various latitudes. Cold-acclimated animals showed a high O_2 consumption at high and low temperatures while warm acclimation resulted in a higher metabolic rate at intermediate temperatures. This metabolic response reflects that obtained after laboratory acclimation of the copepod *Tigriopus japonicus* (Matutani, 1960). Animals reared at 5°, 10°, 20°, and 30°, and studied for survival time at 38·6°, showed the highest heat resistance to be correlated with the highest acclimation temperature. However, heat resistance was not proportional to acclimation temperature, and 5°-reared animals showed higher resistance than those acclimated to either 10° or 20°. The higher metabolic rates at low and high temperature extremes noted for the decapod *Uca* (Vernberg and Vernberg, 1966) correspond in a temperature scale with the heat resistance reported for the copepod *Tigriopus japonicus*. It is unfortunate that no information exists concerning the nature of the metabolic pathways or the ratios of pathways that may have been altered as a result of acclimation to temperature extremes. Limitation in biochemical capacities may account for the species differences shown by Halcrow (1963) from study of the copepod *Calanus finmarchicus*. Responses to acclimation at 4°, 10°, and 20° showed that these animals do not adjust to temperatures beyond those represented by their normal seasonal temperature range. The ecological distribution of a species might be anticipated to reflect the genetic capacity to support fluxes in physiological compensation. Evidence from study of the Australasian barnacle, *Elminius modestus*, (Barnes and Barnes, 1962) supports the view that ecological history influences growth and survival at new locations. While this species demonstrates a considerable eurythermal capacity, its growth rate and reproductive potential are depressed at northern latitudes when compared with populations at lower latitudes. With respect to ecological distribution, it may be emphasized that tolerance and physiological adjustment to temperature ranges of some stage in a life cycle will not necessarily afford a physiological description of species adaptation to an environment.

Variations in physiological capacities at various stages in a life cycle may play a more significant role in successful colonization. Some evidence in favour of this concept is demonstrated by the findings of Barnes (1960) from a study of *Balanus balanoides* in which gametogenesis was shown to have a higher heat sensitivity than was evident in other phases in the life cycle. Thus, this stage is the factor determining the southern extent of the species range. Conversely, the eggs of the branchiopod, *Triops granarius*, withstand temperatures considerably above 40° while this is the upper lethal temperature for mature adults (Cloudsley-Thompson, 1965). The concept of temperature-dependent development of boreo-arctic species and the associated breeding cycles has been presented by Barnes *et al.* (1963).

Capacities for successful acclimatization may exceed those required in the total of seasonal variations which characterize an ecological habitat. In a study of antarctic amphipods, Armitage (1962) demonstrated metabolic compensation between $-1.8°$ and 6° by a vertical displacement (downward) of the R–T curve relating O_2 consumption to temperatures between $-1.8°$ and 12°. It was suggested that evidence for metabolic compensation over a temperature range that is not naturally encountered by circumpolar antarctic species may represent the genetic history of a habitat which once had a wider range of temperature variation. The antarctic euphausid, *E. superba*, has also been shown to follow conventional acclimation patterns through rotation and translation of the R–T curve when held at 0° (McWhinnie, 1964).

The marked sensitivity of these endemic crustacea (Marr, 1962) was evidenced by higher O_2 uptake by animals maintained at 0° in comparison with those held at $1.0°$ for 1.5 days after having been collected from 0.3° seawater. Additionally, animals taken from approximately

1·0° water showed rotation of the rate curve with a concomitant decrease in Q_{10} when held at 0° for 4–5 days. The narrow tolerance range for temperature was represented by a temperature 4·0° being 100% lethal within 24 hours. It is of interest that maximum motor activity occurred at −1·8°, the freezing point of seawater. In contrast to the endemic antarctic euphausid, the sub-antarctic anomuran decapod, *Munida gregaria* (grimothea stage), collected from 8·8° water, showed a higher Q_{10} between 0° and 10° than was found for the euphausid (McWhinnie, 1964). The lower lethal temperature was 0° and maintenance at 2° for 8 days resulted in metabolic compensation expressed by rotation and translation of the R–T curve. These results with southern polar forms are not in complete agreement with those reported by Scholander *et al.* (1953) for arctic crustacea. The northern forms showed little metabolic adaptation when compared with tropical species. However, R–T curves were displaced farther to the left than were those of animals from tropical environments. From this, one can infer adaptation only by increased rates of reactions. It was interpreted that species in regions of low temperature variation, such as polar forms, do not require as broad a competence for physiological adaptation as do those from more widely varying temperature environments.

The temperate decapod, *Orconectes virilis*, showed conventional responses by rotation of the rate–temperature curve after 1 week at 5° (McWhinnie and O'Connor, 1966) but only if the animals were in the intermoult stage (C_3–C_4) of the intermoult cycle. Premoult animals showed no compensation; the response of stage C_3–C_4 animals was lost at 2 weeks and survival at any stage did not exceed 6 weeks at 5°. It is of some significance that stage C_3–C_4 intermoult and stage D premoult crayfish are characterized by measureably different ratios of metabolic pathways (McWhinnie and Kirchenberg, 1962; McWhinnie and Corkill, 1963; McWhinnie and Chua, 1964). Tissue Q_{O_2} values vary with physiological stage, and the pentose phosphate route is operative during intermoult stages while glycolysis is the predominant route during premoult. Simultaneously, whole organism and tissue metabolism are different in animals acclimated to 5° and 18°(McWhinnie and O'Connor, 1966). Thus, the biochemical background of tissue metabolism must represent the matrix of physiological compensation to temperature stress.

2. *Oxygen Level*

Metabolic responses to temperature are measurably influenced by other varying environmental conditions. Wiens and Armitage (1961) have shown that O_2 consumption rises with increasing temperatures and with the level of oxygen saturation. Their results with two species of fresh water crayfish showed an elevation in Q_{O_2} value with increases in temperature to 30–35° and a proportionate decrease in oxygen uptake at any temperature with a reduction in oxygen saturation. Based upon the differences in response to temperature and oxygen availability, it was concluded that the differences in ecological distribution of the two species was based primarily upon the lower capacity of *Orconectes nais* to regulate with respect to stresses of high temperature and low oxygen when compared with *O. immunis*. The degree of oxygen saturation has also been shown to influence heat sensitivity. Matutani (1962a) has reported that the copepod, *Tigriopus japonicus*, has higher resistance to 36·8° after acclimation to 30° when compared with animals acclimated at 20°, but in both groups resistance was higher when the degree of oxygen saturation of the environment was less than 50%. The tropical earthworm, *Pheretima hawayana*, showed no sensitivity to a wide range of oxygen concentrations (down to 15%) and a predictable decrease in Q_{O_2} with a reduction in temperature to 2° (Mendes and Almeida, 1962).

As higher oxygen levels increase the sensitivity of some copepods to high temperatures, so starvation has been reported as a factor influencing thermal sensitivity. The fresh water crab, *Paratelphusa* sp., shows correlation between oxygen consumption, temperature, and body weight. After starvation for 2–3 weeks, there is a decrease in capacity to adjust to high temperatures (as expressed by a decreased Q_{10}) in the 30–35° range which was not observed in fed animals (Rajabai, 1963). Rates of oxidation and the quantity of oxidizable substrate probably account for the influence of both available oxygen and nutritional state, but this must yet be defined at the cellular and biochemical level. Loss and gain of heat tolerance can be varied with acclimation temperature. Spoor (1955) demonstrated a shift in the heat tolerance of crayfish as a consequence of acclimation temperature. Animals maintained at 22–26° showed reduced survival times from 34° to 37°, and transfer to 4° decreased their heat tolerance. Conversely, return to higher temperatures restored their thermal resistance.

In similar studies, Bowler (1963a) showed survival of *Astacus pallipes* to be limited to 34° and 37° for animals acclimated to 8° and 25°, respectively. That is, the lethal high temperature was shifted down with low temperature acclimation. When 8° animals were subseque transferred to 25°, 50% mortality at 35° was reached only after cons ably longer exposure periods. The capacity of physiological compe tion is thereby broad, and dependent upon thermal history. So evidence from this study suggests that a temperature-sensitive region the cephalothorax may be responsible for the onset of death. In subsequent study (Bowler, 1963b), it was shown that tissue respirati continued at temperatures which were lethal to the whole organism. Th conclusion was drawn that metabolic breakdown of tissues could not represent the significant cause of thermal death. Rather was it suggested that, due to changes in circulating sodium and potassium levels and their ratios, death may be a consequence of an alteration in neural co-ordination.

3. Ionic Influences

Other investigators have inquired into ionic influences on metabolic responses to temperature variations among many invertebrates. The heat resistance of the copepod, *Trigriopus japonicus*, to 38·6° after maintenance at 20° in various salinities was measured (Matutani,1962b). Animals in concentrated seawater (150%) showed the highest resistance to 38·6°, while acclimation to dilute seawater (50–75%) for 48 hours was accompanied by an increase in heat resistance. Acclimation to 25% sea water resulted in a significant decrease in resistance. It is clear that, through undefined mechanisms of ionic and osmotic compensations, thermal stress can be decreased. Such adjustments are of adaptational value to organisms encountering environments of changing salinity, but the basis for such compensations remains to be elucidated. Low temperature (4°) has been shown to decrease urinary flow and ion loss in the crayfish, *O. virilis* (Riegel, 1961); exposure of the fresh-water crab, *Paratelphusa* sp., to correspondingly high temperatures (36°) leads to an initial increased exchange in chloride ions with a compensation through decreased ion flux under continued high temperature exposure (Rao and Venkatareddy, 1962). Initially there was a decrease in blood osmotic pressure (Rao and Ramachandra, 1961). Such ion fluxes appear to be associated with changes in cellular-blood balances, and it has been suggested that the interplay of the environmental variables of temperature and ion concentration, coupled with species differences in physiological compensation to these variables, may account for successful colonization of brackish water by competent species (Lockwood, 1960).

Earthworms (*Lampito mauritii*) and mussels (*Lamellidens marginalis*) show similar alterations in the ion concentrations of their body fluids when exposed to low temperatures. Chloride, magnesium, and amino acids decrease in amounts but the cations sodium, potassium, and calcium increase (Rao, 1962, 1963a). These shifts must relate to changes in intracellular concentrations as was suggested by Rao and Ramachandra (1961), for which they inferred an important role in the support of metabolic compensation for temperature changes. However, such measures alone cannot elucidate causal relations between these two responses. It is of interest, from the point of view of general mechanisms, that the addition of Ca^{2+} to environmental water increased the survival of *Paramecium caudatum* at 4° after acclimation to 14°; conversely, these ions increased sensitivity to 29° and 40°. In parallel with the ion changes in earthworms, where the magnesium content decreased during cold acclimation, it was also the least effective ion in influencing sensitivity to temperature extremes by protozoans (Irlina, 1963; Grigoryan, 1964).

More recent studies on the annelid, *Lampito mauritii*, have confirmed the alternate influences of cold and warm temperature acclimation on the levels of inorganic ions and amino acids. It had previously been suggested that cold induces an increase in protein synthesis, and decreased amino acid levels in body fluids were considered to reflect this (Raghupthiramireddy and Rao, 1963). The above view is supported by the evidence that RNA, protein-nitrogen, and dry weight of cold-treated *Lampito mauritii* are increased as is tissue glycogen (Saroja and Rao, 1965). An increase in protein as a result of cold exposure had been demonstrated previously in the fresh-water mussel, *Lamellidens marginalis* (Rao, 1963b, 1963c). While the mechanisms of induction of such changes by cold treatment are not yet well established in poikilothermic animals, it is of particular interest that neurosecretory cell activity of the earthworm brain is differentially increased by cold exposure. Further, transfer of body fluid from cold (19°) to warm (29°, 35°)-acclimated worms increased tissue respiration of the latter. It seems well established, at least in the case of the earthworm, that low temperature induces activation of neurosecretory sites which mediate physiological changes measured through oxygen consumption and protein synthesis (Rao and Saroja, 1963).

B. DEVELOPMENT

Temperature influences on development may have a broader impact on basic biological phenomena and species distribution than upon adult stages. For example, it has been shown that the viability of sperm cells at elevated temperatures (28–40°) is species-specific for three species of the sea urchin, *Strongylocentrotus* (Andronikov, 1963); and that the sex ratio of the copepod, *Macrocyclops albidus*, is temperature-dependent; for, as the temperature rises (10° to 25°), the number of males is significantly increased (Monokov, 1965). Reproductive cycles and growth and maturation of gonads of marine invertebrates have been thoroughly reviewed by Giese (1959).

The temperature dependence of larval development has been reported for the crustacea *Sesarma cinereum* (Costlow et al., 1960) and *Panopeus herbstii* (Costlow et al., 1962). In both species, development to the first crab stage at 30° was complete in approximately one-half the time required to reach the same stage at 20°. However, low and high salinities have a greater influence on development than does temperature. The relationship between developmental time and temperature indicates that a spring brood is favoured by longer development at lower temperatures such that later zoeal and megalops stages would only be reached as environmental temperatures rise. The converse would be unfavourable in fall, and the higher temperatures in early fall would decrease developmental time. The ecological and survival advantages are apparent. Shrimp taken from Gulf of Mexico waters show a low sensitivity to both temperature and salinity (Zein-Eldin and Aldrich, 1965). There was no mortality in post-larval *Pennaeus aztecus* maintained at temperatures of 20–32° in waters having salinities ranging from 5 to 37 p.p.t. However, temperature became critical at a salinity less than 5 p.p.t. Growth was maximal at 32° and zero at 11°. Wide tolerance to these variables is of significance in species which undergo larval development in estuarine waters. Similar temperature influences have been reported for barnacles. Patel (1959) reported that *Lepas anatifera* nauplii are viable at 19° and 25° but not at 15° or 30°, and that developmental rate increases to 25°. Winter adults of several barnacle species were induced to breed by elevation of temperatures to 15° and above (Patel and Crisp, 1960), but it was necessary that food be present. In this study, moulting, an expression of growth in crustaceans, was also temperature-dependent. The blockage of moulting by low temperature has been shown for other crustaceans including crayfish (Kyer, 1942; McWhinnie, 1962) and crabs (Passano, 1960).

A high degree of sensitivity to temperature was shown by the mollusc, *Mytilus edulis*, at high latitudes. Gonadal development and spawning were shown to be confined to animals in water ranging from about 12° to 16° only (Heinonen, 1962). Sastry (1963, 1966) reported that the bay scallop, *Aequipecten irradians*, can be brought to spawn during the winter months by elevation of the temperature to 20° or above. Natural populations initiate spawning in about mid-August off the southeast coast of the United States. The environmental temperature range from May through October is 20–25°, and gametogenesis is initiated in spring (May–June). However, as in the case of the barnacles, gonad growth and maturation are dependent upon nutrient supply also. But scallops maintained at 10° and 15° failed to spawn irrespective of nutritional state. From mature gonads of laboratory-maintained animals spawning was directly related to temperatures between 20° and 30°. Oogenesis is more sensitive to temperature than is spermatogenesis and requires a temperature above 20° for its initiation. Cleavage of fertilized eggs cannot occur below temperatures between 15° and 20°.

In contrast, a wider temperature tolerance was shown for early larvae of *Venus mercenaria* in which the time of setting and size were measured at experimental temperatures of 18° to 30° (Loosanoff, 1959). While time to reach setting was longer at lower temperatures, all groups reached the same developmental size at that time. There was no relation between temperature and size. Similarly animals from widely differing latitudes showed similar growth rates and time for setting. In terms of basic mechanisms in adaptation, the author suggests that *Venus* sp. is unusual when considered among the widely established examples showing that eggs and larvae of southern species develop more slowly than do northern species of the same genus.

While data were not presented on developmental rates at different temperatures, Farmanfarmaian (1963) has shown a wide thermal tolerance for fertilization and development of the eggs of the sea urchin, *Strongylocentrotus purpuratus*. Normal development occurs between 13° and 20°, and previous treatment at 5° does not block fertilization when eggs are transferred to 13°. However, 25° is lethal for adults, and if development is initiated at this temperature, larvae are abnormal. Between 13° and 20° the developmental rate increases with temperature. This species is of interest because its geographical range extends from Mexico (28°N) to Alaska. Survival of the species within this wide thermal gradient may be explained by the behavioural difference in populations at the southern extent of the range. The latter remain subtidal, experiencing smaller temperature fluctuations than do the intertidal populations at more northern latitudes.

Influences of temperature on reproductive processes among invertebrates may be demonstrated by variations in the responses of acellular organisms to temperature. Within the concept of common biochemical alterations resulting from temperature stresses, the possibility remains that information gained from protozoan or metazoan species will illuminate the mechanisms of physiological adjustments in poikilothermic animals in general. Similar to metazoa, *Tetrahymena pyriformis* shows a temperature-dependent reproductive rate. Cultures incubated at temperatures below 20° and above 30° showed a marked increase in generation time, and organisms cultured outside the range of 22–27° were considerably larger (Thormar, 1962a). Evidence for adaptation, however, was obtained since cultures grown at temperatures outside the 17–30° range showed increasingly shorter generation periods after the first division in these temperature extremes. Similar to metazoans, low temperature-treated animals became more heat sensitive and all cell division ceased at 32–33° (Thormar, 1962b). Frankel (1964) confirmed these results and extended the study to alterations in morphogenesis, and observed abnormal membranelle formation at 33° after one division. Morphogenesis is not normal at 33·5° and cell division is totally blocked at 34°. The sensitivity of these developmental phenomena to slight changes in temperature would support a fixed genetic limit for physiological adaptation. The response of *Tetrahymena* sp. to cold shock was considerably less than it was to heat (Gavin, 1965), while *Paramecium aurelia* shows a lower sensitivity to heat (Whitson, 1964).

In *Euglena gracilis* (Buetow, 1962) and in *Chilomonas paramecium* (Johnson, 1962) temperature influences both size and division rate in the same manner as in *Tetrahymena pyriformis*. Reproduction was highest at 25–30° while growth, expressed as dry weight, was more than doubled at 13–17° (Buetow, 1962).

The temperature effect is clearly one separating synthesis and division; a 14-fold increase in activation energy was required for growth at 13·3–17° when compared with 25–28·5°. While the critical incremental energy of activation (the Arrhenius μ value) is an index of a specific catalyst, it must be recognized that in a complex biochemical system a specific temperature characteristic cannot specify a particular catalyst or reaction pathway. None the less, the wide differences in activation energies and in the organismic response at these two temperature ranges point to different biochemical mechanisms (or ratios of metabolic pathways) that support these phenomena differentially at low and high temperatures. Based upon a study of *Trypanosoma ranarum*, a protozoan parasite of the poikilothermic amphibian, Lehmann (1962) has suggested that enzymic systems are differentially sensitive to temperature and that 31° selectively destroys synthetic enzymic systems while those involved in energy release are unmodified. This conclusion was drawn from observations made on cultures which, upon return to 25° after exposure to 31°, showed continued viability but could not resume normal division. The addition of a red blood-cell extract to cultures of the gecko parasite, *Leishmania tarentolae*, stimulated growth at the supranormal temperature of 33°. A deficiency in synthetic capacity for cell multiplication was thereby overcome and may be explained on the basis of differential enzyme inactivation. In *in vitro* culture, 33° is near the upper thermal limit for this species and 37° completely blocks both growth and division (Krassner, 1965).

C. BODY TEMPERATURE OF POIKILOTHERMS

There is some evidence that poikilothermic animals regulate their body temperature to a limited degree as a consequence of physical changes related to environmental variables. Through responses to humidity and by motor activity, the internal body temperature of the crab, *Ocypoda macrocera*, can vary 3–4° from environmental temperatures. At low humidities body temperature is reduced, while in saturated air there is no differential between the organism and its environment. Evaporative heat loss may facilitate survival at high temperatures through this route (Pailey, 1961). Comparable body temperature variations have been reported for isopods in mesic and xeric habitats (Warburg, 1965). Among the crustaceans, this latter group is the most successful in terrestrial adaptation, and a significant step towards this achievement is the capacity to acclimate to a wide temperature differential. Evaporation and convection promote heat loss at high temperatures. Additionally, a behavioural component is employed to increase exposed surfaces for evaporation. In the mesic species, *Armadillidium vulgare*, body temperature decreases 2–3° each time the legs are moved. Mechanisms other than heat loss by evaporation, however, must characterize xeric species. Curves for the xeric *Venezillo arizonicus*, a desert dweller, show low evaporation when compared with the mesic *A. vulgare*, and evaporative loss was low even through long exposure periods. This water conservation in a dry environment breaks sharply at 38–40° in an atmosphere of constant saturation deficiency. At these temperatures, the decrease in body temperature relates closely to evaporation rate.

Body temperature regulation is also related to the reflection or absorption of radiant energy by adaptive colour changes. Wilkens and Fingerman (1965) reported that *Uca pugilator* survives at 40·7° and 45·1–47° when exposed to saturated and dry air respectively. Dark crabs showed a body temperature 2° higher than that of pale ones in bright sunlight, and the rate of evaporative water loss was proportional to the saturation-deficiency of air. Thus, through evaporation and colour adaptation, poikilotherms have some capacity to regulate body temperature. There is additionally a behavioural response to high temperatures characterized as a "feeding retreat" rhythm on hot days when crabs periodically return to their moist, dark burrows. It was interpreted that such an 18 to 24 minute cycle serves to lower the body temperature. A remarkable example of high temperature tolerance has been reported for the high intertidal snail, *Littorina neritoides* (Fraenkel, 1961). This species spends most of its life out of water and was shown to resist 46–47° for 1–2 hours when submerged, and a temperature 2° higher when in air. No behavioural or physiologically adaptive mechanisms were studied but body temperature decrease might occur and could include those means defined for crustacea. This is entirely likely since, in other gastropods, Lewis (1963) observed that the body temperature of *Nerita tesselata* was considerably below that of a black body, due to evaporative water loss. The most effective evaporation rate, among three species studied, was found for the high-tide level *Nerita tesselata*, when compared with the mid-tide level limpet, *Fissurella barbadensis*, and the barnacle, *Tetraclita squamosa*. Efficiency of heat loss was estimated by comparison of tissue temperature with that of a rock surface, an inanimate object, and a black body; relative to the sun–air temperature, these were respectively 4·6°F, 7·8°F, 13·3°F, and 19°F. The limpet and barnacle tissue values were closer to those of the black body. Environmental selection based upon physiological compensations to temperature correlate in these forms with intertidal zonation.

III. Temperature Influences at the Tissue Level

The adaptations of poikilothermic organisms are functions of tissue and cell responses which may adjust as a consequence of direct action of the temperature stress or through a receptor–co-ordinator route. The nature of initiation of metabolic changes is not known in poikilotherms, and may be mediated through both mechanisms. Even in the case of neural regulation, however, direct cellular action cannot be excluded, and this, in turn, could modify or potentiate the effect of a direct action on other cell types. It is of some interest that changes in temperature have been shown by Kerkut and Ridge (1962) to alter resting potentials in nerve cells of the snail, *Helix aspersa*. Increase in temperature increases both the resting potential and the frequency of action potentials; in addition, cooling activated "silent" cells while subsequent elevations in temperature returned the cell to quiet. That a common mechanism involving changes in ionic balance, as a consequence of low temperature, may be responsible for activation of nerve cells, may be inferred from investigations on protozoa. Studying the ciliate *Opalina* sp., Ueda (1961) observed that membrane potentials increase directly with an increase in temperature, though the Q_{10} value for the increase between 8° and 35° was low ($= 1·18°$). In addition, there were cyclic variations in this potential with seasonal change. The previously discussed modifications in ionic ratios in the earthworm, *Lampito mauritii* (Section II. A. 3, p. 360) could be responsible for alteration in nerve excitability.

At the present time, the mechanism of translation of the environmental stress of temperature change to the organismic response is unknown. However, evidence does exist that cells and tissues of poikilotherms show responses to these changes in a fashion that closely resembles that of the intact organism. Using a variety of littoral and sub-littoral marine molluscs, Dzhamusova (1960) demonstrated that the heat resistance of muscle tissue correlated with both vertical and horizontal distribution of the species. Tissue isolated from *Littorina* sp. and *Thais* sp. showed greater heat resistance when taken from the littoral zone of the Sea of Japan than was observed in the same species taken from the more northern Barents Sea. Similar heat resistance of muscle tissue from other species was correlated with latitudinal distribution. The influence of species differences superimposed upon that of latitude was shown by Zhirmunskii and Pisareva (1961) in a study of molluscs, ascidians, and echinoderms. In this study, it was shown that heat sensitivity of ciliary epithelium and muscle excitability were more species-specific than influenced by the different depths and temperatures of their natural environment. The sub-littoral range occupied by these forms was 30–70 metres. However, tissues from four species of gastropods from a narrower geographical range, but having a wider temperature fluctuation, showed both interspecific differences in thermal sensitivity as well as differences in sensitivity based upon intertidal zonation (Zhirmunskii and Chu, 1963). It can be anticipated that the physiological responses of any group will reflect the physiological capacities both genetically and environmentally determined. Comparable heat resistance based upon species differences and vertical distribution has been shown for isolated gills from three pelecypod molluscs (Vernberg et al., 1963). Tissues from the sub-littoral scallop, *Aequipecten irradians*, entered heat narcosis at 37°, while the intertidal *Modiolus demissus* and *Crassostrea virginica* survived at 44° for more than 1·5 hours. Warm acclimation extended survival time at 44° while cold acclimation decreased it.

As survival time of tissue at elevated temperatures reflects the previously described responses of whole organisms acclimated to varying thermal conditions, the Q_{O_2} values are also proportional to temperature. Isolated gills of *Mytilus edulis* studied from 1–45° responded to increasing temperatures by a proportional increase in oxygen consumption with a Q_{10} value of 2·0–2·57 up to 30°. Respiration rate subsequently declined to zero at 40°. These *in vitro* responses correspond in temperature limits to the normal environmental temperature range of the species which is 6·9–28·4° (Hoshi and Hoshiyama, 1963). Entirely comparable responses have been reported for tissues of other invertebrate groups including coelenterates (Dregol'skaya, 1961; 1963), annelids (Gorodilov, 1961) and crustacea (Dehnel and McGaughran, 1964), and have been reviewed recently by Ushakov (1964).

The temperature-mediated changes in isolated tissues and in whole organisms described under Section A, 1, point to a common mechanism of physiological adjustment which is initiated at the cellular level, and may have behavioural modifications superimposed upon them. The latter most probably result from both neural and hormonal regulation, but in this area, knowledge is especially scant for poikilothermic invertebrates.

IV. Biochemical Responses in Thermal Acclimation

Details concerning alterations in metabolism at the cellular and subcellular level induced by extremes in temperature are generally unknown in invertebrate animals. However, increasing attention is being given to this aspect of physiological analysis and will clearly characterize the next phase of investigations into this environmental influence on living systems. Information so gained will elucidate the mechanism(s) by which environmental factors bring about adaptation at the biochemical level.

Changes in physiological measures have been reported for low temperature-acclimated invertebrates and point to alterations in cellular metabolism. For example, it has been shown that there is a reduction in blood glucose levels in the crab, *Uca* sp., after varying periods of exposure to low temperature (Dean and Vernberg, 1965). Acclimation temperatures ranged from 2° to 30°, and blood glucose increases were approximately linear with temperature to 25° followed by a marked rise at 30°. However, crabs acclimated to 10° and 30° showed no difference in glycogen levels in the hepatopancreas. In a similar study with *Uca* sp. it was shown that blood protein decreased approximately 50% and the number of blood cells was reduced to an even greater extent after acclimation to 10° for 21 days. These temperature-induced changes were interpreted as an indication of decreased metabolic activity and correspondingly molecular synthesis (Dean and Vernberg, 1966). Study of the fresh water crayfish, *Orconectes virilis*, maintained at 9° and 24° (M. A. McWhinnie, unpublished data) demonstrated similar responses measured through changes in ^{14}C-glucose distribution after 2 and 3 weeks of acclimation. Carbon-14 activity in blood of 9° animals was less than that of those maintained at 24°, while total hepatopancreas radioactivity was significantly elevated. Simultaneously, as in the case of *Uca* sp., the hepatopancreas glycogen level was unaltered by low temperature through 3 weeks, but muscle glycogen contents decreased significantly. At this time, the protein level of both tissues was greatly increased over the 24°-acclimated animal level. Increased rate of substrate turnover and protein synthesis supported by muscle glycogen input appear to be the consequences of low temperature acclimation. The observation that low temperature-adapted antarctic euphausids show a lower percentage of their tissues to be glycogen (mean = 0·19%) than is present in the temperate crayfish (mean: muscle = 1·44%; hepatopancreas = 3·45%) may represent (in addition to species differences) similar temperature-dependent shifts in metabolic pathways which have, however, become genetically fixed in the endemic antarctic euphausid (McWhinnie, 1964).

At the enzyme level, our information concerning temperature influences is equally scant. However, recent studies on crayfish (McWhinnie and O'Connor, 1966) have produced evidence that low-temperature acclimation results in measurable changes in the ratio of biochemical pathways involved in glucose utilization. Taking advantage of the intermoult cycle, stage-dependent oxidative pathways (Mc-Whinnie and Corkill, 1963; McWhinnie and Chua, 1964), acclimation responses were studied in intermoult and premoult stage animals. These two physiologically different conditions have been shown to be characterized by substrate passing through the hexosemonophosphate shunt and the Embden–Meyerhof route in stages C_3–C_4, and the Embden–Meyerhof route only in stages D_1–D_4. Acclimation to 5° for 1–3 weeks increased substrate utilization in intermoult animals by both routes with a greater increase in glycolysis. Conversely, premoult animals reinitiated hexosemonophosphate oxidations and simultaneously increased glucose utilization through glycolysis. Thus, low-temperature acclimation of this temperate species was expressed by increases in overall metabolic rates and changes in the ratios of substrate utilization and energy production through parallel pathways. These observations provide support for the interpretation offered by Prosser (1958) as the biochemical basis that would account for the classical patterns of acclimation; namely, translation and rotation of the rate–temperature curves obtained with whole organism measurements.

While the taxanomic distance is great between the crustaceans and protozoans, it is of some interest that *Paramacium caudatum* acclimated to 4° (Irlina, 1963b) showed an increase in glycolytic oxidations when compared with animals cultured at 29°. Similarly, low-temperature acclimation induced a shift in respiration with respect to cyanide sensitivity which became measurably decreased. It was concluded that low-temperature adaptation alters the predominant pathway of substrate utilization as well as the ratio of CN^--resistant/CN^--sensitive respiration. A comparable change has been reported for poikilothermic vertebrates acclimated to 10° (Prosser, 1958), and corresponds to that described above for the temperate crayfish. The similarities in responses to low-temperature acclimation by organisms across such widely separated categories points to a common mechanism(s) employed in adaptive adjustments by living systems. Only future research will firmly establish and verify the validity of the interpretations offered in these few studies.

An aspect of low-temperature adaptation which is not clearly related to the previously described biochemical changes may be noted here. In a study of the immediate response to acutely encountered low temperatures, Grainger (1958) reported that significant overshoots and undershoots in gas (O_2 and CO_2) exchange characterized a number of living systems including invertebrates, vertebrates, and yeast. In the study of yeast, sudden introduction to 20° after cultivation at 30° resulted in a significant uptake of carbon dioxide. Within the concept of common biochemical responses to environmental stress, it is of interest that antarctic crustacean amphipods and euphausids consistently absorb inorganic carbon from sodium carbonate. This carbon source has been traced to incorporation into glycogen and lipid as well as into respired carbon dioxide (McWhinnie and Johanneck, 1966). The full meaning of this observation and its relationship to the existing data on biochemical changes occurring in low-temperature adaptation must await further study of these widely occurring phenomena.

It is evident that living systems show wide capacities for adaptation and there is reason to anticipate more similarities than differences in the mechanisms that exist to explain them.

V. Conclusions

Adaptive mechanisms evoked by thermal stress appear to elicit a common type of response in widely differing organisms which is evident at the organismic and the tissue level. While species differences clearly exist, and while differences between thermoregulators and thermoconformers are known, there are, none the less, many evidences for their basic similarities in physiological compensation. Further, while numerous biological phenomena enter into the development of the adapted state, such as neural, hormonal, behavioural, and cellular adjustments, there is evidence that in the wide diversity among organisms there exists also considerable similarity in the characteristics of their responses. The details of the biochemical basis of these responses are presently being pursued with increasing effort and can be expected to add new depth to the understanding of adaptation in living systems.

VI. Acknowledgements

The author is indebted to many colleagues and staff members whose efforts, both patent and silent, have contributed to the completion of this work. In particular, I am indebted to Dr. J. R. Cortelyou, Dr. D. J. McWhinnie, and V. I. Ortner. In addition, gratitude is expressed to the National Science Foundation for grants under which work on the crayfish and antarctic crustacea has been completed.

References

Andronikov (Svinkin), V. B. (1963). *Tsitologiya* **5**, 234.
Armitage, K. B. (1962). *Biol. Bull.* **123**, 225.

Barnes, H. (1960). *In* "Marine Boring and Fouling Organisms", (D. L. Ray, Ed.), pp. 234–248. University of Washington Press, Seattle.

Barnes, H. and Barnes, M. (1962). *Intern. Rev. Ges. Hydrobiology.* **47**, 481.

Barnes, H., Barnes, M. and Finlayson, D. M. (1963). *J. mar. Biol. Ass. U.K.* **43**, 185.

Bowler, K. (1963a). *J. cell. comp. Physiol.* **62**, 119.

Bowler, K. (1963b). *J. cell. comp. Physiol.* **62**, 133.

Buetow, D. E. (1962). *Exp. Cell Res.* **27**, 137.

Bullock, T. H. (1955). *Biol. Rev.* **30**, 311.

Cloudsley-Thompson, J. L. (1965). *Hydrobiologia* **25**, 424.

Costlow, J. D., Jr., Bookout, C. G. and Monroe, R. (1960). *Biol. Bull.* **118**, 183.

Costlow, J. D., Jr., Bookout, C. G. and Monroe, R. (1962). *Physiol. Zool.* **35**, 79.

Dean, J. M. and Vernberg, F. J. (1965). *Biol. Bull.* **129**, 87.

Dean, J. M. and Vernberg, F. J. (1966). *Comp. Biochem. Physiol.* **17**, 19.

Dehnel, P. A. and McGaughran, D. A. (1964). *Comp. Biochem. Physiol.* **13**, 233.

Dill, D. B., Adolph, E. F. and Wilber, C. G. Eds.. (1964). "Handbook of Physiology", Section 4: Adaptation to the Environment. *Publ. Amer. Physiol. Soc., Washington, D.C., U.S.A.*

Dregol'skaya, I. N. (1961). *Tsitologiya* **3**, 475. *Referat. Zhur., Biol., No.* **23A236** (Translation).

Dregol'skaya, I. N. (1963). *Tsitologiya* **5**, 194.

Dzhamusova, T. A. (1960). *Tsitologiya* **2**, 274. *Referat. Zhur., Biol., No.* **7D13** (Translation).

Edney, E. B. (1964). *Physiol. Zool.* **37**, 364.

Farmanfarmaian, A. (1963). *Physiol. Zool.* **36**, 237.

Fraenkel, G. (1961). *Ecology* **42**, 604.

Frankel, J. (1964). *J. exp. Zool.* **155**, 403.

Gavin, R. H. (1965). *J. Protozool.* **12**, 307.

Giese, A. C. (1959). *Annu. Rev. Physiol.* **21**, 547.

Gorodilov, Yu. N. (1961). *Tsitologiya* **3**, 473. *Referat. Zhur., Biol., No.* **23A235** (Translation).

Grainger, J. N. R. (1958). *In* "Physiological Adaptation", (C. L. Prosser, Ed.), pp. 79–91. *Publ. Amer. Physiol. Soc., Washington, D.C., U.S.A.*

Grigoryan, D. A. (1964). *Tsitologiya* **6**, 105.

Halcrow, K. (1963). *Limnol. Oceanogr.* **8**, 1.

Heinonen, A. (1962). *Arch. Soc. Zool. Bot. Fennicae "Vanamo"* **16**, 137.

Hoshi, T. and Hoshiyama, M. (1963). *J. Fac. Sci. Niigata Univ., Ser. II Biol. Geol. Mineral.* **4**, 97.

Irlina, I. S. (1963a). *SB Rabot Inst. Tsitol. Akad. Nauk. S.S.S.R.* **3**, 92. *Referat. Zhur., Biol., No.* **12D44** (Translation).

Irlina, I. S. (1963b). *Tsitologiya* **5**, 183.

Johnson, B. F. (1962). *Exp. Cell Res.* **28**, 419.

Kerkut, G. A. and Ridge, R. M. A. P. (1962). *Comp. Biochem. Physiol.* **5**, 283.

Krassner, S. M. (1965). *J. Protozool.* **12**, 73.

Kyer, D. S. (1942). *Biol. Bull.* **82**, 68.

Lehmann, D. L. (1962). *J. Protozool.* **9**, 325.

Lewis, J. B. (1963). *Biol. Bull.* **124**, 277.

Lockwood, A. P. M. (1960). *J. exp. Biol.* **37**, 614.

Loosanoff, V. L. (1959). *Biol. Bull.* **117**, 308.

McWhinnie, M. A. (1962). *Comp. Biochem. Physiol.* **7**, 1.

McWhinnie, M. A. (1964). In "Biology of the Antarctic Seas", Vol. 1, Antarcti-
Res. Ser., Natl. Acad. Sci. Natl. Res. Counc. Publ. 1190. Pp. 63–72.

McWhinnie, M. A. and Chua, A. S. (1964). Gen. Comp. Endocrinol. 4, 624.

McWhinnie, M. A. and Corkill, A. J. (1963). Comp. Biochem. Physiol. 12, 81.

McWhinnie, M. A. and Johanneck, R. (1966). Antarctic Jour., U.S. (in press).

McWhinnie, M. A. and Kirchenberg, R. J. (1962). Comp. Biochem. Physiol. 6
159.

McWhinnie, M. A. and O'Connor, J. D. (1966). Comp. Biochem. Physiol. (in press)

Marr, J. W. S. (1962). Discovery Repts. 32, 33.

Matutani, K. (1960). Physiol. Ecol. (Japan) 9, 39.

Matutani, K. (1962a). Physiol. Ecol. (Japan) 10, 59.

Matutani, K. (1962b). Physiol. Ecol. (Japan) 10, 63.

Mendes, E. G. and Almeida, A. M. (1962). Bol. Fac. Filosof. Cienc. Letras Univ.
São Paulo Ser. Zool. 24, 43.

Monokov, A. V. (1965). Zool. ZH 44, 606.

Pailey, A. (1961). J. Madras Univ. 31, 109.

Passano, L. M. (1960). Biol. Bull. 118, 129.

Patel, B. (1959). J. mar. Biol. Assoc. U.K. 38, 589.

Patel, B. and Crisp, D. J. (1960). J. Mar. Biol. Assoc. U.K. 39, 667.

Precht, H. (1958). In "Physiological Adaptation", (C. L. Prosser, Ed.), pp. 50–78.
Publ. Amer. Physiol. Soc., Washington, D.C., U.S.A.

Prosser, C. L., Ed. (1958). "Physiological Adaptation", Publ. Amer. Physiol.
Soc., Washington, D.C., U.S.A.

Prosser, C. L. (1964). In "Handbook of Physiology", (D. B. Dill, E. F. Adolph and
C. G. Wilbur, Eds.), Section 4, Chap. 2, pp. 11–26. Publ. Amer. Physiol. Soc.,
Washington, D.C., U.S.A.

Raghupathiramireddy, S. and Rao, K. P. (1963). Proc. Indian Acad. Sci., Section
B 58, 1.

Rajabai, K. G. (1963). Proc. Indian Acad. Sci., Section B 58, 207.

Rao, K. P. (1962). Science 137, 682.

Rao, K. P. (1963a). Proc. Indian Acad. Sci., Section B 57, 290.

Rao, K. P. (1963b). Proc. Indian Acad. Sci., Section B 57, 297.

Rao, K. P. (1963c). Proc. Indian Acad. Sci., Section B 58, 11.

Rao, K. P. and Ramachandra, R. (1961). J. exp. Biol. 38, 29.

Rao, K. P. and Saroja, K. (1963). Proc. Indian Acad. Sci., Section B 58, 14.

Rao, K. P. and Venkatareddy, V. (1962). Comp. Biochem. Physiol. 5, 65.

Riegel, J. A. (1961). J. exp. Biol. 38, 291.

Saroja, K. and Rao, K. P. (1965). Z. Vergleichende Physiol. 50, 34.

Sastry, A. N. (1963). Biol. Bull. 125, 146.

Sastry, A. N. (1966). Biol. Bull. 130, 118.

Scholander, P. F., Flagg, W., Walters, V. and Irving, L. (1953). Physiol. Zool. 26,
67.

Smith, R. E. and Hoijer, D. J. (1962). Physiol. Rev. 42, 60.

Spoor, W. A. (1955). Biol. Bull. 108, 77.

Thormar, H. (1962a). Exp. Cell Res. 27, 585.

Thormar, H. (1962b). Exp. Cell Res. 28, 269.

Ueda, K. (1961). Annot. Zool. Japon 34, 99.

Ushakov, B. (1964). Physiol. Rev. 44, 518.

Vernberg, F. J. (1959). Biol. Bull. 117, 582.

Vernberg, F. J. (1962). Annu. Rev. Physiol. 24, 517.

Vernberg, F. J. and Tashian, R. E. (1959). Ecology 40, 589.

Vernberg, F. J. and Vernberg, W. B. (1966). Amer. Zool. 6, 327 (Abstract).

Vernberg, F. J., Schlieper, C. and Schneider, D. E. (1963). *Comp. Biochem. Physiol.* **8**, 271.

Warburg, M. R. (1965). *Physiol. Zool.* **38**, 99.

Wautier, J. and Troiani, D. (1960). *Ann. Sta. Centr. Hydrobiol. Appl.* **8**, 9.

Whitson, G. L. (1964). *J. cell. comp. Physiol.* **64**, 455.

Wiens, A. W. and Armitage, K. B. (1961). *Physiol. Zool.* **34**, 39.

Wilkens, J. L. and Fingerman, M. (1965). *Biol. Bull.* **128**, 133.

Zein-Eldin, Z. P. and Aldrich, D. V. (1965). *Biol. Bull.* **129**, 199.

Zhirmunskii, A. V. and Chu, Li-Chun. (1963). *Acta Zool. Sinica* **15**, 21.

Zhirmunskii, A. V. and Pisareva, L. N. (1961). *In* "Problems of Cytology and Protistology", pp. 137–142. Institute of Cytology, Academy of Sciences, U.S.S.R. Office of Technical Services, U.S. Dept. of Commerce, Washington, D.C., U.S.A.

Chapter 11

Responses of Vertebrate Poikilotherms to Temperature

F. E. J. FRY

Department of Zoology, University of Toronto,
Toronto, Canada

I. Introduction

With regard to the organism as a whole, the effects of temperature may be discussed under three headings (Fry, 1947). Either a high temperature or a low one may kill the organism in a finite time within what otherwise would be its normal life span. Such an effect of temperature may be termed for obvious reasons, a *lethal* effect. The second effect that temperature may have on the organism is on its activity, an effect which is mediated through the well known influence of temperature on the rate of biochemical reactions and thus on the metabolic rate. The effect of temperature on activity will be termed a *controlling* effect. The controlling effects of temperature are highly diverse and may have morphometric as well as kinetic implications, so that the word activity as used here will be a very general term to indicate any thing an organism does from growing to fighting. Finally, temperature influences the spontaneous movement of organisms, an effect which, for example, may cause them to aggregate in a certain specified region of a temperature gradient when exposed to a wide choice of temperatures. This third effect of temperature will be discussed under *directive* effects.

As is well recognized, the response of a given organism to a given temperature is not a constant one. Its response varies within limits which are appropriate to the species concerned, in a way which is dependent on its history, as well as to any interaction between temperature and other components of the environment. Thus, in the description of a response to temperature, it is as necessary to describe (or to fix in the experimental conditions) the environmental history as it is to identify properly the species concerned. In the present chapter, the state of the organism as determined by its environmental history will be defined by the following three terms, which are used with the restricted meanings given below.

In measuring the effects of temperature in the laboratory, it is a common practice to prepare the organisms for some days or weeks before the experiments by maintaining them at a constant temperature. The term *acclimation* will be applied here to designate such an artificial stabilization of the environmental history. Acclimation may be to a single environmental identity or it may be to a combination of identities such as temperature, photoperiod and salinity. The essence of the word acclimation is that more or less of the immediate environmental history has been artificially controlled by some means or another.

If, on the other hand, the state of the organism before the test has been determined entirely by the natural conditions of the climate in which it exists, then the term used to describe its history will be *acclimatization*. To be "acclimatized", therefore, is to be influenced by all of the subtleties of the natural environment from fertilization up to the point in the annual cycle at which the organism is tested. It is the hope that acclimation can be carried out in a way that permits the response of the acclimatized organism to be described and analysed for all practical purposes, but the limitations of acclimation must always be recognized. Only those processes which are reversible on short term throughout life can be entirely adjusted by acclimation.

Lastly the term *adaptation* will be reserved for the phylogenetic adjustment of the organism to its environment, although no direct reference will be made to the term in this chapter.

By the definitions given above, the species is adapted, the individual is acclimatized, and the subject of a given test may be acclimated.

II. Body Temperature in the Poikilothermic Vertebrates

A. RELATION TO AMBIENT TEMPERATURE

The term "poikilotherm" means literally "many temperatured"; it does not necessarily mean that the body temperature is the same as that of the ambient medium, air or water. Thus, it is essential to determine the relation between the internal temperature of the organism and the temperature of the environment. There is a secondary, but no less important, question as to whether the organism is capable of maintaining any differential between body and ambient temperature that may be found, by means of its own internal regulatory powers. This latter question can be answered by a knowledge of the metabolic rate and by measurements of the rate of change of the body temperature when the subject is transferred from one temperature to another, and will be dealt with in the final section. Three reviews, Gunn (1942) and Brattstrom (1963, 1965), give an extensive account of the body temperatures of the cold-blooded vertebrates.

It is generally agreed that a resting fish has a body temperature that is essentially the temperature of the surrounding water (Gunn, 1942). Even when fish are active, it also seems probable that there is little difference between their general body temperature and the ambient temperature, although few data are available for swimming fish. Recent data obtained by P. Ihssen (personal communication) on goldfish swimming in a rotating chamber show an almost complete identity between the temperature within the stomach and the water temperature. Tuna fish, however, have body-muscle temperatures which have long been known to be elevated above the ambient temperature (Davy, 1816, quoted in Simpson, 1908). Barrett and Hester (1964), whose paper should also be consulted for earlier references, found mean muscle temperatures in the skipjack, *Katsowonus pelamis*, and yellowfin, *Thunnus albacores*, respectively of 8° and 4° above an ambient temperature of 20°. No observations were taken at lower temperatures, and their lines drawn through points recording the observations at higher temperatures converged with the ambient temperature at approximately 40°. The scombroids have a special modification of the vascular system of the lateral muscles (which were the site of the measurements made by Barrett and Hester). Kishinouye (1923), in an interesting paper recently brought to my attention, pointed out that the extensive vascular plexuses of the lateral artery and vein which are characteristic of the scombroids provide a countercurrent system that can conserve the metabolic heat produced by the muscle. Walters (1962) suggested that the enhanced body temperature of the scombroids may function to decrease the kinetic viscosity of the thin film of water adjacent to the fish and thus lessen the drag in swimming. It does not seem, however, that his interpretation is valid in view of the countercurrent system.

However, even in those fish in which body-muscle temperatures have been found to be above ambient, the head must be at the ambient temperature. As Davis (1955) pointed out, it is almost certain that the completeness of the exchange of the respiratory gases between water and blood at the gills means an equally complete equilibration of temperature, and arterial blood thus begins its journey to the tissues at essentially the ambient temperature. Any excess of the body temperature over the ambient temperature must be the result of local production and conservation of heat.

Fish, as gill breathers, face a special problem if any of their tissues are to operate at temperatures much above ambient. If the blood gases are equilibrated with the dissolved gases in the water at the gill, there is the extreme likelihood of supersaturation when the blood takes the temperature of the warmer tissues, and gas bubble disease would ensue. A countercurrent system which could conserve heat would fortunately also tend to desaturate the entering blood.

Both amphibians and reptiles, as aquatic animals, also have body temperatures which closely approximate the water temperature. In air, amphibians may have temperatures well above ambient when they are exposed to radiant heat. In the shade, their body temperatures tend to fall to the dew point (Hall and Root, 1930; Mellanby, 1941) since their skins present a moist surface. Thus, since the dew point fluctuates less than the dry bulb temperature, the terrestrial amphibia have a more constant thermal environment than one would otherwise expect.

The body temperatures of active terrestrial reptiles, usually taken immediately after the animal has been shot, have been measured on many occasions. These body temperatures often diverge markedly from the air temperature and the divergence is ordinarily considered to be brought about by behavioural thermoregulation, particularly since different species in the same region will display different body temperatures (Carpenter, 1961; Schmidt-Nielsen and Dawson, 1964). These data will be discussed in a later section.

B. RATES OF THERMAL EXCHANGE

The exchange of heat by conduction essentially follows Newton's Law of excess temperature. Typical curves for aquatic and terrestrial forms are given in Fig. 1. It is characteristic of the curves that have so far been determined that heating is faster than cooling for a given temperature difference. Assuming such data as are shown in Fig. 1 can be described by a single straight line, we can apply the equation:

$$\frac{dT}{dt} = k(T_{\text{ambient}} - T_{\text{body}})$$

in which we shall take T as the temperature in $°$ and t as the time in minutes. The constant k, thus defined, represents the rate of change of body temperature, in degrees per minute, at a temperature difference of $1°$ between the body and the ambient temperatures. k is a constant

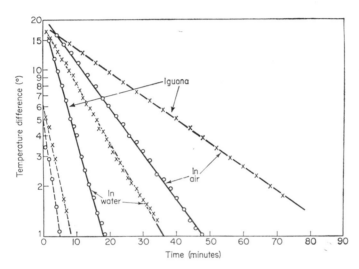

FIG. 1. Rate of temperature change in relation to the difference between body and ambient temperatures in the goldfish, *Carassius auratus* (190 g.; P. Ihssen, personal communication), and the marine iguana, *Amblyrhynchus cristatus* (652 g.; Bartholomew and Lasiewski, 1965). The origin of the curves has no significance, but they are presented in the order of their slopes. × indicates the curve obtained on cooling; ○, the curve obtained on heating. The dotted lines give the data for the goldfish; the continuous lines, those for the iguana.

only under a given set of experimental conditions. For example, movement of the medium relative to the body will affect it considerably. In general, determination of k has been made in apparently still water or in air moving at a stated rate. The size of the organism also has an influence on the value of k. Data for the size-dependence of k are limited. In Harvey's data for small Pacific salmon, illustrated in Fig. 2, k varies approximately as $W^{-0.3}$, where W is the body weight. A similar value for the body weight exponent was found by Bartholomew and Tucker (1964) for various varanids the weights of which ranged from 10 to 10,000 g. Steeper slopes (with exponents of -0.5

13 + T.

and −0·6) were found respectively by DeWitt (1962) for various lizards and by Bartholomew and Lasiewski (1965) for the Galapagos marine iguana. It is possible that the data for the varanids may later be revised, since a correction for metabolism was applied that was derived from data on lizards in general. Tentatively, we may assume that the values of k reported by DeWitt (1962) and by Bartholomew and Lasiewski (1965) may be more typical of lung breathers. The greater size-dependence of k would seem to imply that the loss of heat at the surface of a lung-breathing animal is a function both of the surface area

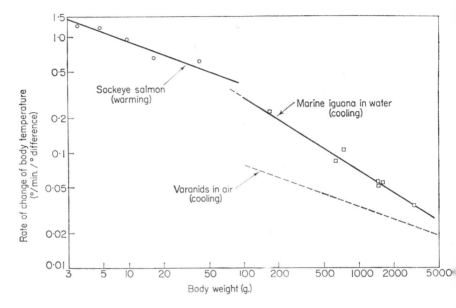

FIG. 2. Relation between the rate of change of body temperature and body weight in the sockeye salmon, *Oncorhynchus nerka* (Harvey, 1964), marine iguana, and varanids (Bartholomew and Lasiewski, 1965).

and the metabolism per unit weight, the latter being taken as an index of the convective transfer of heat. If the latter relation also obeys the surface law, then a temperature change coefficient of −0·6 simply represents the sum of the two indices. The value of k is probably least size-dependent in gill breathers, in which the overwhelming fraction of heat transfer probably takes place at the respiratory surface, and the change in k would then be essentially dependent on the metabolic relation alone.

Assuming that the values of k obtained from the data in Figs. 1 and 2 and otherwise reported in the literature are typical, then the order of the values of k to be expected for the cold-blooded vertebrates will range from 2 to 0·01 for aquatic forms and from 0·5 to 0·005 for terrestrial forms.

Since the exchange of heat between the organism and the environment takes time to reach equilibrium, it is of interest to calculate the rate at which the body temperature would lag behind the ambient temperature at a given rate of temperature change. The question of the lag can be answered in broad terms very simply if we consider a case in which the ambient temperature is undergoing a continuous linear rate of change. Under these circumstances, the difference between the body and the ambient temperatures will reach a limiting value which is the rate of ambient temperature change in degrees per minute, divided by k. Thus, at a rate of change of ambient temperature of 1° per minute, the body temperature of an animal for which k was 0·5 (e.g. a 50 g. salmon) would lag by 2°. If the animal were a 50 g. varanid ($k = 0·1$), the lag would be 10°. Because of the lag alone then, and ignoring the factors of radiation and evaporative cooling, it is essential to make direct measurements of the body temperature of the terrestrial amphibians and reptiles.

III. Lethal Effects

A. MEASUREMENT OF LETHAL TEMPERATURES

The lethal limits of temperature have been determined either by continuously raising the temperature from some non-lethal value, at a rate of 1° per few minutes, or by abruptly exposing the animal to constant temperature and determining its time to death, should the temperature chosen be lethal. Both methods are amenable to statistical analysis and both have their purposes. The method of slow heating is extremely economical with regard to time and material, but it yields results which are less valuable for physiological analysis and which indeed can be predicted from the method of constant exposure. Two recent papers which emphasize respectively the two methods are Hutchinson (1961) and Fry (1957a).

A special use of the method of slow heating has been employed by Hathaway (1927), Cocking (1959b) and Spaas (1959a). These workers have used heating rates of a degree or less per day, whereas the ordinary rate is around a degree per minute. Cocking was concerned with measuring the rate of thermal acclimation. The purpose of Hathaway and Spaas was to obtain an approximation of the ultimate incipient lethal temperature (see below) with as great an economy of material as possible.

By far the greater emphasis has been placed on the upper lethal temperature. The method of slow heating has been the one almost universally applied to the amphibia and reptiles, and offers the immediate ecological index for these organisms, since the terrestrial animals, particularly the desert reptiles, meet upper lethal temperatures as acute fluctuations above their limits of tolerance. Moreover, the rates of heating used approximate the rates at which the body temperature rises when the animal is exposed to the sun, and indeed radiant heat may be employed in the experiment (e.g., Brattstrom and Lawrence, 1962). It has become the custom among American herpetologists to use an endpoint short of death (referred to as the critical thermal maximum; CTM; Cowles and Bogert, 1944), to determine the upper limit of temperature tolerance. The endpoint taken is locomotory disorganization or collapse.

The aquatic animals are subject to much slower changes in temperature and have less chance of finding some adjacent refuge from undue heating, so that determinations of lethal temperatures by the method of continuous exposure have more ecological meaning. Such experiments also provide a firmer basis for physiological analysis in the more detailed pattern of response they provide.

The seasonal history has a profound effect on the lethal temperature (e.g. Brett, 1944). Most but not all of the seasonal range in lethal temperature can be ascribed to thermal history (Davenport and Castle, 1896; Loeb and Wasteneys, 1912; Hathaway, 1927) and the remainder is possibly to be ascribed to the photoperiod (Hoar and Robinson, 1959).

The lethal temperatures of two species of freshwater fish in response to acclimation temperature are shown in Fig. 3. Graphs A and B in the figure show the response of the golden shiner, a minnow of widespread distribution in eastern North America, which has responses typical of temperate freshwater fish (see also Brett, 1952; Hart, 1947). Graph A shows the median time to death of fish acclimated to various temperatures and exposed to temperatures at which at least 50% of the sample died. Each line relating *resistance time* to lethal temperature for a given level of acclimation terminates to the right at a point where no more than 50% mortality was recorded, although the exposure was prolonged well beyond the point indicated. The terminus of each resistance line thus indicates the upper *incipient lethal temperature* (Fry *et al.*, 1946) for that level of thermal acclimation. Graph B shows the upper incipient lethal temperatures calculated from the data in graph A, together with the results of a similar series of experiments done at low lethal temperatures. In addition, graph B gives estimates of the CTM values also calculated from the data in graph A. The highest incipient lethal temperature that can be achieved by acclimation has been termed the *ultimate incipient lethal temperature*. Similarly, by reference to graph B, it can be seen that there is a maximum and an ultimate incipient lower lethal temperature, the latter being often indeterminate because of the freezing point of water. The upper dotted line in graph B connects the CTM values, as estimated by the graphical method (see Fry *et al.*, 1946), assuming that the fish had been heated at the rate of 1° every 4 minutes, a rate employed by Heath (1963) for the cutthroat trout. However, death, rather than the loss of equilibrium which is ordinarily employed in the CTM calculations, is taken as the endpoint.

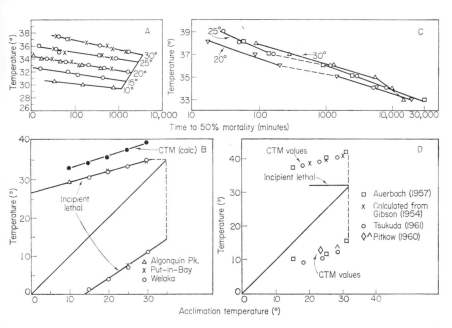

FIG. 3. Graphs A and B: Effect of temperature on the mortality of the minnow, *Notemigonus crysoleucas* (data from Hart, 1952). Graphs C and D: Effect of temperature on the mortality of the guppy, *Lebistes reticulatus* (data from Arai *et al.*, 1963; Auerbach, 1957; Gibson, 1954; Pitkow, 1960; Tsukuda, 1961). The graphical method of Fry *et al.* (1946) was used for calculating CTM values.

In the golden shiner, the CTM value responds to acclimation temperature in approximately the same way as the incipient lethal temperature, and is about 3° higher.

Graphs C and D illustrate some of the lethal temperatures of the guppy. The thermal resistance of the guppy shows a response of the same magnitude as that shown by the golden shiner, but there is not the simple regularity of change of resistance time with lethal and acclimation temperatures. Moreover, in spite of the response in thermal resistance, the upper incipient lethal temperature is virtually unaffected by thermal acclimation. The guppy ultimately succumbs at 33° regardless of the temperature to which it has been acclimated. With the guppy, the CTM value shows a response to acclimation which contrasts markedly with the response of the incipient lethal temperature, reflecting the changes in thermal resistance. The plateau of non-response to thermal acclimation, shown by the upper incipient lethal temperature of the guppy, is the other extreme of the picture shown by the golden shiner in which the plateau is non-existent, except that Hart (1952) suggested the presence of a short plateau beyond the range of his data. Another tropical species, *Tilapia mossambica* (Allanson and Noble, 1964), shows a plateau similar in extent to the guppy. Plateaux of different sizes are shown by various other species (see also Hart, 1947; Cocking, 1959a), and it is at acclimation levels over which the plateau extends that the response of the CTM value to thermal acclimation differs from the response of the incipient lethal temperature.

The rate of thermal acclimation to increasing temperatures is rapid, being ordinarily more than a degree per day per degree increase in temperature (Brett, 1946; Cocking, 1959b), and Brett's (1944) field study showed changes in lethal temperature which reflected short-term changes in the weather. The higher the temperature, the more rapid the rate of thermal acclimation. In consequence, the acclimation temperature reflects the daily maximum rather than the daily mean. Heath (1963) made the interesting observation that a temperature fluctuation which followed a twenty-four hour cycle gave the highest acclimation temperature for a given range of temperature fluctuation. The rate of acclimation of amphibians appears to be particularly rapid (Brattstrom and Lawrence, 1962).

An effect of season on the response of the lethal temperature to acclimation temperature is shown in Fig. 4. The two overlapping areas in this figure represent the shift in the upper lethal temperatures when determined for fish subjected to the same acclimation temperature in mid-winter and mid-summer respectively; these fish had been exposed to the normal photoperiod at approximately 45° N. latitude. Hart (1952) recorded a similar shift in the response of the yellow perch, *Perca flavescens*, in which he also found an approximately 3° difference in the ultimate incipient lethal temperature between winter and summer. Hart also obtained data on the lower incipient lethal temperature. The maximum lower incipient lethal temperature was 3·7° in winter and 8·7° in summer.

Tyler (1966) was not able to reverse completely the seasonal effect by reversing the annual cycle of photoperiod at the autumnal equinox, with tests made at the winter solstice. Thus the annual cycle has a greater effect than can be overcome in that length of time; alternatively, factors other than photoperiod and temperature may be involved.

The responses of the amphibia to lethal temperatures seem to be in general similar to those of fish (Hutchinson, 1961; McFarland, 1955). However, they appear to show somewhat less change in the lethal temperature. For example, the CTM values of the newt, *Diemictylus viridescens*, change one degree for each 5° change in acclimation temperature (Hutchinson, 1961; see also Brooks and Sassman, 1965). Seasonal effects not eliminated by extensive thermal acclimation are also reported by Hutchinson (1961).

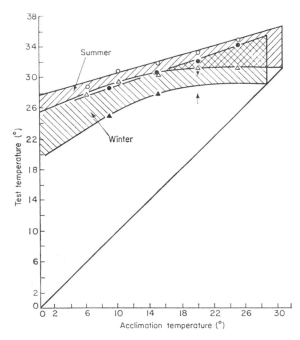

FIG. 4. Seasonal changes in the upper lethal temperature of the red bellied dace, *Chrosmus eos*, in response to acclimation temperature. ○, indicates lethal temperatures giving a median resistance time of 30 min. in summer; ●, lethal temperatures giving a median resistance time of 30 min. in winter; △, secondary effect incipient lethal temperatures in summer; ▲, secondary effect incipient lethal temperatures in winter. From Tyler (1966).

It is also probable that the same principles hold with the reptiles, but attention has been given almost exclusively to the determination of the CTM values. Hutchinson and Kosh (1965) reported a clear-cut example of the effect of photoperiod on the CTM value in the painted turtle, *Chrysemys picta*, in which the difference between acclimation to a 16-hour versus an 8-hour light period changed the CTM value by about the equivalent of a 4° increase in acclimation temperature. The lethal temperatures of the three orders cover essentially the same ranges, and some forms in each order have upper lethal temperatures approximating those of mammals and birds

Data on the lethal temperatures of fish have been tabulated by Brett (1956) and Fry (1964), and the few more recent values (e.g. Alabaster, 1963; Allanson and Noble, 1964) do not extend the limits known earlier. The goldfish has an ultimate upper incipient lethal temperature of 40° and appears to be as heat-resistant as any other species in this respect. Morris (1962) indicated that the cichlid, *Aequidens portalgrensis*, also has a similar ultimate lethal temperature. The salmonoids have ultimate lethal temperatures of the order of 25° and, while it is probable (Wohlschlag, 1964) that there are Antarctic species with upper lethal temperatures considerably below that value, no measurements appear to have yet been made.

The maximum lower lethal temperatures recorded for fish vary from approximately 0° for some of the salmonoids to 20°, and it appears that the characteristic difference between tropical and temperate species lies in the lower and not the upper lethal temperature. However, it should be emphasized that, in summer, the lower lethal temperatures of most temperate species that have been investigated are well above the freezing point of water. In winter, temperate species have lower lethal temperatures down to freezing point, and some marine species are supercooled to the freezing point of seawater or have the freezing point of their blood depressed (Gordon *et al.*, 1962). However, many marine fishes, which normally winter in the temperate zone, cannot withstand the lowest temperatures that seawater can reach (see Woodhead, 1964, for additional references). Sudden chilling often kills fish that might otherwise be hardy if they had time to acclimate (e.g. Gunter, 1941, 1947).

Brattstrom (1963) gave the CTM values for various species of amphibia including some from his own observations and some from the literature. Most of these values lie between 30° and 40°. There appear to be only four records of ultimate incipient lethal temperatures. Hutchinson (1961) observed that the newt, *Diemictylus viridescens*, could not be acclimated above 35°, at which point the CTM value was 41°. In the same way, Hutchinson also found approximately 35° to be the ultimate upper lethal temperature of the salamander, *Ambystoma opacum*. Hathaway (1927) determined the ultimate upper incipient lethal temperature of *Bufo americanus* to be approximately 40°. The ultimate CTM value for *Rana pipiens* is approximately 36° (Brattstrom and Lawrence, 1962) so that the ultimate incipient lethal temperature for this species is probably around 32°. With regard to the lower lethal temperatures of the amphibia, little can be said except that the subtropical species investigated die well above freezing point, and that temperate species can be undercooled by rapid cooling to around −8°.

It is not likely, however, that such undercooling represents a long-term state (Weigmann, 1930; Mullaly, 1952) and the overwintering of temperate species most probably depends on refugia, either under water or in the soil, where the temperature drops little if any below 0° (Bailey, 1949; Carpenter, 1953; Fitch, 1956, Stebbins, 1954). It is doubtful whether any vertebrate can withstand extensive freezing of its tissues (Scholander et al., 1953; Hansen, 1954).

The CTM values for reptiles are of the order of 40° for turtles and snakes, and around 45° for lizards. The lowest CTM value for a reptile that Brattstrom (1965) recorded was 34° for the legless lizard, *Anniella pulchra*, a soil-dwelling species, and the highest was approximately 48° for the iguanid, *Uta stansburiana*. Brattstrom largely confined his review to the American literature, but reports on old-world species (e.g. Adensamer, 1934) show a similar range of values. The CTM value responds to the acclimation temperature in reptiles also (Lowe and Vance 1955), the degree of response being of the order of one degree in seven for the painted turtle, *Chrysemys picta* (Hutchinson and Kosh, 1965). Most of the reports in the literature on the lower lethal temperatures of reptiles concern overwintering in the temperate zone. The most thorough experiment reported is probably that of Bailey (1949), who overwintered garter snakes in sealed burrows at various depths. He found survival in burrows where the temperature reached − 2° for some days, but not at lower temperatures.

B. CAUSES OF THERMAL DEATH

The primary question is whether all thermal deaths are brought about by the same type of metabolic breakdown in all living organisms. If there were a single cause, then one would look for a homogeneity in response at a given lethal temperature and a regularity of change in resistance time from one temperature to another. The time-mortality response (Bliss, 1937) yields a single straight line on a probability verus logarithmic grid (e.g. Brett, 1952; Arai et al., 1963) with sufficient frequency to suggest that the basic response of a population is unimodal and fits the normal probability curve when the logarithmic transformation of time is used. However, at certain temperatures, there may be a decided heterogeneity in the statistical response. Figure 5 gives examples of such heterogeneity to support similar data already in the literature.

Gibson's data in Fig. 5 are further examples taken from her thesis (Gibson, 1953) which can be compared with data in Gibson (1954). Her data show that three different batches of fish showed the same type of statistical response when exposed at a given temperature, with some displacement of the means. If the data in Fig. 5A are compared with Fig. 1 of Arai et al. (1963), it will be seen that the same type of variability was displayed by the two batches of fish at each lethal temperature. In Fig. 5A, the probit lines for males and females are shown separately at the highest temperature, and it will be seen that fish of each sex behaved statistically like the combined plot. Finally, the probit lines for

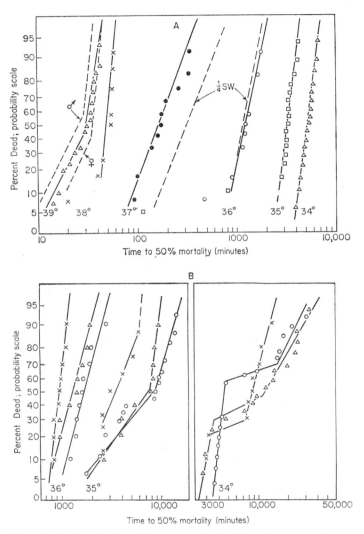

FIG. 5. A statistical analysis of heterogeneity in the time-mortality pattern of upper lethal temperatures of the guppy, *Lebistes reticulatus*, in fresh water. Graph A indicates patterns for fish reared and acclimated at 25°. (From Arai *et al.*, 1963; and unpublished observations.) Graph B indicates patterns for fish reared at 20° (crosses), 25° (circles), or 30° (triangles), and acclimated at 30° before test. From Gibson (1953). Note that the effect of rearing history cannot be completely eliminated by acclimation.

the times to death in one-quarter strength sea-water ($\frac{1}{4}$ SW) are indicated for 37° and 36°. It will be seen that a change takes place so that, at 36°, dilute sea-water no longer prolongs life. Thus, at 36°, some effect which shortens life at the higher temperatures in fresh water no longer operates.

The heterogeneity in the guppy data suggests at least three loci of response to an upper lethal temperature (Gibson, 1954), but the precise sites of breakdown have not been suggested. One site (affected above 36° in the example quoted) is probably related to osmoregulation as the investigations of Arai et al. (1963), Allanson and Noble (1964) and Craigie (1963), together with the classical work of Loeb and Wasteneys (1912) on Fundulus, suggest. Heat rigour at very high lethal temperatures was long ago associated, in Rana temporaria, with a rapid accumuation of lactic acid in the muscles (Woodrow and Wigglesworth, 1927). The primary effect, however, was on the central nervous system since there was no such rapid increase in lactic acid in the muscles of pithed frogs exposed to the same temperature (38°). At some temperatures (Brett, 1952; Cocking, 1959a), the symptoms of heat death are reminiscent of asphyxia. There appears little else specific that can be said at the present time.

With regard to the mode of operation of lower lethal temperatures the ultimate cause of death at temperatures below freezing is most probably destruction of the tissues by the formation of ice. The transition from death by chill coma to death by freezing is clearly demonstrated in the data of Brett and Alderdice (1958) for the chum salmon, Oncorhynchus keta, in which the two effects are separated by an interval of several hours at −1·0°. Primary chill coma, which was defined by Doudoroff (1942), is considered by Pitkow (1960) as the failure of the respiratory centre, on the basis of experiments which showed guppies to be less susceptible to chilling when provided with increased oxygen. At somewhat higher but still lethally low temperatures, fish may recover spontaneously from primary chill coma and, after a period of apparently normal behaviour at that temperature, ultimately succumb. Doudoroff termed the second entry into coma, "secondary chill coma". The statistical distinction between primary and secondary chill coma is well illustrated by Brett's (1952) data on Pacific salmon. Secondary chill coma can sometimes (Doudoroff, 1945; Brett, 1952) be at least partially prevented by decreasing the osmotic stress, and Doudoroff concluded that the cause was a failure in the osmoregulatory system. Wikgren (1953) showed that carp are subject to excessive loss of ions at low temperatures, and Woodhead and Woodhead (1959) suggested that the cod is in osmotic imbalance below 2°.

Another approach to the analysis of the causes of thermal death has been to examine the death points of tissues (see Precht, 1964; Prosser, 1962; Ushakov, 1964). Such work in general has suffered from being done only by the method of slow heating, so that the opportunities for observing gradations in response are limited. But the general conclusion that has been reached, namely that the animal dies through the breakdown of some central regulatory activity rather than from the collapse of its cells, seems valid.

However, the thermal breakdown of isolated tissues does sometimes take place at temperatures associated with the death of the whole organism. Wolf and Quimby (1962) found the ultimate upper lethal temperature of a culture of the cells of the rainbow trout, *Salmo gairdneri*, to be 26°, which is within a degree of the ultimate incipient lethal temperature of the whole organism.

C. LETHAL TEMPERATURES OF AQUATIC EGGS

While there is probably little difference in the lethal temperatures of the free-living stages of a cold-blooded vertebrate throughout its life (McCauley, 1963), the responses of aquatic eggs are quite different. In these eggs, the range of thermal tolerance is narrowed. There are interesting racial differences in the thermal tolerance of eggs (Hubbs, 1964; Moore, 1949; Ruibal, 1955), and in these cases it would be interesting to have some knowledge of the thermal tolerance of the adults. It is possible that, through evolution of the size of the egg and the nature of the egg mass, there have been changes in the response of this critical stage without any change in that of the adult. The thermal tolerance of the adult tends to be a conservative property (Hart, 1952).

IV. Controlling Effects

A. RELATION OF TEMPERATURE TO ACTIVITY

Just as there is a wide spectrum of lethal temperatures among invertebrates, so various species are adapted each to be active at various temperatures over a wide range. Figure 6 illustrates this phenomenon for fish. The data shown are all from species of the north temperate zone, but it is clear that the variety of thermal adaptation they show spreads over the range of water temperatures available during the season of open water. The inclusion of polar species would extend the graph since it would embrace species active in the range of $-2°$ to $0°$ (Wohlschlag, 1960).

In amphibia and reptiles, the relation between activity and temperature has rarely been determined by any experimental procedure similar to the measurement of speeds of forced continuous swimming which has been applied to fish (but see Moberly, 1965). With these orders, the evidence for a range of temperatures for activity which vary according to the species, comes from direct observations of the temperature of the animals, taken while active in nature. Extensive summaries of such measurements are given by Brattstrom (1963, 1965) and comparable material is to be found for old-world reptiles (see Saint-Girons and Saint-Girons, 1956). The amphibia in general have a range of activity

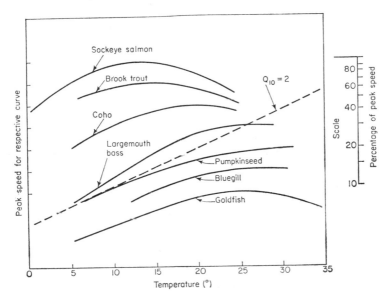

FIG. 6. Relative cruising speeds of various fish in relation to temperature when acclimated to the test temperature. The data for the sockeye salmon, *Oncorhynchus nerka*, and coho, *O. kisutch*, are from Brett *et al.* (1958); those for brook trout, *Salvelinus fontinalis*, from Graham (1949); for largemouth bass, *Micopterus salmoides*, from Johnson and Charlton (1960); for goldfish, *Carassius auratus*, from Fry and Hart (1948); for pumpkinseed, *Lepomis gibbosus*, from the unpublished data of B. E. Pearson and F. E. J. Fry; for bluegill, *L. macrochirus*, from the unpublished data of E. C. Bousefield. The percentage of peak speed scale is set to the peak of the topmost curve.

temperatures similar to those of the temperate and tropical species of fish. With regard to reptiles, the data in Brattstrom (1965), based on more than 10 observations, are plotted in Fig. 7.

The tuatara, *Sphenodon punctatum*, has a mean activity temperature of approximately 12° which corresponds to the optimum for trout, and there are no doubt other island species with similar values. An indirect experimental approximation of the temperature for maximum activity is the thermal preferendum (see p. 399).

The response of activity to thermal acclimation is shown in Fig. 8.

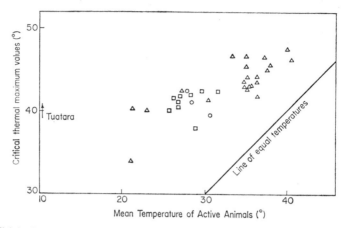

FIG. 7. Critical thermal maxima of reptiles in relation to mean body temperature of active animals measured in the field. Data from Brattstrom (1965), Bogert (1953), and Dawbin (1962). ○, represent data for turtles; □, for snakes; △, for saurians.

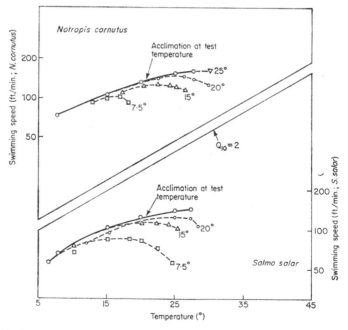

FIG. 8. Influence of temperature on the cruising speeds of the young Atlantic salmon, *Salmo salar*, and the minnow, *Notropis cornutus*, in relation to acclimation temperature. Redrawn from McCrimmon (1949).

These previously unpublished data of McCrimmon show the same type of response to acclimation as seen previously (Ferguson, quoted in Fry, 1964; Fry and Hart, 1948), namely that, at a given temperature, the animal performs at its best when acclimated to that temperature. However, it is only at the extremes that thermal history shows a major effect, a circumstance which may account for the failure of Grainger and Goldspink (1964) to see an effect of acclimation on the performance of the frog.

Some activities of the organism may, if necessary, be satisfied at the expense of others. Thus Henderson (1963) found complete temperature independence in the development of the ova of the eastern brook trout, *Salvelinus fontinalis*, at 8° and 16°. The rate was controlled entirely by the photoperiod, there being presumably adequate energy available at either temperature. On the other hand, Brown (1946) found a still more complex situation in the growth of the brown trout, *Salmo fario*. She found two optima for growth (8° and 18°) with a decided minimum between them. Her explanation was that the directive effect of temperature brought about more spontaneous activity in the region of the temperature preferendum, so that maintenance requirements rose sharply between 8° and 15° while food intake was more or less constant.

As the two latter examples indicate, it is difficult to discuss the effects of temperature on activity independently of other concurrent environmental effects, but I have chosen to do so here to keep within the confines of the subject matter of the chapter. For a general discussion of the interaction of environmental factors, see Fry (1947), and for more detailed analyses of the effects of low oxygen and high carbon dioxide concentrations on fish in relation to temperature, see Beamish (1964b, c) and Basu (1959). Kinne (1964) has reviewed the effects of temperature-salinity combinations.

B. METABOLIC RATE IN RELATION TO TEMPERATURE

At any given temperature, the metabolic rate of an animal can show wide fluctuations. An example of such diversity is shown in Fig. 9 for the goldfish. For the present purposes, the following points may be noted: (1) under conditions of spontaneous activity, with the fish guarded from outside stimuli, a wide variety of rates of metabolism may be found up to almost the maximum rate to be determined under forced activity; (2) the maximum increase in the metabolic rate is some tenfold; (3) at low swimming speeds, there may be extensive oxygen consumption which is not accounted for by the activity measured. On the basis of such data, it has become customary to recognize three levels of oxygen consumption of fish (Fry, 1957b). (a) *Standard*—the minimum rate, preferably extrapolated to zero activity by determining some relation between activity and oxygen consumption (Spoor, 1946; Ruhland and Heusner, 1959; Blazka *et al.*, 1960; Beamish and Mookherji, 1964; Brett, 1964; Muir *et al.*, 1965; Smit, 1965; Wohlschlag, 1962), but approximated by taking the low point of metabolism in the daily cycle (e.g. Job; 1955; Schultze, 1965), or by the use of anaesthesia or operative immobilization: (b) *Routine*—the mean oxygen consumption

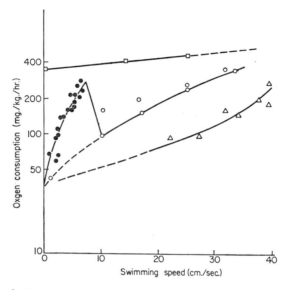

FIG. 9. Relation between oxygen consumption and swimming speed of goldfish, as affected by spontaneous and forced activity. Squares give unpublished data, from C. Cook, on forced acute activity. The remaining data are from Smit (1965). Solid dots indicate spontaneous activity; circles are for data on fish undisturbed except for rotation of the chamber; triangles are for data on fish that spent 7–8 hr. in Blazka's respirometer (Blazka *et al.*, 1960). Fish weights were approximately 80 g. Smit's fish were 18 cm. long. All fish were acclimated and tested at 20°.

as ordinarily measured with precautions against outside stimuli impinging on the fish (e.g. Stroganov, 1956): (c) *Active*—the maximum steady rate of oxygen consumption under continuous forced activity. In the past, this value has usually been approximated in acute experiments (e.g. Basu, 1959) such as those of Cook, illustrated in Fig. 9. Entry into a large segment of the literature relating the metabolism of fish to temperature can be made through Winberg (1961).

Figure 10 shows the influence of temperature on the standard, routine, and active metabolic rates of yearling sockeye salmon. These data were obtained in an apparatus in which the fish could be maintained at various steady swimming speeds, and the standard rate was determined by extrapolation. The routine rate shown is perhaps not entirely typical, since it is the level of spontaneous activity after recovery from severe fatigue, and the values may possibly be low on that account. At some temperatures, Beamish (1964a) found routine rates which were two to four times the standard rate. The active rates in Fig. 10 are the maximum levels attained in experiments lasting 5–7 hours, and in which the speed was increased in steps of approximately 10 cm./sec. at the end of every 75 min.

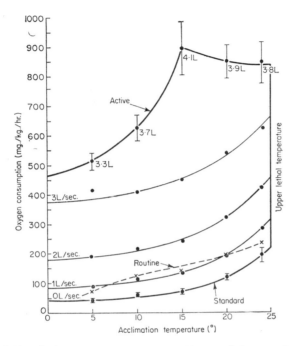

FIG. 10. Relation between oxygen consumption and temperature at various swimming speeds for yearling sockeye salmon (18 cm. long; 50 g.). Standard and active rates are indicated as mean ± 2 S.E. The 60 min. "critical speed" accompanying each active rate is shown. Swimming speeds of 1–3 lengths L/sec. were obtained by interpolation; those at 0 L/sec. were obtained by extrapolation. Modified from Brett (1964). The dashed line represents the routine rate from Brett's Fig. 10.

The standard rate of metabolism of the sockeye salmon increases slightly faster than a simple geometric progression, and a tangent to the curve at about 12° would have a Q_{10} of 2·0. Up to 15°, the active curve is essentially a multiple of the standard curve, the ratio being approximately 12:1. Brett interprets the drop in the active curve beyond 15° as being due to the limiting effect of the concentration of dissolved oxygen in air-saturated water. He was able to obtain a value of approximately 1200 mg./kg./hr. at 20° by increasing the oxygen concentration to 14·0 p.p.m. (water saturated with air contains about 9 p.p.m.). He thus extrapolated the trend shown below 15°. The routine rate shows a convex curve which deviates most from the standard curve around 10–15°.

Brett's data display the various characteristics that appear to be typical of the three levels of metabolism as defined. The standard rate accounts for the repair reactions required to keep the protoplasm at a given level of irritability for a given temperature, and this reflects the basic relation of biochemical processes to temperature. In Brett's data, standard metabolism includes the cost of respiration which probably

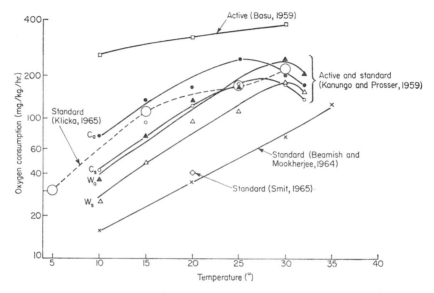

Fig. 11. Effect of temperature and thermal acclimation on the metabolism of the goldfish as measured by oxygen consumption. Data from Basu (1959), Beamish and Mookherji (1964), Kanungo and Prosser (1959), Klicka (1965) and Smit (1965).

accounts for the Q_{10} value increasing slightly with increasing temperature. Beamish, whose apparatus probably accounted for respiratory movements as well as swimming, obtained standard curves with a constant or decreasing Q_{10} value. The convexity, or possibly slight sinuosity, of the routine curve reflects the directive effect of temperature on the degree of spontaneous activity, which is also illustrated for goldfish in Fig. 11. On the basis of the usually held hypothesis that increasing irritability permits increasing response, active metabolism would be a multiple of standard metabolism and, in this instance, appears to be so when no limit intervenes.

Performance (level of activity, which in this case is the speed of steady swimming) is related to the difference between standard and active metabolism (scope). With physical activity, the relation is geometric so that the scope goes up as the power of the speed attained. Hence swimming speed varies much less with temperature than does the metabolic rate. In the sockeye salmon, the speed is virtually constant from 10–25° although this constancy is achieved above 15° by the limiting effect of oxygen. From the point of view of ecology, it may be said that the emphasis that physiologists have placed on standard metabolism has been undue. The poikilothermic animal, although subject to the laws relating chemical reactions to temperature, nevertheless can achieve a major level of constancy of activity over a range of temperatures.

References in Brett (1964) will lead the reader to the majority of the work on activity and metabolism in fish, except for the paper by Spaas (1959b) who measured the oxygen consumption of *Tilapia melanopleura* and *T. macrochir* at rest and when spontaneously active.

The measurement of standard and active metabolism has only recently been given consideration for reptiles. Bartholomew and Tucker (1963) worked with the Australian agamid, *Amphibolurus barbatus*, taking as the maximum activity in that animal the maximum observed in spontaneous struggling. Since the maximum declined over the range 20–40°, its course with temperature may possibly be due to the directive effect of temperature (p. 402), so that their finding of a maximum scope at 20° probably bears no relation for the temperature for peak activity in this reptile, whose mean activity temperature was found to be 35°.

In a later paper (Bartholomew and Tucker, 1964), the active level of oxygen consumption in four species of varanids was elicited by electric shock, and the scope increased up to 40°. The same authors, together with Lee (Bartholomew *et al.*, 1965), measured the scope activity in the skink, *Tiliqua scincoides*, and found little difference between 30° and 40°. Finally Moberly (1965) has measured the activity of *Iguana iguana* on a treadmill. He reported that they can maintain three times the speed at 36° as compared with that at 20°.

Licht (1965) measured the heart rate during rest and after electrical stimulation in three iguanids and a skink. He found maximum temperatures for differences between the resting and active rates to be as follows: *Dipsosaurus dorsalis* (42°), *Uma notata* (39°), *Sceloporus graciosus* (37°) and *Tiliqua rugosa* (35°). For the first three of these species, the mean body temperatures of free animals, as summarized by Brattstrom (1965), agree within a degree or so with Licht's findings for maximum scope.

No reports of the limits of metabolism in relation to temperature could be found for the amphibia.

C. EFFECTS OF ACCLIMATION ON METABOLIC RATE

It is an observation of long standing that the metabolic rate of an animal acclimated to a low temperature is higher, often over a range of temperatures, as compared with the rate of another of the same species acclimated to a higher temperature, and there have been numerous attempts to relate this phenomenon to differences in the metabolic rate of excized tissues. The problem will not be dealt with exhaustively here, and discussion will be largely confined to Precht's two-temperature experiment with the eel (Precht, 1961), recently brought to a definitive conclusion by Schultze (1965). Precht placed an eel in a special chamber so that its anterior portion was maintained at one temperature and the posterior at another. Schultze maintained eels in such chambers under four different temperature regimes. He then measured their oxygen consumption at 18° after each acclimation period. His results are summarized in Table I. The eels behaved according to the thermal

TABLE I. *Effect of Subjecting the Anterior and Posterior Regions of Eels to Different Acclimation Temperatures, on the Relative Oxygen Consumption of the Animals (From Schultze, 1965).*

Acclimation temperature (°)		Relative oxygen consumption at 18°
Anterior	Posterior	
14	14	100
14	25	100
25	25	69
25	14	69

history of their heads. In the same experiments, the respiratory activity of muscle slices was also measured, and each showed the behaviour characteristic of the temperature to which it had been subjected. Prosser *et al.* (1965) concluded, from the number of electrical spikes produced in the body muscle of eels acclimated in Precht's two-temperature apparatus, that the nervous system, by its tonic discharge, can cause enzymic changes that persist in isolated muscle, and that part of the metabolic compensation during temperature acclimation may result indirectly from acclimative changes in the nervous system. Thus, the general conclusion is that the phenomenon of temperature compensation, as seen in the metabolism of the whole animal, is under some central regulation. It appears impossible at the present time to make acute measurements of standard metabolism in fish. There is no means of being certain that all of the results of the central stimulus of the temperature change can be removed from the measurement (see Fig. 15, p. 404).

Meaningful acute measurements of active respiration appear to have been made only by Kanungo and Prosser (1959), who found little difference, at 30°, in goldfish acclimated either at 10° or 30°, but that, at 10°, the active rate for the cold-acclimated fish was about double that for the warm-acclimated individuals. Their data, together with recent data for standard and active metabolism of goldfish acclimated to the respective temperatures before measurement, are shown in Fig. 11. The scatter of the data indicate the difficulty in drawing sound physiological conclusions from such measurements. Figure 11 also shows the most recent measurements of the routine metabolism of the goldfish used as the comparison for acclimative changes in the metabolic rate (Klicka, 1965). It is obvious that these latter measurements contain a large component of metabolism above the standard level.

V. Directive Effects

Motile organisms ordinarily respond to a temperature gradient by congregating with some degree of precision about a temperature which is characteristic of the species concerned. In the English literature, the terms *preferred temperature* or *temperature preferendum* have been commonly used, and the latter term will be used in this chapter. But there are many synonyms, and in particular the term "eccritic temperature" is often applied with respect to reptiles in the American literature. The pioneer student of temperature preferenda in tetrapods was Herter (Herter, 1941, 1943). His bar-gradient apparatus (Herter, 1925, 1934) has been widely used with many modifications. Studies on temperature selection in fish go back to the same period, possibly beginning with the use of Shelford's two-choice apparatus (Wells, 1914). A review and classification of the various types of gradient apparatus used in the study of fish have been given by Fry (1958).

Temperature selection is under central nervous system control (Sullivan, 1954), and goldfish have been trained to adjust the temperature in their aquarium with about the same precision as rats perform a similar task (Rozin and Mayer, 1961). Temperature selection is achieved by exploration if the medium (water) is essentially opaque to infrared, or in air by orientation to a source of radiant heat.

The relation of thermal history to the temperature preferendum has been explored most widely in fish, and it has been found that the response is most diverse (Fig. 12). As Fig. 12 indicates, there is a positive correlation between acclimation temperature and the temperature preferendum in some species. In other species, the thermal history has no effect on the temperature preferendum, while in still others there is a slight negative correlation. The causes of such diversity are still unknown, but Zahn (1962) has provided a classification of the various responses based on the angle with which the line describing the relation between acclimation temperature and temperature preferendum crosses the line, drawn in Fig. 12, with a slope of 45°.

The response of the temperature preferendum to acclimation temperature has been little explored in amphibia and reptiles. Strübing (1954), who has made almost all the measurements available for amphibia (but see also Reichling, 1957), notes some changes between spring and summer. Scott (1943) found the temperature preferendum of tadpoles of *Rana clamitans* to shift from 20° to 25° with a change in acclima-

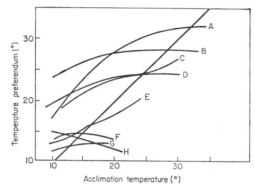

FIG. 12. Temperature preferenda of various fish. Data from Ferguson (1958) and Zahn (1962). A, indicates data for *Cyprinus corpio*; B, for *Carassius auratus*; C, for *Perca flavescens*; D, for *Girella nigricans*; E, for *Salvelinus fontinalis*; F, *Oncorhyncus nerka*; G, for *O. tshawytscha*; H, for *Salmo gaindneri*. Reprinted from Fry (1964).

tion temperature from 11° to 25°. With respect to reptiles, Herter (1940) usually found little difference between various batches of the same species, and Wilhoft and Anderson (1960) found no change or a slight negative shift, at the highest acclimation temperature, in the temperature preferendum of *Sceloporus occidentalis*.

If the relation between the thermal acclimation and the temperature preferendum is known, the temperature at which these two values are the same, the *final preferendum*, can be calculated and may be taken as an index for the species. Such final preferenda are known for several fishes, but for the reptiles and amphibia we can only assume that the preferenda as measured correspond to the final preferenda.

There may be seasonal shifts of the temperature preferendum that are not related to thermal history. Sullivan and Fisher (1953) found a sudden increase in the temperature preferendum of the eastern brook trout, *Salvelinus fontinalis*, in late winter, and Mantleman (1958) reported a decrease of the temperature preferendum value in the rainbow trout, *Salmo irideus*, during the fall.

The value of the final preferendum appears to be an index of two properties of the free organism. In fish, it appears to be an indicator of the temperatures in nature at which the species will be found during its active season (Ferguson, 1958). It also appears to indicate the optimum temperature for activity in those organisms in which activity and the

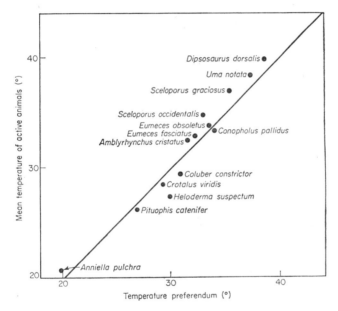

FIG. 13. Experimentally determined preferred body temperatures in reptiles in relation to the temperatures of active animals observed in the field. From Bogert and del Campo (1956), Brattstrom (1965), Licht (1965), Wilhoft (1958), and Wilhoft and Anderson (1960).

temperature preferendum have been measured in relation to the acclimation temperature (e.g. see references in Fry, 1964). This latter relation, however, has by no means been explored to any sufficient degree.

In reptiles also, the temperature preferenda show good agreement with the activity temperatures in nature (Bogert and del Campo, 1956; Wilhoft and Anderson, 1960; Brattstrom, 1965; Licht, 1965; Fig. 13). Licht (1965) also obtained a peak increment of the stimulated heart rate over the resting rate in four lizards at temperatures which corresponded closely to the temperature preferenda.

There is also a relation between the temperature preferendum and spontaneous activity as has been mentioned earlier (p. 396). The relation is a complex one (Fry, 1964) and opposite effects are obtained according to whether the spontaneous activity is measured in animals acclimated to the temperature concerned or whether the measurements are made with relatively rapid changes of temperature. The first circumstance (Sullivan, 1954; see also her data in Fry, 1957b) leads to maximum spontaneous activity in the region of the temperature preferendum. It is this type of spontaneous movement which influences the course of

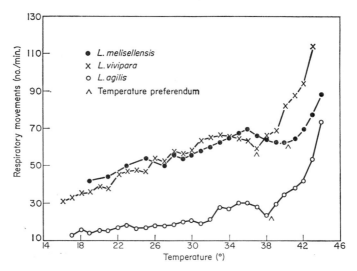

FIG. 14. Respiratory movements in lizards exposed to continuous temperature changes. From Herter (1941).

routine metabolism with temperature as mentioned earlier (p. 396). A thorough investigation of this subject was made by Schmein-Engburding (1953).

If, however, activity is observed in a steadily changing temperature, then there is a decrease in activity at the preferendum as compared with activity at adjacent temperatures (Ivlev, 1960). The metabolic rate also reflects these changes, and a change in metabolic rate may even be seen without overt movement. The examples given in Fig. 15 show changes in the rate of respiratory movements of two lizards resting on a substrate that was being steadily warmed. C. M. Sullivan (personal communication; quoted in Fry, 1964) pointed out that a sojourn in changing temperature gives the animal the same experience as moving in a temperature gradient and, in her experiments, movement in a gradient is influenced by the change of temperature encountered in a single translocation. Thus, as Ivlev (1960) also pointed out, the activity displayed under changing temperature is related to the mechanism of temperature selection.

A. TEMPERATURE REGULATION IN REPTILES

Cowles (1962), who has long been a student of the reptiles, proposes the abandonment of the word "poikilotherm". He suggests that *ectotherm* be used instead on the grounds that the poikilotherm does, by behavioural regulation, really control its body temperature. Two extensive articles on the subject are by Bogert (1959) and the Saint-Girons (1956). The desert reptiles are the most efficient in achieving this regulation (Schmidt-Nielsen and Dawson, 1964), whereas certain tropical reptiles have little ability in this respect (Bogert, 1959). The extent

TABLE II. *Body Temperatures of Active* Uta stansburiana *Observed in Nature* (*From Brattstrom, 1965*).

Month	Temperature (°)			No. of Observations
	Minimum	Maximum	Mean	
February	—	—	33·0	1
March	32·0	37·5	33·6	26
April	28·0[a]	38·4	35·6	46
May	31·0	38·2	36·0	45
June	34·0	38·0	36·7	5
July	31·2	40·0	35·9	15
September	29·0	36·7	33·0	4

[a] One record of 24·5 was not included.

to which reptiles can regulate their body temperature is indicated by Brattstrom's data for *Uta stansburiana*, given in Table II. In this animal, the mean body temperature of active individuals changes less than 4° from March to September. Another example of a narrow range of body temperature during periods of activity is given in Fig. 15, in which it is seen (Panel C) that the total range of body temperatures in active animals covered only 10° throughout the season. The range of air temperatures at which the racerunners were active was twice as large, and the total seasonal range of temperatures, though not given, was greater still.

However, to achieve the regulation of body temperature shown in Fig. 15, the racerunner must withdraw from the environment to a large degree. In Kansas, this species spends about two-thirds of the year in hibernation, and its activities, when not hibernating, are restricted to favourable periods of the day, the lengths of which vary with the season. Thus the source of heat is exogenous, either the sun's rays or a warm substrate, and control is largely by behaviour.

Heliothermic reptiles must be of a relatively small size. Strong insolation can warm a 1 cm. cube of water about one-half to one degree in a minute, depending on the air mass. An animal more than a few centimetres thick would therefore warm very slowly, so that large reptiles thus could not be heliotherms.

Reptiles show a limited amount of physiological temperature regulation. Many species pant at high temperatures (e.g. Colbert *et al.*, 1946; Dawson and Templeton, 1962; Fitch, 1956), and achieve at least a limited amount of evaporative cooling (e.g. Langlois, 1902). It is characteristic

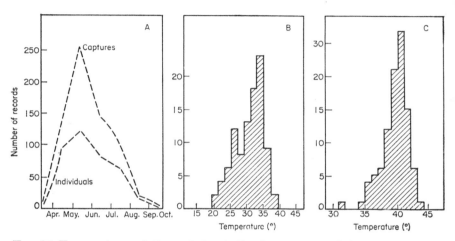

FIG. 15. Temperature relations of the six-lined racerunner. A indicates data for active animals observed in the open field; B air temperatures for sightings of active animals; C body temperatures of active animals. From Fitch (1958).

of reptiles, when exposed to a new temperature, that they heat faster than they cool (see the examples in Fig. 1). Bartholomew and Tucker (1963) pointed out that this differential is associated with changes in heart rate, so that there is a circulatory adjustment (see also Cowles, 1958). Later (Bartholomew *et al.*, 1965) it was found that the differential between the rates of heating and cooling in the Australian skink, *Tiliqua scincoides*, could be attributed to the production of metabolic heat. However, such heat could not produce a useful excess of body temperature over air temperature because of the conductivity coefficient of the animals concerned (approximately 0·04). If the heat production were taken to be 0·05 cal./g./min., equivalent to about the highest oxygen consumption these authors recorded, the excess of body temperature over ambient would be of the order of 1·2°.

There is now good evidence (Dowling, quoted in Pope, 1961; Hutchinson *et al.*, 1966) that the brooding Indian Python, *Python molurus*, can achieve a substantial level of physiological thermoregulation by spasmodic muscular contractions. In the study of Hutchinson *et al.* (1966), the body temperature and the rate of oxygen consumption were measured in a 14 kg., 2·7 m. python coiled about a clutch of 23 eggs. Figure 16 shows the relation of oxygen consumption to the ambient temperature and to the rate of muscular contraction. The maximum temperature differential achieved was 5° above the ambient, and the apparent desired body temperature was 32°, which could only be maintained down to an ambient of 27°. Below that temperature, body temperature was maintained approximately at the maximum differential

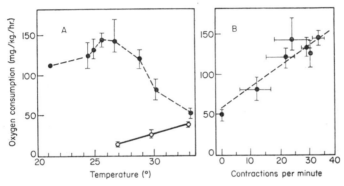

FIG. 16. Oxygen consumption of an Indian python, *Python molurus*. A indicates oxygen consumption in relation to temperature, the upper curve for brooding, the lower curve for non-brooding animals; B indicates oxygen consumption while brooding in relation to the frequency of muscular contraction. From Hutchinson *et al.* (1966).

down to an ambient temperature of 21°. From Fig. 16, it will be noted that the peak metabolic rate was a little more than twice the standard, being about 100 mg./kg./hr. This rate can hardly be the peak for physical activity which, while it has not apparently been measured for snakes, is of the order of 1000 mg./kg./hr. for saurians and fish. Thus, in its muscular thermoregulatory activity, the python probably keeps well within the limits of physical exhaustion, as indeed it demonstrates it does.

It is of some interest to calculate the coefficient of temperature exchange for the coiled python since the data for heat production are available. In round numbers, the python observed by Hutchinson *et al.* (1966) produced enough heat to raise its temperature 0·01°/min. To achieve a temperature differential of 5°, k must be 0·002. However, since some heat would inevitably be dissipated by evaporation, it is more probable that k approximated to 0·001, a value about one-tenth that for a varanid of similar size. Posture alone could perhaps account for this difference.

With the ability of the brooding python to maintain a limited degree of constancy in its body temperature by metabolic regulation, it would seem that the reptiles have achieved all but the last step towards homo-eothermism and that physiological regulation of body temperature has evolved from the behavioural response. The last step is the evolution of an insulating coat. However, it should be pointed out that the brooding python achieves about the same economy of heat in air as the seal does in water. The coefficient of heat exchange for a 30 kg. seal is also about 0·001, on the basis of maintaining a body temperature of 37° in water at 0°. The greater temperature differential in the seal is obtained by about a five-fold greater expenditure of metabolism. These estimates are based on data in Hart and Irving (1959).

References

Adensamer, E. (1934). *Z. vergl. Physiol.* **21**, 642.

Alabaster, J. S. (1963). *Int. J. air wat. Poll.* **7**, 541.

Allanson, B. R and Noble, R. G. (1964). *Trans. Amer. fish. Soc.* **93**, 323.

Arai, M. N., Cox, E. T. and Fry, F. E. J. (1963). *Canad. J. Zool.* **41**, 1011.

Auerbach, M. (1957). *Z. Fischeri u.d. Hilfswiss. N. F.* **6**, 605.

Bailey, R. M. (1949). *Ecology* **30**, 238.

Barrett, I. and Hester, F. J. (1964). *Nature, Lond.* **203**, 96.

Bartholomew, G. A. and Lasiewski, C. (1965). *Comp. Biochem. Physiol.* **16**, 573.

Bartholomew, G. A. and Tucker, V. A. (1963). *Physiol. Zool.* **36**, 199.

Bartholomew, G. A. and Tucker, V. A. (1964). *Physiol. Zool.* **37**, 341.

Bartholomew, G. A., Tucker, V. A. and Lee, A. K. (1965). *Copeia,* 169.

Basu, S. P. (1959). *J. fish. Res. Bd. Canada* **16**, 175.

Beamish, F. W. H. (1964a). *Canad. J. Zool.* **42**, 177.

Beamish, F. W. H. (1964b). *Canad. J. Zool.* **42**, 355.

Beamish, F. W. H. (1964c). *Canad. J. Zool.* **42**, 847.

Beamish, F. W. H. and Mookherji, P. S. (1964). *Canad. J. Zool.* **42**, 161.

Blazka, P., Volf, M. and Cepela, M. (1960). *Physiol. bohemoslov.* **9**, 553.

Bliss, C. I. (1937). *Ann. appl. Biol.* **24**, 815.

Bogert, C. M. (1953). *Zoologica, N.Y.* **38**, 63.

Bogert, C. M. and del Campo, R. M. (1956). *Bull. Amer. Mus. nat. Hist.* **109**, 1.

Bogert, C. M. (1959). *Scientific American* **200**, 105.

Brattstrom, B. H. (1963). *Ecology* **44**, 238.

Brattstrom, B. H. (1965). *Amer. Midland Nat.* **73**, 376.

Brattstrom, B. H. and Lawrence, P. (1962). *Physiol. Zool.* **35**, 148.

Brett, J. R. (1944). *Univ. Toronto Stud. Biol. Ser.* **52**, 1.

Brett, J. R. (1946). *Univ. Toronto Stud. Biol. Ser.* **53**, 9.

Brett, J. R. (1952). *J. fish. Res. Bd. Canada* **9**, 265.

Brett, J. R. (1956). *Quart. Rev. Biol.* **31**, 75.

Brett, J. R. (1964). *J. fish. Res. Bd. Canada* **21**, 1183.

Brett, J. R. and Alderdice, D. F. (1958). *J. fish. Res. Bd. Canada* **15**, 805.

Brett, J. R., Hollands, M. and Alderdice, D. F. (1958). *J. fish. Res. Bd. Canada* **15**, 587.

Brooks, G. R. and Sassman, J. F. (1965). *Copeia*, 251.

Brown, M. E. (1946). *J. exp. Biol.* **22**, 145.

Carpenter, C. C. (1953). *Ecology* **34**, 74.

Carpenter, C. C. (1961). *Proc. Oklahoma Acad. Sci.* **41**, 72.

Cocking, A. W. (1959a). *J. exp. Biol.* **36**, 203.

Cocking, A. W. (1959b). *J. exp. Biol.* **36**, 217.

Colbert, E. H., Cowles, R. B. and Bogert, C. M. (1946). *Bull. Amer. Mus. nat. Hist.* **86**, 327.

Cowles, R. B. (1958). *Evolution* **12**, 347.

Cowles, R. B. (1962). *Science* **135**, 670.

Cowles, R. B. and Bogert, C. M. (1944). *Bull. Amer. Mus. nat. Hist.* **83**, 265.

Craigie, D. E. (1963). *Canad. J. Zool.* **41**, 825.

Davenport, C. B. and Castle, W. E. (1896). *Roux. Arch. f. Entwicklungsmech* **2**, 227.

Davis, E. R. (1955). *Copea*, 207.

Dawbin, W. H. (1962). *Endeavour* **21**, 16.

Dawson, W. R. and Templeton, J. R. (1962). *Physiol. Zool.* **36**, 219.

De Witt, C. B. (1962). *Amer. Zool.* **2**, 517.

Doudoroff, P. (1942). *Biol. Bull.* **83**, 219.

Doudoroff, P. (1945). *Biol. Bull.* **88**, 194.

Ferguson, R. G. (1958). *J. fish. Res. Bd. Canada* **15**, 607.

Fitch, H. S. (1956). *Univ. Kansas Publ. Mus. Nat. Hist.* **8**, 417.

Fitch, H. S. (1958). *Univ. Kansas Publ. Mus. Nat. Hist.* **11**, 11.

Fry, F. E. J. (1947). *Univ. Toronto Stud. Biol. Ser.* **55**, 62 pp.

Fry, F. E. J. (1957a). *Ann. Biol.* **33**, 205.

Fry, F. E. J. (1957b). *In* "The Physiology of Fishes", (M. E. Brown, Ed.), vol. 1, pp. 1–63. Academic Press, New York.

Fry, F. E. J. (1958). *Proc. Indo-Pacific Fish. Coun.* **III**, 37.

Fry, F. E. J. (1964). *In* "Handbook of Physiology, 4: Adaptation to the Environment", (D. B. Dill, E. F. Adolph and G. C. Wilber, Eds.), pp. 715–728. Amer. Physiol. Soc., Washington.

Fry, F. E. J. and Hart, J. S. (1948). *J. fish. Res. Bd. Canada* **7**, 169.

Fry, F. E. J., Hart, J. S. and Walker, K. F. (1946). *Univ. Toronto Biol. Ser.* **54**, 9.

Gibson, M. B. (1953). M.A. Thesis: University of Toronto.

Gibson, M. B. (1954). *Canad. J. Zool.* **32**, 393.

Gordon, M. S., Amdur, B. H. and Scholander, P. F. (1962). *Biol. Bull.* **122**, 52.

Graham, J. M. (1949). *Canad. J. Res. D.* **27**, 270.

Grainger, J. N. R. and Goldspink, G. (1964). *Helgol. Wiss. Meeresunters.* **9**, 420.

Gunn, D. L. (1942). *Biol. Rev.* **17**, 293.

Gunter, G. (1941). *Ecology* **22**, 203.

Gunter, G. (1947). *Science* **106**, 472.

Hall, F. G. and Root, R. W. (1930). *Biol. Bull.* **58**, 52.

Hansen, R. M. (1954). *Herpetologica*, **10**, 200.

Hart, J. S. (1947). *Trans. Roy. Soc. Can. 41*, Ser. *III*, Sec. 5, 57.

Hart, J. S. (1952). *Univ. Toronto Stud. Biol. Ser.* **60**, 79 pp.

Hart, J. S. and Irving, L. (1959). *Canad. J. Zool.* **37**, 447.

Harvey, H. H. (1964). *Verh. Internat. Verein. Limnol.* **15**, 947.

Hathaway, E. S. (1927). *Bull. U.S. Bur. Fish.* 169.

Heath, W. G. (1963). *Science* **142**, 486.

Henderson, N. E. (1963). *J. fish. Res. Bd. Canada* **20**, 859.

Herter, K. (1925). *Z. vergl. Physiol.* **1**, 221.

Herter, K. (1934). *Biol. Zentralbl.* **54**, 487.
Herter, K. (1940). *Z. vergl. Physiol.* **28**, 105.
Herter, K. (1941). *Naturwiss.* **29**, 155.
Herter, K. (1943). *Biol. generalis* **17**, 243.
Hoar, W. S. and Robinson, G. B. (1959). *Canad. J. Zool.* **37**, 419.
Hubbs, C. (1964). *Ecology* **45**, 376.
Hutchinson, V. H. (1961). *Physiol. Zool.* **34**, 92.
Hutchinson, V. H. and Kosh, R. J. (1965). *Herpetologica* **20**, 233.
Hutchinson, V. H., Dowling, H. G. and Vinegar, A. (1966). *Science* **151**, 694.
Ivlev, V. S. (1960). *Zool. Zhurn.* **39**, 494.
Job. S. V. (1955). *Univ. Toronto Stud. Biol. Ser.* **61**, 39 pp.
Johnson, M. G. and Charlton, W. H. (1960). *Prog. Fish-Culturist, Wash.* **22**, 155.
Kanungo, M. S. and Prosser, C. L. (1959). *J. cell. comp. Physiol.* **54**, 265.
Kinne, O. (1964). *Oceangr. Mar. Biol. Annu. Rev.* **2**, 281.
Kishinouye, K. (1923). *J. Coll. Agric. (Imperial Univ. Tokyo)* **8**, 293.
Klicka, J. (1965). *Physiol. Zool.* **38**, 177.
Langlois, J. P. (1902). *J. Physiol. Pathol. gén.* **4**, 249.
Licht, P. (1965). *Physiol. Zool.* **38**, 129.
Loeb, J. and Wasteneys, H. (1912). *J. exp. Zool.* **12**, 543.
Lowe, C. H. and Vance, V. J. (1955). *Science* **122**, 73.
Mantleman, I. I. (1958). *Isvest. Vsesiuznovo Nanechno-Isselovatelskovo Instituta Ozernovo i Rechnovo Rybnovo Khoz* **47**, 1. (*Fish. Res. Bd. Canada. Trans. Ser.* **257**, 1960.)
McCauley, R. W. (1963). *J. fish. Res. Bd. Canada* **20**, 483.
McCrimmon, H. R. (1949). Ph.D. Thesis: Univ. Toronto.
McFarland, W. N. (1955). *Copeia*, 191.
Mellanby, K. (1941). *J. exp. Biol.* **18**, 55.
Moberly, W. R. (1965). *Amer. Zool.* **5**, 706.
Moore, J. A. (1949). *Evolution* **3**, 1.
Morris, R. W. (1962). *Amer. Nat.* **98**, 35.
Muir, B. S., Nelson, G. J. and Bridges, K. W. (1965). *Trans. Amer. fish. Soc.* **94**, 378.
Mullaly, P. (1952). *Copeia*, 274.
Pitkow, R. B. (1960). *Biol. Bull.* **119**, 231.
Pope, C. H. (1961). "The Giant Snakes", 289 pp. Knopf, New York.
Precht, H. (1961). *Z. vergl. Physiol.* **44**, 451.
Precht, H. (1964). *Helgol. Wiss. Meeresunters.* **9**, 392.
Prosser, G. L., Precht, H. and Jankowsky, H. D. (1965). *Naturwiss.* **52**, 168.
Prosser, G. L. (1962). *In* "Comparative Physiology of Temperature Regulation. Part I", (J. P. Hannon and E. Viereck, Eds.), pp. 1–44. Arctic Aeromed. Lab. Fort Wainwright, Alaska.
Reichling, H. (1957). *Zool. Jb. allg. Zool.* **67**, 1.
Rozin, P. N. and Mayer, J. (1961). *Science* **134**, 942.
Ruhland, M. L. and Heusner, A. (1959). *Compt. rend. Soc. Biol.* **153**, 161.
Ruibal, R. (1955). *Evolution* **9**, 322.
Saint-Girons, H. and Saint-Girons, M. C. (1956). *Vie et Milieu* **7**, 133.
Schmein-Engburding, F. (1953). *Z. Fischeri u. d. Hilfswiss.* **2**, 125.
Schmidt-Nielsen, K. and Dawson, W. R. (1964). *In* "Handbook of Physiology. Vol. 4. Adaptation to the Environment", (D. B. Dill, E. F. Adolph and G. C. Wilber, Eds.), pp. 467–480. Amer. Physiol. Soc., Washington.
Scholander, P. F., Flagg, W., Hock, R. J. and Irving, L. (1953). *J. cell. comp. Physiol.* **42**, Suppl. 1: 1.

Schultze, D. (1965). *Z. wiss. Zool.* **172**, 105.

Scott, G. W. (1943). Ph.D. Thesis: University of Toronto.

Simpson, S. (1908). *Proc. Roy. Soc. Edin.* **28**, 66.

Smit, H. (1965). *Canad. J. Zool.* **43**, 623.

Spaas, J. T. (1959a). *Biol. Jaarb. Dodonaea, Ghent* **21**, 21.

Spaas, J. T. (1959b). *Hydrobiologia* **14**, 155.

Spoor, W. A. (1946). *Biol. Bull.* **91**, 312.

Stroganov, N. S. (1956). Izatel'stvo Akademii Nauk SSSR Moskva, (Trans. OTS 61 31038, Office of Technical Services, U.S. Dept. Comm. Washington, 1962).

Strübing, H. (1954). *Z. Morph. Ökol. Tiere* **43**, 357.

Sullivan, C. M. (1954). *J. fish. Res. Bd. Canada* **11**, 153.

Sullivan, C. M. and Fisher, K. C. (1953). *J. fish. Res. Bd. Canada* **10**, 187.

Tsukuda, H. (1961). *J. Biol. Osaka City Univ.* **12**, 15.

Tyler, A. V. (1966). *Canad. J. Zool.* **44**, 349.

Ushakov, B. (1964). *Physiol. Rev.* **44**, 518.

Walters, V. (1962). *Amer. Zool.* **2**, 143.

Weigmann, (1930). *Z. wiss. Zool.* **136**, 195.

Wells, M. M. (1914). *Trans. Illinois Acad. Sci.* **7**, 48.

Wikgren, B. J. (1953). *Acta Zoologica Fennica* **71**, 1.

Wilhoft, D. C. (1958). *Herpetologica* **14**, 161.

Wilhoft, D. C. and Anderson, J. D. (1960). *Science* **131**, 610.

Winberg, G. G. (1961). *Voprosy Ikhtiologii* **1**, 157. Fish. Res. Bd. Canada Trans. Serv. 362.

Wohlschlag, D. E. (1960). *Ecology* **41**, 287.

Wohlschlag, D. E. (1962). *Science* **137**, 1.

Wohlschlag, D. E. (1964). *In* "Biology of the Antarctic Seas", Amer. Geophys. Un., Antarct. Res. Ser. Vol. 1, pp. 33–62.

Wolf, K. and Quimby, M. C. (1962). *Science* **135**, 1065.

Woodhead, P. J. M. (1964). *Helgol. Wiss. Meeresunters.* **10**, 283.

Woodhead, P. J. M. and Woodhead, A. D. (1959). *Proc. Zool. Soc. Lond.* **133**, 181.

Woodrow, C. E. and Wigglesworth, V. B. (1927). *Biochem. J.* **21**, 812.

Zahn, M. (1962). *Zool. Beitr. N.F.* **71**, 15.

Chapter 12

Resistance to Cold in Mammals

S. A. BARNETT AND L. E. MOUNT

Department of Zoology, University of Glasgow, Scotland, and
Institute of Animal Physiology, Agricultural Research
Council, Babraham, Cambridge, England

14+T.

I. Foundations

It is customary to name the maintenance of deep body temperature "homeothermy", while heterothermous (poikilothermous) animals are those in which deep body temperature follows the temperature of their environment. In a homeotherm, a regulated flow of *heat* determines body *temperature*. Hence the term "homeothermy" can mislead, since it may seem to mean "steady heat", instead of "steady temperature", and in this way perpetuate the confusion between heat and temperature which has bedevilled the growth of animal energetics. Mendelsohn (1964) shows how the subject remained undeveloped until the concepts of heat and temperature were separated. Heat as a quantity of energy, and temperature as a measure of the ratio of heat content to heat capacity, are rarely separated in general usage, and are still confused even in some scientific contexts.

The most convenient definition of a "homeotherm" is an animal which maintains a steady internal temperature in a wide range of external temperatures. A heterothermous animal, on the other hand, has a nearly constant temperature only in an environment which has itself an almost unvarying temperature.

General reviews of thermoregulation have been published by Hardy (1961), Thauer (1961), von Euler (1961) and Bligh (1966). Constancy of core temperature in a fluctuating environment demands regulated heat production and heat flow. A brief exposure to cold requires only a temporary increase in heat production or thermal insulation; the latter may be brought about by behaviour such as nest-making. Long-lasting exposure entails structural changes as well, as part of a chronic adaptation which can occur only if there is plenty of food. Usually, if the thermal demand of the environment (Burton and Edholm, 1955) for long exceeds the temperature-maintaining ability of the organism, the animal dies. But there are part-time homeotherms, such as the humming-birds, Trochilidae (Lasiewski, 1963), which develop a regular nocturnal hypothermia; this is an energy-saving process in animals that need a high metabolic rate to maintain their body temperature. Similarly, seasonal hibernation, with its accompanying hypothermia, is a means of evading the consequences of food shortage in winter.

These special cases excepted, the outcome of a homeotherm's struggle against cold depends on the relation between three quantities: heat production, thermal insulation, and the temperature difference between the animal's core and the environment. The three main sorts of outcome of exposure to cold—metabolic, insulative (Hart, 1963,

1964a,b), and hypothermic (Hammel, 1964)—reflect these primary factors.

II. Heat Production and Loss

A. THERMAL NEUTRALITY

The basal metabolic rate is conventionally defined as the metabolic rate of an animal (a) resting, (b) post-absorptive, (c) in a thermally neutral environment; but this concept has some defects. Giaja (1938) points out that, to obtain a "true" basal metabolic rate, the animal should first be for a time in an environment which does not call for any change in heat production. However, ignoring such refinements, a resting rate can be determined, for many species, of about 40 kcal./hr. m.^{2} body surface.

A thermally neutral environment, then, is one in which an animal produces heat at the minimum rate. When the environment cools, a point comes at which the metabolic rate begins to rise; this is the *critical temperature*. The lower the critical temperature, the greater is the possible economy in energy expenditure. In some arctic species, this is realized to a remarkable degree. An extreme is the very low critical temperature of − 40° in the arctic fox, *Alopex lagopus* (Scholander *et al.*, 1950); this is due to a thick coat of hair.

Heavy insulation makes it difficult to dissipate heat arising from activity. Yet the arctic fox, despite its thick fur, can run for long periods without pause. In general, heat can be lost by radiation and convection (and, to a small degree, by conduction), and by evaporation (reviewed by Mount, 1966a). The non-evaporative heat loss from a heavily coated animal is small, and takes place mainly from the poorly insulated head and legs (Irving *et al.*, 1955; and see Section II.B. 5). An Eskimo dog, *Canis*, does not melt snow on which it lies down to sleep (Hammel, 1964). But evaporative heat loss can be increased considerably through panting (Hardy, 1955), and such loss is independent of temperature gradients or thermal insulation. Some of the extra heat produced during activity may be dissipated in this way.

In a resting mammal at thermal neutrality, body temperature is maintained mainly by control of the circulation in the skin, and by sweating—the so-called "physical thermoregulation". As the temperature rises, heat is lost increasingly by sweating or, in animals such as the pig (Mount, 1963a; Ingram, 1964a) and sheep (Brockway *et al.*, 1965) which sweat little, by increased respiratory movements. A further rise in ambient temperature produces a rise in body temperature. The fully fleeced sheep, with a respiration rate of 90–120/min. at 20° ambient temperature, seems often to be near this point. After shearing, the rate falls to 16–20/min. (Bligh, 1963), a rate more usual for a mammal of this size. However, if the metabolic rate does not rise above the minimum characteristic of thermal neutrality, the animal is by definition still within that zone, in spite of the work being done by thermoregulatory mechanisms.

Peripheral vasoconstriction also contributes to insulation. It does not, however, always coincide with a rise in metabolic rate. The metabolic rate of fat men in a water bath rises when the bath temperature is lowered below 33°, although the maximum tissue insulation is not

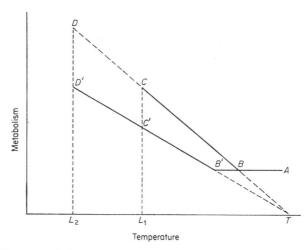

Fig. 1. A diagram of the relationship between an animal's metabolic rate and the ambient temperature. As the animal's insulation increases, the slope moves from BC to B^1C^1, pivoting on the animal's deep body temperature, T. The critical temperature falls at the same time from that opposite B to B^1, and the cold limit falls from L_1 to L_2, at the same maximum metabolism; this is insulative adaptation to cold. In "metabolic" adaptation, the curve BC is extended to BCD; at this point, the cold limit is extended from L_1 to L_2 by a rise in metabolic rate from $C = D^1$ to D. Variation in the level of minimal metabolism A, would move B relative to the temperature scale, and thus change the critical temperature. (After Hart, 1964a)

achieved until the temperature is much lower (Cannon and Keatinge, 1960). Since the metabolic and vasomotor responses do not occur at the same water temperature, these authors suggest calling the first the "metabolic threshold temperature"; they calculate a "theoretical critical temperature", that is, the lowest water temperature in which a man could in theory achieve thermal stability without an increase in metabolic rate. It is, however, probably better to give two critical temperatures, based on metabolic rate and skin circulation, respectively. For thin men, these temperatures are not far apart; and the same applies to another bare-skinned mammal, the young pig (Mount, 1959, 1964a).

The reciprocal of the insulation conferred by superficial tissues, that is, the thermal conductance, is proportional to the skin blood flow (Hensel, 1956). In a bare-skinned mammal (man: Miller and Blyth, 1958; pig: Irving, 1956; Mount, 1963b) subcutaneous fat enhances the control of insulation achieved by changes of peripheral blood flow. When the blood vessels of the skin are dilated, the subcutaneous fat can have little effect, since warm blood is moving through it to the surface, where heat exchange with the surroundings can take place. After vasoconstriction, this shunt no longer exists, and heat exchange must then take place through the fat. In the new-born pig, which has no subcutaneous fat but in which peripheral vasoconstriction does occur in the cold, the effect of vasomotor control on tissue insulation is relatively small (Mount, 1964a). In the older pig, which has subcutaneous fat, the effect is much greater (Ingram, 1964b). Vasomotor changes in animals with thick hair are probably less significant: little of the skin is in direct contact with the environment; hence skin temperature is closer to that of the core (Bligh, 1963).

While the white fox has a very low critical temperature, bare-skinned mammals such as naked man (Burton and Edholm, 1955), the young pig (Mount, 1960) and the shorn sheep (Graham *et al.*, 1959) have high critical temperatures. Hence critical temperature, thermal insulation and deep body temperature are intimately related (Fig. 1).

B. HEAT FLOW AND ENVIRONMENT

1. *Modes of Cold Adaptation*

When a mammal is exposed to cold, there are usually changes both in heat production and in insulation. Sometimes the response is almost wholly either one or the other. The effect on laboratory rats, of exposure to cold in the laboratory, is a rise in metabolic rate; but wild rats, exposed to the more complex situation of winter out of doors, also improve their insulation (Héroux, 1962). In a discussion on differences of insulation between individuals, Kleiber (1947) quotes an experiment carried out by Hoesslin in 1888. Hoesslin reared two dogs from the same litter, one at 32° and the other at 5°. Kleiber points out that the animal in the cold had to cope with a temperature difference between body and environment six times as great as that to which the other dog was exposed; yet the cold-exposed dog's metabolic rate was only 12% higher. The cold-exposed dog's hair, however, weighed three times that of its litter mate.

This is an example of chronic adaptation to cold. The acute response to cold must always be primarily metabolic. Even in the acute case, however, an insulative component enters in the form of changes in posture, pilo-erection and, if exposure to thermal neutrality preceded the cold, peripheral vasoconstriction as well.

2. Heat Flow

Heat flow from an animal to its environment obeys Fourier's law, which states that heat flow between two regions is proportional to the temperature difference and to the thermal conductance (Kleiber, 1961). Kleiber disagrees with the commonly held view that heat loss takes place according to Newton's law of cooling, which states that the rate of cooling is proportional to the temperature difference between the body's surface and the surroundings. He points out that, since the body's temperature is regulated, a simple law of cooling does not apply. In practice, the difference between these laws is not great; but when, for example, thermal insulation is changing, Fourier's law is superior, since it deals with a regulated flow rather than one which is diminishing as the body cools.

3. Maximum Metabolic Rate

In theory, the limit of thermoregulation in the cold is set by the animal's maximum metabolic rate. In practice, such high levels of heat production, which can be kept up for short periods on sudden exposure, have little relevance to cold resistance, because the animal cannot maintain them.

This situation has been examined in young pigs in the first week after birth (Mount, 1961, 1963c). A new-born pig weighs rather more than 1 kg. at birth and is unusually mature. It has little thermal insulation; subcutaneous fat is absent, and there is little hair. The animal's defence against cold must therefore be primarily metabolic (Mount, 1959); but it may also be helped by postural changes, huddling with its litter-mates (Mount, 1960, 1964b), and by nesting material.

The metabolic rate of pigs less than 1 week old approaches a maximum at about 5° environmental temperature at low air movement (10 cm./sec.). In these conditions, the highest rate observed in any pig was 162 kcal./m.^{2}hr.; the mean maximum for 31 pigs was 133 kcal./m.^{2}hr. (Mount, 1963c). About half the animals managed to maintain their body temperatures, by means of a high metabolic rate, when they were kept at 5° singly for up to 6 hours. The temperatures of the others fell progressively.

The reciprocal of the rate of fall of rectal temperature gives a measure of the thermoregulatory capacity or cold resistance, in terms of the time taken for body temperature to fall 1°. The longer this time, the greater is the animal's cold resistance. Only about two-thirds of the variance of this estimate of cold resistance in young pigs can be accounted for by variation in age and body weight. The correlation of rectal temperature change with cold resistance increases markedly if the individual "metabolic capability" is taken into account (L. E. Mount, unpublished observations). Metabolic capability is estimated as the metabolic rate when the rectal temperature is 36° and falling. It is argued that, when the rectal temperature is falling, the animal's metabolic rate is at the maximum, since added to the metabolic stimulus provided by a low environmental temperature is the effect of a falling deep body temperature (Mount, 1961). The pig's normal deep body temperature is close to 39°; when it has fallen to 36°, owing to cold exposure, the metabolic rate is held to be the maximum for that deep body temperature, *and to be limited by that temperature*. This is an important consideration for the comparison of maximum metabolic rates between animals, either of the same or of different species.

When the deep body temperature of a young pig begins to fall below about 37°, the metabolic rate has passed its maximum and is beginning to decline. As the body temperature falls still further, the decline follows a slope corresponding to a Q_{10} value of about 2. A similar Q_{10} value was found by Graham *et al.* (1959) in mature sheep above thermal neutrality. But often a considerable change of body temperature entails little change in metabolic rate. Adamsons *et al.* (1965) found similar metabolic rates in new-born human babies with deep body temperatures from 33·5° to 37·5°. This could be related to the incomplete development of the thermoregulatory mechanisms at birth less complete than in the pig.

A Q_{10} value for the whole animal might hold only at minimum or maximum metabolic rates; at intermediate rates, no simple correlation would be expected between metabolic rate and body temperature, since regulatory mechanisms alter the relationship. At minimum and maximum rates, however, there is no regulation. Young pigs at 4° have a mean Q_{10} value of about 2·9, with 95% confidence limits of 1·5 to 5·3; at 30° the Q_{10} value is 4·8, with limits 2·4 to 9·7 (Mount and Rowell, 1960). The critical temperature for these pigs is about 34° (Mount, 1959); hence the metabolic rate is regulated at 30°; at 4° the rate approaches the maximum, and therefore unregulated, level.

The observations of Silverman and Agate (1964), on small new-born human infants, are in accordance with those on pigs: the body temperatures of all infants fall in air temperatures controlled at 32° and 34°. Some infants prevent a marked fall in deep body temperature by increasing oxygen consumption, but others do not. Evidently there is considerable variation in metabolic capability, as in pigs.

The human baby and the piglet are good subjects for the investigation of cold resistance, since they have such low thermal insulation. Mature mammals have a subcutaneous layer of fat, a capacity for peripheral vasoconstriction and, in some species, a highly insulating coat. Even pigs have considerable thermal insulation, when resident in the Arctic (Irving, 1956). The other important feature of a mature mammal is that the cold must be intense before it induces a maximum metabolic rate. Iampietro *et al.* (1960) managed to achieve high rates in naked men by the use of wind in a cold environment. In a coated species, Alexander (1962) achieved maximum rates for lambs in an apparatus in which he could not only lower the temperature but also produce a wind and wet the animal as well. The cold had to be more severe than for young pigs, since a lamb's thermal insulation is about twice that of a piglet. The rectal temperature was made to fall at about 3°/hr., and oxygen consumption was then measured for 20 min. Wet lambs in a wind produce heat at rates as high as 250 kcal./m.²hr, compared with the piglet's upper limit of 162 kcal./m.²hr. The higher metabolic capacity and higher thermal insulation of lambs allow them to tolerate about three times the cold stress which can be withstood by young pigs. This is matched by the considerably greater cooling to which the lamb is exposed in its usual outdoor habitat, as compared with the young pig which, in natural conditions, lives in a nest with its litter-mates and the sow.

4. *Metabolic Body Size*

The "summit" or maximum metabolism of lambs is roughly proportional to body weight (Alexander, 1962). In this case the rectal temperature has no effect. In the young pig, however, there are clear effects of rectal temperature on the metabolic rate measured at 4°, that is, near the animal's cold limit (Mount and Rowell, 1960). When the effect of rectal temperature has been allowed for, metabolic rate is proportional to body weight raised to the power 0·56. The figure of 0·56 is not significantly different from the 0·67 power corresponding to the so-called "surface law". Alexander's value of 1·0 is, on the other hand, significantly different from 0·67. For maximum metabolism, Alexander's figure for lambs is a more probable one than that of Mount and Rowell for pigs, since an exponent of body weight of 1·0 means that the maximum metabolism is proportional to the active body mass, assuming that all the animals have similar body compositions.

The same reasoning may be applied to the reference base for the minimum metabolic rate at thermal neutrality. The standard metabolism of normal human infants between eight days and one year is proportional to body weight (Karlberg, 1952). In older infants and children, however, the relationship is closer to the 0·75 power of the body weight used for comparisons between species (Kleiber, 1947). Karlberg suggests that the higher exponent in infancy is due partly to the influence of growth on energy metabolism. At minimum or maximum metabolic rates, the heat production of mature animals may be proportional to active body mass. Between these limits, proportionality is likely to be some function of body size which takes into account the areas, shapes and insulation of all the parts of the organism.

This relationship between metabolic rate and body structure has been called the "metabolic body size" (Kleiber, 1947). Some workers have denied that there is any unifying type of function which could apply to different species. Benedict (1938) considered it futile to try to find one. However, as Kleiber has pointed out, a large animal produces more heat per unit time than a small animal, and a basis for comparing animals of different sizes is a rational objective. Many measurements of the metabolic rates of different species have been made. They show that the metabolic rate of both large and small homeotherms is more nearly proportional to body surface area than to body weight (Kleiber, 1947).

This is the basis of the "surface law", first postulated in 1839. It was held that an animal's heat production was proportional to its surface area, and hence for animals of the same shape and density it must be proportional to the 0·67 power of the body weight. Surface area, calculated from various equations, has been used in a great deal of metabolic work. However, several authors, notably Brody (1945) and Kleiber (1947), have been concerned rather with that function of body weight which has the most general application to metabolic rate.

For the equation $H = aW^b$, where H = rate of heat production, W = body weight, and a and b are constants, Brody eventually settled on the value of 0·70 for the body weight exponent, b. Kleiber determined the value of b as 0·75, and recommended this power of body weight as representative of metabolic body size. In standard conditions, he found that the metabolic rate of adult homeotherms, from mice to cattle, averaged 70 kcal./kg.$^{0·75}$ day. To determine whether the metabolic rate was proportional to W or to $W^{0·75}$, it was necessary that the heaviest animals weighed at least three times as much as the lightest. This was a consequence of the great variation in the figures used. Similarly, the 0·67 and 0·75 powers could not be distinguished unless there was a ninefold weight range.

A fixed value of the exponent is useful only in a given set of conditions—for example, with standard metabolism in mature animals. Mount and Rowell (1960) give an analysis of the variance of metabolic rate for pigs in relation to age, body weight and rectal temperature. The effect of age is not significant during the first week, but the effect of rectal temperature is significant. The exponent of body weight which gives proportionality to metabolic rate is 0·86 ± 0·05 at 4° and 30° ambient temperatures, when the effects of age and rectal temperature

14*

are ignored, but 0.60 ± 0.06 when age and rectal temperature are allowed for. This represents a considerable difference.

The same problem has recently been considered by Gridgeman and Héroux (1965) in relation to measurements of oxygen consumption in rats. They show that the body weight exponent can be an unstable parameter, although they have no ground for opposing Kleiber's (1947) recommendation of the use of the 0.75 power for homeotherms in normal conditions. They find, however, that the exponent can be influenced by exceptional conditions, particularly of temperature. Their general recommendation is to use analysis of covariance to allow for the effect of body weight on oxygen uptake, and so derive experiment-specific values of the exponent. This involves no assumptions about the exponent, and allows for ancillary factors which may vary from experiment to experiment.

5. *Insulation*

Body temperature in cold conditions is maintained most economically, that is, with the lowest heat production, when the insulation is high. The effective insulation is, however, not a simple, unvarying quantity. It most closely approaches fixity in an animal such as the arctic fox, in which the very high insulation of the coat determines the non-evaporative heat loss. The same is true for the fully fleeced sheep. More usually, however, the coat is only one component of insulation, and may itself change by pilo-erection and as a result of penetration by wind.

The factors which determine the efficiency of insulation may be divided into two groups: (i) those which affect the insulation per unit area of the animal's surface, that is, the specific insulation (Kleiber, 1947), and (ii) those which affect the total insulation.

a. Specific insulation. The effects due to peripheral vasoconstriction and subcutaneous fat have already been discussed (Section II.A, p. 413). The hair or wool coat, when it is present, however, is the major factor in specific insulation. The presence of a coat has a clear effect on the skin-air temperature gradient. The thermal impedance which it offers depends on the air trapped between the fibres: a smoothed coat offers less insulation than the same coat with hairs raised and a thicker layer of air. Blaxter and Wainman (1961) conclude that in steers pilo-erection is responsible for a large part of the difference in measured insulation above and below the critical temperature.

The density of the hair fibres is also important. Berry and Shanklin (1961) used a heat-flow meter applied to the coat surface to measure the total hair-coat insulation of dairy calves. The insulation was linearly related to the hair weight per unit area of body surface. Mount (1964a) recorded the metabolic rates of shaved and unshaved new-born piglets, and so estimated the insulation conferred by their sparse hair coats. He found a total hair insulation of $0\cdot03°m.^2hr./kcal.$ The corresponding figure for the calf is $0\cdot08°m.^2hr./kcal.$ The hair density of a calf is about $9\cdot8$ mg./cm.^{2}, however, and that of a piglet only $1\cdot5$ mg./cm.^{2}. For a given amount of hair, therefore, a pig's hair insulation is about $2\cdot5$ times greater than that of a calf's. Hence, although Berry and Shanklin (1961) find a linear relation between hair density and degree of insulation among calves, this relation does not necessarily extend to comparisons between species. Barnett (1959) measured the thermal insulation of excised mouse skin, shaved and unshaved. From his figures, it is possible to calculate, with certain assumptions, that the hair density of the mouse skin is about $0\cdot6$ mg./cm.^{2}, and that at a density of 1 mg./cm.^{2} the thermal insulation is $0\cdot08°m.^2hr./kcal.$ At the same hair densities, this is about four times the insulation of pig hair, and ten times that of calf hair. Hence mouse coat, per unit weight, is better than either pig or calf hair. This may be because a great density of fine hairs provides a better trap for still air.

Blaxter *et al.* (1959) made a study of the insulation offered by the fleece of the sheep. Values derived from measurements on excised pelts may, however, not apply in the living animal. The growth of wool increases the area available for heat exchange; it allows spreading of fibres at the periphery and so permits greater heat loss by convection; and it leads to "cracking" of the fleece, that is, the appearance of divisions in the fleece as the sheep moves its body. However, fleece does not cover the whole of the sheep. When allowance is made for this by including estimates of the areas not covered, *in vivo* estimates of fleece insulation do not differ greatly from those determined on excised pelts. The insulation of fleece and hair falls within the range $0\cdot16–0\cdot20°m.^2hr./kcal.$ per cm. length of coat.

The penetration of fleece by wind decreases the thermal insulation of the coat (Joyce and Blaxter, 1964). In sheep with different fleece lengths, impairment of coat insulation is detectable over the whole range of wind speeds from 27 to 430 cm./sec. At 430 cm./sec., it is 42%. It can be calculated that, at 430 cm./sec., a closely clipped sheep loses 55% of the insulation that it possesses in a wind speed of 27 cm./sec. The corresponding loss for a sheep with a 30 mm. fleece length is 44%, but the fleeced animal has a much higher insulation initially. The figures indicate the greater susceptibility of the bare-skinned mammal (in this case the closely clipped sheep) to increments of wind speed, compared with the coated animal. Even so, the influence of wind speed on a newborn pig is less than that on a stationary, heated model, perhaps owing to the effects of posture (Mount, 1966b).

b. Total insulation. The total thermal insulation may be defined as the ratio of the body-environment temperature difference to the total non-evaporative heat flow. Although a heavy coat may be a dominant component of a mammal's insulation, no one component determines by itself the total non-evaporative heat loss. In the resting animal this is shown by the effect of postural changes on heat flow (Benzinger and Kitzinger, 1963). Lowering the ambient temperature leads a young pig to decrease its effective radiating surface area; but it probably increases the convective heat loss by inducing shivering (Mount, 1964b). Grouping animals together (Kleiber, 1961; Mount, 1960) or providing nesting material (Sørensen, 1962) decreases heat loss. When animals move about and leave the group, heat loss increases considerably. An active animal exposes an increased body surface area and increases air movement over its surface; hence there is a rise in metabolic rate from this cause, as well as that resulting from muscular action.

The rate of cooling of a body in air is proportional to its surface area, that is, to $W^{0.67}$, if other conditions remain constant; and it is inversely proportional to the heat capacity, that is to W, if the mean specific heat remains constant. Combining these effects, the cooling of a given body is then proportional to $W^{-0.33}$ (Kleiber, 1961); the larger the body, the more slowly it cools. For an animal of 1 kg. body weight, $W^{-0.33}$ is 1; for 8 kg., it is 0·5; for 27 kg., 0·33, and so on. By the same reasoning, the heat input, required *per unit body weight* to maintain the body temperature, falls progressively as body size increases. This is a reflection of the "surface law" discussed earlier, and shows how the thermal insulation of an animal rises simply as body size increases; no change in the specific insulation is required to bring about the rise. Usually, animals grow, and also increase their specific insulation by coat and subcutaneous fat, at the same time, so that the cold tolerance of older and larger animals is increased out of proportion to the increase in size. Another effect of size depends on the radius of curvature of parts of the animal: fingers lose more heat, both per unit area and also per unit of temperature gradient, than does the trunk (Hardy, 1949). The disposition of limbs in relation to the body, the control of posture, and the proportion of time in which the animal is active and therefore exposing more of its appendages, have a marked effect on the total thermal insulation and therefore on cold resistance.

Hart (1964a) refers to the presence of thinly furred tissues in the appendages of heavily insulated mammals as solving the problem of exercise heat on the one hand, and conserving heat by cooling on the other. There is considerable variation in skin temperature in the appendages; this is in contrast to the skin under thick fur, which remains uniformly warm. Hart points out that the cooling of peripheral tissues has an insulating effect. This is accompanied by a remarkable ability to withstand changes of temperature, and by the presence of structures which allow alterations in the rate of heat loss.

Heat exchange in homeotherms has also been discussed by Scholander (1958). Mammals in the cold are protected from heat loss largely by their fur, yet the legs and other appendages of arctic mammals are poorly insulated, and seals, for example, swim about in very cold water with hairless flippers. If these appendages were kept warm, the heat loss would be very great. In fact, they are at rather low temperatures, and it is by a remarkable degree of local cold adaptation that the tissues maintain normal function and irritability. Other tissues do not function at these temperatures. Hart (1964a) refers to the ability of peripheral nerves in the legs of cold-adapted gulls to conduct at lower temperatures, and to cell division in the peripheral tissues of cold-adapted rats. Cell division in the peripheral tissues, however, occurs only in animals that have been exposed to cold for some days (Héroux, 1959a). It depends on the resumption of a normal blood supply to the skin; this in turn requires a substantial increase in the rate of heat production (discussed below in Section II.C, p. 424).

Scholander (1958) discusses the way in which the extremities of cold-adapted mammals are held at a low temperature. Heat from arterial blood is shunted back into the veins before the blood reaches the periphery. The testicle of most mammals is provided with a counter-current vascular system, and this no doubt contributes to keeping it at a temperature lower than that of the body core (Waites and Moule, 1961). A simpler form of thermal shunting may regulate heat dissipation, in exercise and rest, from the poorly insulated limbs of the arctic fox. In man, the temperature in the brachial artery can fall by as much as 0·3°/cm. through transmission of heat to the veins (Bazett et al., 1948). Scholander considers this simple system to be rudimentary compared with the multichannel arteriovenous rete systems (networks of blood vessels) which have been described in the manatee (*Manatus*), whales (Cetacea), and tall wading birds, among others. The retes are usually at the bases of limbs, tail or fins. They probably not only aid in conserving heat, but also contribute to heat loss. Heat loss, rather than conservation, is evidently a main function of the hairless tail and feet of rats (Thompson and Stevenson, 1965) and presumably of other Muridae.

6. *The Effective Environment*

The metabolic effort required to maintain body temperature is not a simple function of air temperature alone. Although lowering the air temperature raises the metabolic rates of exposed men, the highest rate is observed in a wind at an air temperature higher than the lowest a man can stand (Iampietro et al., 1960).

The "thermal demand of the environment" is the total heat loss through radiation, convection and conduction (Burton and Edholm, 1955). In cold conditions, evaporative heat loss continues, mainly from the respiratory tract, but it is relatively slight. Air movement and radiant temperature have a marked influence on heat loss. Air at 20°, moving at 30 cm./sec., produces greater heat loss from the backs of pigs than nearly still air at 15° (Mount and Ingram, 1965). Thirty cm./sec. is not a high air speed, but it is equivalent in this case to a 5° difference in ambient temperature. For lightly dressed persons, the subjective effect of an increase in air temperature of 1° can be nullified by a decrease of 1·39° in the mean radiant temperature (Koch, 1962). Determinations of heat loss in new-born pigs have shown similar effects of air and radiant temperatures on metabolic rate (Mount, 1964b, 1965).

There have been many attempts to find a way to express in a single term the effects of the environment on an animal's heat loss. Yaglou (1949) came to the conclusion that such a concept was unrealistic, and that it was necessary to make separate estimates of heat exchange through the four channels of radiation, convection, conduction and evaporation; a unitary estimate would not be useful for different subjects under different conditions. Burton and Edholm (1955) have examined the "equivalent still air temperature" as applied to man, and have shown how a thermal wind decrement and a radiation increment may be calculated in the form of temperature differences to be added algebraically to the air temperature to give the "still shade temperature". Although these calculations are suitable for man in specified conditions, they do not necessarily apply to other mammals (Mount, 1965).

To sum up, the effective environment comprises a number of factors, the combined effects of which cannot be stated for all mammals by any single universally applicable quantity. The influence of each factor must be assessed separately.

C. PHYSIOLOGICAL ADAPTATION TO COLD

1. Metabolic Rate

The most important recent contributions to the study of metabolic rate in cold adaptation have been on "non-shivering thermogenesis". When a mammal is first exposed to cold, if the cold is severe enough the animal shivers and so produces more heat. The blood supply to the periphery is also decreased. After some days the shivering and peripheral vasoconstriction decline, but heat production remains high. This sequence is well substantiated in laboratory animals (Cottle and Carlson, 1956; Davis et al., 1960); it has also been recorded in wild animals, for instance by Pohl and Hart (1965) in a ground squirrel, *Citellus tridecemlineatus*; and it has been demonstrated in man (Davis *et al.*, 1959). The important sites of non-shivering heat production are not yet fully known, but evidently include the viscera and still more the skeletal muscles and brown adipose tissue (Smith, 1964; and see Section VII.A). In cold-adapted animals, noradrenalin stimulates thermogenesis (Leduc, 1961). Men living in a cold environment are more sensitive to noradrenalin (Joy, 1963), and this is indirect evidence for cold adaptation in man. The same applies to rats (Héroux, 1963).

The experiments of Scholander and his colleagues (1958a) on the effects on man of exposure to cold also illustrate the "metabolic" type of adaptation to cold in man. Eight young men lived for 6 weeks in the autumn in primitive conditions in the Norwegian mountains. They wore only light summer clothing during the day, and took exercise by hiking and hunting. Each slept in a simple wind-proof blanket bag under a shelter open on one side, at an air temperature of about 4°. The oxygen consumption of these men was higher than that of controls; their skin temperatures too tended to be higher. They resemble those of the thinly clad Alacaluf of Tierra del Fuego (Hammel, 1964). Hammel points out that the response of these men to moderate cold represents a clear example of metabolic adaptation, and that Arctic Indians and Eskimo behave in a similar way.

2. *Enzymic Changes*

The extra "non-shivering" heat produced by a cold-adapted homeotherm is an index of intracellular changes in catabolism. This large subject has been reviewed, with full bibliographies, by Sellers (1957), Depocas (1961), Smith and Hoijer (1962) and Hannon (1963). As Depocas (1961) remarks, thermoregulation provides a convenient means of studying the control of the release of energy.

It might be expected that, once shivering had ceased, it would be possible to detect a changed but stable pattern of enzymic activity in, for instance, the liver of a cold-adapted animal. This is not the case. Substantial changes continue, even between 30 and 150 days of exposure, in the livers of laboratory rats kept at 4° (Fig. 2). Hence, even in this one situation, there are evidently at least two phases of cold adaptation without shivering. For this, as for other aspects of adaptation to cold, the precise conditions of experiment, especially the duration of exposure, must be clearly specified. This requirement is illustrated, not only by changes in enzyme activity, but also by the rates of oxygen consumption of liver slices *in vitro* (summarized by Smith and Hoijer, 1962). The rate of oxygen uptake rises during the first 30 days of cold exposure, but after this it declines; by about 120 days there may be no decisive difference from the control figure. Yet, in some experiments, the rate of oxygen uptake by the whole animal remains indefinitely more than 2·5 times that of controls at about 23°. The discrepancy may be related to the enlargement of the liver and other heat-producing tissues (discussed below in Section V, p. 442), partly to a belated increase in heat production by other organs, especially muscles; or changes in the intact animal may not be fully reflected in the metabolism of isolated tissues. A quantitative expression of all these effects is needed, but is not yet available, even for laboratory rats.

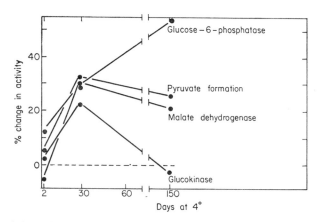

Fig. 2. Activity of liver enzymes during exposure of laboratory rats to cold. (After Hannon, 1963)

Specific changes in enzyme activity have been reviewed especially by Hannon (1963). Most of the scattered information concerns carbohydrate metabolism. After two days at 4°, the activity of liver lactate dehydrogenase, measured by lactate formation, has risen by about 50%. This is only a temporary phenomenon, possibly related to the increased heat production by shivering. After thirty days' exposure, lactate dehydrogenase activity is back to normal, but other changes in enzyme activity have become evident.

The activity of glucokinase, which catalyses the phosphorylation of glucose, is increased by 20%. The activity of other enzymes involved in the Embden-Meyerhof pathway is also increased; these include phosphoglyceromutase, phosphopyruvate hydratase (enolase), and pyruvate kinase. Hence the rate of formation in the liver of pyruvate from dietary glucose is evidently increased at this stage of cold adaptation. At the same time, the activity of liver dehydrogenases that catalyse reactions involved in the tricarboxylic acid cycle is increased.

A special case, evidently, is that of glucose-6-phosphatase (Fig. 2). The activity of this enzyme, measured by phosphate formation, increases in the liver during the first days of cold exposure, and by thirty days is raised by about 35%. But the increase continues even after thirty days. This enzyme is involved in the reversed Embden–Meyerhof pathway. Its increased activity may signify a greater rate of glucogenesis.

These observations concern the use of dietary carbohydrate as the source of energy. As for alternative sources, a few facts bear on the use of protein. During only two days' cold exposure, the activity of liver (and muscle) transaminases rises, and the new level is evidently maintained for many weeks. Hence, it is supposed, the rate at which amino acids can be used for heat production is increased. This is accompanied by a temporary cessation of growth or even by a loss of body weight (Fig. 5, p. 436). This topic, and observations on fat metabolism, are discussed in Section V, p. 442.

3. Endocrine Changes

Until recently, nothing could be said about the intracellular enzymic changes described above, but the endocrine adjustments during cold exposure have been known for decades. Hormones are now seen as the agents which provoke the cellular changes. Lowered temperature of the skin and colon induce not only shivering but also, by way of the hypothalamus, increased secretions of pituitary and other hormones (Hsieh et al., 1957; von Euler and Söderberg, 1958; Anderson et al., 1963; Benzinger, 1964).

On exposure to cold there is an immediate increase in the secretion of catecholamines by the adrenal medulla. Of these, noradrenalin is especially important. This hormone activates liver phosphorylase reactions, and so increases the rate of production of glucose 1-phosphate from glycogen. This is evidently part of a mechanism for the prompt mobilization of reserves of energy. Noradrenalin probably continues to play an important part in cold-adapted animals, for—as we saw above—the responsiveness of the tissues of these animals to noradrenalin is increased (Carlson, 1960).

The response of the thyroid is less rapid. Brown–Grant (1956), for example, exposed laboratory rats to a temperature of 6–12°, and observed increased thyroid secretion within 8 hours. But more severe cold sometimes led to a decrease. Brown–Grant (1960), Keller (1960), Knigge (1960) and Anderson (1963) have discussed the control of thyroid secretion. The necessary part played by the pituitary has been demonstrated in several species. The increased secretion of thyroid-stimulating hormone (TSH) on exposure to cold depends in turn on the hypothalamus: suitably placed injuries in the hypothalamus can result in diminished thyroid secretion, and electrical stimulation can increase it. If the pituitary stalk is cut, there is no thyroid response to cold. The action of thyroid hormone is usually said to be on catabolism: the effect of noradrenalin in increasing heat production is enhanced (e.g. Carlson, 1960; Smith, 1963). The role of thyroid hormone is, however, not simple. Fregly *et al.* (1961) confirm the importance of the thyroid for the survival of rats in severe cold, but show that cold can induce a rise in metabolic rate in the absence of the thyroid (cf. Hsieh and Carlson, 1957). But thyroidectomized rats lose heat at a greater rate than controls, evidently owing to loss of the ability to constrict peripheral blood vessels. The thyroid response to cold has also been observed in guinea-pigs, *Cavia*, (Yamada *et al.*, 1965): in them, too, it is necessary for the acute phase of cold adaptation.

Finally, there are the steroid hormones of the adrenal cortex. Since adrenocorticotrophin (ACTH) secretion by the pituitary increases immediately on exposure to cold, so also does the secretion of adrenal cortical hormones. The little relevant information on the action of these hormones is reviewed by Smith and Hoijer (1962). At least in adaptation to cold, their most important function probably concerns protein metabolism. The breakdown of keto acids for oxidation is accelerated by them. This is evidently a temporary measure to meet the demands for extra energy before food intake has increased. There is, however, even in a cold-adapted animal, a rise in protein turnover of the order of 50%. The additional deamination in the liver probably depends in part on the activation of enzymes. The breakdown of arginine to urea is evidently similarly regulated by adrenal steroids.

The recent rapid developments in knowledge of the chemistry of release of energy in cells, and its regulation by hormones, have made it possible to present in outline a causal chain from the first stimulus of cold to the final production of heat. Cold receptors, probably both peripheral and central, initiate reflex responses and also very rapid changes in the secretion of a number of hormones. The hormones in turn act on the cells which produce the extra energy. To what extent the various endocrine effects are confined to the period during which cold adaptation is taking place is not yet clear.

4. *Insulation*

Adaptation to cold, by increasing the metabolic rate, puts heavy demands on the food supply. Increasing thermal insulation, and hence the range of ambient temperatures which allow minimum metabolism, is a less hazardous mode of cold adaptation. Well known work on wild rats

(Héroux, 1959b; Héroux, 1962; Hart and Héroux, 1963; Héroux, 1963) has shown that the cold resistance of rats caught in the winter is superior to that of summer rats, and that this difference is related to the higher metabolic rates of which winter rats are capable. Winter rats tolerate ambient temperatures about 20° lower than summer rats. However, this metabolic adaptation is accompanied by changes in thermal insulation; winter rats have more fur and lower skin temperatures under the fur.

A larger species, the varying hare, *Lepus americanus*, has been studied by Hart *et al.* (1965). Animals caught in winter have 27% more hair than those caught in summer. Correspondingly, the critical temperature of winter hares is −5°, but that of summer hares is 10°. Evidently, in this species, seasonal adjustments are largely or wholly in insulation.

5. *Hypothermia and Hibernation*

The third group of ways in which homeotherms can adapt to cold involves lowering the body temperature. This decreases the level of metabolism required for a given degree of thermal insulation.

A distinction must be made between tolerance of environmental cooling, and tolerance of hypothermia. Tolerance of environmental cooling is achieved by increasing the metabolic rate or thermal insulation, or both, and so by maintaining deep body temperature. This may be accompanied by cooling of peripheral tissues, well demonstrated in pigs kept in arctic conditions (Irving, 1956). Tolerance of hypothermia, that is, a lowering of the body core temperature, does not necessarily accompany this. The two forms of tolerance do, however, go together in, for example, Australian aborigines (Scholander *et al.*, 1958b): these men undergo both a cooling of the body shell and a fall in deep body temperature during cold exposure at night, without an increase in metabolic rate. Europeans in similar circumstances feel cold, shiver violently and have a raised metabolic rate; they do not tolerate hypothermia.

As a rule, only when metabolic capacity is exceeded by the thermal demand of the environment does the animal succumb to an imposed and progressive hypothermia. In hibernating animals, by contrast, active thermoregulation is replaced by tolerance of hypothermia when the ambient temperature falls below a certain value. Hibernation has been reviewed by Kayser (1961) and Hoffman (1964). The heterothermic type of response, which occurs during hibernation, takes place only within a certain range of ambient temperatures: arousal occurs if the temperature falls below about −2° or above about 30°. Burton and Edholm (1955) quote the ground-hog's emergence from its burrow on or about 2 February ("ground-hog day") as a probable example of the protective arousal which occurs when conditions become too cold. Soil temperature at burrow depth lags behind that of the surface, and is likely to reach its minimum at this time of year.

The metabolic rate during hibernation is about 1–3% of the basal value whilst awake. Basal heat production in summer varies directly with the surface area of the body, but during hibernation heat production varies with body weight (Kayser, 1959). These two "metabolic body sizes" may be related to the presence and absence, respectively, of nervous control. Kayser considers that thermoregulation of hibernators is deficient mainly through poor control of heat loss. When they are awake, their heat production, however, is higher in the cold than is that of other homeotherms, and their maximum metabolic rate during arousal by cold is higher than the peak reached during the summer.

Hoffman (1964) points out that, if they are not exposed to cold, animals which would otherwise hibernate behave as typical homeotherms. They do not prepare for hibernation until cold weather begins. For an animal with poor regulation of heat loss, hibernation is a means of solving the annual problem of food scarcity and other adversities.

III. Food Consumption

A. AMOUNT EATEN

Other things equal, to produce more heat an animal must eat more. The need for extra food, on exposure to cold, is especially marked in small mammals, owing to their high rate of heat loss from a relatively large body surface. Hence their food intake must be assumed to fluctuate with season, unless they hibernate. Campbell (1945) recorded a small rise, during several successive winters, even in laboratory rats, Rattus norvegicus, kept indoors. Stevenson and Rixon (1954) carried out more conventional experiments on laboratory rats: they exposed rats to 2–5°, and observed an increase in calorie intake, relative to body weight, of 40–50% over that in an ordinary laboratory temperature. Sellers et al. (1954) exposed albino rats to 1·5° for 6–7 weeks, and fed them on mixtures of constant protein content but with fat varying from 5 to 44% by weight. The raised calorie intake of the rats that survived was constant, at the low temperature, regardless of diet; growth was always less than at room temperature.

When a laboratory rat is transferred suddenly to a room at, say, 4°, it loses weight, much of it in the form of adipose tissue, as described below. Hence, during this initial phase, food consumption does not keep pace with heat production. However, laboratory rats exposed to *seasonal* cold in *groups* do not lose weight; and healthy *wild* rats have more adipose tissue during winter (in Canada) than during summer (Héroux, 1963). This is evidence that a small mammal, unchanged by domestication, is able not only to eat and digest enough food in winter to maintain heat production, but can even "over-eat" and so increase the amount of its food reserves and possibly its insulation.

It has been supposed that large, well-insulated mammals do not have to eat more in winter, since they do not lose more heat in cold weather than in warm. This is evidently true for clothed man (Consolazio, 1963). The question has also been tested by Durrer and Hannon (1962) on domestic dogs, *Canis familiaris*. They kept five Alaskan husky dogs, each weighing 30–40 kg., out of doors in Alaska: in summer, their calorie intake was 49 kcal./kg.day but, by November, it was 87 kcal./kg.day, or 77% more, despite an extra growth of hair when cold weather began; body weight was, however, lower in winter than in summer (Fig. 3). In very cold weather, activity was much reduced: the dogs lay curled up, and were difficult to arouse; they got up to feed for only brief periods. Once the huskies were cold-adapted, more severe cold did not make them eat still more; but it did so in beagle dogs weighing 11–13 kg.

It is sometimes assumed that there is a simple, fixed relationship between the amount of food eaten, on the one hand, and heat production plus growth and storing of reserves, on the other. This relationship holds only if the efficiency of food utilization is constant. In some situations, an appearance of superior efficiency in a cold environment can be misleading. Andik *et al.* (1963) kept male laboratory rats at about 21°, and gave them a diet with only 4·3% protein. The rats stopped growing, and died within about 6 weeks. Other rats on this diet, kept at 5°, survived and grew; but return to the warm arrested growth and led to death in a few weeks. The primary effect of the cold environment was to double food intake. This incidentally increased the protein eaten to a level which permitted growth. Klain and Vaughan (1963), however, have described changes in enzyme activity in rats adapted to 7° for 3–4 weeks: these changes made possible growth on diets which, owing to an unbalanced amino acid content, did not support growth in rats kept in a warm environment. Here is authentic evidence of improved metabolic efficiency.

Work on inbred laboratory mice, too, has raised the question of food utilization, especially during pregnancy and lactation. Barnett and Little (1965) compared virgin, pregnant and lactating mice at 21° with similar mice at − 3°. The latter had been born and reared in the cold environment; all mice had cotton wool nests. Relative to body weight, virgin mice ate about 70% more in the cold environment than in the

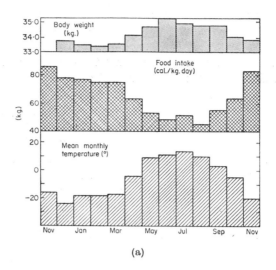

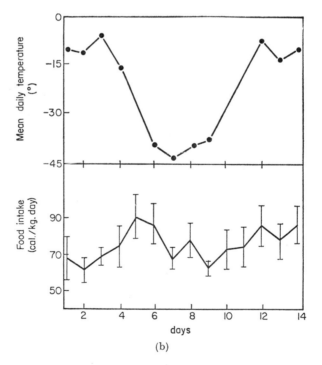

Fig. 3. Food intake and season in the dog, *Canis familiaris*. (a) Rise in food consumption of husky dogs in winter. Body weight falls. (b) Absence of correlation between food intake and brief fluctuations in external temperature (cf. Fig. 5). (After Durrer and Hannon, 1962)

warm, but the difference was less during pregnancy, and during lactation there was no difference (Fig. 4). Lactation is the most exacting test of a female's metabolism; probably, at this stage, food consumption was limited by the capacity of the gut (Barnett and Widdowson, 1965). Fewer young were born and reared at $-3°$ than at $21°$. The cost of rearing 10 g. of young to ten days, in terms of extra food consumed during the last 10 days of lactation, was about 18 g. at $21°$ but, in mice

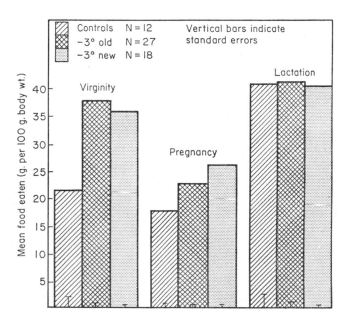

FIG. 4. Environmental temperature, and food consumption by female mice. The controls were kept at an ambient temperature of $21°$. The new stock were first or second generations bred at $-3°$; the old stock was of the 17th. to the 19th. generations at $-3°$. Virginity: mean daily weights of food eaten during the 9th. week after birth. Pregnancy: daily consumption during the last three days of pregnancy. Lactation: daily consumption during the first ten days after the birth of a litter. (After Barnett and Little, 1965)

of the same strain but of long ancestry in the cold, only 11 g. This suggests superior food utilization by the cold-adapted mice.

However, the ability of mice to breed in such a cold environment, on such a modest increase of food, probably depends partly on a decrease in the need for food through lowered activity, as we shall see later (Section IV.A, p. 437). Another means of reducing the need for food would be improved thermal insulation, but this cannot be an important factor for a small mammal (Section V.D.1, p. 449). Resort to a nest must, however, reduce heat loss (Section IV.B, p. 438). Probably, time spent outside the nest is minimized in a cold environment, as Strecker (1955) observed in wild house mice, *Mus musculus*. Rapidly eaten meals at rather long intervals can promote a higher growth rate, and deposition of more tissue fat, than frequent meals, at least in laboratory rats (Cohn and Joseph, 1960; Hollifield and Parson, 1962a,b); hence, up to the limit imposed by the capacity of the gut, a "stuff and starve" regime may be no disadvantage.

B. COMPOSITION OF THE DIET

Studies have been made of the effects of varying the fat content of the diet on performance in a cold environment, but the results have been conflicting. Evidence in favour of a fatty diet comes from Dugal *et al.* (1945): the survival and growth of their rats, at $-2°$, was improved by a fat-rich diet. Pagé (1957) has reviewed work from his laboratory in which laboratory rats grew better when given extra fat; at room temperature the extra growth was due to formation of adipose tissue, but at $3°$ it was not. Giaja and Gelineo (1934) exposed rats to cold and fed them on protein, or fat, or carbohydrate alone. Judged by survival, a purely protein diet was little better than starvation; fat was less effective than carbohydrate. Similarly, Lang and Crab (1946) studied rats kept at $6°$, on diets containing 10–50% of the calories as fat. The resistance of these rats to cold declined with increasing fat content of the diet. Bobek and Ginter (1966) too find that a diet high in fat and cholesterol retards the growth of rats exposed for 8hr./day to $2°$. The many factors, which might influence the ability of animals to use fat and other dietary components, preclude any confident explanation of the difference of the observations from those of Dugal, Pagé and their colleagues.

Another of the factors is again efficiency of food utilization. For example, Templeton and Ershoff (1949) found that addition of fat (margarine) to the diet reduced mortality due to cold only after the rats had undergone cold-adaptation by being exposed to $2°$. Similarly, Pagé (1957) quotes work in which laboratory rats kept at $11°$ gained less weight than controls during their first month of exposure, owing to fat depletion; but, during the second month, there was a great increase in weight due to fat deposition. Such work shows that much information can be lost if experiments are restricted to only a few days or weeks.

Increase in metabolic efficiency on cold exposure is also illustrated by the work of Beaton (1963a,b). He observed the growth, body fat content and other features of young laboratory rats for a week at $22°$ and $2°$. On a diet containing 40% protein, the cold-exposed rats maintained body weight and synthesized fat, whereas others, on 20%

or 5% protein, did not. This suggests that, contrary to other reports, a high protein diet is advantageous for a rapidly growing rat in a cold environment. The differential effects of the various diets were, however, less in rats kept at 2°: for instance, (i) the rats fed on 40% protein ate the most of the three groups while at 22° but, on transfer to 2°, the others increased their food intake to the level of the 40% group (which did not change); (ii) the 5% group had a lower blood glucose than the other two groups at 22° but not at 2° at which temperature it was raised in all three groups. Beaton and Sangster (1965) have recently given further evidence of increased efficiency of protein utilization in cold-adapted rats.

C. SELECTION OF DIET

The experiments in which foods are forced on animals still leave open the question of the best diet for a cold environment; but mammals themselves, given a choice, might be able to select an optimum diet for survival or growth. Laboratory rats, at least, can, at ordinary temperatures, adjust their intake to their needs for certain salts and vitamins, as well as calories (reviewed by Barnett, 1963).

Donhoffer and Vonotzky (1947) gave laboratory mice a choice of three mixtures containing predominantly carbohydrate (starch), protein (casein), and fat (lard) respectively. At room temperatures, all three diets were eaten regularly, but more of the protein mixture than of the others. After 2–3 weeks, the mice were transferred to 10–11°. The consequent increase in food eaten was drawn almost entirely from the carbohydrate mixture. Görner (1956) found a similar preference for carbohydrate, rather than fat, at a low temperature, not only in house mice, but also in the wood mouse, *Apodemus sylvaticus*.

Little is known of the physiology of the change in appetite in an altered temperature. Animals do not change their intake at once to match the ambient temperature. Durrer and Hannon's (1962) dogs displayed no day-to-day correlation of calorie consumption with temperature (Fig. 3b). The rats studied by Donhoffer and Vonotzky took some days, after transfer to the cold, to reach their raised level of intake. Nevertheless, very brief, intermittent exposures to cold can influence food intake. Weiss (1958) exposed rats to 0° for only 20 min./day; controls were at 21°. Food consumption of the cold-exposed rats, during the hour after exposure, was low for the first 1–3 days; but, by about the eleventh day, it was much above that of the controls. A similar sequence in mice transferred to a cold environment is illustrated in Fig. 5. The low initial food intake of Weiss's rats was accompanied by decreased activity.

D. PROBLEMS OF FOOD CONSUMPTION

We now list some of the main factors which influence food intake in cold-exposed mammals. The first is genotype. Not only different species, but varieties of the same species, have different dietary needs, as Fenton (1960) has shown for mice. Secondly, age may alter needs; in particular, the demands of a rapidly growing young mammal differ from those of an adult. The same applies to pregnant and

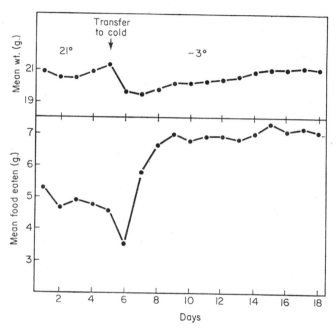

FIG. 5. Mean food consumption and body weights of ten mice, aged 5 weeks, transferred from 21° to −3°. There was a delay in the adjustment of food consumption to need.

lactating females. Little is known about the effects of any of these.

A further source of variation are the conditions experienced by the animal, from fertilization on. Uterine effects are discussed later (Section VI.C, p. 457). Adult laboratory rats or mice, transferred to a cold environment, go through a sequence of metabolic changes already described (Section II.C.2, p. 425). These changes may influence dietary needs. Moreover, mammals adapt their behaviour to circumstances: they may alter the amount eaten, the number of meals taken and their food preferences. Even for the much studied laboratory rat, nearly everything remains to be learnt on all these features of adaptation to cold.

IV. Behaviour

A. "ACTIVITY"

Three features of behaviour concern us in this review: (i) feeding, which has been discussed in the previous section; (ii) "activity", which here means any movement of the whole body or of the trunk or limbs; and (iii) any behaviour which tends to reduce heat loss.

Decreased activity on exposure to cold is a general finding. The example of husky dogs (Durrer and Hannon, 1962) has been mentioned in Section III.A. p. 431. Ostermann (1956) observed a decline in activity during winter of four species of Muridae and three Gliridae. Zollhauser (1958) studied wild and laboratory mice (*Mus musculus* and *Apodemus sylvaticus*) in the laboratory, in cages each on a suspended platform. A temperature of 8°, instead of that of the animal house, reduced activity especially when there was no nest. Barnett and Scott (1964) compared the movements of mice at 21° with others at −3° and fully adapted to the cold; the latter were less active.

The decrement in activity due to cold is a function of the extent to which an animal is adapted to the cold. Hart (1953) showed this by recording wheel-running in deer mice, *Peromyscus leucopus*: by adapting some of his animals to 10° instead of 21°, he increased their rate of running at temperatures below 0°. This illustrates the fact that gross locomotor movements do not necessarily contribute to the extra heat needed at low temperatures. Hart and Héroux (1955) demonstrated this also for lemmings, *Dicrostonyx groenlandicus*, and rabbits, *Oryctolagus cuniculus*, and Hart and Jansky (1963) for laboratory rats.

The *effect* of exercise, too, is influenced by cold adaptation: rats kept at 4° for four weeks, and then exercised, display greater vaso-dilation in tail and colon than controls kept at 4° for only one day (Thompson and Stevenson, 1966).

The term "decline in activity", used with reference to the researches quoted above, has a precise significance in each case; but it is not always the same significance. The presence of a running wheel or treadmill stimulates more movement than would be displayed in its absence (Eayrs, 1951; Zollhauser, 1958); hence the same animal might display a different effect of cold in a treadmill from that in a tambour-mounted cage. "Activity", as defined in the first paragraph of this section, varies with general exploratory behaviour, specific "appetitive" movements (provoked, for example, by hunger), and stereotyped activities such as hoarding objects in the nest (reviewed by Barnett, 1963). Ross and Smith (1953) record a decline in hoarding in laboratory mice exposed to cold. Barnett and Scott (1964) observed two kinds of stereotyped behaviour, in both inbred and hybrid laboratory mice, at 21° and − 3°. In the warm, the mice gnawed food in excess of their need, and also gnawed wood, in an apparently futile way; at − 3°, though fully adapted, they did no such useless gnawing. Even nest-building with unfamiliar material (paper strips) was less efficient in the cold, though with cotton-wool (which was familiar) it was more efficient (Barnett, 1956).

There are vast gaps in our knowledge of the relation of activity to cold adaptation. It is not known how total activity (as defined) is related, in any natural or seminatural situation, to temperature and the competing demands of (i) economizing in heat loss and (ii) getting food. It is not clear how different forms of activity interact. In a given situation, with declining temperature, the intensities of different sorts of behaviour evidently diminish at different rates. The earliest to disappear are those which make no immediate contribution to survival.

B. THERMOREGULATORY BEHAVIOUR

Although activity (as defined) does not necessarily contribute to thermoregulation by producing extra heat, specific movements may put the animal in a warmer, or better insulated, place.

Herter (1941) has reviewed a long series of experiments on the "thermotactic optimum" of various land animals. The mammals he used were laboratory mice. In a passage with a temperature gradient, the mice settled at a preferred floor temperature of 34–37°. Stinson and Fisher (1953) put deer mice, *Peromyscus maniculatus*, in an aluminium tube. When it was at a uniform temperature, they settled at the ends; in a gradient from 6° to 50° they did not respond very uniformly, but their preferred temperatures were between 20° and 30°; individuals, however, were fairly consistent when tested several times. This, like some aspects of feeding behaviour (Section III.A, p. 430), is an example of the way in which behaviour is sometimes unequivocally homeostatic in function: a mouse (or other mammal—the domestic cat is a familiar example) is restless if the temperature of its skin departs from a certain range. This is another instance of so-called "appetitive" behaviour; it can lead the animal to a warmer place (or a cooler one) in which it settles; hence the animal achieves a "consummatory state".

No doubt there are species differences in the thermotactic optimum. Herter (1941) even reports genetically determined differences between strains of laboratory mice. But we know little about the extent or causes of variation in preferred temperature. Temperature certainly influences behaviour early in life. Mount (1963d) finds that infant pigs,

Sus scrofa, prefer a temperature of about 30°. Nestling rats are pro-voked to squeaking by lowered temperature, as when they stray or fall from the nest (Wiesner and Sheard, 1933). An obvious gap in our knowledge is the effects of exposure to a cold environment on preferred temperature. Since we do not know how "thermotactic" behaviour develops, it would be rash to assume that it is highly stable in develop-ment and constant within each species.

There is some information on the ways in which adaptive behaviour can contribute to the achievement of an optimum temperature. Clearly, once an animal has discovered a warm or insulated place, it will tend to return to it, but laboratory rats can learn to do more than this. Weiss and Laties (1960, 1961) have observed rats in a modified Skinner box, in which pressing a lever switches on a source of heat for a fixed period. At a low temperature, the animals spent most of the first 5 hours or so crouching in a corner and shivering; they occasionally pressed the lever, but only casually. Then there was a sudden change in behaviour, and the heat was switched on regularly, at intervals determined by the amount of heat given and the surrounding temperature. This sort of behaviour is also adjusted to internal state: rats short of pantothenic acid, and hence with a low tolerance for cold, press the bar correspond-ingly more often (Weiss, 1957). In a similar situation pigs, *Sus scrofa,* too, will press a lever to turn on a source of heat, but a steady response rate is established more quickly (B. A. Baldwin and D. L. Ingram, personal communication). Here we have trial-and-error be-haviour contributing to homeostasis.

A special case of apparently thermotactic behaviour is huddling. Probably all small mammals, and many large ones, sleep and rest in contact with others, when they can. Huddling is crucial for the survival of the young of small mammals when the temperature outside the nest is low (Section VIII, p. 465). It can also contribute to thermo-regulation, or at least reduce the amount of food needed, in adults. Prychodko (1958) recorded food consumption in laboratory mice at $-3°$, $4°$ and $25°$; some mice were alone, some in pairs and some in groups of five. In the warm there was only a slight effect of grouping; but at the low temperatures the sparing effect on food consumption was very marked: at $-3°$ the presence even of a single companion decreased food consumption by about 18% (Fig. 6). Pearson (1960) estimated calorie and oxygen consumption in a harvest mouse, *Reithrodontomys megalotis*: oxygen consumption was at a minimum of 2·5 ml./g.hr. at an ambient temperature of 33°; below thermal neutrality, each decline of 1° led to an increase in oxygen consumption of 0·27 ml./g.hr.; but if three mice were put together at 1°, there was a decrease in oxygen consump-tion of 28%. Mount (1960) found a reduction, due to huddling, of about

30% in the oxygen consumption of piglets. Sealander (1952) observed the contribution of huddling to the survival at low temperatures of the deer mice, *Peromyscus leucopus* and *P. maniculatus*. At $-23°$ the presence of a single companion greatly prolonged survival.

Many mammals display not only thermotactic behaviour but also what Darwin called "architectural instincts": nest-making is especially important for small mammals. Kinder (1927) gave laboratory rats strips of paper: the weight of paper used for making a nest increased as the ambient temperature was lowered. Barnett (1956) recorded the nests (made of cotton wool) constructed by laboratory mice fully adapted to,

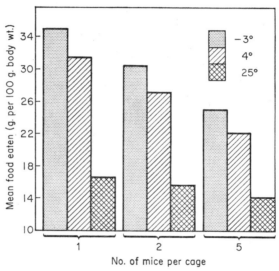

FIG. 6. Effect of ambient temperature and huddling on the daily food consumption of mice. (After Prychodko, 1958)

and breeding in, a room kept at $-3°$: as expected, they were superior to those of controls living at $21°$. Important features of good nests were (i) the extent to which they were covered in; (ii) a domed shape; and (iii) fluffing of the cotton wool. Pearson (1960), in his work on harvest mice, found that a nest allowed a decline in heat production of about 20%. Thorne (1958) analysed one feature of nest-making in *Peromyscus maniculatus*, namely, the shredding of material (paper); these rodents shredded much more paper at $8°$ than at $21°$. Hayward (1965) has illustrated the extent to which the burrowing habit of this species protects it from the fluctuations of the outside temperature (Fig. 7).

Nest building is influenced not only by outside conditions but also by internal state. A pregnant or parturient female, of a nest-making species, always builds a good nest, but this affects the thermoregulation of the young rather than the mother. Interference with the endocrine system can, however, increase the nest-building even of males, by reducing ability to adapt to cold by other means. Richter (1937) reviews early work on the effects of thyroidectomy or hypophysectomy, both of which impair cold resistance and also induce laboratory rats to make better nests. Stone and Mason (1955) confirmed these observations on hypophysectomized male laboratory rats: assessed on an elaborate scale, these rats, at 15°, made much better nests than controls.

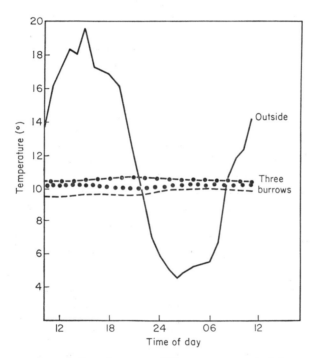

FIG. 7. Temperatures in three burrows of *Peromyscus maniculatus*, compared with those recorded outside in a 24-hr. period. (After Hayward, 1965)

Apart from maternal nest building, these observations all suggest a rather simple relation between huddling or nest-making on the one hand, and the thermal demands of the environment on the other. But in fact these two kinds of behaviour may be performed in the absence of the need to conserve heat: they are stereotyped activities, characteristic of many species and, like many other such activities, have a certain autonomy. The huddling of laboratory rats makes, in ordinary conditions, no contribution to conserving energy (Benedict, 1938).

Nevertheless, the immediate stimulation which induces huddling is probably the contact with a warm surface; huddling may, in fact, be an example of thermotactic behaviour even when it is not heat-conserving. The surface temperature of a mouse is near that chosen by mice in a gradient, for in air at 21° the temperature on the surface of the hair of a mouse is about 34°, while in air at −3° it is about 31° (Barnett, 1956). Features of a companion other than surface temperature could help to provoke contact but, if so, they are probably common to many species. Members of different species huddle together: an example is the association of *Rattus rattus* and *R. norvegicus* (Barnett, 1963).

The partial independence of heat conservation, displayed by nest-building, is even clearer. There are two aspects to this, one special and one general. The special aspect appears in the work of Gelineo and Gelineo (1952) on the ambient temperature preferred by lactating laboratory rats: this is 16°, far below thermal neutrality; if the ambient temperature rises to about 20°, the female moves the nest.

The general aspect is the autonomy (already referred to) of species-characteristic behaviour such as nest making, that is, the performance of the behaviour even when it has no homeostatic effect. Barnett and Scott (1964) gave mice 24 paper strips which could be drawn into the cage. This was done, on the average, more readily when there was already a well constructed cotton wool nest in the cage: the existing nest was then lined with paper, sometimes after shredding. Low temperature, in the conditions of these experiments, did not increase the rate of nest-building with paper; often it diminished it. This was perhaps due to the unfamiliarity of the paper strips, for the mice had had no experience of using them to conserve heat.

Although, therefore, the behaviour described in this chapter is all homeostatic in function, it does not follow that it is directly and simply related to need on every occasion. In the example just given, a learning process was evidently needed, before the standard patterns of drawing material to a nest site, shredding it and arranging it, could be performed in a way which corresponded to need. The obverse of this is the fact that nest-making and huddling may both occur in the absence of the need to conserve temperature.

V. Growth and Body Composition

A. NATURE OF "TROPHIC" RESPONSES

Exposure to cold below the critical temperature usually entails an alteration of body weight or of the rate of total growth. These effects are always accompanied by less evident changes in the relative weights of organs and in body composition. Three types of process are involved. First, material may be diverted from anabolism to heat production. This applies both to food and also to reserves already in the tissues. Second, certain organs may enlarge, evidently as a result of the extra work thrown upon them by the increased metabolic rate. Such enlargement may be expected in, for example, liver and gut, and some endocrine organs. Third, some structures are provoked to extra growth by cold, though not, presumably, as a result of having to do more work. This applies to some of the components of skin (Section II.C.4, p. 428). All these adjustments are reflected by changes in body composition, of which those in fat content are among the most obvious.

The changes in individual mammals after exposure to cold must be distinguished from differences between species or varieties which influence resistance to cold. If animals of one type have, for instance, a lower ratio of surface area to volume than those of another then, other things equal, the latter will be at a disadvantage in the cold. "Bergmann's rule" states that members of a taxon tend to be larger in the colder regions of its distribution (Bergmann, 1847); according to "Allen's rule", the colder the environment, the shorter the appendages and the more compact the body. Scholander (1955) has critically reviewed these beliefs. In this section, we discuss, not genetically determined differences in growth, but those imposed on individual mammals making their own physiological adjustment to a cold environment.

The scattered information on this topic has been reviewed by Hart (1957), Héroux (1961, 1963), Smith and Hoijer (1962), and Kleiber (1963). Héroux and Gridgeman (1958), and Angervall and Carlström (1963), have discussed some of the statistical hazards of the analysis of relative growth. Here we try to bring out the principles which underlie the facts.

B. BODY WEIGHT AND FOOD RESERVES

1. Changes in Total Weight

Assuming a constant shape, an adaptive change in total weight on exposure to cold must be an increase. Sealander (1951) found one species of *Peromyscus* to be heavier by about 2·5 g. in winter than in summer; but another species was unchanged in weight; and Hayward (1965), in an extensive study of *Peromyscus* from north-eastern North America, recorded lighter weights in winter (the winter mice may have been younger than the summer ones). *Rattus norvegicus* evidently keeps the same mean weight, summer and winter, in Canada (Héroux, 1963). For large animals, loss of weight is less serious than for small

15+T.

ones. Sheep lose weight in winter, especially if kept out of doors (Armstrong *et al.*, 1959). The still larger Brahman cow, however, at two years, exposed to winter temperatures down to − 13°, merely reduces her growth rate (Ragsdale *et al.*, 1950).

Most of the information on the effects of cold on body weight is from work on small laboratory mammals. Below we distinguish five groups of relevant facts.

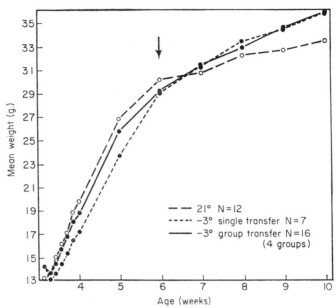

FIG. 8. Changes in the body weights of random-bred mice after exposure to cold. Controls were kept singly in an ambient temperature of 21°. Experimental mice were transferred at three weeks to − 3° (with bedding) either singly (···) or in groups of 4 (——). At six weeks, the experimental mice were returned to 21°. The curves show the immediate effect of the cold on growth, the effect of grouping, and a favourable effect of cold exposure on subsequent capacity for growth.

(i) Héroux (1961) has summarized the literature on the effects of transferring laboratory rats from around 20° to about 4°, cavies, *Cavia cobaya*, to a rather higher temperature, and hamsters, *Mesocricetus auratus*, to 6°. In these experiments, the animals are usually caged singly without a nest, and they have no opportunity to make a gradual adjustment to cold. The immediate effect is loss of weight, but survivors may begin to make up the loss after a few days. Figure 5, p. 436, illustrates this sequence from laboratory mice, and also shows the typical accompanying changes in food consumption.

(ii) Adults may never completely make up the initial loss of weight on cold exposure, but young, rapidly growing, mammals, if they survive the first few days, may be expected to resume growth, though at a lower rate (e.g. Barnett et al., 1960). Figure 8 illustrates the responses of just-weaned laboratory mice to two kinds of cold exposure.

(iii) Barnett and Scott (1963) and S. A. Barnett (unpublished observations) have recorded the effects on body weight of breeding mice permanently in an environment at $-3°$. The mice made nests of cotton wool. When growth is recorded from birth, or from weaning, one may study the relationship between maternal performance and development of the young. The masses of litters at birth and weaning, in a polytocous mammal such as the mouse, may indeed be used as indices of maternal performance. Body weight, at least in early life, is influenced not only by the physical environment, uterine conditions, milk supply and maternal care but also by number in litter. Usually, body weight at weaning declines with an increase in size of litter. This effect of "competition" (presumably for milk) among litter mates (Biggers et al., 1958) may be enhanced by cold (Barnett and Manly, 1959). Hence a full account of the effects of cold on body weight in the early life of a small mammal requires a statement of the regression of body weight on number in litter.

After weaning, the course of growth in a cold environment reflects that in the nest: mice already slightly stunted by very early exposure to cold continue to grow at a lower rate than controls (Barnett and Scott, 1963; but contrast Fig. 8).

(iv) This raises the question of the effects of cold in early life on later growth in a more favourable environment. Barnett and Scott (1963) transferred some of their mice from $-3°$ to $21°$, where they kept them in small groups. There was no compensatory growth. The mice, initially lighter than controls reared at $21°$, remained so. However, much more information is needed on the effects of exposure at different ages, as Fig. 8 shows. After a period of undernourishment, a mammal may or may not make up the lost weight, according to (i) the severity of the deprivation, and (ii) the age at which it occurred (reviewed by Wilson and Osbourn, 1960). At certain ages, an unfavourable environment may set an animal's growth capacity for life (e.g. Widdowson and Kennedy, 1962). Exposure to cold in early life may have effects very similar to those of food shortage.

(v) There may be substantial genetical variation, within a species, in growth in a cold environment. Most laboratory mice, if reared at an ambient temperature of $-3°$, would probably be lighter than controls of the same strain reared at $21°$. However, C57BL mice display no such difference (Barnett and Scott, 1963). More important, the same authors crossed inbred mouse strains. The growth of the three types of F_1 mice produced in this way was not depressed by cold; and at $-3°$ all three were heavier than parent strains, that is, they displayed "luxuriance" or "growth heterosis".

Genetical variation allows selection for resistance to cold, and this may have an effect on body weight (Fig. 9). A genetically mixed stock of laboratory mice was selected for ability to breed in the cold; after twelve generations these mice were heavier than controls kept at 21° (Barnett and Scott, 1963).

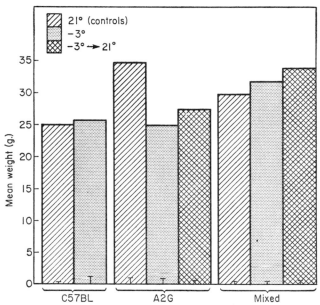

FIG. 9. Effect of environmental temperature on the body weights of male laboratory mice aged sixteen weeks. Mice at $-3°$ were born and resident in that ambient temperature. Mice moved from cold to warm (21°) were reared at $-3°$ for their first three weeks. Low environmental temperature had no effect on the body weight of the highly inbred C57BL mice, but a large effect on the A2G mice (also highly inbred); A2G mice transferred to 21° at three weeks did not recover from the effect of being reared at $-3°$ (Contrast Fig. 8.). The genetically mixed stock at $-3°$ had been selected for twelve generations for reproductive success at that temperature; this resulted in their being heavier than the controls bred at 21°. Vertical lines represent standard errors. (After Barnett and Scott, 1963)

2. Energy Reserves

Changes in gross body weight are accompanied by changes in the relative weights of tissues and organs; hence body weight is only a crude index of physiological function. The most labile structure is adipose tissue. It is not only metabolically active, but is also capable of changing enzymically in response to demand (reviewed by Shapiro, 1963; Masoro, 1963, 1966). Accordingly, in this section we are concerned, not with its insulative role in cold-adapted species, but with its function as a reserve of energy. It is, however, not the only tissue reserve of energy: during cold adaptation, reduction in the mass of the muscles may lead to a substantial loss of body weight, at least in laboratory rats (Héroux and Gridgeman, 1958).

The body fat of some species alters seasonally. *Peromyscus leucopus* may have more than three times as much fat, relative to body weight, in winter as in summer (Sealander, 1951). Wild *Rattus norvegicus* in Canada may increase their abdominal and subcutaneous adipose tissue by 30% in winter (Héroux, 1963). These accumulations perhaps have some insulative or heat-storing function, but they are probably most important as food reserves. Certainly, fat stores are rapidly depleted on sudden exposure to severe cold, as well as in starvation: this depletion can be responsible for a large part of the loss of weight which follows exposure of laboratory mammals (reviewed by Héroux, 1961).

Pagé and Babineau (1953) exposed laboratory rats to a temperature between 3° and 10°; energy expenditure was nearly doubled, and there was loss of fat which accounted for about 30% of the total weight loss. Male laboratory rats were studied by Héroux and Gridgeman (1958): after four weeks at 6°, they had about half the body fat of rats kept for four weeks at 30°; this represented about one-fifth of the difference in total body weight. This was by far the largest percentage loss of any tissue or organ. Hart and Héroux (1956) exposed laboratory mice to −7° or −13° for four days; 85–89% of the *reserve* of energy used came from fat. Nevertheless this source provided only 15–20% of total energy needs during that period. Most of the heat produced still came from the combustion of the carbohydrate in the food.

The loss of fat on cold exposure does not necessarily persist. For instance, adult laboratory rats exposed to 11° lose fat during the first month, but later restore it (Babineau and Pagé, 1955). This sequence may be compared with that of the enzymic changes described in Section II.C.2, p. 425.

Continued exposure may, however, reduce the growth of adipose tissue after cold adaptation has taken place. Young and Cook (1955) put male Swiss mice at 4° for about seven weeks. These mice stopped growing, and ended with fat weighing about 4·8% of the whole body; the figure for controls at 24° was 10·5%. Barnett *et al.* (1959) and Barnett and Widdowson (1965) studied A2G mice breeding at −3°; these mice were kept in groups and had nests. Females of the first or second generations in the cold weighed less than controls at 21°; the decrement corresponded to the difference in body fat content (Table I) but, as we shall see later, there were other differences in the constitution of the body. In males, although the difference in body weight of the A2G mice was even greater, the difference in fat content was less. This may be related to the fact that control females had about twice as much fat as control males. This strain is probably typical of laboratory mice. The C57BL strain, already mentioned as differing in total growth, also has a quite different fat metabolism (Table I).

TABLE I. *Body Weight and Fat Content of Virgin Female Mice Aged 16 Weeks: Means with Standard Errors (Barnett and Widdowson, 1965 and Unpublished Observations)*

Strain	Temperature (°)	No. of Mice	Body Wt. (g.)	Body Fat	
				(g.)	(g./100 g.)
A2G	21	16	24·4 ± 0·2	3·5 ± 0·2	14·1 ± 0·7
	−3	13	21·8 ± 0·3	1·8 ± 0·1	8·5 ± 0·3
C57BL	21	12	21·5 ± 0·4	1·8 ± 0·2	9·2 ± 0·8
	−3	9	21·6 ± 0·6	1·9 ± 0·2	8·7 ± 0·9

A disadvantage of estimations of total fat content is that they take no account of the different types of adipose tissue. An important distinction is between brown and white adipose tissue (reviewed by Johansson, 1959; Smith, 1964). These are not readily distinguished by the naked eye, but the former differs from white tissue in the following ways. (i) The yellowish colour, which turns to brown if much fat is lost, is due to a high content of respiratory pigments. (ii) It is present in the rat especially in the interscapular region of the back, in the neck, and dorsal to the kidneys. (iii) It is exceptionally labile: the fat, which within each cell forms many small vacuoles surrounded by mitochondria, is quickly converted to fatty acids; these are readily oxidized. The heat so produced is evidently an important means of thermoregulation in small mammals suddenly exposed to cold. (iv) During prolonged exposure to cold, brown fat undergoes hyperplasia, and heat production from this source rises correspondingly.

Brown adipose tissue is active in young mammals. Dawkins and Hull (1963) and Hull and Segall (1964, 1965) state that it is an important site of heat production in new-born rabbits. It may also contribute largely to thermogenesis in human infants (Aherne and Hull, 1964). Chaffee *et al.* (1964) find that the brown adipose tissue of cold-adapted hamsters, *Mesocricetus auratus*, has a greater heat-producing capacity than that of controls; this is accompanied by changes in enzyme activity.

Emphasis on brown fat should not lead to a neglect of white adipose tissue. This too constitutes a reserve of energy. Indeed, within the brown tissue there are cells with the structure typical of the white and, during cold exposure, these give up their fat as well; in a laboratory rat exposed to 6° for four days, they have almost disappeared from the interscapular tissue (Cameron and Smith, 1964). No doubt the larger masses of plain white adipose tissue give up their fat over a still longer period, if an energy deficit persists.

C. GROWTH OF APPENDAGES

Loss of fat, or of weight from any other cause, is disadvantageous in a cold environment, but other changes in bodily proportions seem to be adaptive.

The length of the tail and the ears, and the length of the body relative to body weight, may all be reduced by rearing laboratory rats or mice in a cold environment (Sumner, 1909, 1915; Przibram, 1923; Emery et al., 1940; Chevillard et al., 1962; Barnett, 1965b). Moreover, the mouse tail lengthens in a hot environment (e.g. Harrison, 1963). Harrison (1958) cut off the tails of mice and found that this lowered their tolerance to an ambient temperature of 32°. There is also now no doubt that the rat tail is an organ of thermoregulation: its blood vessels dilate in a warm environment, and this greatly increases heat loss from the surface; the same thing happens in the feet, but not the ears (Rand et al., 1965; Thompson and Stevenson, 1965).

Much remains to be discovered about the growth of the hairless Murid tail in different environments, and also the effects of selection on it. Barnett (1965b) found a shortening effect of cold, not only in mice with tails of typical length, but also in mice with genetically short tails. There was a decrease in size without a major change in proportions; but cold evoked a slight reduction in the number of tail vertebrae. However, he also studied mice of a genetically mixed stock selected in a cold environment for eighteen generations; these mice, already mentioned as being heavier than controls after twelve generations, developed *longer* tails than the controls at 21°. Probably the shorter tails in cold environments are an incidental result of the action of the low temperature during development, with little or no adaptive significance.

D. ADAPTIVE GROWTH

1. *The Organs Affected*

The increased respiration, food consumption, intermediary metabolism and excretion, which result from exposure to cold below the critical temperature, must require certain organs to do much more work.

Endocrine organs, especially thyroid and adrenals, constitute a special case of adaptive growth in cold-exposed mammals, and they are referred to separately (Section II.C.3, p. 427). Of the larger organs, there is no good evidence that the lungs are affected (Héroux and Gridgeman, 1958), but the heart, gut, liver and kidneys all tend to enlarge. The evidence for this, mostly from laboratory rats, has been summarized by Héroux (1961). Since then Chaffee *et al.* (1963) have observed a 30% rise in absolute kidney weight in hamsters, *Mesocricetus auratus*, exposed (without nests) for about nine weeks to 5°. Barnett and Widdowson (1965) have reported on the weights of organs of mice of the first or second generations breeding (with nest material) at −3°: regressed weights of stomach, small intestine, liver and kidneys were, as expected, greater than those of controls at 21°; there were, however, some differences in detail between the sexes.

In the usual type of laboratory experiment, the animals are inbred or at least domesticated; and they are suddenly exposed to cold alone and without protection. In nature, the onset of cold is usually gradual; and a wild population is genetically very different from a domestic one. These differences certainly influence the effects of cold on rats (Table II). The significance of the failure of wild rats to have enlarged livers or kidneys in winter is uncertain: perhaps these organs are more efficient per unit weight than those of laboratory rats, at least in winter; in more severe cold they might enlarge, as do those of the laboratory strains.

One other large organ undergoes changes on exposure to cold, namely, the pelt. In large arctic mammals, such as the wolf, *Canis lupus*, and the black bear, *Euarctos americanus*, insulation improves in winter (Hart, 1956). Durrer and Hannon (1962) find that husky dogs have a thicker hair coat in winter. In small mammals there is little scope for improvement in insulation from skin or hair, since a great increase in either would immobilize a mammal the size of a mouse. Nevertheless, mammals evidently have a general capacity to grow thicker hair in cold conditions; but this does not apply to the skin, since this is liable to become lighter on exposure to cold: indeed, total insulation from skin and hair may decrease in a cold environment in the laboratory (Hart, 1957; Barnett, 1959). Here again Héroux has demonstrated a difference between the effects of laboratory experiments and those of seasonal cold (Table II).

A general effect of prolonged exposure to cold is a proportionate increase in actively metabolizing tissues, such as liver and gut. Hence cold-adapted laboratory mammals usually contain more water than controls: this holds for rats (Deb and Hart, 1956; Baker and Sellers, 1957), hamsters (Farrand, 1959) and mice (Barnett and Widdowson, 1965). There is a corresponding decline in the proportion of nitrogen

TABLE II. *Changes in Rats Exposed to Cold (after Héroux, 1963)*

| | Laboratory Rats | | Wild Rats |
	indoors	outside	natural habitat
Total growth	−	−	+
Adipose tissue	−	○	+
Liver weight	+	+	○
Kidney weight	+	+	○
Heart weight	+	○	+
Pelt insulation	○	+	+
Resting metabolic rate at 30°	+	○	+

The laboratory rats were exposed, in groups, either (a) to continuous cold indoors or (b) to seasonal cold outside. The wild rats were trapped. ○, indicates no difference; −, a decline in cold; +, an increase in cold.

(that is, in effect, protein) in the body. The connective tissues also bulk rather less; this is reflected in a lowered collagen content. The relative weight of the skeleton, too, indicated by the calcium content of the body, tends to be lower; but in this there is a difference between the sexes, since virgin females are less affected than males (Barnett and Widdowson, 1965).

There are also shifts in electrolyte balance (Baker, 1960a,b). During the early stages of cold adaptation, rats retain some sodium and, to a smaller extent, potassium. There is a very brief initial period of chloride loss. In man, the blood also becomes more concentrated. After some weeks the picture is different, just as it is in other respects: blood volume is raised above the control level, and plasma potassium and chloride have returned to the normal range; but plasma sodium remains high. The significance of these changes is not yet clear: they need to be linked with the other processes of cold adaptation.

2. Problems of Function

Differences in the gross weights of organs, or in total body composition, can only hint at the means by which a mammal becomes adapted to cold. Their limitations include the following: (i) an organ can become more efficient without an alteration in weight; (ii) total weight does not indicate which tissues are changed by cold.

The fact that an organ, such as the kidney or thyroid gland, can become more efficient per unit weight has been discussed by Abercrombie (1957) and by Goss (1964). The evidence comes from experiments in which compensatory growth occurs after removal of tissue; if a large part of a kidney is removed, regeneration follows, but the original weight is not fully restored though function is. Something of the sort may occur

15*

during adaptation to cold. Barnett and Widdowson (1965) give the weights of the kidneys of three classes of A2G mice: (a) controls at 21°, (b) mice of the first or second generations reared at −3°, (c) mice of the fourteenth generation at −3° (Table III). Absolute weights were lower in both experimental groups, and even the relative weight was lower in the mice of long ancestry in the cold. Yet the latter were the better adapted to the cold environment (reviewed by Barnett, 1965a).

In a complex organ, hypertrophy or hyperplasia may occur in only some of the component tissues. In the kidneys of hamsters exposed to 5°, large numbers of mitoses appear after two days; this hyperplasia, which persists for some weeks, occurs principally in the proximal tubules: there is no general enlargement of the organ, and no new

TABLE III. *Weights of Bodies and Kidneys of Male A2G Mice aged 16 Weeks: Means with Standard Errors*

Temperature	No. of Mice	Body Wt. (g.)	Kidney Wt.	
			(g.)	(g./100 g. body wt.)
(°)				
21	14	28·7 ± 0·72	0·573 ± 0·014	2·00 ± 0·04
−3 (generations 1 or 2)	17	24·0 ± 0·77	0·498 ± 0·037	2·07 ± 0·05
−3 (generation 14)	12	27·5 ± 0·57	0·478 ± 0·015	1·73 ± 0·04

nephrons are formed (Chaffee *et al.*, 1963). Another example of (evidently) histological complexity is provided by the small intestines of the three classes of mice mentioned in the previous paragraph. The intestines of one group of mice in the cold were heavier than those of the controls, but not much longer; hence the amount of tissue per unit length was increased. But the mice of long ancestry in the cold had much the longest intestines. These differences require more detailed study.

Another kind of special hyperplasia occurs in the capillary systems of some organs (Héroux and St. Pierre, 1957). After four weeks at 6°, rats have about twelve times as many capillaries in their skeletal muscles as have controls kept at 30°. The capillaries of the ears undergo a similar increase, but—surprisingly—not those of the heart or liver.

3. *Problems of Morphogenesis*

The enlargement of organs, which constitutes a part of cold adaptation, raises difficult problems of the regulation of growth. The control of compensatory regeneration and hypertrophy has been principally studied in animals from which large masses of tissue have been removed; and the control of skin growth has been investigated after wounding (e.g. Sandblom, 1949). These operations produce changes on a massive scale. Those of cold adaptation are by comparison small, but they may be of the same sort. This notion is supported by the observations of Chaffee *et al.* (1963), mentioned above, on the hamster kidney during cold adaptation. The distribution of mitotic figures, and the time of their onset, resemble those described by Williams (1961) during compensatory hyperplasia in the kidney of the rat. The "trophic" changes which take place during exposure to cold perhaps deserve investigation from this point of view.

VI. Reproduction

A. BREEDING SEASONS

Most mammals breed seasonally: young are born in spring or summer, and reproduction ceases in colder weather. In mammals, as in birds, the onset of breeding is probably unaffected by the temperature of the environment: day length is often crucial (reviewed by Fraps, 1962). Cold may induce a prolonged anoestrus, for instance in the golden hamster, *Mesocricetus auratus* (Grindeland and Folk, 1962); exposing laboratory rats to outdoor winter temperatures lengthens the oestrous cycle (Lee, 1926); and in the laboratory mouse, dioestrus is lengthened by environmental temperatures around 0° (Parkes and Brambell, 1928) or −3° (Barnett and Coleman, 1959).

In nature, small mammals which have no fixed breeding season perhaps stop breeding in autumn or winter as a result of a decline in the food supply. Little is known about such seasonal influences. Barnett and Coleman (1959) and Perrault and Dugal (1965) have suggested that the effects of cold and of food shortage are often similar. Perrault and Dugal, in a study of testicular function in cold and shortage of food, distinguish a systemic action from a specific endocrine effect. But there is little information on the effects of cold on the reproductive powers of males. A prolonged study has, however, been made of the reproductive performance of laboratory mice at −3° (reviewed by Barnett, 1965a), and this at least makes clear that males of several inbred strains can be fertile at that temperature. Most of this work, however, concerns females, and the rest of this section is confined to them.

B. REPRODUCTIVE PROCESSES IN FEMALES

The general effect of a cold environment on female reproductive processes is to slow them down (Figs. 10 and 11). The vaginae of random-bred mice, born in a room kept at 5°, open later than those of controls at 21° (Biggers *et al.*, 1958). Inbred A2G mice of a stock breeding at − 3° had a mean age of vaginal opening of 33 days, while the control figure was 26 days; in both groups, mean body weight at opening was 13 g. (Barnett and Coleman, 1959). There is evidently a correlation between vaginal opening and the processes which regulate total growth.

The effects of cold on the oestrous cycle are less simple. A2G mice have a mean age of onset of typical oestrus of 38 days at 21°, but of 61 days at

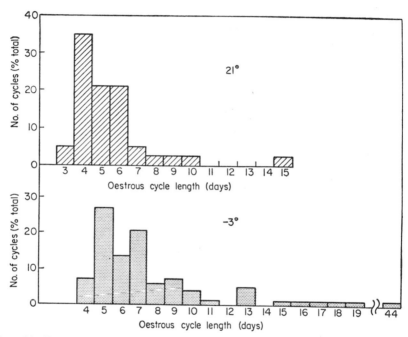

FIG. 10. Lengthening of the oestrous cycle of virgin female A2G mice by a cold environment. The mice at − 3° were born in that ambient temperature. Based on 79 cycles at 21°, and 82 cycles at − 3°. (After Barnett and Coleman, 1959)

− 3°. Thereafter, females kept in groups have mean cycle lengths of 4·8 and 8·5 days, respectively (Barnett and Coleman, 1960). Emery *et al.* (1940) recorded longer oestrous cycles, and briefer oestrus, in laboratory rats exposed to 1·6° for 16 hr. each day. These facts fit into the picture of slower reproductive processes in the cold (Fig. 10), but those concerning mice transferred to the cold as adults do not. Transfer does lead to lengthened oestrous cycles, but only at first; after many weeks, the control length of 4·8 days is restored. Parkes and Brambell (1928) reported a similar finding in mice transferred to an environment at about 0°. These observations suggest that cycle length in a cold environment with plenty of food reflects, not the temperature to which the adult is subjected, but that in which it was reared. Perhaps there is an early sensitive period during which cycle length is determined for life.

Corresponding to the late onset of oestrus, the first parturition is delayed in a cold environment; in two inbred strains the mean age for controls is about eleven weeks, while at −3° it is about seventeen

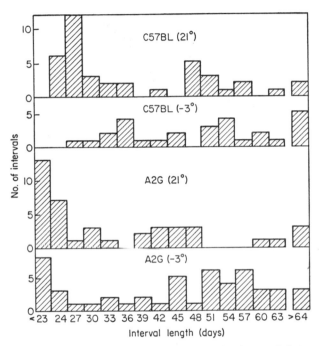

FIG. 11. Effect of low ambient temperature on the interval between parturitions of mice of two inbred strains. The mice in the cold were members of stocks bred in a room at −3°, and were in permanent male–female pairs.

weeks (Barnett and Coleman, 1960). Furthermore, when each female is kept permanently with one male, the interval between parturitions is longer in the cold; in strain A2G at 21°, about 60% of conceptions (apart from first ones) take place at post-partum oestrus, but at −3° about two-thirds occur around three weeks later, at post-lactation oestrus (Fig. 11).

Inevitably, the rate at which young are produced in a cold environment is lower than that in a warm one. From the facts just given, this would hold even if the number of young born and weaned per litter were

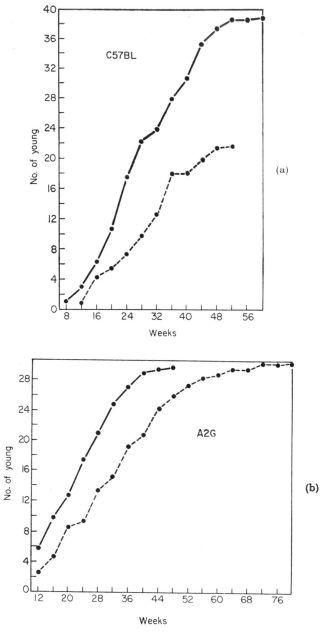

FIG. 12. Effect of low temperature on the number of young mice born per mated pair. Continuous lines indicate controls at 21°; broken lines, mice at −3°. (a) C57BL mice are shown to stop breeding at about the same age at both temperatures, and to be less fertile at −3°. (b) A2G mice, after many generations in the cold, continue to breed for about twice as long as controls, and so produce eventually as many young. (From Barnett, 1962)

unaffected by cold. It does not, however, follow that the total number of young produced per pair must be reduced. This is illustrated by a study of mice of strains C57BL and A2G which were allowed to breed until their reproductive capacity was exhausted (Fig. 12). The C57BL mice stopped breeding, in both temperatures, at about fifty weeks; hence their fertility at $-3°$ was much lower than in the warm environment. The A2G mice at $21°$ stopped at about forty weeks; but, at $-3°$, they continued to about eighty weeks. Hence their total output of young was the same at the two temperatures. These A2G mice were of the eighth or ninth generations in the cold environment; had they been of the first or second generations, the outcome would have been different, as we shall see below. Unfortunately, there is not yet any information on the total performance of random bred mice in a cold environment.

C. THE MATERNAL ENVIRONMENT

The first environment of a mammal is a uterus, and the second—which is often a nest or lair—is one in which the mother remains the only source of food. The environment provided by a female for her foetal and nestling young is in turn affected by (i) the environment in which she lives; (ii) the environments in which she was reared; and hence (iii) the environments in which her mother lived. There is only the barest beginning of information on these relationships: for instance, the optimum ambient temperature for reproduction is not known even for laboratory mice. C57BL mice, given nest material, wean more young per pair at $10°$ than at $21°$, though other strains do better at $21°$ (Barnett and Manly, 1956, 1959; Barnett, 1964).

From the works just quoted, a summary may be made of the effects on fertility of transferring mice from $21°$ to $-3°$ at puberty. The number of young born per litter is reduced, often by about one-third. This probably reflects conditions *in utero*, rather than ovulation rate; but on this more needs to be found out. Much the same applies to breeding among the *offspring* of mice transferred in this way, that is, of the first generation born and reared in the cold. There is, however, one important qualification: maternal performance in this generation is inferior to that of the females of the transferred generation; this is evident from the weights of the young at three weeks (Table IV). Correspondingly, mice reared at $-3°$ and transferred to $21°$ at mating have lighter young than controls at $21°$ (Barnett and Manly, 1959). Other evidence of such maternal effects is summarized by Barnett (1965a). Clearly, in the conditions of the experiments on these mice, it is a disadvantage for a female mouse to be reared in a cold environment. Chevillard and Cadot (1963) have observed an analogous decline in fertility in laboratory rats bred for three generations at 5°. Their animals, however, gave no evidence of recovery: there was therefore no possibility of continued breeding in the conditions they used.

TABLE IV. *Maternal Effect in A2G Mice: Advantage Resulting from Parents Having Been Reared in a Warm Environment. Means with Standard Errors. (From Barnett, 1961)*

	(a) Transferred from warm to cold at mating	(b) Offspring of (a)
Fecund pairs	8	5
Born per pair	16·6 ± 2·8	12·2 ± 2·5
Born per litter	5·5 ± 0·5	5·5 ± 0·6
Weaned per weaned litter	5·4 ± 0·3	5·0 ± 0·7
Weights of young at 3 weeks (g.) $\{ \substack{\male \\ \female}$	9·3 ± 0·2 8·7 ± 0·1	7·7 ± 0·2 7·6 ± 0·3
Barren pairs	1	4

D. GENETICAL VARIATION

The laboratory animals most used in physiological experiments are often highly inbred. Members of such strains may be referred to as "the mouse", "the rat" and so on, but this is misleading. First, inbred strains differ among themselves; second, laboratory animals always differ genetically from the wild forms of their species; third, inbred populations offer little scope for genetical change due to selection; and fourth, homozygosis, due to inbreeding, generally reduces fertility and other components of fitness. These matters have been more fully discussed elsewhere (Barnett, 1965a).

Some minor effects of selection for fertility at −3° have been observed in a mixed stock of laboratory mice (Barnett, 1961; Barnett and Scott, 1963). Body weight increased, but adipose tissue declined. The number of young born and weaned per pair rose substantially over twelve generations. Mortality in the nest declined from over 40% to below 10%. We shall see in the next section that not all these changes were necessarily due to selection of favourable genotypes; but some of them probably were.

A slightly less obvious genetical principle is illustrated by the performance in the cold of F_1 mice, produced by mating two inbred strains. Such mice display "hybrid vigour" in an ordinary environment; and this superiority over inbred animals may be enhanced in unfavourable conditions. For example, mice of the cross C57BL × A2G at 21° rear twice the weight of young produced by their parent strains; but at −3°

they rear nearly five times the weight produced by the parent strains (Barnett and Coleman, 1960). Hence heterozygosis may be especially important in an adverse environment. This is also exemplified by the resistance to cold of young mice: among all possible crosses between four inbred strains, nearly all the F_1 types were superior to the inbred parent strains (Barnett, 1964).

E. CUMULATIVE EFFECT OF COLD

It would be expected that, after one or two generations, inbred animals in a cold environment, unlike the mixed stock of mice referred to above, would show no progressive change in reproduction or growth. But in fact, a progressive decline in nestling mortality, over several

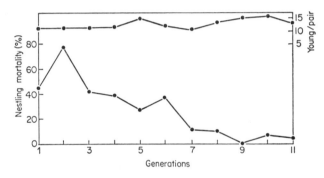

FIG. 13. Decline in nestling mortality among A2G mice bred for eleven generations in an ambient temperature of $-3°$. The total number of pairs was 57. The number of young born per pair remained steady. Controls bred at $21°$ did not display any such improvement. (After Barnett, 1961)

generations, has been observed among mice of inbred strains A2G and C57BL at $-3°$ (Barnett, 1961). These mice differed from the mixed stock (referred to above) in retaining a steady rate of number of young *born* over the generations (Fig. 13). There was no corresponding improvement among the controls at $21°$. Mice transferred to a cold room on later occasions again had a high nestling mortality; hence the decline in mortality was a property of the permanently cold-bred stock, and not a temporary consequence of the conditions in which they were kept, or of any factor acting at both temperatures.

The A2G mice bred for many generations in the cold differ from recently introduced mice also in growth properties (Table V) and in several aspects of maternal efficiency (Barnett and Little, 1965; Barnett and Widdowson, 1965). A progressive, adaptive change in an adverse environment, such as this, suggests selection of favourable genotypes, but there is little scope for this in inbred strains. There are in fact

TABLE V. *Effects on Male Mice (Strain A2G) of Long Ancestry in a Cold Environment (After Barnett and Widdowson,* 1965).

[○ *Indicates no Difference from Controls; +, an Increase; − a Decrease*]

	Generations 1 or 2	Generation 14
Body weight	−	○
Body fat	○	+
Body water	+	−
Nitrogen	−	○
Collagen	−	○
Calcium	−	○
Heart	+	+
Stomach and intestine	+	○
Liver	+	○
Kidneys	○	−
Testes	+	○

overwhelming reasons for rejecting a genetical explanation of the change (Barnett, 1960, 1961). Improbable though it seems, a cumulative maternal effect must be sought, to account for the secular changes in at least the two inbred strains.

The principal fact is that inbred mice have become better adapted to a cold environment as a result of breeding there for a number of generations. This unexpected observation, whatever the detailed explanation, shows that the cold adaptation of mammals may have features which cannot be fully revealed by short-term experiments.

VII. Ontogeny

A. HOMEOTHERMY AND HETEROTHERMY

The homeothermic powers of new-born mammals vary greatly (reviewed by Gelineo, 1959). One of the smallest, the mouse, at birth completely fails to respond to cooling by a rise in metabolic rate (Fitzgerald, 1953). However, the new-born mouse displays a corresponding tolerance of hypothermia which is characteristic of mammals immediately after birth (McCance, 1959). The same applies to new-born rats (Campbell and Riccio, 1966). At the other end of the scale, the reindeer calf, *Rangifer tarandus*, is born while the herd is moving towards the sea in the spring; and it is so resistant to cold and so mature that, within minutes, it is accompanying its mother and keeping up with the rest of the herd.

Hart *et al.* (1961) have investigated the metabolic rates and body temperatures of the closely similar infant caribou, also *R. tarandus*, in diverse conditions of temperature, wind and wetting of the fur. Thermoregulation is well established at birth. The metabolic rate is doubled by exposure to 0°, but a low temperature together with wind and wetting raise the metabolic rate to over five times the resting value. If, however, the calves have no protection, they can be made hypothermic, and so can die, if they are exposed to the extreme conditions prevailing during storms in northerly latitudes.

Most other animals lie between mice and caribou in this respect. The rat has been much investigated, notably by workers in Prague (see Hahn *et al.*, 1961). The rat was once thought to be heterothermous at birth (Fairfield, 1948), since it evidently does not increase its oxygen consumption on exposure to cold until it is 3–4 days old. But even new-born rats increase their oxygen consumption if they are moved from an environment at 36° to one at 29° or 30° (Gelineo and Gelineo, 1951). If they are kept at 30° for longer than about 30 min., oxygen consumption begins to fall. Taylor (1960) confirmed these findings, and commented that the large and abrupt drop from 35° to 20° in Fairfield's experiments led to cooling of the tissues and so prevented an increase in oxygen consumption. Taylor found that, during the first six days after birth, the critical temperature is between 33° and 38°. There is always a rise in oxygen consumption when the environmental temperature is lowered from 35° to 29°. The rise is small in unfed rats: the greatest metabolic response occurs soon after the rats have begun to feed. Barić (1953) had already found that, when rats of 4–5 days of age are fed, they behave like homeotherms in the ambient temperature range 30–37°; but when fasted they behave like heterotherms at the same temperature. Nevertheless their oxygen consumption at 37° is 1,800 ml./kg.hr. whether they are fed or fasted. At 30°, the rate increases to 3,100 when the rats are fed, but falls to 1,250 ml./kg.hr. when they are fasted.

Gelineo (1959) points out that the puppy, too, loses its capacity for homeothermy when starved, whereas starvation of a fully grown dog, even to the point of death, does not change the type of thermoregulation. More surprising, the new-born guinea-pig, *Cavia*, remains a homeotherm when starved. These rodents are born in a much more mature state than most others. Gelineo (1957) finds that thermoregulatory ability at birth increases in the order: rat, rabbit, dog, guinea-pig; the corresponding cold limits are 29°, 23°, 19° and 7° ambient temperature.

In some species, noradrenalin greatly increases heat production in the newborn. Moore and Underwood (1963) found this to be so in kittens, rats and rabbits; the effect declines with advancing age. Non-shivering thermogenesis in the new-born (Brück and Wünnenberg, 1965a) may be related to the presence of brown fat (Dawkins and Hull, 1964; Dawkins and Scopes, 1965; Brück and Wünnenberg, 1965b; Hull, 1966; and see Sections II.C.1 and V.B.2, pp. 425 and 446).

B. METABOLIC RATE

Metabolic rate increases after birth, in thermally neutral and in cold conditions. This is true for the rat (Gelineo and Gelineo, 1951; Taylor, 1960), dog (Gelineo, 1957), ox (Roy et al., 1957), pig (Mount, 1959), sheep (Dawes and Mott, 1959; Alexander, 1961), rhesus monkey (Dawes et al., 1960), and perhaps in man. In our own species, however, the increase has been unequivocally shown only in cool conditions. Some workers have recorded a rise at thermal neutrality (Hill and Rahimtulla, 1965) but others have not (Brück, 1961; Karlberg, 1952). The increase in metabolic rate in the rat is rapid during the first 24 hours, and thereafter is more gradual up to three weeks. The most striking increase in response to cold occurs soon after a new-born rat begins to feed (Taylor, 1960). Correspondingly, Mourek (1962) found a large decrease in oxygen consumption in rather older rats at 26° after a 24-hour fast. The gradual rise in metabolic rate during the three weeks after birth is associated with improved thermoregulation.

In the new-born pig, there is a vigorous metabolic response, with shivering, when the environment is cooled; this increases as the temperature falls towards 0° (Mount, 1959). The cold limit for a solitary new-born pig, as opposed to a litter of huddled pigs, is about 5° when air movement is low (Mount, 1963a). The highest rate of heat production observed in any single pig is 162 kcal./m.^{2}hr.; this was in an animal during the first week after birth. During the first few post-natal hours, however, the pig cannot approach this level. Oxygen consumption rises, over a wide range of ambient temperatures including thermal neutrality (above 34°), during the first 1–2 days after birth. This rise is accompanied by an increase in rectal temperature from a mean of 38·0° for the first post-natal day to 39·0° later.

The metabolic rate of new-born pigs, at the neutral temperature (34°), nearly doubles during the first two days after birth (Mount, 1961). In lambs, the corresponding increase is nearly threefold during the first day (Dawes and Mott, 1959). The oxygen consumption rate of rhesus monkeys at thermal neutrality nearly doubles during the first week; this is associated with a steady rise in rectal temperature during the first 3–4 days (Dawes et al., 1960). These authors calculate that, in the lamb and the monkey, oxygen consumption per unit surface area in a thermally neutral environment rises during the early post-natal period, to a figure almost identical with that of an adult female. The same is true for the pig.

Brück (1961), Hill and Rahimtulla (1965) and Adamsons *et al.* (1965) found that the new-born full-term human baby responds to a cold environment by increasing its heat production. The figure for oxygen consumption rate at thermal neutrality just after birth found by Brück was similar to those obtained by Hill and Rahimtulla (4·8 ml./kg.min.) and by Adamsons *et al.* (4·6 ml./kg.min.). The basal metabolic rate of Hill's babies increased to 6·6 ml./kg.min. at 18–30 hours of age, and to 7·0/ml.kg.min. at 6–10 days, whereas Bruck found no increase. Hill found the critical temperature to decrease from 36° at birth (a value close to that found by Adamsons *et al.*, 1965) to 32° at the end of the first week. In view of the results obtained with other species, the human infant's basal metabolic rate probably does rise in the days after birth. Both Hill and Brück found that metabolic rates in the cold increased with age.

A baby often remains at the same body weight for several days after birth; and it usually takes about six months to double its birth weight. The young of other species grow much more rapidly (Brody, 1945): even the new-born pig doubles its birth weight in about a week. Hence the metabolic rate of the baby clearly increases with age, since body weight changes only slowly; but the relation of metabolic rate to the post-natally rising body temperature is less certain (Hill and Rahimtulla, 1965). The situation is still more complicated in the new-born pig, since here body weight is changing as well. Mount and Rowell (1960) therefore applied multiple regression analysis to the oxygen consumption rates of pigs during the first five weeks after birth, in relation to body weight, rectal temperature and age. This allowed the relation of each of these variables to be assessed, while the other two were held constant. At ambient temperatures of 30° and 4° (that is, close to thermal neutrality and around the cold limit, respectively) heat production per unit body weight decreased with increasing body weight; but calculated per unit surface area it remained more uniform. Both body weight and rectal temperature had large effects on oxygen consumption in the first five weeks after birth. The effect of age was less marked: indeed, in pigs less than one week old there was no significant effect at all. In older pigs, oxygen consumption fell slightly but significantly with increasing age. This result does not mean that oxygen consumption decreases as the pig grows older; this is clearly not so, since the animal is increasing in size. It does suggest, however, that, among a number of pigs of the same body weight and rectal temperature, the older pigs will have a lower oxygen consumption. This may be related to better thermal insulation in the older animals.

The small effect of age indicates that thermogenesis in the pig is well developed at birth. In other species, time since birth has a marked effect on the response to environment. In the rat, during the early post-natal period, age is an indication of the level of development of nervous control and consequently of the degree of metabolic response which the animal can make to changes in its environment (Adolph, 1957).

In the puppy, *Canis familiaris*, heat production increases during the first two weeks of postnatal life, but mechanisms of heat conservation lag behind (McIntyre and Ederstrom, 1958). This lag occurs in the pig as well. It may be related to the lack of subcutaneous fat at birth (Widdowson, 1950), coupled with the absence of an effective hair coat, since peripheral vasoconstriction in the cold does occur in the new-born pig (Mount, 1964a). Vasoconstriction in the absence of a fat layer has little effect (Section II.A, p. 414). A similar state of affairs exists in the human infant (Brück, 1961). The critical temperature falls in the first weeks of life in the pig (Mount, 1960), dog (Gelineo, 1954), rabbit (Hull, 1965) and baby (Hill and Rahimtulla, 1965). An animal born in a relatively mature state, such as the calf (Roy *et al.*, 1957) or lamb (Dawes and Mott, 1959), has a high rate of heat production from birth, like the pig. In addition, the calf and lamb have thick coats which conserve heat and so give them a substantial advantage over bare-skinned mammals such as pig and man.

C. HYPOTHERMIA AND RECOVERY

The body temperature of a new-born mammal falls immediately after birth. The extent and duration of this fall are determined by the species and the external conditions. The body temperature of a new-born pig often falls by 2–3° during the first 20 min. or so after birth, and then rises towards the mature level (Newland *et al.*, 1952; Pomeroy, 1953; Mount, 1959). The rise takes 1–10 days according to the ambient temperature. Although the new-born pig greatly increases heat production on exposure to, say, 5°, the rectal temperature nevertheless tends to fall if the piglet is alone and unprotected. The fall depends in part on body weight and age (Mount, 1961, 1963a) but there is much individual variation which cannot be accounted for in this way.

Other species undergo analogous changes, but the details depend on body size and maturity at birth. A new-born rat's body temperature falls several degrees when the mother leaves the nest exposed to an ambient temperature of 15° for 30 min.; but, if the nest is in a room at 28–30°, the difference between rats feeding from the mother, and those left exposed by the mother's absence, is not significant (Gelineo, 1959). The puppy, too, is thermally unstable at birth (Jensen and Ederstrom, 1955). By contrast, the temperature of a new-born guinea-pig remains at about 38° even if it is kept at an ambient temperature of 10°; but, if the ambient temperature falls to 6°, body temperature falls rapidly to 16° and the animal may die (Gelineo, 1959). New-born rats, however, can be subjected to these low temperatures and still recover.

Adolph (1951) and McCance (1959) have discussed the way in which new-born animals can survive a much greater fall in body temperature than adults of the same species. Adolph found that the guinea-pig could survive cooling only to around 15°, whereas new-born kittens and rabbits could recover after experiencing body temperatures of 6°, and rats survived after having been as low as 0°. By any standards—open eyes, thermal insulation, feeding—the guinea-pig is more mature at birth than the other species mentioned. It is also a much better homeotherm, but this evidently entails a lower tolerance of cold.

D. EARLY EXPOSURE AND COLD-RESISTANCE

The conditions in which mammals are reared can have a considerable influence on their later response to cold. This is one aspect of a larger phenomenon: early exposure to slightly adverse conditions probably improves subsequent resistance, not only to cold but to other "stressors" (Levine, 1962; Hutchings, 1963; Schaefer, 1963). Early exposure of female mice to cold may also improve their reproductive performance (Barnett and Burn, 1966).

The rate at which thermoregulation develops in new-born rats depends on the temperature of the nest (Gelineo and Gelineo, 1951). Rats may be reared at nest temperatures below 10–12°. At the end of the first post-natal week, such rats have a higher oxygen consumption at 21° than at 30°; but those with a nest temperature of 23–23·5° do not respond in this way until about 10 days, and those with a nest temperature of 28–30°, only towards the end of the second week. If a litter of rats, with the mother, is exposed four times a day for 1 hour to 0°, the oxygen consumption at an environmental temperature of 29·5° is increased earlier than in controls (Capek et al., 1956, quoted by Hahn et al., 1961). Correspondingly, if rats are reared from birth with their mother at a temperature of 34°, the development of thermoregulation is delayed; but this delay does not occur if the animals are exposed to a temperature of 0° for 1 hour daily between the fourteenth and the eighteenth day after birth. Eighteen days is the time at which a homeothermic response usually develops. Hahn et al. (1961) suggest that the effects of a rat's early environment probably persist throughout life.

VIII. Some Problems

A. MULTIVARIATE ANALYSIS

Most of the observations we have quoted have been on animals suddenly exposed alone to moderate cold. The syndrome of cold adaptation then includes increased heat production, improved thermal insulation, changed behaviour and altered proportions by weight of organs, tissues and substances. All these entail the operation of negative feedbacks which keep the core temperature and certain chemical features of the body at steady values. Among the feedbacks are those of the nervous and endocrine systems; but there is also intracellular regulation; and compensatory growth is controlled in ways which are still obscure.

A major problem of the immediate future is to analyse just how these many processes, hitherto examined piecemeal, interact and regulate each other. For this, more factual raw material is needed; but, once obtained, it will present problems of multivariate analysis which can be solved only by modern computing methods. The time has come when research programmes may be planned to provide material for computer analysis.

The need for these methods is increased by the temporal sequence of cold adaptation (Section II.C, p. 424). A change of environmental temperature does not merely require a resetting of the rates of a number of regulated processes: there is a series of stages, in each of which there are characteristic settings of, for instance, the rates of hormone secretion and enzyme activity.

B. GENOTYPE AND ENVIRONMENT

The seasonal changes, to which mammals in temperate and arctic regions are exposed, differ from the exposures used in laboratories: (1) they are gradual and fluctuating, and (ii) they are usually ameliorated by the protection of a nest and of huddling with companions. These differences, as Héroux has shown, can certainly influence the course of cold adaptation, even in laboratory rats. Moreover, the response to cold of a wild mammal may be different from that of laboratory strains of the same species (Héroux, 1963). Under genetical differences within species, two general types of effect have to be considered (Barnett, 1965a): (i) heterozygosis alone can confer superior cold resistance; (ii) selection of particular genotypes, in accordance with the demands of the environment, is inevitable in any large, heterogeneous population. Little is known about the detailed operation of either of these.

A more specific question is suggested by the work on wild and laboratory rats just quoted. If isolated wild rats were subject to more severe cold than those observed by Héroux, would their response more closely resemble that of laboratory rats to moderate cold? This sort of question arises also for other species.

C. ONTOGENY AND CROSSED RESISTANCE

Much work has been done on the development of homeothermy in young mammals, but remarkably little is known of the effects on later development of differing degrees of exposure in early life. This sort of question has so far been the concern more of students of behaviour than of physiologists. Early stimulation, involving exposure to cold, can influence later resistance to adverse conditions (Section VII.D, p. 465); it may also affect behaviour and maternal efficiency. The age of exposure is important, for there are sensitive periods in development, during which stimulation by hostile conditions produces more profound changes than at other times.

The multiplicity of the effects of early stimulation raises the question of the effects of exposure to one kind of adversity on resistance to others. For example, if laboratory rats have tourniquets on both hind limbs for 4 hours, most of them die after the bandages are taken off. Previous exposure to cold increases resistance to the hind limb ischaemia so produced; but the relationship between the two types of "stress" is not symmetrical, for previous ischaemia lowers resistance to cold (Schachter et al., 1959; Stoner, 1963). An obvious difference between the two conditions is that cold-adaptation is a slow process which can leave the animal in good health, while ischaemia is not.

An attempt was made in the 1940s to construct a unitary theory of the response to a hostile environment. It was based, in part, on the increased activity of the adrenal cortex resulting from such diverse agencies as cold, infection and wounding (Selye, 1946). Today, adrenal and other endocrine effects are seen as only peripheral: attention is increasingly turned to the brain, especially the hypothalamus, as the source of all adaptive responses to adverse conditions such as cold (e.g. Ganong, 1959; Ganong and Forsham, 1960; Vogt, 1960). Quite separately, the studies of the consequences of early stimulation have led to the notion that, to be effective, stimulation has to be stressful, in the sense of activating the hypothalamus and the pituitary and other endocrine organs (Levine, 1962).

Accordingly, general questions which need to be investigated by experiment now include the following: (i) To what extent does adaptation to one kind of adverse conditions increase or diminish resistance to others? (ii) What are the changes—neural, endocrine and so on—which produce crossed resistance or sensitization? (iii) To what extent does age at exposure to unfavourable conditions influence the later consequences of the exposure? (iv) When there is a prolonged improvement in resistance, what intracellular changes in nervous and other tissues are responsible?

D. PREGNANCY AND MATERNAL EFFECTS

The normal life history of a female mammal includes, in pregnancy and lactation, states which, like exposure to cold, raise the rates of flow of matter through the body. Two general questions are: (i) to what extent does adaptation to cold influence maternal efficiency? (ii) to what extent does pregnancy (or lactation) influence resistance to cold? These questions would have to be made more specific to provide a basis for an experimental programme. First, there is the matter of the precise temperature: what is "cold" to a laboratory mouse would not necessarily be so to a polar bear, *Ursus maritimus*. Second, temperatures which allow survival sometimes preclude breeding: does prior adaptation to cold lower the temperature at which, say, a rat or mouse can reproduce? Third, when a mammal does breed in an ambient temperature much below the optimum, how do the physiological effects of cold and pregnancy (or lactation) interact?

After some pioneering work by Parkes and Brambell (1928), remarkably little work was done on the reproduction of mammals in cold environments for a quarter of a century. But we now know that even laboratory mice can breed at freezing temperatures, given nest material (Section VI, p. 453). Hence a large and almost new area of study of cold adaptation in mammals has been opened. The questions which have consequently to be asked concern not only maternal performance in a hostile environment but also the effects on the young of cold-exposed females. In general, the body weight (for example) of a mammal reflects the maternal genotype (and the environmental influences which have acted on the mother) up to birth or even to weaning; after this, the genotype of the offspring, and the action of the environment in which it is living, become effective (McLaren, 1960). But maternal influences may still be evident in the adult, for instance in the reproductive performance of females. Hence, effects of exposure to cold can be passed, by non-genetical means, to a second generation (Barnett, 1961, 1965a); but the scope of the information so transmitted, and the number of generations which can be measurably influenced, have still to be discovered.

IX. Summary

Mammals are homeothermous in the sense that their deep body temperature remains steady while the outside temperature changes. Thermal neutrality is the range of temperature at which resting metabolism is minimum. The critical temperature is that at which heat production increases, and so maintains body temperature, despite greater heat loss from the surface.

Insulation. The greater the insulation, the lower the critical temperature: the range is from about 30° for small tropical mammals, to − 40° for arctic species. Many mammals grow thicker hair in winter, and some put on more fat. All mammals which have been tested, regardless of insulation, can increase heat production when stimulated by cold. This increase depends on the thermal demand of the environment, or the total heat loss from radiation, convection and conduction.

Immediate Response to Cold. When a mammal is suddenly moved to an environment well below the critical temperature, its first response is peripheral vasoconstriction (which reduces loss of heat) and shivering (which increases heat production). There is also an immediate increase in the secretion of hormones by the adrenal medulla. There follows greater activity by the pituitary, thyroid and adrenal cortex. The metabolic roles of these hormones are not yet clear.

Metabolism. If the cold persists, shivering ceases but extra heat production is still maintained. The development of this "non-shivering thermogenesis" is accompanied by a sequence of changes in the enzymic activities of the muscles, liver and other organs. The cold-adapted tissues are more responsive to noradrenalin.

Eating. In winter, or on experimental exposure to cold, a mammal, even up to the size of a large dog, eats more. But intake is not adjusted to brief fluctuations of temperature. Cold-adapted animals probably also utilize their food more efficiently. The extra food evidently need consist only of carbohydrate, but the optimum diet for severe cold is not known for any species. Rodents, given a choice, take extra carbohydrate rather than protein or fat.

Behaviour. Mammals are less active in a cold than in a warm environment, especially before cold adaptation is complete. Nest-making species make better nests, and select warm surfaces to sit on; huddling by species ranging from mice to pigs can be an important means of conserving heat. Efficient nest building may require a gradual learning from experience. Rats and pigs can learn to push a switch to turn on a source of heat.

Growth. Heat conservation is aided by an increase in body weight in a cold environment, but such an increase rarely, if ever, occurs in an individual mammal on exposure to cold. Laboratory mammals usually lose weight on exposure to about 4°, but young ones may later restore it. Exposure to cold in early life may result in permanent stunting; but later exposure can have an opposite effect. Selection for resistance to cold, over several generations, can result in a genetically determined increase in body weight.

Body shape may be influenced by the temperature of the environment during growth. The appendages, especially the tails of rodents, are shortened by cold.

Adaptation to cold is accompanied, at least in laboratory animals, by the enlargement of organs that do more work, namely, heart, gut, liver and kidneys, and thyroid and adrenal glands. In addition, hair usually grows longer during prolonged exposure.

Changes in body weight, or in the weights of organs, only crudely reflect alterations of function. Organs can become more efficient without increase in size.

Body Composition. On sudden exposure to cold, there is a marked loss of adipose tissue and there may be loss of muscle. These can sometimes be made up after shivering has ceased, but living in a cold environment may entirely prevent the deposition of the amount of fat present in a warm environment. "Brown fat" is a special type of adipose tissue, even more labile than white fat, which produces much heat on sudden exposure to cold. It is important in young mammals. Both types of adipose tissue undergo enzymic changes, evidently adaptive, during prolonged exposure.

Other chemical changes in cold-adapted small mammals include an increase in the proportion of water, and a decline in nitrogen, calcium and collagen.

Reproduction. Usually, mammals stop breeding in the cold season. This may be due to shortage of food, rather than low temperature. Even laboratory mice, given excess food and bedding, can breed in an environment at −3°. In them, low environmental temperatures delay reproductive maturity in the female, lengthen the oestrous cycle, and postpone the birth of the first litter. The effect of cold on reproductive performance depends on whether the animals have been transferred to a cold environment, or reared there. Mice transferred from 21° to −3° (with bedding) as young adults are less fertile; but their offspring are usually less fertile still. The third generation may, however, partly recover. The full scope of such maternal effects has still to be determined, but there is evidence of the possibility of a non-genetical, cumulative adaptation to cold over several generations.

Ontogeny. Small mammals, and some large ones, are virtually heterothermous at birth, but some newborn artiodactyls, at least, are homeothermous. The newborn laboratory rat has some capacity to increase heat production if the outside temperature falls slightly, especially just after a meal; and the guinea-pig, *Cavia*, has greater powers of thermoregulation. Larger mammals respond more effectively: the hairless piglet, *Sus*, can shiver virtually at birth. There is a rapid change towards the adult form of homeothermy during the first days or weeks. Newborn mammals can survive degrees of hypothermia which would kill adults.

Early exposure to moderately adverse conditions, such as cold, can probably improve resistance to stressful conditions in later life.

Problems. The many, changing processes, reflex, behavioural, enzymic and "trophic", involved in adaptation to cold, present problems which can be solved only by multivariate analysis.

Genetical problems include the relationship of hybrid vigour with resistance to cold, and the differences between wild and laboratory varieties of the same species.

Little is known about the effects of early exposure to cold on subsequent development. Exposing an adult to cold can improve its resistance to other adverse conditions, but the mechanism of this crossed resistance (and of the opposite, crossed sensitization) is not known.

A complete account of cold-adaptation in mammals requires information on the effects of cold on reproduction, and on the characteristics of the young of cold-exposed females.

References

Abercrombie, M. (1957). *Symp. Soc. exp. Biol.* **11**, 235.
Adamsons, K., Gandy, G. M. and James, L. S. (1965). *J. Pediat.* **66**, 495.
Adolph, E. F. (1951). *Amer. J. Physiol.* **166**, 75.
Adolph, E. F. (1957). *Quart. Rev. Biol.* **32**, 89.
Aherne, W. and Hull, D. (1964). *Proc. Roy. Soc. Med.* **57**, 1172.
Alexander, G. (1961). *Austral. J. agric. Res.* **12**, 1152.
Alexander, G. (1962). *Austral. J. agric. Res.* **13**, 100.
Anderson, B. (1963). *Acta Physiol. Scand.* **59**, 12.
Anderson, B., Gale, C. C. and Sundsten, J. W. (1963). *In* "Olfaction and Taste", (Y. Zotterman, Ed.). Pergamon Press, Oxford.
Andik, I., Donhoffer, S., Farkas, M. and Schmidt, P. (1963). *Brit. J. Nutr.* **17**, 257.
Angervall, L. and Carlström, E. (1963). *J. theoret. Biol.* **4**, 254.
Armstrong, D. G., Blaxter, K. L., Graham, N. M. and Wainman, F. W. (1959). *Anim. Prod.* **1**, 1.
Babineau, L. and Pagé, E. (1955). *Canad. J. Biochem. Physiol.* **33**, 970.
Baker, D. G. (1960a). *Fed. Proc.* **19**, 125.
Baker, D. G. (1960b). *Canad. J. Biochem. Physiol.* **38**, 205.
Baker, D. G. and Sellers, E. A. (1957). *Canad. J. Biochem. Physiol.* **35**, 631.
Barić, I. (1953). *Bull. Acad. serbe Sci.* **12**, 71.
Barnett, S. A. (1956). *J. exp. Biol.* **33**, 124.
Barnett, S. A. (1959). *Quart. J. exp. Physiol.* **44**, 35.
Barnett, S. A. (1960). *Nature, Lond.* **188**, 500.
Barnett, S. A. (1961). *Proc. Roy. Soc. B.* **155**, 115.
Barnett, S. A. (1962). *J. Reprod. Fert.* **4**, 327.
Barnett, S. A. (1963). "The Rat: A Study in Behaviour", Aldine Press, Chicago. Methuen, London.
Barnett, S. A. (1964). *Quart. J. exp. Physiol.* **49**, 290.
Barnett, S. A. (1965a). *Biol. Rev.* **40**, 5.
Barnett, S. A. (1965b). *Quart. J. exp. Physiol.* **50**, 417.
Barnett, S. A. and Burn, J. (1966). *Nature, Lond.*, in the press.

Barnett, S. A. and Coleman, E. M. (1959). *J. Endocrin.* **19**, 232.

Barnett, S. A. and Coleman, E. M. (1960). *Genet. Res., Camb.* **1**, 25.

Barnett, S. A. and Little, M. J. (1965). *Proc. Roy. Soc. B*, **162**, 492.

Barnett, S. A. and Manly, B. M. (1956). *J. exp. Biol.* **33**, 325.

Barnett, S. A. and Manly, B. M. (1959). *Proc. Roy. Soc. B*, **151**, 87.

Barnett, S. A. and Scott, S. G. (1963). *J. Embryol. exp. Morph.* **11**, 35.

Barnett, S. A. and Scott, S. G. (1964). *Anim. Behav.* **12**, 325.

Barnett, S. A. and Widdowson, E. M. (1965). *Proc. Roy. Soc. B*, **162**, 502.

Barnett, S. A., Coleman, E. M. and Manly, B. M. (1959). *Quart. J. exp. Physiol.* **44**, 43.

Barnett, S. A., Coleman, E. M. and Manly, B. M. (1960). *Quart. J. exp. Physiol.* **45**, 40.

Bazett, H. C., Love, L., Newton, M., Eisenberg, L., Day, R. and Forster, II, R. (1948). *J. appl. Physiol.* **1**, 3.

Beaton, J. R. (1963a). *Canad. J. Biochem. Physiol.* **41**, 139.

Beaton, J. R. (1963b). *Canad. J. Biochem. Physiol.* **41**, 161.

Beaton, J. R. and Sangster, J. F. (1965). *Canad. J. Physiol. Pharmac.* **43**, 241.

Benedict, F. G. (1938). "Vital Energetics", Carnegie Institution of Washington, Publication 503, Washington, D.C.

Benzinger, T. H. (1964). *Symp. Soc. exp. Biol.* **18**, 49.

Benzinger, T. H. and Kitzinger, C. (1963). *In* "Temperature—its Measurement and Control in Science and Industry", (C. M. Herzfeld, Ed.), Vol. 3, Part 3, pp. 87–109. Reinhold, New York.

Bergmann, A. (1847). *Göttingen Studien* **1**, 595.

Berry, I. L. and Shanklin, M. D. (1961). *Res. Bull. Mo. agric. Exp. Sta.* 802.

Biggers, J. D., Ashoub, M. R., McLaren, A. and Michie, D. (1958). *J. exp. Biol.* **35**, 144.

Blaxter, K. L. and Wainman, F. W. (1961). *J. agric. Sci., Camb.* **56**, 81.

Blaxter, K. L., Graham, N. McC. and Wainman, F. W. (1959). *J. agric. Sci. Camb.* **52**, 41.

Bligh, J. (1963). *J. Physiol.* **168**, 764.

Bligh, J. (1966). *Biol. Rev.* **41**, 317.

Bobek, P. and Ginter, E. (1966). *Brit. J. Nutr.* **20**, 61.

Brockway, J. M., McDonald, J. D. and Pullar, J. D. (1965). *J. Physiol.* **179**, 554.

Brody, S. (1945). "Bioenergetics and Growth", Reinhold, New York.

Brown-Grant, K. (1956). *J. Physiol.* **131**, 52.

Brown-Grant, K. (1960). *Brit. med. Bull.* **16**, 165.

Brück, K. (1961). *Biol. Neonat.* **3**, 65.

Brück, K. and Wünnenberg, B. (1965a). *Pflügers Arch. ges. Physiol.* **282**, 362.

Brück, K. and Wünnenberg, B. (1965b). *Pflügers Arch. ges. Physiol.* **283**, 1.

Burton, A. C. and Edholm, O. G. (1955). "Man in a Cold Environment", Arnold, London.

Cameron, I. L. and Smith, R. E. (1964). *J. cell Biol.* **23**, 89.

Campbell, B. A. and Riccio, D. C. (1966). *J. comp. physiol. Psychol.* **61**, 234.

Campbell, H. L. (1945). *Amer. J. Physiol.* **143**, 428.

Cannon, P. and Keatinge, W. R. (1960). *J. Physiol.* **154**, 329.

Carlson, L. D. (1960). *Fed. Proc.* **19**, 25.

Chaffee, R. R. J., Clark, R. T., Reynafarje, B., Cunningham, M. D. and Bartlett, W. L. (1963). *Proc. Soc. exp. Biol. N.Y.* **113**, 115.

Chaffee, R. R. J., Allen, J. R., Cassuto, Y. and Smith, R. E. (1964). *Amer. J. Physiol.* **207**, 1211.

Chevillard, L. and Cadot, M. (1963). *C. R. Seanc. Soc. Biol.* **157**, 1388.

Chevillard, L., Cadot, M. and Portet, R. (1962). *C. R. Seanc. Soc. Biol.* **156**, 1043.

Cohn, C. and Joseph, D. (1960). *Amer. J. clin. Nutr.* **8**, 682.

Consolazio, C. F. (1963). *Wld. Rev. Nutr. Diet.* **4**, 55.

Cottle, W. H. and Carlson, L. D. (1956). *Proc. Soc. exp. Biol. N.Y.* **92**, 845.

Davis, T. R. A., Johnston, D. R. and Bell, F. C. (1959). Report 386, Envtl. Med. Div., U.S. Army Med. Res. Lab., Fort Knox, Kentucky.

Davis, T. R. A., Johnston, D. R., Bell, F. C. and Cremer, B. J. (1960). *Amer. J. Physiol.* **198**, 471.

Dawes, G. S. and Mott, J. C. (1959). *J. Physiol.* **146**, 295.

Dawes, G. S., Jacobson, H. N., Mott, J. C. and Shelley, H. J. (1960). *J. Physiol.* **152**, 271.

Dawkins, M. J. R. and Hull, D. (1963). *J. Physiol.* **169**, 101.

Dawkins, M. J. R. and Hull, D. (1964). *J. Physiol.* **172**, 216.

Dawkins, M. J. R. and Scopes, J. W. (1965). *Nature, Lond.* **206**, 201.

Deb, C. and Hart, J. S. (1956). *Canad. J. Biochem. Physiol.* **34**, 959.

Depocas, F. (1961). *Brit. med. Bull.* **17**, 25.

Donhoffer, S. Z. and Vonotzky, J. (1947). *Amer. J. Physiol.* **150**, 329.

Dugal, P. L., Leblond, C. P. and Thérien, M. (1945). *Canad. J. Res. E.* **23**, 244

Durrer, J. L. and Hannon, J. P. (1962). *Amer. J. Physiol.* **202**, 375.

Eayrs, J. T. (1951). *J. Endocrin.* **7**, 349.

Emery, F. E., Emery, L. M. and Schwabe, E. L. (1940). *Growth* **4**, 17.

Euler, C. von (1961). *Pharmacol. Rev.* **13**, 361.

Euler, C. von and Soderberg, U. (1958). *Acta physiol. scand.* **42**, 112.

Fairfield, J. (1948). *Amer. J. Physiol.* **155**, 355.

Farrand, R. L. (1959). *Stud. Nat. Hist. Ia. Univ.* **20** (*iii*) 1.

Fenton, P. F. (1960). *Postgrad. med. J.* **28**, 173.

Fitzgerald, L. R. (1953). *J. exp. Zool.* **124**, 415.

Fraps, R. M. (1962). *In* "The Ovary", (S. Zuckerman, Ed.), Vol. 2. Academic Press, New York.

Fregly, M. J., Iampietro, P. F. and Otis, A. B. (1961). *J. appl. Physiol.* **16**, 127.

Ganong, W. F. (1959). *In* "Comparative Endocrinology", (A. Gorbman, Ed.), Wiley, New York.

Ganong, W. F. and Forsham, P. H. (1960). *Annu. Rev. Physiol.* **22**, 579.

Gelineo, S. (1954). *C. R. Seanc. Soc. Biol.*, **148**, 1483.

Gelineo, S. (1957). *Bull. Acad. serbe. Sci.* **18**, 97.

Gelineo, S. (1959). *Usp. Sovrem. biol.* **47**, 108.

Gelineo, S. and Gelineo, A. (1951). *C. R. hebd. Seanc. Acad. Sci., Paris* **232**, 1031.

Gelineo, S. and Gelineo, A. (1952). *Bull. Acad. serbe Sci.* **4**, 197.

Giaja, J. (1938). *Actual. scient. ind.* **576**, 577.

Giaja, J. and Gelineo, S. (1934). *C. R. hebd. Seanc. Acad. Sci., Paris* **198**, 2227.

Görner, G. (1956). *Z. vergl. Physiol.* **38**, 317.

Goss, R. J. (1964). "Adaptive Growth", Academic Press, New York.

Graham, N. McC., Wainman, F. W., Blaxter, K. L. and Armstrong, D. G. (1959). *J. agric. Sci., Camb.* **52**, 13.

Gridgeman, N. T. and Héroux, O. (1965). *Canad. J. Physiol. Pharmac.* **43**, 351.

Grindeland, R. E. and Folk, G. E. (1962). *J. Reprod. Fert.* **4**, 1.

Hahn, P., Koldovský, O., Křeček, J., Martínek, J. and Vaček, Z. (1961). *In* "Somatic Stability in the Newly Born", (G. E. W. Wolstenhome and M. O'Connor, Eds.), pp. 131–148. Churchill, London.

Hammel, H. T. (1964). *In* "Handbook of Physiology. Section IV. Adaptation to the Environment", (D. B. Dill, Ed.), pp. 413–434. American Physiological Society, Washington, D.C.

Hannon, J. P. (1963). *Fed. Proc.* **22**, 856.

Hardy, J. D. (1949). *In* "Physiology of Heat Regulation", (L. H. Newburgh, Ed.), p. 78. Saunders, Philadelphia.

Hardy, J. D. (1955). *Harvey Lect.* **49**, 242.

Hardy, J. D. (1961). *Physiol. Rev.* **41**, 521.

Harrison, G. A. (1958). *J. exp. Biol.* **35**, 892.

Harrison, G. A. (1963). *Fed. Proc.* **22**, 691.

Hart, J. S. (1953). *Canad. J. Zool.* **31**, 117.

Hart, J. S. (1956). *Canad. J. Zool.* **34**, 53.

Hart, J. S. (1957). *Revue canad. Biol.* **16**, 133.

Hart, J. S. (1963). *In* "Temperature—its Measurement and Control in Science and Industry", (C. M. Herzfeld, Ed.), Vol. 3, Part 3, pp. 373–406. Reinhold, New York.

Hart, J. S. (1964a). *Symp. Soc. exp. Biol.* **18**, 31.

Hart, J. S. (1964b). *In* "Handbook of Physiology. Section IV. Adaptation to the Environment", (D. B. Hill, Ed.). American Physiological Society, Washington, D.C.

Hart, J. S. and Héroux, O. (1955). *Canad. J. Biochem. Physiol.* **33**, 428.

Hart, J. S. and Héroux, O. (1956). *Canad. J. Biochem. Physiol.* **34**, 414.

Hart, J. S. and Héroux, O. (1963). *Canad. J. Zool.* **41**, 711.

Hart, J. S. and Jansky, L. (1963). *Canad. J. Biochem. Physiol.* **41**, 629.

Hart, J. S., Héroux, O., Cottle, W. H. and Mills, C. A. (1961). *Canad. J. Zool.* **39**, 845.

Hart, J. S., Pohl, H. and Tener, J. S. (1965). *Canad. J. Zool.* **43**, 731.

Hayward, J. S. (1965). *Canad. J. Zool.* **43**, 341.

Hensel, H. (1956). *Klin. Wschr.* **34**, 1273.

Héroux, O. (1959a). *Canad. J. Biochem. Physiol.* **37**, 811.

Héroux, O. (1959b). *Canad. J. Biochem. Physiol.* **37**, 1247.

Héroux, O. (1961). *Revue canad. Biol.* **20**, 55.

Héroux, O. (1962). *Canad. J. Biochem. Physiol.* **40**, 537.

Héroux, O. (1963). *Fed. Proc.* **22**, 789.

Héroux, O. and Gridgeman, N. T. (1958). *Canad. J. Biochem. Physiol.* **36**, 209.

Héroux, O. and St. Pierre J. (1957). *Amer. J. Physiol.* **188**, 163.

Herter, K. (1941). *Naturwissenschaften* **29**, 155.

Hill, J. R. and Rahimtulla, K. A. (1965). *J. Physiol.* **180**, 239.

Hoffman, R. A. (1964). *In* "Adaptation to the Environment", (D. B. Dill, Ed.), pp. 379–403. American Physiological Society, Washington, D.C.

Hollifield, G. and Parson, W. (1962a). *J. clin. Invest.* **41**, 245.

Hollifield, G. and Parson, W. (1962b). *J. clin. Invest.* **41**, 250.

Hsieh, A. C. L. and Carlson, L. D. (1957). *Amer. J. Physiol.* **188**, 40.

Hsieh, A. C. L., Carlson, L. D. and Gray, G. (1957). *Amer. J. Physiol.* **190**, 247.

Hull, D. (1965). *J. Physiol.* **177**, 192.

Hull, D. (1966). *Brit. med. Bull.* **22**, 92.

Hull, D. and Segall, M. M. (1964). *J. Physiol.* **175**, 58.

Hull, D. and Segall, M. M. (1965). *J. Physiol.* **177**, 63.

Hutchings, D. E. (1963). *Trans. N.Y. Acad. Sci.* **25**, 890.

Iampietro, P. F., Vaughan, J. A., Goldman, R. F., Kreider, M. B., Masucci, F. and Bass, D. E. (1960). *J. appl. Physiol.* **15**, 632.

Ingram, D. L. (1964a). *Res. vet. Sci.* **5**, 348.

Ingram, D. L. (1964b). *Res. vet. Sci.* **5**, 357.

Irving, L. (1956). *J. appl. Physiol.* **9**, 414.

Irving, L., Krog, H. and Monson, M. (1955). *Physiol. Zoöl.* **28**, 173.

Jensen, C. and Ederstrom, H. E. (1955). *Amer. J. Physiol.* **183**, 340.

Johansson, B. (1959). *Metabolism* **8**, 221.

Joy, R. J. T. (1963). *J. appl. Physiol.* **18**, 1209.

Joyce, J. P. and Blaxter, K. L. (1964). *Brit. J. Nutr.* **18**, 5.

Karlberg, P. (1952). *Acta Paediat., Stockh.* **41**, Supplement 89, 11.

Kayser, C. (1959). *C.R. Seanc. Soc. Biol.* **153**, 167.

Kayser, C. (1961). "The Physiology of Natural Hibernation", Pergamon, Oxford.

Keller, A. D. (1960). *Fed. Proc.* **19**, 30.

Kinder, E. F. (1927). *J. exp. Zool.* **47**, 117.

Klain, G. J. and Vaughan, D. A. (1963). *Fed. Proc.* **22**, 862.

Kleiber, M. (1947). *Physiol. Rev.* **27**, 511.

Kleiber, M. (1961). "The Fire of Life", Wiley, New York.

Kleiber, M. (1963). *Fed. Proc.* **22**, 772.

Knigge, K. M. (1960). *Fed. Proc.* **19**, 45.

Koch, W. (1962). *Nature, Lond.* **196**, 587.

Lang, K. and Crab, W. (1946). *Klin. Wch.* **24**, 37.

Lasiewski, R. C. (1963). *Physiol. Zoöl.* **36**, 122.

Leduc, J. (1961). *Acta Physiol. Scand.* 53, suppt 183, p. 5.

Lee, M. O. (1926). *Amer. J. Physiol.* **78**, 246.

Levine, S. (1962). *In* "Experimental Foundations of Clinical Psychology", A. J. Bachrach, Ed.), pp. 371–402. Basic Books, New York.

McCance, R. A. (1959). *Archs. Dis. Childh.* **34**, 459.

McIntyre, D. G. and Ederstrom, H. E. (1958). *Amer. J. Physiol.* **194**, 293.

McLaren, A. (1960). *Proc. 1st. Int. Conf. on Congenital Malformations, Lond.* pp. 211–222.

Masoro, E. J. (1963). *Fed. Proc.* **22**, 868.

Masoro, E. J. (1966). *Physiol. Rev.* **46**, 67.

Mendelsohn, E. (1964). "Heat and Life", University Press, Harvard.

Miller, Jr, A. T. and Blyth, C. S. (1958). *J. appl. Physiol.* **12**, 17.

Moore, R. E. and Underwood, M. C. (1963). *J. Physiol.* **168**, 290.

Mount, L. E. (1959). *J. Physiol.* **147**, 333.

Mount, L. E. (1960). *J. agric. Sci., Camb.* **55**, 101.

Mount, L. E. (1961). *In* "Somatic Stability in the Newly Born", (G. E. W. Wolstenholme and M. O'Connor, Eds.), pp. 117–130. Churchill, London.

Mount, L. E. (1963a). *Fed. Proc.* **22**, 818.

Mount, L. E. (1963b). *J. Physiol.* **168**, 698.

Mount, L. E. (1963c). *Anim. Prod.* **5**, 223.

Mount, L. E. (1963d). *Nature, Lond.* **199**, 122.

Mount, L. E. (1964a). *J. Physiol.* **170**, 286.

Mount, L. E. (1964b). *J. Physiol.* **173**, 96.

Mount, L. E. (1965). *In* "Energy Metabolism", (K. L. Blaxter, Ed.), pp. 379–386. European Association for Animal Production Publication, no. 11. Academic Press, London.

Mount, L. E. (1966a). *Brit. med. Bull.* **22**, 84.

Mount, L. E. (1966b). *Quart. J. exp. Physiol.* **51**, 18.

Mount, L. E. and Ingram, D. L. (1965). *Res. vet. Sci.* **6**, 84.

Mount, L. E. and Rowell, J. G. (1960). *J. Physiol.* **154**, 408.

Mourek, J. (1962). *J. Physiol., Paris* **54**, 384.

Newland, H. W., McMillen, W. N. and Reineke, E. P. (1952). *J. anim. Sci.* **11**, 118.

16 + T.

476　　S. A. BARNETT AND L. E. MOUNT

Ostermann, K. (1956). *Jber. Zool.* **66**, 355.

Pagé, E. (1957). *Revue canad. Biol.* **16**, 269.

Pagé, E. and Babineau, L. M. (1953). *Canad. J. med. Sci.* **31**, 22.

Parkes, A. S. and Brambell, F. W. R. (1928). *J. Physiol.* **64**, 388.

Pearson, O. P. (1960). *Physiol. Zool.* **33**, 152.

Perrault, M. J. and Dugal, L. P. (1965). *Canad. J. Physiol. Pharmacol.* **43**, 809.

Pohl, H. and Hart, J. S. (1965). *J. appl. Physiol.* **20**, 398.

Pomeroy, R. W. (1953). *J. agric. Sci., Camb.* **43**, 182.

Prychodko, W. (1958). *Ecology* **39**, 500.

Przibram, H. (1923). "Temperatur und Temperatoren im Tierreiche", Deutige, Leipzig.

Ragsdale, A. C., Thompson, H. J., Worstell, D. M. and Brody, S. (1950). *Res. Bull. Univ. Missouri*, no. 460.

Rand, R. P., Burton, A. C. and Ing, T. (1965). *Canad. J. Physiol. Pharmacol.* **43**, 257.

Richter, C. P. (1937). *Cold Spr. Harb. Symp. quant. Biol.* **5**, 258.

Ross, S. and Smith, W. (1953). *J. genet. Psychol.* **62**, 299.

Roy, J. H. B., Huffman, C. F. and Reineke, E. P. (1957). *Brit. J. Nutr.* **11**, 373.

Sandblom, P. (1949). *Ann. Surg.* **129**, 305.

Schachter, H., Sidlofsky, S., Baker, D. G., Hamilton, J. R. and Haist, R. E. (1959). *Canad. J. Biochem. Physiol.* **37**, 211.

Schaefer, T. (1963). *Trans. N.Y. Acad. Sci.* **25**, 871.

Scholander, P. F. (1955). *Evolution* **9**, 16.

Scholander, P. F. (1958). "Counter Current Exchange; a Principle in Biology", Hvalrådets Skrifter. Scientific results of marine biological research, no. 44. 1 Kommisjon Hos. H. Aschehong and Co., Oslo.

Scholander, P. F., Hock, R., Walters, V., Johnson, F. and Irving, L. (1950). *Biol. Bull. mar. biol. Lab., Woods Hole* **99**, 237.

Scholander, P. F., Hammel, H. T., Andersen, K. L. and Løyning, Y. (1958a). *J. appl. Physiol.* **12**, 1.

Scholander, P. F., Hammel, H. T., Hart, J. S., Lemessurier, D. H. and Steen, J. (1958b). *J. appl. Physiol.* **13**, 211.

Sealander, J. A. (1951). *J. Mammal.* **32**, 122.

Sealander, J. A. (1952). *Ecology* **33**, 63.

Sellers, E. A. (1957). *Revue canad. Biol.* **16**, 175.

Sellers, E. A., You, R. W. and Moffatt, N. M. (1954). *Amer. J. Physiol.* **177**, 367.

Selye, H. (1946). *J. clin. Endocr. Metab.* **6**, 117.

Shapiro, B. (1963). *Wld. Rev. Nutr. Diet.* **4**, 81.

Silverman, W. A. and Agate, Jr., F. J. (1964). *Biol. Neonat.* **6**, 113.

Smith, R. E. (1963). *Fed. Proc.* **22**, 738.

Smith, R. E. (1964). *Science* **146**, 1686.

Smith, R. E. and Hoijer, D. J. (1962). *Physiol. Rev.* **42**, 60.

Sørensen, P. H. (1962). In "Nutrition of Pigs and Poultry", (J. T. Morgan and D. Lewis, Eds.), pp. 88–103. Butterworths, London.

Stevenson, J. A. F. and Rixon, R. H. (1954). *Revue canad. Biol.* **13**, 91.

Stinson, R. H. and Fisher, K. C. (1953). *Canad. J. Zool.* **31**, 404.

Stone, C. P. and Mason, W. A. (1955). *J. comp. Physiol. Psychol.* **48**, 456.

Stoner, H. B. (1963). *Fed. Proc.* **22**, 851.

Strecker, R. L. (1955). *J. Mammal.* **36**, 460.

Sumner, F. B. (1909). *J. exp. Zool.* **7**, 97.

Sumner, F. B. (1915). *J. exp. Zool.* **18**, 325.

Taylor, P. M. (1960). *J. Physiol.* **154**, 153.

Templeton, H. A. and Ershoff, B. H. (1949). *Amer. J. Physiol.* **159**, 33.

Thauer, R. (1961). *Arch. des Sciences Physiol.* **15**, 95.

Thompson, G. E. and Stevenson, J. A. F. (1965). *Canad. J. Physiol. Pharmacol.* **43**, 279.

Thompson, G. E. and Stevenson, J. A. F. (1966). *Canad. J. Physiol. Pharmacol.* **44**, 139.

Thorne, O. (1958). Thorne Ecol. Res. Stat. Boulder, Colorado Bull., no. 6, 1.

Vogt, M. (1960). *Biochem. Soc. Symp.* **18**, 85.

Waites, G. M. H. and Moule, G. R. (1961). *J. Reprod. Fert.* **2**, 213.

Weiss, B. (1957). *J. comp. Physiol. Psychol.* **50**, 481.

Weiss, B. (1958). *Science* **127**, 467.

Weiss, B. and Laties, V. G. (1960). *J. comp. Physiol. Psychol.* **53**, 603.

Weiss, B. and Laties, V. G. (1961). *Science* **133**, 1338.

Widdowson, E. M. (1950). *Nature, Lond.* **166**, 626.

Widdowson, E. M. and Kennedy, G. C. (1962). *Proc. Roy. Soc. B* **156**, 96.

Wiesner, B. P. and Sheard, N. M. (1933). "Maternal Behaviour in the Rat", Oliver & Boyd, Edinburgh.

Williams, G. E. G. (1961). *Brit. J. exp. Path.* **42**, 386.

Wilson, P. N. and Osbourn, D. F. (1960). *Biol. Rev.* **35**, 324.

Yaglou, C. P. (1949). *In* "Physiology of Heat Regulation", (L. H. Newburgh, Ed.), p. 286. Saunders, Philadelphia.

Yamada, T., Kajihara, A., Onaya, T., Kobayshi, I., Takemura, Y. and Shichijo, K. (1965). *Endocrinology* **77**, 968.

Young, D. R. and Cook, S. F. (1955). *Amer. J. Physiol.* **181**, 72.

Zollhauser, M. (1958). *Z. vergl. Physiol.* **40**, 642.

Chapter 13

Resistance to Heat in Man and Other Homeothermic Animals

HARWOOD S. BELDING

*Graduate School of Public Health, University of
Pittsburgh, Pittsburgh, Pennsylvania, U.S.A.*

I. Introduction

The statement that mammals and birds are homeotherms implies that they possess successful mechanisms for the maintenance of relative internal thermal constancy under climatic conditions which have the potential for lowering or elevating body temperature. It has long been recognized by biologists that the capacity to adjust heat losses from the body so that they balance metabolic and other potential gains imparts a special advantage (Cannon, 1939). The basic chemical reactions of metabolism are temperature-dependent as are all chemical reactions, approximately doubling in rate for each 10° rise in temperature over the range 0–40°. The ability to maintain a stable body temperature over a range of environmental temperatures and of metabolic activity permits predictable responses of the receptor, integrating and effector mechanisms of the body. The homeotherm is thus free, within broad limits, to determine his own activities rather than have them determined for him by environmental conditions.

This chapter is restricted to one aspect of the range of thermal stress, namely heat stress. It would appear that almost all birds and mammals cope with heat stress at one time or another, particularly when they are active. The argument that this is so is based on the concept of *critical* temperature, which is defined as that environmental temperature below which resting metabolism is raised in defence against body cooling. The critical temperature varies with the natural habitat, as has been demonstrated by Scholander *et al.* (1950a,b); in other words, the resting metabolic rate and the amount of insulation provided by the skin and its natural covering are in approximate balance in the usual habitat of a species.

Heat stress may be considered to exist whenever physiological mechanisms, such as an increase in dermal blood flow, sweating, or panting, must be activated to bring heat loss into balance with metabolic heat production. This being so, animals like the arctic fox or bear, which have heavy insulation, may be under heat stress in an environment at 0°, even while inactive, whereas the tropical raccoon or man may not be under such stress until a temperature of at least 30° is reached.

But the purpose of this chapter is not simply to state the thermal conditions that are critical for the appearance of heat stress. We are interested in physiological responses which result from various intensities of imposed heat stress, the mechanisms for maintaining thermal homeostasis, and the factors which determine the tolerance limits and the types and manifestations of overstrain. This chapter gives consideration to all of these phenomena as they apply to man. Man is chosen as the principal model partly because we know more about his responses, but also because his capacity for maintaining homeothermism under heat stress is relatively highly developed.

The literature on the responses and adaptations of man to heat stress is voluminous. For more detailed information the reader is referred to a number of comprehensive treatments each of which contains a large list of references to original articles. Dill (1964) assembled chapters by several authorities, as did Hardy (1963). McPherson (1960) reviewed and interpreted a long series of studies that were sponsored by the British Medical Research Council. Newburgh's (1949) book summarized much of the work on man performed in the U.S.A. prior to and during World War II. Hardy (1961) provided a long, critical review on temperature regulation. It is obvious that in preparing this chapter it has been necessary to exercise a high degree of selectivity in making literature citations. And it is only fair to admit that, when illustrating the findings on men, the author has found it convenient to cite the studies in which he and his colleagues have been involved over the past 25 years.

Certain responses of other mammals and birds are indicated at the end of the chapter. In these accounts, the emphasis is on deviations from the pattern described for man.

II. Resistance to Heat in Man

A. MAN AS A TROPICAL ANIMAL

Man is a tropical animal. This statement is based not only on the negative reasoning that his critical temperature is higher than that of

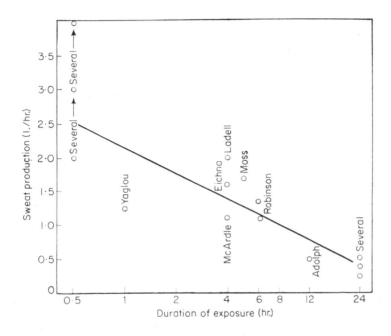

FIG. 1. Rates of sweating observed in studies of various investigators, plotted as a function of the duration of exposure to heat. Note that a sweat production of 3–4 litres per hour has been recorded for brief periods. The highest average rates observed for 24 hours involve turnover of about 12 litres of body water per day. From Belding and Hatch (1956).

most other animals because of his relative lack of hairy insulation. There is the positive reason that he has a well developed capacity to sweat, as indicated in Fig. 1. Under favourable circumstances, man can produce sweat at a rate of one litre an hour for several hours, and by so doing achieve evaporative cooling to the extent of nearly 600 kcal./hr. This is sufficient to remove the metabolic heat he produces at sustained hard work in an environment at 35°. It can also remove his metabolic heat when walking at the rate of 5 km./hr., together with the heat impinging on him from an environment at 50°, provided that the ambient conditions are dry enough to permit full evaporation of the sweat which he produces. The capacity is sufficient to permit survival in the hottest natural climates on the earth, if he is protected from direct insolation.

B. HEAT STRESS

The heat load which results from the exposure of a nude man may be estimated from a knowledge of his metabolic rate, M, and of the environmental conditions which establish gain (or loss) by radiation, R, and convection, C, by:

$$M + R + C = \text{heat load}$$

The heat load is the evaporative equivalent of the sweat required to maintain thermal balance, E_{req}. Thus,

$$M + R + C = E_{req}$$

The statement is simplified in that it omits consideration of the fraction of M which is going into external work, and which, therefore, does not appear as part of the heat to be dissipated. E_{req} includes heat of vaporization of water from the lungs as well as from the skin. Woodcock and Breckenridge (1965) provided a detailed theoretical model of thermal exchange for the nude man in hot environments.

1. *Coefficients of Heat Exchange*

Hatch (1963) has recently provided a revision of the coefficients which he originally developed with others to describe heat exchanges of nude men by radiation and convection, and the potential for the removal of heat by evaporation, E_{max}. Four environmental measurements provide the necessary data; these are air temperature, t_a; the equilibrium temperature of a 15·2 cm. (6 in.) blackened globe, t_g; the wet bulb temperature, t_{wb}; and the air speed, V. The temperature of the skin, t_s, and the amount of body surface area exposed for transfer must also be known. Hatch has shown how t_s values may be estimated from a knowledge of M and of the environmental factors, but he also pointed out that the assumption that $t_s = 35°$ provides an acceptable approximation under many circumstances of exposure. He used this value, and the further assumption that the surface area is that of a 70 kg. *standard man*, namely 1·86 m.², to provide specific coefficients for R, C and E_{max}. These coefficients are given below.

Radiation exchange is a fourth-power function of the gradient between the temperature of the solid surround, t_w, and t_s. However, unless the radiation load is very large, a first power relationship can be used for estimating R. Thus:

$$R = K_r(t_w - t_s)$$

For the standard man:

$$R = 11(t_w - 35) \text{ kcal./hr.}$$

To obtain t_w, one applies the equation:

$$t_w = t_g + 0.24 V^{0.5}(t_g - t_a)$$

where V is in m./min. The coefficient assumes that the skin is exchanging radiation as a black body, which is true for long-wave radiation. When exposed to direct sunlight, some of the energy is reflected. This has the effect of decreasing the value of K_r from 11 to about 7 kcal./hr. if the skin is light, and to about 9 kcal./hr. if it is dark.

Exchange by convection is a function of V and t_a, as given by the equation:

$$C = K_c . V^{0.6}(t_a - t_s)$$

For the standard man:

$$C = 1.0 V^{0.6}(t_a - 35) \text{ kcal./hr.}$$

The calculation of the heat load, $M + R + C$, allows an estimate of the rate of sweat production required for heat balance. Within the physiological capacity for sweat production (Fig. 1), and under ambient conditions in which free evaporation is possible, it has been shown that sweat will be produced in an amount sufficient to balance the load. Actually, there is always an insensible loss of water from the skin and lungs. Thirty g./hr. is a representative amount for a resting man, and this amount would account for 18 kcal./hr. of the evaporative heat loss. Evaporative loss from the lungs is proportional to the ventilatory volume and to the difference in water vapour pressure between the inspired and the expired air. Thus:

$$E_l = (0.6) . (\text{no. mm.}^3 \text{ respired}) . (VP_l - VP_a) \text{ kcal.}$$

where VP_l is the vapour pressure in the lungs. VP_l may be assumed to be the vapour pressure of saturation at body core temperature; e.g. at 37° it would be 47 mm.Hg. The equation given for E_{max} includes a nominal assessment of E_l. The evaporative equivalent of sweat is approximately 0.58 kcal./g.

To estimate whether the necessary evaporative capacity is available

16*

in a given environment requires a consideration of the effective gradient of water vapour pressure and V. Thus:

$$E_{max} = K_e . V^{0.6}(VP_s - VP_a)$$

where VP_s is the water vapour pressure at the skin when fully wetted; at 35° it is 42 mm.Hg. The vapour pressure of the ambient air, VP_a, is

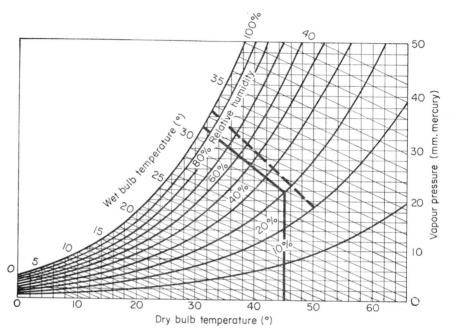

FIG. 2. A psychrometric chart. The superimposed heavy lines indicate the calculated prediction of limiting conditions for maintaining heat balance at a normal level, using the assumptions stated in the text. The vertical segment indicates the limit when sweat production is 1 litre per hour and evaporation from the skin is unrestricted. The diagonal extension denotes the limit as determined by evaporative capacity. The broken line indicates the limiting conditions for maintaining heat balance as reported by Robinson et al. (1945) for conditions nearly the same as those used in the calculated prediction.

obtainable from a psychrometric chart, at the intercept of t_a and t_{wb} (Fig. 2). For the standard man:

$$E_{max} = 2.0 V^{0.6}(42 - VP_a) \text{ kcal./hr.}$$

The equation for the heat exchanges of the standard man can be used to predict the limiting conditions for maintaining heat balance. The results of such a prediction may be shown on a psychrometric chart an example of which is given in Fig. 2. The question to be answered with this experiment was what are the limiting conditions for a man who is walking at 6 km./hr. at a cost of 350 kcal./hr.? It is necessary to know the air speed and, in this case, we assume it is 90 m./min. For simplicity, we also assume that the air temperature and the temperature of the solid surround (effective radiant temperature) are equal. The subject cannot be expected to sweat more than about 1 litre/hr.; thus, his potential evaporative cooling will not exceed 600 kcal./hr.

What conclusions can be drawn? First, the sum of the contributions from radiation and convection cannot exceed 600 minus 350, i.e. 250 kcal./hr. Calculations show that $R + C = 250$ when t_a and t_w are 44·7°. The heavy vertical line on Fig. 2 depicts this limit. Second, at what point does the capacity for evaporation become just equal to 600 kcal./hr.? Using the equation for E_{max} to solve for VP_a, we find that the limit is reached when $VP_a = 21·9$ mm.Hg. Thus, the vertical line at 44·7° terminates at that intercept. Third, what line describes the condition for heat balance when E_{max} is less than 600 kcal./hr.? Values for $R + C$ must be less by the same amount. For example, when $R + C = 0$ (i.e. at 35°), the heat load is represented by M alone (350 kcal./hr.). By calculation, $E_{max} = 350$ kcal./hr. at $VP_a = 30·2$ mm.Hg. This point and the upper end of the 44·7° line can be used to define the position of the diagonal line representing $E_{req} = E_{max}$.

It is of interest to compare such a line with actual experience. Robinson et al. (1945) showed that fit men, dressed in shorts, could maintain heat balance at $M = 350$, under the combinations of conditions indicated by the broken line in Fig. 2. The slope of the diagonal is somewhat steeper, and the position is displaced upward by about 3–5 mm.Hg. Robinson showed no vertical line in his data because he was not exploring responses to low humidities at the limits of sweating of his men. The discrepancy between the two limit lines may partially be accounted for. Robinson's men were walking up a moderate grade, so that about 23 kcal./hr. of the metabolic cost went into external work of climbing and did not appear as heat to be lost through the skin. Also, the skin temperatures of Robinson's subjects averaged 0·6° higher than the 35° assumed in the use of the equations. Consequently, the potential vapour pressure gradient was 1·5 mm.Hg higher. If these factors are taken into account, the predicted limits for Robinson's men are different by only 0·5–2·0 mm.Hg from those which he actually observed. Incidentally, the slope of these lines is only a little steeper than that for the wet bulb lines. Long before systematic data were available, Haldane (1905) noted that heat strain is better related to wet bulb temperatures than to dry bulb temperatures.

A word of caution is indicated against interpreting the calculated limits as being safe for prolonged exposures. The fact that the limits for maintaining heat balance can be predicted does not mean that the strain for some individuals will not be excessive under those conditions. Nor does it indicate that more severe conditions will be intolerable if the exposure is brief.

2. *Role of Clothing*

Clothing imposes a barrier against heat transfer by all three of the available avenues. By interfering with air motion across the skin, i.e. by lowering the value for V, it decreases convection and the potential for evaporation. A decrease of convective transfer when under heat stress is a disadvantage if air temperatures are lower than the skin temperature, and an advantage if the gradient is in the opposite direction. The effect of clothing in decreasing the evaporative potential is usually not critical unless the ambient vapour pressure is high, as in the wet tropics, or the clothing material is relatively impermeable. It has been suggested tentatively that the decrease in the values for C and E_{max} attributable to the wearing of ordinary work clothing is of the order of 30–40%, but data to support this estimate are incomplete.

The wearing of clothing also decreases transfer by radiation. When the radiant temperature is high, as for example near industrial furnaces, ordinary work clothing such as cotton khaki shirt and trousers, has been found to decrease the amount of energy impinging on the skin by as much as 30–40% (Belding *et al.*, 1960b). Adolph *et al.* (1947) estimated that the solar heat gain for seminude men in the desert was about 200 kcal./hr. The wearing of clothing of light colour decreased the gain by about half. The effect was to decrease the demand on the sweating mechanism by about 170 g./hr.; this is equivalent to decreasing the values for both t_a and t_w by 4–5°.

The relatively thick, loose fitting, light coloured clothing used by natives of the Middle East is appropriate in that it provides protection against desert extremes of heat in daytime and of cold at night. In coastal areas, where the ambient water vapour pressure is high, the clothing can be adjusted to permit the necessary evaporation of the sweat. In the wet tropics, where air temperatures rarely exceed 33° and the evaporative potential is small, the wearing of any clothing would appear to be disadvantageous.

The physical properties of clothing fabrics which are related to thermal transfer, the physiological effects of wearing clothing and the clothing customs of primitive peoples are considered in chapters in Newburgh's (1949) book.

3. *Tolerance Time*

Tolerance time, under conditions too hot for prolonged exposure, is a subject of interest to the so-called hot industries, e.g. glass and metal production, to military commanders, and to those responsible for lifting man into space. Students of the subject of heat tolerance have been courageous as well as curious, the challenge being to bring subjects, often themselves, as closely as possible to the point of collapse. Blagden (1775) and his colleague Fordyce were pioneers. In one experiment, they exposed themselves in a room heated to 125°. Their observations emphasized the separate effects of the air temperature, the radiant heat from a stove, and the humidity on physiological strain. They attributed their endurance of such high temperatures in part to the evaporation of sweat. For the benefit of sceptics, they "overdid" a beefsteak in one of the environments which they tolerated.

Robinson *et al.* (1945) studied the effects of various combinations of air temperature and humidity on men at three levels of activity, with and without clothing. They contrived an *Index of Physiological Effect* to measure the severity in terms of pulse rate, rectal temperature, skin temperature and sweat rate. Concurrently, the London "Queen Square group", sponsored by the Medical Research Council and led by B. McArdle (see McPherson, 1960), carried out similar work. They decided that sweat rate offered the best single criterion of physiological strain, and suggested the *Probable Four Hour Sweat Rate* (P4SR) as an index of the severity of exposure conditions.

Wyndham *et al.* (1952) explored the endurance of wet heat, at three levels of activity, and of wind speed. Men endured for up to 4 hours the highest level of work (400 kcal./hr.) at a wet bulb temperature of 32°; the same tolerance time was found for the lowest level of work (175 kcal./hr.) at 35°. However, in both cases, rectal temperatures rose to about 39°. High air speed had a favourable physiological effect, as would be expected under conditions where E_{max} is limiting.

Goldman *et al.* (1965) described the endurance of men while at rest in even hotter wet environments. Wet bulb temperatures up to 36° were endured for the limit of 3 hours. However, at 46°, the tolerance time averaged only 19 min. It is reasonable to suppose that, under these last circumstances, sweating was completely ineffective and that some heat was gained by the condensation of ambient water vapour on the skin.

Figure 3 was assembled by Lind (1963b) to show the tolerance time as found by various investigators (under conditions where $t_w = t_a$). He equated heat load and humidity by using the weighting factor:

$$0 \cdot 85 t_{wb} + 0 \cdot 15 t_a = WD$$

where t_{wb} is the wet bulb temperature and WD is the *Wet, Dry Index*. The system is a simplification of that originally suggested by Yaglou as being applicable when radiant heat is present, namely:

$$0{\cdot}7t_{wb} + 0{\cdot}2t_g + 0{\cdot}1t_a = WBGT$$

where $WBGT$ is the *Wet Bulb, Globe Temperature Index*. These formulae yield index numbers which approximate those of the commonly used *Effective Temperature and Corrected Effective Temperature Scales*, respectively.

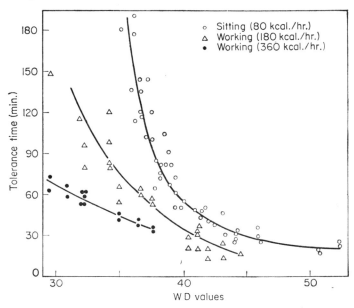

FIG. 3. Average tolerance times for different groups of men as affected by the degree of heat stress (expressed in terms of Wet, Dry (WD) Index values). The men experienced three different levels of activity: ◯ indicates data for men sitting (80 kcal./hr.); △ for men working (180 kcal./hr.); and ● for men working (360 kcal./hr.). From Lind (1963b).

As indicated later in this chapter, the tolerance time may be limited by an overstrain of any of the mechanisms of compensation. However, for fit individuals, it is usually relatable to the rate and the amount of heat storage in the body. Belding and Hatch (1956) selected a storage value of about 64 kcal. as a conservative limit for intermittent exposures of the standard man. In their experience, a 1·1° rise in temperature was readily and safely tolerated. The specific heat of the body is usually taken to be 0·83, so that:

$$70 \text{ kg.} \times 0{\cdot}83 \times 1{\cdot}1° = 64 \text{ kcal.}$$

In single exposures, the limit of endurance may not be reached until the body temperature has increased by about 3° (equivalent to the storage of 175 kcal.). The rate of storage may be predicted from the calculation of the moment-to-moment excess of $M + R + C$ over E.

The tolerance of high environmental temperatures will sometimes be limited by dermal pain. Pain may first be felt when small areas of skin are elevated to about 44° and when larger areas reach 42°. The rate of rise in skin temperature is a factor in the sensation; adaptation of the receptors is such that pain that has initially been incurred may subside.

A summary description of most of the indices of heat stress referred to above has been provided by Leithead and Lind (1964).

C. PHYSIOLOGICAL MECHANISMS WHICH REGULATE HEAT LOSS

When heat balance is threatened, corrective homeostatic responses are evoked. Figure 4 shows the changes that are operative when the body is under heat load. The events associated with breakdown of the regulatory mechanism (broken lines in Fig. 4) will be dealt with in a later section.

1. *Dermal Conductivity and Dermal Blood Flow*

By adjustment of dermal blood flow, the conductivity of the skin may be increased several-fold. At low grades of heat load, this mechanism alone may suffice to maintain heat balance, and accordingly it has been called the *first line of defence* of homeothermism.

The immediate result of dermal vasodilation is a rise in skin temperature. This increases the temperature gradient between the skin and the environment, and thus favours the unloading of metabolic heat by radiation and convection (or decreases heat gain by these avenues). The data of Robinson (1949) have been adjusted by a nominal 10% for metabolic heat loss via respiration to produce estimates of dermal conductivity for the standard man. This reveals that the conductivity, while at rest in a cool environment, may be as little as 16 kcal./hr./° of core-to-skin temperature gradient; in a hot environment, it may be as high as 60 kcal./hr./°. During moderate work in a hot environment, it may rise to 120 kcal./hr./°. The increase accompanying work is facilitated by a rise in blood pressure.

If it be assumed that the skin is 100% efficient as a heat exchanger, which it is not, then 1 litre of blood flow would be required to remove 1 kcal. of metabolic heat per degree of core-to-skin gradient. Under equilibrium conditions, the smallest gradient reported at rest was 1·3°, and at moderate work it was 1·7°. The minimum requirements for dermal flow would appear to be 1 l./min. and 2 l./min. respectively. That the actual volume is considerably higher is suggested by the observation of

Kraning *et al.* (1966). Using a dye dilution technique, they found an increment of 2 l./min. due to heat when at rest, and of about 3 l./min. at moderate work. This is in addition to such diversion of flow as may occur from splanchnic or other central areas. A schematic representation of the effects of heat on cardiac output and on the distribution of blood flow is given in Fig. 5.

The hands, and to a lesser extent the feet, are especially well adapted

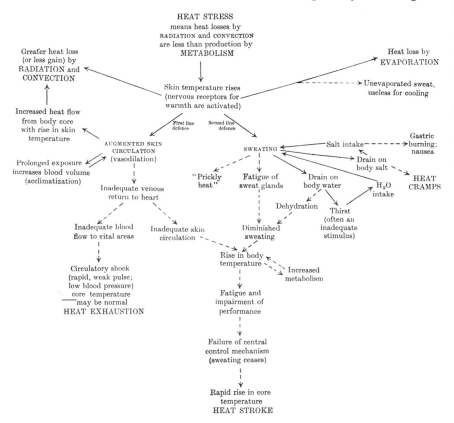

Fig. 4. A chart indicating the physiological responses to heat stress in man. Solid lines indicate usual responses, and the directions of the arrows show cause and effect relationships. Broken lines denote events leading to injury.

to serve as heat exchangers. They have a large surface area and produce relatively little metabolic heat. Direct arteriovenous shunts increase the potential for achieving a high rate of blood flow. In fact, by means of venous occlusion plethysmography, Forster *et al.* (1946) found flows of 80 ml./min. for each hand in resting men, which projects to a rate of about 4 l./min. for the full surface area of a standard man.

The increased dermal flow is attributable to the reflex release of dermal arteriolar tone by cholinergic vasodilator influences (Robinson, 1963) and to compensatory adjustments of the circulation. The latter include the diversion of blood flow from the splanchnic bed by vasoconstriction. It has been reported that the volume of blood plasma

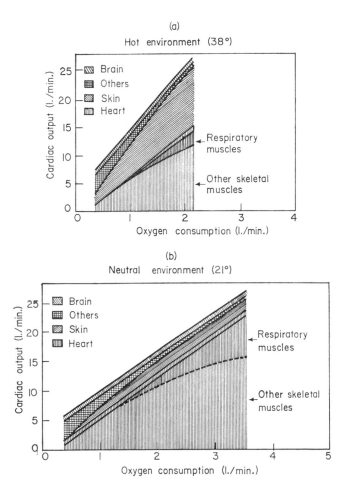

FIG. 5. Distribution of total cardiac output to various organs of the body as a function of oxygen consumption (metabolic cost), (a) under heat stress at 38° and (b) in a thermally neutral environment at 21°. The values quoted are approximate. Visceral blood flow, which is designated as "others", is markedly decreased with moderate to heavy exercise, and practically all of the increase in total blood flow goes to the muscles. Under hot conditions, the extra blood flow to the skin will decrease the work capacity achievable at maximum cardiac output. The data are adapted from Brouha and Radford (1960).

increases significantly during a single exposure (average 13%) and as a result of acclimatization. Obviously, this would represent an advantage, but the extent and permanence of this effect have been questioned by Bass (1963). The elevation of blood pressure which accompanies muscular exercise also favours an increase in dermal blood flow.

2. *Circulatory Strain*

It is clear that the increment in dermal circulation evoked by exposure to heat is accomplished at a cost in cardiac work. It may also be at the expense of vital circulation of blood to other body regions, as described in the later section on heat injury (p. 504).

Hatch (1963) regards circulatory responses as the primary strain of exposure to heat. In fact, under conditions where either the sweating capacity or the E_{max} value is limiting, the circulatory demands may become greater than the capacity to deliver blood. The cost may be regarded as due to the conflict between the attempt of the body to maintain its normal core temperature, and the fact that the skin temperature is increased by external thermal conditions. The resulting "squeeze" on the temperature gradient can only be compensated by increasing the blood flow to the skin and, to the extent that this is not possible, the body temperature must rise.

The demands of heat and work on the cardiovascular system are competitive. Those seeking a criterion of the relative cost of various combinations of the two demands have examined the validity of measuring the rate of heart beat (Brouha and Radford, 1960). At rates of 100 beats/min. and above, an increase in metabolic rate brings about a proportionate increase in the cardiac output and heart rate (Fig. 6). This relationship has recently been confirmed, (a) with a rising level of work at a fixed total heat stress (i.e. with $R + C$ decreased to compensate for rising values of M), and (b) with an increasing heat stress at a fixed level of work (Kraning *et al.*, 1966). It therefore appears reasonable that, when men are active, the circulatory strain of combinations of heat stress and work are manifested in the heart rate. Christensen (1953) attributed some significance to heart rates. He characterized work as "unduly heavy" when it demanded a heart rate of 175 beats/min. or higher, "heavy" at 150/min., and "light" at a rate below 100/min. Such rates do not always have the same meaning when at rest as they do at work. For example, a rate of 130 beats/min. when at rest in the heat may signify excessive strain. Under these conditions, the support afforded by the return flow of blood to the heart may be the missing critical factor. An acceleration of the heart rate without a proportionate rise in the venous pressure may not increase cardiac output sufficiently to satisfy the total needs of the organ systems.

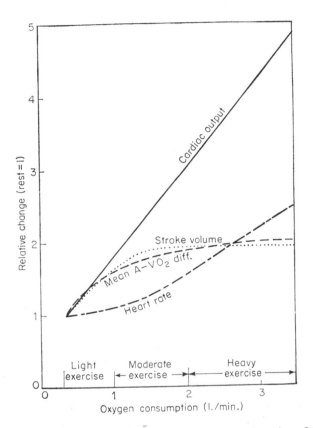

FIG. 6. Relative changes in cardiovascular responses as a function of the intensity of work expressed by oxygen consumption. With light exercise, changes in the stroke volume of the heart account for most of the increase in cardiac output. With heavier exercise, the stroke volume becomes relatively constant and the cardiac output is proportional to the heart rate. These relative changes apply only after cardiovascular responses reach steady values. "A-V" indicates arteriovenous. Data reproduced from Brouha and Radford (1960).

Caution is also suggested in using the single function, $M + R + C$, to predict circulatory strain. Kraning et al. (1966) have indicated that the cardiac cost of a unit of M, which requires circulation of blood to the active muscles as well as to the skin, is about twice as great as that of a unit of $R + C$. $R + C$ does not affect the requirements of muscle, only those of the skin.

3. *Body Core Temperature*

Body core temperature refers to a supposed average temperature of the body mass underlying the skin and representing about 70–80% of the body mass. At any particular moment, the separate organs will have temperatures higher or lower than the average, depending on their individual levels of metabolic activity and the rate of removal of their heat by blood flow. Minard and Copman (1963a) catalogued the temperatures recorded at various sites by different investigators; for men at rest, they deviated by 0·4° to −0·6° from the rectal temperature. Robinson *et al.* (1965b) found that the temperature of active muscles sometimes exceeded the rectal temperature by as much as 1°.

Certain orifices of the body represent the most convenient sites for the routine measurement of body core temperature. However, differences between the values obtained must be recognized. Minard and Copman (1963a) have shown that, when body temperatures are in equilibrium, at rest or at work, the rectal temperature is 0·2–0·3° higher than temperature at the tympanic membrane of the ear canal and in the oesophagus. When the body temperatures are changing, as for example upon first entering or leaving a hot environment or upon initiating or terminating a bout of physical work, the rectal temperature change lags behind that in the ear or oesophagus. The rectal wall may be slower to respond because it is relatively ischaemic when the body is coping with heat stress.

The best site for measuring body core temperature in human studies appears to be the ear canal, as close as possible to the tympanic membrane, as suggested by Benzinger (1959). The blood flow to that general region is large, and the response to a change in blood temperature is rapid. The good correspondence between values for the ear temperature and those recorded in the oesophagus (in close proximity to the heart) suggests that the ear temperature gives a good estimate of the temperature of blood in the large vessels of the body core.

Nielsen (1938) first showed that a controlled elevation of body core temperature occurs during work. The magnitude of the rise resulting from this is dependent on the value of M, and is largely independent of the environment over the broad range of thermal and work conditions within which physiological compensation is effective. If 37·0° is accepted as being representative of the body core temperature at rest, an upward reset of approximately 0·6° may be expected when the value of M is 300 kcal./hr., and of about 1·2° when M is 900 kcal./hr. (Robinson, 1949). A thermal advantage during work in heat accrues from the establishment of increased core-to-skin and skin-to-environment temperature gradients.

When the heat load exceeds that which is being dissipated, either because the E_{max} value or sweating is insufficient, then the t_s value rises and the body core temperature is forced above the normal level for the activity. Even though a thermal balance may be found at a higher core temperature, experience indicates that work will be performed with increasing discomfort and difficulty. This has led Lind (1963a) and others to suggest that the limiting conditions for prolonged exposures should be those which can just be sustained without such a rise in body core temperatures.

Voluntary tolerance may be exceeded at 39–40°, and the risk of injury increases sharply beyond these temperatures. Minard and Copman (1963a) suggested that hyperthermia resulting from causes such as those described above should not be designated as "fever". They would reserve use of the term fever to describe the elevation of body temperature which accompanies certain disease states. The elevation experienced during fever is controlled in that the mechanisms of thermal adjustment seem to be intact; the threshold for their operation simply becomes higher.

4. *Sweating*

Three important aspects of the response of the sweating mechanism have already been mentioned. First, is the observation that, within its capacity, the sweating mechanism will respond with the production of sufficient sweat to maintain thermal balance. Second, that the capacity apparently falls with the duration of exposure. Third, that the effectiveness of sweat for skin cooling is dependent on its evaporation; sweat which drips off is useless and that which is blotted up by clothing and evaporated at some distance from the skin is worth less for skin cooling than the nominal 0·6 kcal./g.

The first aspect deserves further attention. How is the level of sweating adjusted? Evidence from many sources indicates that the mechanism is responsive both to the elevation of dermal temperature and to the elevation of body core temperature above the normal values. When the M value is greater than the loss by $R + C$, the temperature of the skin, or of the body core, or both rises. Within limits, the response of the sweating mechanism is sufficient to cool the skin and thereby bring the equation into balance. Assuming adequate evaporation, the resultant drop in body temperatures decreases the demand. This negative feedback loop establishes sweating at a level appropriate to the requirement for thermal balance.

If the circumstances of exposure do not permit adequate evaporation, body temperatures rise further, with a resultant increase of sweating beyond the nominal need to balance the heat load. To the extent that this assures further wetting of the skin, the extra sweat is useful, even though its efficiency for cooling is lower. That the driving mechanism does not achieve a "run-away" increase of sweating under these circumstances is remarkable. Some years ago Robinson (1949) observed that conditions of humid heat, sufficient initially to evoke the same sweating as those in dry heat, soon resulted in a marked fall in sweating. Subsequent studies during immersion in warm baths (where sweating is useless) have substantiated this so-called hidromeiosis (Hertig et al., 1962). While wetting of the skin is responsible for the decline, the mechanism is unknown.

The morphological characteristics, distribution and innervation of sweat glands have been studied by Kuno (1956) and his colleagues. The total number of glands on the human body surface has been estimated at about 2·4 million. The palmar surface of the hand, the sole of the foot and the head are most abundantly supplied. Thermal sweating is primarily a function of the eccrine glands. These are supplied by cholinergic fibres of the sympathetic nervous system. The apocrine glands, which are associated with the hair follicles, are not considered to be supplied by nerves, but do respond to adrenaline in the blood stream.

Sweat production is ultimately dependent on an adequate intake of water. It has been demonstrated that a moderate deficiency of intake does not significantly alter the sweat rate. In fact, during heat exposure, drinking in accordance with the dictates of thirst frequently does not prevent dehydration to the extent of 1–2% of the body weight. This "voluntary deficit" is usually incurred during the first hour or two of exposure, after which intake and output are more nearly balanced. That men can work better when not seriously dehydrated is well established. The doctrine that a fit man can do as well in hot weather if he rations his drinking water is ill-founded. In fact, Moroff and Bass (1965) found a significant benefit from overhydration prior to exposure. When dehydration occurs, urine volume is markedly decreased to 500 ml. per day or less, whereas, if water intake is maintained in the heat, urinary volume is largely unaffected.

Adolph et al. (1947) studied the ability of men to walk in the desert in relation to water deprivation. The men claimed that they were unable to maintain hiking pace at air temperatures between 35° and 45° when their water loss equalled 4–8% of their initial weight. In emergencies, and under cooler conditions in which little sweat is required to maintain core temperature, it was predicted that work might be performed until a 10 or 12% deficit was incurred. Men required to travel on foot in the desert, with insufficient drinking water, will travel farther if they do their walking in the relatively cool desert night, and rest in the shade during the day.

Survival without water, in contradistinction to performance, is another matter. Records indicate that dehydration of up to 20% of the body weight may be endured without loss of life. McGee (1906) reported that a hardy 40 year-old prospector, Pablo, was stranded with one day's water, yet survived eight days in the Arizona desert in August; he walked or crept 100–150 miles, mostly at night. The temperatures during the period varied between a maximum of 35° in the shade during the day to a minimum of 28° at night. During the period he lost 25% of his body weight, which normally was 70 kg.

The normal dietary intake of NaCl, 8–10 g. per day, is far more than is needed to meet the metabolic needs of the tissues, which are estimated at about 1 g. per day. The remainder is available for sweat, but otherwise is excreted in the urine. The concentration of NaCl in the sweat varies widely, but usually lies between 0·1 and 0·3%(w/v), the lower value being more generally found in acclimatized men. This indicates that men who are required to sweat profusely for prolonged periods need extra salt. For example, a sweat production of 10 litres per day, at a concentration of 0·2%, will require 20 g. NaCl per day. Lee (1964) has provided a tabular guide to supplemental intake. While salt tablets have been used with some success for this purpose, present views favour augmentation of intake by heavier salting of food when sweating is expected to be profuse. An awareness among military and industrial leaders of the need for extra salt is believed to have substantially lowered the incidence of heat cramps.

5. *Acclimatization*

A subjective improvement in well-being occurs after days or weeks of habituation to hot environments. While this phenomenon has long been common knowledge, it was not established until relatively recently whether it was simply accustomization, in terms of feeling better, or had a demonstrable physiological basis. Dill (1938) reported a lowering of the NaCl content of the sweat as a feature of acclimatization to a hot, desert climate. Dreosti (1935), and later others, observed that the heart rates and body core temperatures accompanying hard physical work were lower after acclimatization to a hot environment. In a typical study of the phenomenon (Robinson *et al.*, 1943), unacclimatized subjects approached a state of collapse in 1–1½ hours, with rectal temperatures of 39·2–40·0°, heart rates of 165 to 195 beats/min., and skin temperatures of 36·4–37·3°. Figure 7 shows that, when these exposures were repeated daily, the final rectal temperatures were less by 0·9–1·6°, heart rates by 25–50 beats/min., and skin temperatures by 1·1–1·6°. The 1½ hour exposures were considered to be very difficult on the first day, yet two of the subjects succeeded in walking for 4½ hours with relative ease after acclimatization. Some reasons for the large improvement were sought. Increased sweat production seemed a likely explanation, but this proved not to be consistent enough or large enough. It

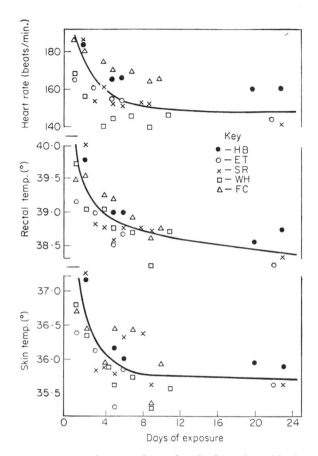

FIG. 7. Acclimatization to heat as shown by the lowering of body temperatures and heart rates of men in a standard work experiment (room temperature 40°; humidity 23%). On some of the days of exposure, the men wore clothing which differed from the standard costume, and the resulting data are omitted from this figure. The key refers to the initials of the subjects involved in the experiment. From Robinson *et al.* (1943).

now appears (Belding and Hatch, 1963) that a key change during acclimation is the 1–2° downward shift in the skin temperature at which the sweat glands are activated. As a result, sweating is initiated somewhat earlier in the exposure, but the important advantage is that the rate of sweating necessary for establishing heat balance is achieved at a lower skin temperature. The decreased circulatory strain, as reflected in the heart rate and the lower core temperature, are results of the increased latitude for the removal of metabolic heat. The mechanism which enhances the responsiveness of the sweating mechanism is not understood.

It is also reasonable to postulate that acclimatization brings an improved efficiency in the circulatory transfer of heat to the skin. This is the most plausible explanation for the improvement that is observed in humid heat, in which enhanced responses of the sweating mechanism do not appear to offer much advantage. However, such a change in dermal conductivity remains to be demonstrated.

Conn et al. (1946), and Robinson and Macfarlane (1958), have imputed changes in the concentrations of pituitary adrenocorticotropic hormone and adrenal steroid hormones, particularly aldosterone, in the blood during the adjustments of acclimatization. A supposed role is the conservation of salt in the sweat. Bass (1963) and Ladell (1964) have reviewed the evidence, and it must be admitted that the role played by such hormonal changes is still far from clear.

The general subject of acclimatization, or adaptation, to a hot environment has been intensively studied in recent years. Many of the findings have been reported in the proceedings of two recent international symposia (Smith, 1963, 1966).

6. Differences Related to Age, Sex, and Weight

Quantitative observations on human tolerance and responses to heat have largely been limited to relatively fit, young men. A few recent observations on women suggest that they acclimatize, but that they tolerate moderate work in the heat less well than men (Hertig and Sargent, 1963). This probably is related to the smaller stroke capacity of the female heart. Hardy et al. (1941) suggested that, during rest, women may tolerate heat better than men. It appears that the tolerance of children has not yet been studied.

Infants at birth are said to have incompletely developed thermoregulation. Kuno (1956) reported that, in a series of 66 full-term infants briefly exposed in an overly warm incubator, none sweated on the day of birth. Within 5 days, sweating could be elicited from about half of the group. Eighteen days passed before all responded.

A restudy 20 years later of men who had participated in the study of acclimatization described in the previous section revealed that those who had not taken on too much extra weight could again become acclimatized to the same conditions, and had not lost tolerance (Robinson et al., 1965a). However, to the extent that ageing results in a loss of cardiovascular capacity, less tolerance is to be expected. The large numbers of excess deaths in the 1934 heat wave in the midwestern part of the U.S.A. were mostly among elderly persons with established cardiovascular or respiratory impairment, and to a lesser extent among infants (Collins, 1934).

The tolerance of women and of overweight men to cold is considered to be enhanced by subcutaneous fat, which acts as extra insulation. It has been argued that this fat represents a handicap to heat transfer under hot conditions, but in fact the dermal vascular bed effective for augmenting heat loss is mostly external to the adipose tissue. Thus, in a hot environment, the handicaps attributable to being overweight may only be that more energy is required to do work, and that the amount of extra surface area for heat removal does not increase proportionally.

D. CENTRAL CONTROL OF RESPONSES

The mechanisms for maintaining thermal homeostasis are so diverse and well integrated that they are frequently chosen for consideration in the introductory or the final lecture of formal courses in mammalian physiology. During thermal homeostasis, major organ systems, including the central and autonomic nervous, muscular (in shivering), and circulatory systems, work together. Hardy (1961) has provided a diagram, which here appears as Fig. 8, to show most of the main organs involved and their interrelations in control. The same author (Hardy, 1961) discussed current theories of central control and the underlying evidence for them.

The anterior hypothalamus has long been identified as the principal centre for the control of heat loss. Direct heating of the anterior hypothalamus using a thermode (Fusco, 1963), or warming the entering blood supply, brings about dermal vasodilatation and sweating or panting. The temperature of the skin and perhaps the temperature at other body loci affect this centre, apparently via afferent nervous pathways. The control of sweating has been the subject of vigorous debate and intensive experimentation as a result of Benzinger's (1959) conclusion that the hypothalamic temperature alone determines sweat rate. Belding and Hertig (1962), Randall (1963) and others have provided evidence that skin temperature also plays a role, a point later partially accepted by Benzinger.

E. EFFECTS OF HEAT ON PERFORMANCE

It is reasonable to suppose that exposure may affect performance at levels of heat stress below those which result in injury. We have already indicated the competitive demands of muscle and skin for the cardiac output during the performance of physical work. The result may be a decrease in work capacity, or M value, as indicated previously (Fig. 4, p. 490). Also, as stated earlier, a decrease in work capacity may result because of a rise in body temperature.

Strydom *et al.* (1963) studied the work output of miners subjected to various intensities of wet heat. At a wet bulb temperature of 32° and

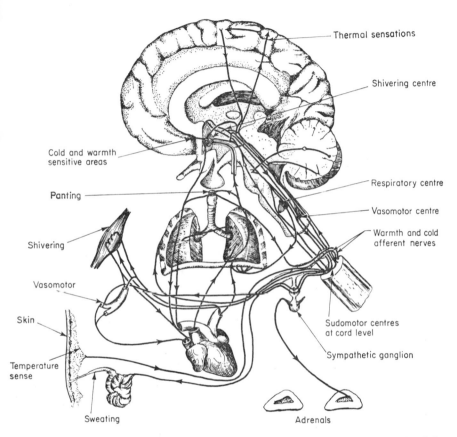

FIG. 8. Diagrammatic representation of the control mechanisms involved in maintaining thermal homeostasis in man. Reproduced from Hardy (1961).

above, the work output began to fall off sharply. This was despite good effort on the part of the workers, as attested by their high heart rates and rectal temperatures. At a wet bulb temperature of 35·5°, the productivity of the workers declined almost to nothing.

Heat may also affect mental work, or manual dexterity, neither of which involves an appreciable increase in the value of M. This might be the result of a diversion of blood flow from the brain, or of a distraction because of discomfort, or even indirectly because heat has interfered with the normal pattern of sleep. Lassitude has long been associated with living in the tropics. Lee (1957) stated: "There is no gainsaying the importance of the psychological effects of tropical climates. Most new-comers from temperate climes experience a disinclination to work, mentally as well as physically. This may have a physiological basis and may subside to a certain extent with adaptation. But there are those who question whether the customary level of activity and initiative is ever restored, or whether those born and raised in tropical climates ever aspire to the degree of activity characteristic of cooler environments".

Attempts to collect comparable evidence on human productivity at light work under moderate heat stress and under comfortable conditions have not yielded any very certain differences. Experiments have usually been invalidated by changes in the motivation of those being studied, or by problems in obtaining quantitative data on work output. Pepler (1963) has summarized some of the findings in this difficult area of study.

Mackworth (1946) appears to have avoided some of these pitfalls. He studied the accuracy of eleven telegraph operators in decoding Morse Code when subjected to different intensities of heat exposure. His results are shown in Fig. 9. The 3-hour performance of the most skilled men of this group was little affected, even under the hottest conditions, whereas that of the less skilled fell off very markedly. This was inter-preted to mean that the effects of two concurrent stresses may be compounded; the task itself represented a considerable stress for those who were less skilled. Considering the performance of all of the subjects, a significant decrement did not occur except under conditions worse than those ordinarily encountered under shelter in hot climates. However, the fact that the impairment was not observed in a 3-hour test does not mean that the climatic conditions are acceptable. The brain is a stern taskmaster, and may sustain performance, at a cost, if motivation is high!

Industrial accident frequency may be considered as an indirect measure of performance. Belding et al. (1960a) noted that, over a period of four years, the accident frequency in a large steel plant near Chicago had been nearly twice as great in the summer as in the winter. On a percentage basis, the seasonal effect was not different from department to department, regardless of the degree of exposure to process heat. The association with season does not prove that heat caused the summer increase, but it invites speculation. Accident frequency is partly a function of human alertness. When workers are under a 24-hour heat duress, as they are in this region during summer, the general "tonus" of bodily activity may decrease significantly.

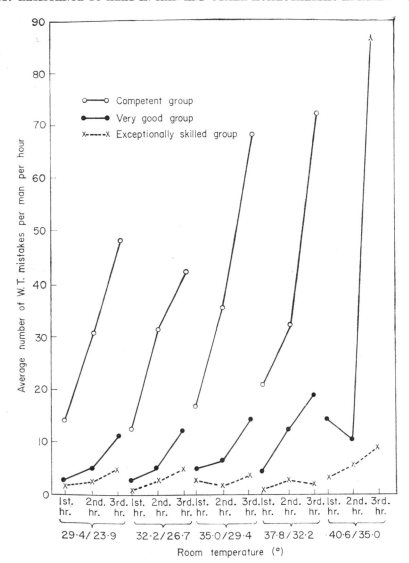

FIG. 9. Effect of different intensities of heat exposure on the performance of three groups of wireless telegraph operators. From Mackworth (1946).

F. OVERSTRAIN OF MECHANISMS OF RESISTANCE TO HEAT

Whereas man in general is to be regarded as a tropical animal capable of surviving naturally occurring hot climates on the earth, the spectrum of individual abilities to cope with heat is broad. It may even vary from day to day with health status; for example, diarrhoea may temporarily hamper the operation of the sweating mechanism of an otherwise fit person. Furthermore, the overexposure of groups of individuals has sometimes been ordered by a non-participant, as in the infamous imprisonment in the "Black Hole of Calcutta". Or it has been inflicted unwittingly by someone who is himself exposed, but who is physiologically more fit than his followers, as in military operations or in pilgrimages to Mecca. Many such events have been recorded (Leithead and Lind, 1964). The result is heat injury for those who are less fit. Commonly, this takes the form of simple exhaustion, or a temporary inability to continue. Far less frequently, "stroke" involving injury to the thermal control mechanism is incurred.

Attempts to classify heat illness are complicated by the number and interdependence of the demands on the thermal regulatory mechanisms, as illustrated in Fig. 4, (p. 490). In this figure, broken lines are used to indicate the sequences of the failures that may occur.

1. *Heat Exhaustion*

The presenting symptoms of heat exhaustion are weakness, a feeling of inability to continue, faintness or actual fainting, and sometimes breathlessness. Objective examination reveals signs of circulatory shock, shown by a rapid, thready pulse, arterial hypotension, paleness, and unsteadiness. It may be helpful to know that, in laboratory studies, the symptoms and signs offer a quite dependable forewarning of collapse from heat exhaustion.

It has been stated that the primary strain of heat exposure is circulatory. Heat exhaustion is attributed to the progressive failure of the circulatory system to fulfill the combined demands of the brain, vital organs including skeletal muscle, and the skin. This may reflect a deficiency of cardiac output or just an improper distribution of the output that is achieved. For whatever reason, those who have a well-developed cardiovascular capacity and those who are acclimatized are less susceptible.

Heat exhaustion may be self-limiting if it has been acquired during work and if the subject stops and lies down. A decrease in the value of M to the resting level decreases the heat load and simultaneously lowers the circulatory demands of the muscles. However, whether the subject is active or inactive at the time that exhaustion occurs, complete removal of the heat load is desirable. This may sometimes be accomplished by taking a neutral or cool bath or shower, which brings about dermal vasoconstriction. If removal to a thermally neutral environment is not feasible, relief may be achieved by the application of water to the skin; fanning will enhance evaporative cooling. The object of these measures is to achieve dermal vasoconstriction. Dehydration is often a factor in heat exhaustion; this and possible salt lack can be corrected by drinking lightly salted water (a teaspoonful of salt per gallon) or by intravenous injection of physiological saline.

2. *Hyperthermia and Heat Stroke*

Hyperthermia is used in this section to mean elevation of the body core temperature above the value which is usual for the particular grade of activity. Minard and Copman (1963b) have recently reviewed this subject in some detail. Three factors may contribute to the development of hyperthermia. The first has been dealt with previously, namely, the failure to achieve heat balance at normal body core temperature, because the value for E_{req} exceeds that for E_{max}.

The second potential contributor is diminished sweating. The sweating mechanism fails to produce at the level required for thermal balance. Apparently this can occur despite the ingestion of adequate amounts of water and NaCl, though it is more apt to be a result of gradual dehydration. A contributory factor may also be the actual plugging of substantial numbers of sweat ducts, a condition known as "prickly heat".

A third factor in the development of hyperthermia may be the inability of the body to sustain adequate dermal circulation to meet the needs for the transfer of heat from the core to the skin.

Whatever the causes of a particular case of hyperthermia, the condition warrants strict observation, because an equilibrium may not be achieved at a physiologically acceptable level without a decrease in the stress. Positive feedback contributes to the problem in that a rise in body temperature itself increases the total heat load through its effect on the M value.

When hyperthermia has been sustained for some time, and/or when some critically high core temperature has been reached, the homeostatic mechanism may be overwhelmed. It is reasonable to assume that the proximate cause of this is thermal damage to the hypothalamic control centre. At this point, a sharp diminution in sweating occurs, and the body temperature rises rapidly. Collapse and coma usually occur, sometimes with convulsions. When first measured, the body core temperature is usually still rising and may be 41° or higher. Rapid cooling is required to avoid permanent or lethal damage. Because the control mechanism has been affected, subsequent treatment requires special precautions, often extending over weeks, to stabilize body temperatures within normal limits.

3. *Heat Cramps*

The muscular cramps which sometimes result from prolonged, severe heat exposures have been attributed to a disturbance of the electrolyte balance, particularly to a loss of NaCl in the sweat. Relief is obtained by ingestion, or more immediately by an intravenous injection, of a solution containing NaCl (see Section II.F.1, p. 504).

III. Resistance to Heat in Other Homeothermic Animals

A. MAMMALS

The observations of the previous sections regarding heat exposure and its effects have been specific to man. Other mammals have been studied far less extensively, but differences and similarities are evident.

1. *Heat Stress*

The Schmidt-Nielsens (1952) pointed out that heat load represents a greater immediate hazard to small mammals than to large ones. This arises from the fact that the surface area relative to the weight of small mammals is large, so that a unit of heat gained via the surface means a larger rise in body temperature. They have also noted how behaviour serves to decrease the effective heat load of desert environments. Small animals burrow into the ground, where temperatures are much lower, and remain there during daytime. The camel has been observed to orient his body parallel to the sun's rays and remains in one spot on the ground, thus minimizing his exposure. The camel is further protected by the fur on his back. Other mammals of all sizes presumably benefit from the insulation of fur whenever they are exposed at temperatures above skin temperature.

2. *Tolerance and Mechanisms of Adjustment*

Among different species of mammals, the tolerance to an elevation of body core temperature seems to be similar; body temperatures above about 40° represent a threat to survival, and above 42–44° are not consistent with survival (Spector, 1956).

Schmidt-Nielsen *et al.* (1957) observed diurnal fluctuations of as much as 6° (34–40°) in camels that had been deprived of drinking water. This indicated that much of the daytime heat load was stored, to be lost in the form of $R + C$ during the night. By this means, a substantial amount of water was conserved. Only when body temperature neared 40° did sweating become copious. The camel can also endure a greater degree of dehydration than man. This can be up to 30% of his body weight, as compared with 10 to 12% for man.

Thermal sweating is made use of only by a limited number of the larger mammals. In addition to man and the camel, these include the horse, donkey, marmot, monkey and sheep. Sheep and cattle both sweat and pant. The cat, dog, guinea pig, rabbit and pig apparently make use of panting alone to achieve augmented evaporative cooling. Desert rodents have been observed to salivate and to spread the saliva over their fur when body temperatures have risen above 40° (Schmidt-Nielsen and Schmidt-Nielsen, 1952).

B. BIRDS

Birds are also homeothermic. A compilation of body temperatures of various species of birds, when active, shows mean values between 40·5° and 43·3°, with a minimum value of 39·4° and a maximum of 44·9° (Dawson and Schmidt-Nielsen, 1964). A body temperature of 45° apparently may be sustained over considerable periods of time without injury; generally, a rise above 47° is lethal.

Birds do not sweat but, like many mammals, they pant. They also have the capacity to alter dermal conductivity. Naturalists have observed that, under daytime heat, birds often seek shade. They also have noted that larger soaring birds take advantage of updrafts to attain higher, cooler altitudes at a minimum cost in terms of the M value.

Birds may raise their ventilation rates three- or four-fold by panting and thereby enhance evaporative loss (Dawson, 1958). However, the heat production of panting offsets the loss by as much as 40%. For small birds, the water of oxidation does not go far toward meeting the requirements for evaporation. Large birds require proportionately less evaporative cooling, and water of oxidation may nearly balance the requirement of water for the purpose.

Some birds apparently estivate. By lowering the value for M, they minimize the problem of achieving heat balance and, at the same time, conserve food and water stores. Students of avian thermal physiology have been few, and quantitative aspects of thermal responses have received little attention. More or less comprehensive statements of the little that is known and the questions which remain unanswered have been provided in articles by Randall (1943), Bartholomew (1960), and King and Farner (1964).

The original intent of the author was to conclude this chapter with a summary. However, as it turns out, it has been necessary to yield to pressures of space to the point where the chapter itself is only an abridged treatment of the subject of resistance to heat among homeotherms. Instead of imposing on the reader a summary of what is already a summary, it seems more appropriate to offer apologies, (a) to the heat-transfer biophysicists, and (b) to the organ system and cellular physiologists, whose meaningful contributions to this field have not been directly cited in this chapter.

IV. Acknowledgements

The author acknowledges partial support by the Medical Research and Development Command, U.S. Army, and Research Grant OH-00048 from the National Institutes of Health for services in preparation of this manuscript.

References

Adolph, E. F. and Associates (1947). "Physiology of Man in the Desert", 357 pp. Interscience Publ. Inc., New York.

Bartholomew, G. A. (1960). *Anat. Record* **137**, 338.

Bass, D. E. (1963). *In* "Temperature, its Measurement and Control in Science and Industry", (J. D. Hardy, Ed.), Vol. 3, pp. 299–306. Reinhold Publ. Corp., New York.

Belding, H. S. and Hatch, T. F. (1956). *Trans. Amer. Soc. heat vent. Eng.* **62**, 213.

Belding, H. S. and Hatch, T. F. (1963). *Fed. Proc.* **22**, 881.

Belding, H. S. and Hertig, B. A. (1962). *J. appl. Physiol.* **17**, 103.

Belding, H. S., Hatch, T. F., Hertig, B. A. and Riedesel, M. L. (1960a). *Proc. 13th. Int. Congr. Occ. Hlth.* 839.

Belding, H. S., Hertig, B. A. and Riedesel, M. L. (1960b). *Amer. ind. Hyg. Assoc. J.* **21**, 25.

Benzinger, T. H. (1959). *Proc. nat. Acad. Sci. Wash.* **45**, 645.

Blagden, C. (1775). *Philos. Trans.* **65**, Pt. 1, 484.

Brouha, L. and Radford, E. P. (1960). *In* "Science and Medicine of Exercise and Sports", (W. R. Johnson, Ed.), pp. 178–206. Harper and Brothers, New York.

Cannon, W. B. (1939). "The Wisdom of the Body", 333 pp. W. W. Norton and Co., New York.

Christensen, E. H. (1953). *In* "Symposium on Fatigue", (W. F. Floyd and A. T. Welford, Eds.), pp. 93–108. H. K. Lewis, London.

Collins, S. D. (1934). *Publ. Hlth. Repts. (U.S.A.)* **49**, 1015.

Conn, J. W., Johnstone, M. W. and Louis, L. H. (1946). *J. clin. Invest.* **25**, 912.

Dawson, W. R. (1958). *Physiol. Zool.* **26**, 37.

Dawson, W. R. and Schmidt-Nielsen, K. (1964). *In* "Handbook of Physiology", (D. B. Dill, Ed.), pp. 481–492. Amer. Physiol. Soc., Washington.

Dill, D. B. (1938). "Life, Heat and Altitude", 211 pp. Harvard Univ. Press., Cambridge, Massachusetts.

Dill, D. B., Ed. (1964). "Handbook of Physiology, Section 4, Adaptation to the Environment", 1056 pp. Amer. Physiol. Soc., Washington.

Dreosti, A. O. (1935). *J. chem. Met. Min. Soc., So. Afr.* **36**, 102.

Forster, R. E., Ferris, B. G. and Day, R. (1946). *Amer. J. Physiol.* **146**, 600.

Fusco, M. M. (1963). *In* "Temperature, its Measurement and Control in Science and Industry", (J. D. Hardy, Ed.), Vol. 3, pp. 589–596. Reinhold Publ. Corp., New York.

Goldman, R. F., Green, E. B. and Iampietro, P. F. (1965). *J. appl. Physiol.* **20**, 271.

Haldane, J. J. (1905). *J. Hyg., Camb.* **5**, 494.

Hardy, J. D., Milhorat, A. T. and DuBois, E. F. (1941). *Brit. J. Nutr.* **21**, 383.

Hardy, J. D. (1961). *Physiol. Rev.* **41**. 521.

Hardy, J. D. Ed. (1963). "Temperature, its Measurement and Control in Science and Industry", Vol. 3, Pt. 3, 683 pp. Reinhold Publ. Corp., New York.

Hatch, T. (1963). *In* "Temperature, its Measurement and Control in Science and Industry", (J. D. Hardy, Ed.), Vol. 3, pp. 307–318. Reinhold Publ. Corp., New York.

Hertig, B. A. and Sargent, F. (1963). *Fed. Proc.* **22**, 810.

Hertig, B. A., Riedesel, M. L. and Belding, H. S. (1962). *Advanc. Biol. Skin* **3**, 213.

King, J. R. and Farner, D. A. (1964). *In* "Handbook of Physiology", (D. B. Dill, Ed.), pp. 603–624. Amer. Physiol. Soc., Washington.

Kraning, K. K., Belding, H. S. and Hertig, B. A. (1966). *J. appl. Physiol.* **21**, 111.

Kuno, Y. (1956). "Human Perspiration", 268 pp. Charles C. Thomas, Springfield, Illinois.

Ladell, W. S. S. (1964). *In* "Handbook of Physiology", (D. B. Dill, Ed.), pp. 625–660. Amer. Physiol. Soc., Washington.

Lee, D. H. K. (1957). "Climate and Economic Development in the Tropics", 182 pp. Harper and Brothers, New York.

Lee, D. H. K. (1964). *In* "Handbook of Physiology", (D. B. Dill, Ed.), pp. 551–582. Amer. Physiol. Soc., Washington.

Leithead, C. S. and Lind, A. R. (1964). "Heat Stress and Heat Disorders", 304 pp. Cassell, London.

Lind, A. R. (1963a). *J. appl. Physiol.* **18**, 51.

Lind, A. R. (1963b). *In* "Temperature, its Measurement and Control in Science and Industry", (J. D. Hardy, Ed.), Vol. 3, pp. 337–345. Reinhold Publ. Corp., New York.

Mackworth, N. J. (1946). *Brit. J. industr. Med.* **3**, 143.

McGee, W. J. (1906). *Interstate Med. J.* **13**, 279.

Macpherson, R. K. (1960). "Physiological Responses to Hot Environments", 323 pp. Brit. Med. Res. Counc. Spec. Rept. No. 298. H.M.S.O., London.

Minard, D. and Copman, L. (1963a). *In* "Temperature, its Measurement and Control in Science and Industry", (J. D. Hardy, Ed.), Vol. 3, pp. 527–543. Reinhold Publ. Corp., New York.

Minard, D. and Copman, L. (1963b). *In* "Temperature, its Measurement and Control in Science and Industry", (J. D. Hardy, Ed.), Vol. 3, pp. 253–273. Reinhold Publ. Corp., New York.

Moroff, S. and Bass, D. E. (1965). *J. appl. Physiol.* **20**, 267.

Newburgh, L. H. Ed. (1949). "Physiology of Heat Regulation and the Science of Clothing", 457 pp. W. B. Saunders Co., Philadelphia.

Nielsen, M. (1938). *Skand. Arch. Physiol.* **79**, 193.

Pepler, R. D. (1963). *In* "Temperature, its Measurement and Control in Science and Industry", (J. D. Hardy, Ed.), Vol. 3, pp. 319–336. Reinhold Publ. Corp., New York.

Randall, W. C. (1943). *Amer. J. Physiol.* **139**, 56.

Randall, W. C. (1963). *In* "Temperature, its Measurement and Control in Science and Industry", (J. D. Hardy, Ed.), Vol. 3, pp. 275–286. Reinhold Publ. Corp., New York.

Robinson, K. W. and Macfarlane, W. V. (1958). *J. appl. Physiol.* **12**, 13.

Robinson, S. (1963). *In* "Temperature, its Measurement and Control in Science and Industry", (J. D. Hardy, Ed.), Vol. 3, pp. 287–297. Reinhold Publ. Corp., New York.

Robinson, S. (1949). *In* "Physiology of Heat Regulation and the Science of Clothing", (L. H. Newburgh, Ed.), pp. 193–231. W. B. Saunders Co., Philadelphia.

Robinson, S., Turrell, E. S., Belding, H. S. and Horvath, S. M. (1943). *Amer. J. Physiol.* **140**, 168.

Robinson, S., Turrell, E. S. and Gerking, S. D. (1945). *Amer. J. Physiol.* **143**, 21.

Robinson, S., Belding, H. S., Consolazio, F. C., Horvath, S. M. and Turrell, E. S. (1965a). *J. appl. Physiol.* **20**, 583.

Robinson, S., Meyer, F. R., Newton, J. L., Ts'ao, C. H. and Holgersen, L. O. (1965b). *J. appl. Physiol.* **20**, 575.

Schmidt-Nielsen, B. and Schmidt-Nielsen, K. (1952). *Physiol. Rev.* **32**, 135.

Schmidt-Nielsen, K., Schmidt-Nielsen, B., Jarnum, S. A. and Houpt, T. R. (1957). *Amer. J. Physiol.* **188**, 103.

Scholander, P. F., Walters, V., Hock, R. and Irving, L. (1950a). *Biol. Bull.* **99**, 225.

Scholander, P. F., Hock, R., Walters, V. and Irving, L. (1950b). *Biol. Bull.* **99**, 237.

Smith, R. E., Ed. (1963). *Fed. Proc.* **22**, 687.

Smith, R. E., Ed. (1966). *Fed. Proc.*, in press.

Spector, W. S., Ed. (1956). "Handbook of Biological Data", 584 pp. Div. of Biol. and Agric., Nat. Acad. Sci, and Natl. Res. Counc., Washington.

Strydom, N. B., Wyndham, C. H., Cooke, H. M., Maritz, J. S., Bredell, G. A. G., Morrison, J. F., Peter, J. and Williams, C. G. (1963). *Fed. Proc.* **22**, 893.

Woodcock, A. H. and Breckenridge, J. R. (1965). *Ergonomics* **8**, 223.

Wyndham, C. H., Bouwer, W. v. d. M., Devine, M. G. and Paterson, H. E. (1952). *J. appl. Physiol.* **5**, 290.

Chapter 14

Medical Applications of Thermobiology

BRYAN BROOM

Beit Memorial Research Fellow, Department of Physiology,
Middlesex Hospital Medical School,
London, W.1, England

I. Introduction

"The great difficulty which men have in all ages experienced in the acquisition of knowledge, has arisen from the promptitude of the human mind to decide in regard to causes. . . . The most eminent physicians in every period of the world, impatient of observing and delineating, have been eager to explain and even to systematize; and the science of life owes its corruptions more to the misapplication of learning, than even to the dreams of superstition" (Currie, 1798).

"The design of a fully controlled experiment in the classical sense, in which one or a few components of the system are varied in an otherwise static system, is unlikely to be achieved in work on hypothermia. A comparison of various authors' work on the same aspect of the circulation, under conditions of body-cooling, is further bedevilled by the use by a wide variety of anaesthetic, narcotic, analgesic, muscle-relaxant and other agents. A perusal of the literature on this subject has been a salutary lesson to the author of this paper on the need for really careful planning of experiments on hypothermia, and for much more extensive reports of the experimental details than is usually the case" (Cooper, 1961).

In the last twelve years, over a dozen symposia, monographs and review articles have appeared on various medical aspects of thermobiology, embracing thousands of communications published before and during this period (Burton and Edholm, 1955; Virtue, 1955; Dripps, 1956; Allen, 1958; Gollan, 1959; Taylor, 1959; Boba, 1960; Cooper and Ross, 1960; Horvath, 1960; Parkes and Smith, 1960; Starkov, 1960; Lewis, 1961; Smith, 1961; Blair, 1964; Leithead and Lind, 1964). The brief account which follows is an attempt to highlight some of the more interesting and important features of a field which is expanding at a confusing rate. In man, as in other mammals, there is a homeostatic mechanism that maintains the temperature of the body between 36° and 38° despite wide fluctuations in environmental temperature. However, there are many established medical practices in which part or all of the human body is subjected to elevated or decreased temperatures. In this chapter, the diagnostic and therapeutic uses of heat and cold will be considered, and mention will also be made of the effects of environmental temperature on man. The medical applications of thermobiology lie chiefly in the effects of temperature upon blood flow and oxygen uptake, at the local cell and general body levels of activity. The role of hypothermia, the reversible depression of body temperature and hence of oxygen uptake, in medicine and surgery is the chief theme of this account of the medical applications of thermobiology.

The rapid growth of low temperature biology over the past two decades has indicated clearly the economic and medical advantages that the use of lowered temperatures confer, both in prolonging or shortening life, according to the circumstances. In situations of actual or potential lack of oxygen supply, or of excessive demands upon energy turnover, the lowering of the oxygen requirements of either the isolated tissue or whole animal, by reversible depression of tissue or body temperature, is a practicable method of forestalling the otherwise inevitable cell death that will result when energy demand exceeds supply.

Though both local and general hypothermia have been in clinical use for some 25 years, there is far from complete agreement or understanding as to what constitute the optimum conditions for the production and use of generalized hypothermia, the causes of the complications that can result from its use, and whether, in the short term, the artificial augmentation of oxygen supply is preferable to the artificial lowering of oxygen requirements. That this somewhat unsettled and uncertain state of affairs has arisen is due to no especial lack of knowledge or foresight on the part of the clinician, but reflects the difficulties of standardizing the clinical situation. The solution of a given clinical problem is commonly urgent, evidence is often inadequate, variables are either unknown or uncontrollable, and there is lack of detailed knowledge of the natural history of the major clinical conditions.

Much has already been accomplished, but it is to the future that one must look for the solution of this basic medical problem. The statistical treatment of medical data is coming into fashion with advantages that are apparent, and the advent of the computer, and agreed data processing, may provide many of the answers to problems raised by the use of hypothermia, if allied to sufficient educational and financial investment in medical technology.

II. Effects of Increased Temperatures

A. SPECIFIC EFFECTS

1. *Local Applications*

The application of heat to areas of inflammation has been practised since antiquity. The action of heat, whether applied as infrared radiation, short-wave diathermy, wax baths, or poultices, is beneficial in its soothing and pain-relieving properties and, allegedly, by its action in increasing local blood flow to the area of inflammation, with consequent hastening of the recovery processes and resolution of the inflammatory response. Extensive burns are satisfactorily treated, along with other specific measures, in conditions of dry heat which may minimize the considerable transudation of plasma which can result and threaten life by dehydration and electrolyte depletion. A similar argument is put forward by the advocates of the use of cold in this context. The administration of warm, moist air or oxygen is a valuable adjunct to the treatment of severe respiratory infections which are associated with copious, thick secretions that narrow or actually block the respiratory passages.

The direct application of diathermy heat for surgical incisions and haemostasis (the arrest of surgical wound haemorrhage) has an established place in surgical technique. The use of heat deliberately to destroy tissue is a feature of the stereotactic surgery of Parkinson's disease and of other conditions, such as the relief of intolerable and incurable pain, in which the neurosurgeon wishes to inactivate small areas of the brain for therapeutic purposes. However, the use of cold is now considered more satisfactory than thermocoagulation. The application of temperature selectively to destroy circumscribed areas of brain tissue may, however, be supplanted by the use of ultrasonic vibrations, which dispenses with the need to open the skull.

The use of heat for the sterilization of surgical instruments in an autoclave is routine. Chemical methods and gamma irradiation of disposable items of equipment are, however, coming to the fore, on the grounds of convenience, cost and efficiency.

In diagnosis, the detection and delineation of localized areas of increased temperature are of considerable clinical use. Localized increase of temperature is, in general, a reflection both of increased metabolism and increased blood flow, and may indicate the presence of an underlying new growth, infection, varicose vein, or venous or arterial occlusion (Williams, 1964a,b). In the case of venous occlusion, the raised temperature is due to the relative overheating of the limb from defective venous drainage, whereas, in arterial occlusion, the skin temperature is lowered owing to the impairment of blood flow to the limb or digit.

2. General Applications

The diagnostic implications of a raised body temperature (pyrexia) are known to most people as usually signifying bacterial or viral infection. While it is seldom now necessary to procure a classical temperature chart before starting antibiotic treatment, the presence of fever during treatment still retains its prognostic significance, as an indication of the need for additional treatment. The causes of pyrexia are many and varied. Fever may result from basal brain disturbances, which carry a grave prognosis unless treatment is fairly rapidly effective. Pyrexia may occur in the rare form of so-called mesencephalic epilepsy. Dehydration, anaemia, and factitious fever from hysteria or malingering may cause diagnostic difficulties, as may certain kinds of new growth. Rare cases of fever are found to be due to the increased secretion of etiocholanolone, a product of sterol metabolism (Kappas et al., 1961).

Sterols are known to affect body temperature. A rise in 17-hydroxy-corticosteroid secretion, resulting from pituitary stimulation and adrenocorticotrophic hormone (ACTH) release, is the basis of the pyrogen (bacterial lipopolysaccharide from Proteus vulgaris) test of pituitary-adrenal function. Pyrogen administration also increases urinary leucocyte excretion in pyelonephritis. Other sterols have antipyretic or fever-reducing properties, and the diminution of the normal inflammatory response during prolonged sterol treatment is a hazard to the patient who is deprived both of the normal defensive response to infection and an awareness of its initiation. The slight mid-cycle, intermenstrual, rise of body temperature in the healthy woman indicates normal ovulation due to the thermogenic action of progesterone. The role of sterols in the control of body temperature has, however, not been fully investigated.

Instability of temperature control and excessive sweating are features of familial dysautonomia, an inherited recessive metabolic block in the pathway from catechol precursors to adrenaline and noradrenaline, that is associated with an increased excretion of homovanillic acid and a decreased excretion of vanillylmandelic acid. The implications of this recently described syndrome in the normal physiology and pharmacology of temperature control have yet to be studied.

The type of treatment required in accidental hypothermia after cold exposure is a moot point. The rate and duration of cooling prior to treatment are probably critical factors. Cases treated by gradual rewarming, after what has presumably been gradual cooling, have most often recovered from the lowest temperatures that have been recorded, and vigorous attempts at rewarming have usually been reported to have failed (Duguid et al., 1961). However, victims of acute cold exposure are best subjected to rewarming at an ambient temperature of about 40° (Alexander, 1946). This important aspect will be further considered in the section on hypothermia (see p. 520).

B. NON-SPECIFIC EFFECTS

1. *General Applications*

The non-specific therapeutic uses of increased temperature are of historical interest. Thus certain skin conditions, neurosyphilis and type II nephritis were once thought to benefit from fever; also warmth is a feature of Spa treatments. Acclimatized men are capable of normal or nearly normal work in water-saturated temperatures up to about 29°. Despite the great efficiency of human thermoregulation, the neglect of basic principles, or undue exposure to extreme heat, may cause ill health or death. The upper limit of body temperature compatible with survival is probably of the order of 45°.

The effects of undue or prolonged heat exposure may not be as dramatic as to cause acute symptoms, but the great improvement in health following the institution of air-conditioning in the Royal Navy is suggestive of the fact that chronic heat and humidity are prejudicial to the enjoyment of full health. There is a significant correlation between the development of kidney stones and the duration of tropical service in the Royal Navy, which would suggest that chronic heat exposure may be associated with chronic mild dehydration, or a relative deficiency of water intake to balance losses by sweating. Skin disorders may feature in chronic heat exposure. However, the biology of temperature control in human heat exposure is not yet clarified, largely owing to the wide variety of conditions and criteria of testing that have been reported.

The prevention and treatment of heat disorders is discussed in the section of this chapter dealing with hypothermia (p. 520). The basis of the clinical symptoms of heat disorders is either a relative or absolute deficiency of sweating, resulting in a dangerous rise in body temperature (heat stroke), or excessive sweating without replacement, leading to excess water and/or salt loss (heat exhaustion). Ultimately, peripheral

17*

circulatory failure from dehydration will occur, unless treated, and this is commoner in heat exhaustion than in heat stroke.

III. Effects of Decreased Temperatures

A. SPECIFIC EFFECTS

1. *Local Applications*

Local cooling of injured, infected, or burnt extremities has been recommended since ancient times, both for the pain relief that it undoubtedly provides, and for its beneficial action in decreasing the absorption of toxic metabolites from the diseased area. There is experimental evidence that the procedure is beneficial, though attempts to establish this mode of treatment have not met with much success. Certainly, undue heating of diseased extremities should be avoided, with the possible exception of burns, where dry heat may help to diminish the transudation of plasma.

The treatment of peripheral areas of cold injury, such as frostbite or "trench foot", is another moot point, despite their military importance which has prompted considerable experimental and clinical activity. Rapid rewarming may be successful experimentally, but it is usually impracticable in the circumstances of cold injury. Moderate rewarming is positively harmful, as the increased rate of metabolism in local tissue is not matched by the ability of the blood supply to furnish additional oxygen to the damaged cells. Intense vascular stasis is the dominant pathology. Under these conditions, initial pharmacological measures to increase the local tissue blood flow are probably desirable, followed at a later stage by the careful application of indirect heat to encourage reflex vasodilatation.

In addition to the death of local tissue that results from undue cold exposure, certain clinical conditions of undue cold hypersensitivity exist (Shafar, 1965). These cold hypersensitivity states are associated with a pathological intolerance to cold. Cryoglobulinaemia signifies the presence of abnormal quantities of a globulin in the blood which precipitates on cooling and redissolves on warming. Cold urticarial states are thought to be due to histamine release producing local and possibly generalized reactions. A third type of hypersensitivity to cold depends on the presence of cold agglutinins and haemolysins. Changes in vascular tissue, involving the smooth muscle of blood vessels or their blockage by precipitated proteins, predominate in cryoglobulinaemia, which may prove distressing or fatal, depending upon which tissues are involved. The avoidance of cold is essential, and sterol treatment may be tried in cases of cryoglobulinaemia. Desensitization may help some patients with cold urticaria. The term cryopathy has been used to describe such states as peripheral arterial disease, myopathies, and myxoedema, in which existing diseases are exacerbated by cold.

Before modern gastric surgery was established, morphia by subcutaneous injection and ice-water by mouth was the standard treatment for acute haemorrhage from the stomach and duodenum. Recent work has tended to support the therapeutic efficiency of local gastric cooling in arresting haemorrhage by local vasoconstriction, though as an alternative to the excision of a chronic or complicated ulcer, gastric cooling is probably not indicated owing to the anatomical and functional changes that local cold injury may produce in the gastric mucosa (Smith *et al.*, 1964). Moreover, controlled trials have shown no lasting clinical benefit from gastric cooling (Wangensteen *et al.*, 1964).

Brain surgery involving the deliberate destruction of small areas of tissue for therapeutic purposes (stereotaxis) can be accomplished by the local injection of alcohol or by heating or cooling with the aid of suitable probes and X-ray control. The use of cold is attractive to the neurosurgeon operating with local anaesthesia, as the initial injury produced by cold may be entirely reversible. Detailed clinical and electrophysiological testing of the patient before the definitive lesion is made is a considerable aid to the exact anatomical and functional localization necessary. Such information also makes the clinical response to treatment more predictable.

There is experimental and some clinical evidence that hypothermia, both local and general, may assist the radiotherapy of certain tumours (Bloch *et al.*, 1961; Weiss, 1961). Profound hypothermia will ultimately decrease the oxygen supply to the tissues with the result that their radiosensitivity will be decreased. This permits normal tissues to tolerate a considerable increase of X-irradiation, and abnormal tissues, which have relatively greater radiosensitivity, are then likely to suffer more irradiation damage. At the present time, a temporary increase in tissue oxygenation, and hence increase in tumour radiosensitivity, can be accomplished by hyperbaric oxygenation (Churchill-Davidson *et al.*, 1955). The clinical success of using hyperbaric oxygenation during radiotherapy, and the difficulties of controlling radiation dosage and hypothermic technique, have precluded the general adoption of hypothermia in this context, though the simultaneous or alternate combination of both techniques might be a useful development.

The refrigeration of organs and tissues has been practised for some 200 years. In 1935, blood transfusion was introduced as a standardized procedure, and by 1943 storage of blood in an acid-citrate-glucose solution at 5° for three weeks was possible, with the preservation of cell viability sufficient for transfusion. Over the last two decades, considerable progress has been made in low-temperature biology, and the survival of several tissues after storage at $-79°$ (the temperature of solid carbon dioxide) to $-196°$ (liquid nitrogen), for periods ranging from an hour to a year, has been accomplished. Fundamental to these exciting developments was the discovery, in 1949, of the protective effects of the hydrophilic non-electrolyte glycerol in preventing undue ionic imbalance, during the cellular dehydration of freezing and rehydration of rewarming this being the chief cause of cell damage during profound cooling. The use of glycerol, and more recently dimethyl-sulphoxide, enables the return of normal function after storage at subzero temperatures of isolated organs and transplanted tissues. The pharmacological responses of smooth muscle, uterus and heart muscle, the electrical activity of peripheral nerves, the functions of profoundly cooled spermatozoa and blood cells, and the endocrine functions of transplanted glandular tissues (testis, ovary, adrenal, thyroid) have all been restored to their precooling levels of activity, in a variable but high percentage of cases, after return to normal temperatures.

The utilization of tissues after storage at subzero temperatures has an increasing medical importance. Skin, bone, cornea, bone marrow, blood vessel and heart valve grafts are already stored at low temperatures, and used to replace damaged or diseased parts in patients, with satisfactory results. The developing experimental potentialities of cartilage grafting are opening up new possibilities for the treatment of arthritis, perhaps the commonest non-fatal, physical affliction in the Western hemisphere. Grafted skin will ultimately slough unless it is obtained from an identical twin, but even this limited viability on the host may be life-saving after severe burns. Bone marrow transfusion, after total irradiation of the leukaemic host bone marrow, has produced some striking remissions of an apparently fatal outcome. Encouraging results are being obtained in the technique of human kidney grafting, and experimental transplantation of the lungs, heart and liver has been performed with some success. One case of human lung transplantation, with survival of more than a week, has been reported.

The ethical and aesthetic difficulties of the removal of young healthy tissues from the fatal victims of accidents, for cold storage and subsequent grafting, have not proved insuperable, but the technical problems, both of long-term organ storage and of the host rejection of the graft by the immune response, are not yet solved. The complex biophysical problems of the osmotic and ionic changes induced by cooling tissues and organs are being intensively studied, and the future possibility of organ storage after perfusion with dimethyl sulphoxide or some other protective substance, seems feasible. The use of hyperbaric oxygenation is the latest technique being explored with some success

(Blumenstock *et al.*, 1965). A great amount of immunological research is being done in an attempt to attenuate or abolish the primary and secondary host rejection of donor graft material from genetically dissimilar sources. X-Irradiation and various antimitotic drugs are being used, with increasing effect, to diminish the immune response while the donor cells function sufficiently long to permit their eventual acceptance, or replacement, by host cells.

These problems do not arise with relatively inert tissues such as cornea, bone, cartilage and blood vessels. Low immunological specificity and low metabolic turnover may explain the comparative ease with which these tissues can be grafted; also the inhibition of DNA synthesis at low temperatures may be a relevant factor. The decreased immune responses of certain tissues and experimental animals at low temperatures have a possible clinical application, and there is evidence of a decreased immunological response in the human at 30° as compared with 37° (Bloch, 1963). Complete, or sufficient, immunological suppression may prove impracticable, but the theoretical basis for immunological typing has already been established and suitable cold storage of appropriately typed organs in a bank could enable avoidance of undesirable immune reactions, in a manner analogous to that in which blood transfusion reactions are avoided, by "cross-matching" compatible cell types.

It is to be hoped that sufficient time and resources will soon be available to permit the solution of these problems, for the replacement of diseased or injured parts will probably prove less difficult than either the early diagnosis or cure of the processes of ageing and cancer.

2. *General Applications*

Heat stroke (hyperpyrexia) is fatal unless treated. The diagnosis is made from the history of heat exposure, the signs of central nervous system disturbance, delirium or coma, and lack of sweating. In hyperpyrexia, the body temperature is 40·6° or above. The causes of death in heat stroke include damage to the central nervous system and diffuse hypoxic changes; haemorrhage and congestion are seen in the major organs at autopsy (Malamud *et al.*, 1946). During heat stroke, measures may sometimes be necessary to combat concomitant circulatory failure due to dehydration from salt and water depletion. But the urgent necessity is to lower the body temperature to near normal values as quickly as possible. Vigorous convective and evaporative cooling of the patient, such as by the combination of a fine spray of cold water and a fan, using a special bed designed in the form of a grille to permit maximum exposure, is the treatment of choice. Cooling in a bath of ice-chips and water is a practicable alternative. Many drugs have been used and recommended in the treatment of heat stroke, but the efficacy of none of them is established. Administration of salt and water by mouth or intravenous infusion may on occasions be necessary. The average mortality of the treated condition is in the region of 35%; however, its prevention is perfectly possible, by avoidance of excessive exposure, provision of air-conditioning, and adequate intake of salt and water.

B. NON-SPECIFIC EFFECTS

1. *Principles Underlying the Application of Hypothermia*

Below about 30°, the rate of chemical and physiological reactions in the human body decreases in an approximately linear manner with decreasing temperature. Below 20°, "cold narcosis" supervenes in non-hibernating animals, and this condition correlates with the disappearance of the normal electrical activity of the brain. Below about 15°, oxygen uptake, cardiac output and organ functions in general are greatly decreased, to less than 10% of their basal values, and may be "suspended" in the human for up to 55 min. In 80% or more of cases, there is complete recovery. The increasing tolerance to hypoxia (decreased oxygenation) and ischaemia (diminished blood flow) that decreasing temperatures permit is a general phenomenon in all cells and organs, and contrasts with a maximum safe tolerance of about 5 min. cardiorespiratory arrest at normal body temperature (37°).

In a period of 5 min., at a body temperature of 37°, there is a basal oxygen uptake of approximately 250 ml./min., from an available store of 1 litre of oxygen contained in 5 litres of air in the lungs. This corresponds to a tolerable diminution of arterial oxygen tension from 90 to 20 mm.Hg. In normal conditions, the heart and brain receive, respectively, 4% and 13% of the total cardiac output of some 5·8 litres/min., and their corresponding oxygen uptake is about 11% and 20% of the total.

Since the regulation of blood flow and oxygen uptake form the basis of the application of hypothermia, it is necessary, firstly, to consider these factors as they operate in the normal and abnormal human being before going on to consider how these functions are affected by hypothermia.

There is a great functional reserve capacity of both the respiratory and cardiovascular systems in health and in disease. There is a virtually linear relationship between the amount of work done in exercise and the oxygen uptake, the pulse rate, the cardiac output and the increase in the difference between the venous and arterial oxygen saturation, below the limits of tolerance as determined by training and age. In the suitably trained athlete, an increase of up to twenty times the resting oxygen uptake may occur (Åstrand and Christensen, 1964), and the blood flow and oxygen uptake of the exercising muscles may increase by as much as twenty times (Wade and Bishop, 1962). For less healthy humans threatened by disease, there is a safety factor of about nine which comprises, usually, the ability to treble the pulse rate, and the ability to treble the difference in arteriovenous oxygen saturation. Tissue oxygen uptake normally equals the difference between an arterial oxygen content of 19 ml./100 ml. blood (95 mm.Hg) and a mixed venous oxygen content of 15 ml./100 ml. blood (40 mm.Hg). The "tissue" oxygen tension is of the order of 35 mm.Hg, but the tension in the mitochondrion of the cell, the major site of oxygen metabolism, is probably less than 1 mm.Hg. There is thus a considerable physical pressure gradient causing oxygen transport from the lungs, at about 100 mm.Hg, to the mitochondrion within the cell. Arterial oxygen tensions as low as 20 mm.Hg have been recorded in patients with respiratory diseases. Symptoms of oxygen deficiency do not become manifest in the healthy person until there is a decrease from the normal 21% inspiratory oxygen percentage down to 14% (alveolar $pO_2 = 65$ mm.Hg), and it is not until about 10% oxygen is breathed (alveolar $pO_2 = 45$ mm.Hg), that central nervous system dysfunction becomes apparent. However, the acclimatized Andean native can perform hard physical work with an alveolar pO_2 of 50 mm.Hg, at an altitude of 4,540 metres, a degree of hypoxia intolerable to the acutely exposed individual. Also the Korean diving woman tolerates, without loss of consciousness, a decrease of her alveolar pO_2 to 40 mm.Hg, after a minute of work on the seabed, and this is followed by a further decrease to 25 mm.Hg during and immediately after ascent. The basis of these changes is the adaptability of the respiratory and circulatory systems to meet altering and increasing demands by increasing transport of oxygen to, and carbon dioxide and waste products from, the tissue cell. The heart, brain and exercising muscles do not have sufficient stores of glucose or oxygen for more than resting requirements, and they are thus critically dependent upon the rates at which these essential ingredients are provided.

Cellular respiration is enhanced by increasing the dissociation of oxyhaemoglobin and the local rate of tissue blood flow. Both of these effects are brought about by increasing the body temperature, by raising the acidity and carbon dioxide tension of the blood, and possibly by the accumulation of vasodilator metabolites. Increases in respiratory rate and depth are chiefly dependent upon the stimulatory effects of increasing carbon dioxide tensions and acidity on the reflex nervous control of ventilation. A positive feedback mechanism thus operates in a system with a storage capacity of about 1 litre of oxygen and about 20 litres of carbon dioxide, in which the metabolic production of acids and carbon dioxide is largely responsible for the local and general uptake of oxygen and output of carbon dioxide, hydrogen ions and metabolic acids. The circulatory changes occurring in response to abrupt or extreme general alterations of gas exchange chiefly comprise selective lowering in splanchnic (gut), renal and skin blood flow (which normally account for some 50% of the cardiac output), with a preferential maintenance of blood flow to the heart and brain and, in the case of exercise, a considerable increase of blood flow to the muscles, with an intermediate increase of skin blood flow (Wade and Bishop, 1962). In the resting state, the oxygen uptake of muscles comprises about 30% of the total body uptake, and that of the gut and kidneys some 40%. During maximum exercise, as much as 90% of the total oxygen uptake may be utilized by the muscles. The control of this circulatory redistribution is effected by autonomic initiation of selective vasoconstriction, with blood flow consequently being decreased to those tissues not actively consuming much oxygen and increased to actively metabolizing tissues. With the exception of frank heart failure and certain cases of chronic lung disease, in which latter situation ventilatory insufficiency may lead to carbon dioxide retention and an increase in the cerebral and skin circulation, all types of relative or absolute oxygen deficiency that result from respiratory and circulatory impairment are associated with initial changes of blood flow resembling those of exercise, and with a relative decrease of blood flow to the guts, kidney and skin with preferential maintenance of blood flow to the heart and brain. Whether this series of adjustments is sufficient to meet the needs of the altered conditions depends upon the nature and duration of the alteration, the age of the patient, the state of health or otherwise of the systems involved, and the temperature at which the situation occurs. Whereas the healthy person has the ability to increase both ventilation and circulation, the diseased patient may be unable to do either.

Diminished oxygen transfer from the lungs to the blood, due either to a decrease of inspiratory oxygen tension or an impairment of diffusion from the alveoli, is known as hypoxic hypoxia. Lowered oxygen carriage in the blood, due to a decreased haemoglobin concentration, is known as anaemic hypoxia. Decreased oxygen transport due to circulatory stasis is known as stagnant hypoxia. Histotoxic hypoxia is the term reserved for the impairment of oxygen uptake resulting from cell damage. A mixed disturbance is commonly encountered in diseases of the heart, lungs and circulation. The energy demands of exercise, which can be excessive, may be met by temporary anaerobiosis and glycolysis in the muscles, with lactacidosis, a state of affairs tolerable for brief periods, with the establishment of an "oxygen debt" to be paid off on the resumption of normal blood flow. The acidosis which results from a blood flow insufficient for metabolic needs is a fundamental feature of states of hypoxia, about which more must be said later. Selective vasoconstriction is the basic primary response of the human body to situations calling for a selective increase of blood flow to some organs and a decreased flow to others, with a fixed or decreasing circulating blood volume. When the circulating blood volume, or its rate of flow, or degree of oxygenation, is diminished, there is a limit to which compensatory mechanisms can remain effective. A mean arterial blood pressure of about 100 mm.Hg is the peak of a pressure gradient that reaches − 5 mm.Hg in the veins returning to the heart. Prolonged vasoconstriction at the arteriolar level will penultimately decrease the amount of blood returning to the heart. This diminishes the cardiac output, and local tissue damage with cellular swelling finally decreases local tissue blood flow and respiration.

The muscle mass forms about half of the body weight, while the venous system comprises some two-thirds, and the pulmonary venous system approximately a quarter of the circulating blood volume. Alterations of blood flow in these compartments of the vascular system are of fundamental importance in compensatory circulatory changes, though their dynamics have not been sufficiently studied. Inequalities of the ratio of the volume of perfusing pulmonary blood to the volume of alveolar ventilation are a feature of all states of hypoxia, and underventilation of perfused alveoli or underperfusion of ventilated alveoli results in diminished arterial oxygen tensions. Hyperventilation is the first line of defence against insufficient oxygenation. But this too has limitations, for eventually carbon dioxide tensions in the blood will fall as a result of excessive ventilation and this predisposes to peripheral vasoconstriction and decreased flow rates of blood, unless it is balanced by the active production of carbon dioxide that maintains the *status quo*, as in muscular exercise.

Thus, in health, a linear relationship exists between oxygen consumption and blood flow. An increase in oxygen consumption is limited by the capacity of the circulation to increase volume and flow rates, and may temporarily be supplemented by the anaerobic glycolysis of glucose. Acidosis has an initial stimulatory action on local cell blood flow and respiration and on general oxygen uptake and circulation, but progressive or sustained impairment of oxygenation or circulation will ultimately lead to cellular metabolic failure, with marked acidosis. With hypothermia, increasing peripheral resistance to blood flow from vasoconstriction (above 26°) is associated with decreasing oxygen uptake and cardiac output, and at temperatures in the region of 1°, "tissue" oxygen tensions reach levels of 0–2 mm.Hg, as measured by the oxygen cathode. At these temperatures, the transport of oxygen by haemoglobin can become superfluous and life may temporarily be supported by the dissolved oxygen in solution in the plasma.

From the foregoing account, it will be clear that cell death may be described as a permanent inability to utilize oxygen, and that a virtually complete, but at the same time temporary, suspension of oxygen uptake of the whole animal is compatible with recovery, under the conditions of an appropriately lowered temperature. If an animal is to survive a period of hypothermia, satisfactory control of circulation and oxygenation during the cooling and rewarming periods is necessary. It is now possible to review the literature on the applications of hypothermia.

2. *Applications of Hypothermia*

In 1862, Walther reported the survival of rabbits after surface cooling to 20° for up to 12 hours. Sixteen years later, detailed measurements of oxygen uptake were made by Pflüger (1878) during the cold exposure of the unanaesthetized rabbit after administration of curare. In 1902, Simpson reported the cooling of the monkey to 15° using ether anaesthesia during surface cooling, with subsequent survival after rewarming. Experimental and clinical interest remained sporadic until 1940, when Fay reported the lowering of the body temperature of humans to about 30° for up to five days, by surface cooling and initial anaesthesia, in an attempt to treat certain forms of cancer. In 1953, the successful closure of an atrial septal defect under hypothermia was performed by Lewis and Taufic using surface cooling. As long ago as 1798, cold immersion had been used by Currie to decrease unduly high fevers resulting from infections, but it was not until Potts (1949) and McQuiston (1950) reported the prevention of fever by surface cooling during operations on children with congenital heart defects to be beneficial that interest in hypothermia was re-awakened. Impetus was given by the experimental work of Bigelow and his associates (1950a,b), and in less than a decade the maintenance of a body temperature of 15°, with the suspension of respiration and circulation for 55 min., had been achieved. Artificial oxygenation was found to be dispensable in profound hypothermia. The patient's own lungs may be used during cooling, and a pump is needed only to circulate the blood through a heat exchanger (Drew and Anderson, 1959). The maintenance of the circulation by means of a pump had been demonstrated in 1937 by Gibbon, but it was not until about 1955 that the development of bloodstream cooling with a pump-oxygenator was sufficiently advanced for its utilization in cardiac surgery (Gollan *et al.*, 1955). Reports of the experimental and clinical use of pump-assisted oxygenation and bloodstream cooling soon followed (Brock and Ross, 1955; Sealy *et al.*, 1959). Hyperbaric oxygenation, involving the administration of oxygen under 3 atm. pressure, was first utilized experimentally in 1956 by Boerema and his associates. Since then, however, the clinical development of hyperbaric oxygenation has chiefly been at normal temperatures, though it is still being employed in conjunction with hypothermia in certain cardiac operations (Vermeulen-Cranch, 1965).

This profusion of techniques is a reflection both of the realization that hypothermia offers definite therapeutic advantages, and of the difficulties and complications that surround use of the procedure. It is perhaps understandable, though possibly unfortunate, that academic physiologists have in general preferred the experimental steady state to the unsteady clinical situation, while the clinician has had to cope with problems as best he could. The rapid advances in technology over the past two decades should soon enable a shift of emphasis from an unavoidable pre-occupation with instrumentation to an investigation of the complex co-ordinated changes of circulation and respiration that occur both in health and disease states. So far, progress in this direction is encouraging.

While oxygen deficiency may be lethal if unrelieved, so may oxygen excess, and the administration of oxygen at one or more atmospheres pressure produces a diminution both of cardiac output and peripheral blood flow, and cannot be withstood indefinitely by the spontaneously breathing human or animal; after a period, pulmonary and cerebral oedema (tissue swelling and damage) will occur. The duration of tolerance to the administration of excess oxygen may be appreciably lengthened by artificial ventilation, or by a decrease in oxygen enrichment to about 35% of the inspiratory concentration. At the present time, increasing oxygen supply by artificial oxygenation and circulation enables the cessation of spontaneous respiration and circulation for over an hour at normal temperatures, and decreasing oxygen uptake by hypothermia, with or without similar mechanical aids, enables cardiorespiratory arrest for about an hour at temperatures in the region of 15°. In either situation, important disturbances of function may lead to mortality. Whereas most experimental animals are healthy, none of the patients subjected to either normothermic or hypothermic perfusion, or hyperbaric oxygenation, has been healthy, and it is possible that a certain mortality is unavoidable. However, when one considers how well the unaided healthy body can sustain severe hypoxia, given time, it is not unreasonable to suggest that attempts to improve upon natural processes might profitably imitate them as closely as possible. At the present time, it is not possible clearly to separate those complications due to perfusion techniques from those due strictly to lowered temperatures. Nevertheless, in certain centres, extensive practice seems to have made the technique nearly perfect.

In those patients that succumb after surviving operative intervention, mortality has been attributed to low output circulatory failure, widespread brain damage, embolism (migratory clots) in the cerebral arterial field, and vascular and parenchymal lung damage, individually or in combination (Ehrenhaft *et al.*, 1961; Brierley, 1963; Patrick *et al.*, 1958; Muller *et al.*, 1958; Dodrill, 1958; Willman *et al.*, 1958). Omitting factors such as inoperability, the unsatisfactory repair of defects, and associated vascular or cardiac pathology prejudicial to survival after operation, there are several factors that have been shown favourably to influence the outcome after hypothermic cardiorespiratory arrest.

High rates of perfusion of blood flow have been found to diminish metabolic acidosis and to favour survival after perfusion (Kirklin *et al.*, 1958; Senning, 1958; Bernhard *et al.*, 1961; Yeh *et al.*, 1961). It is interesting to compare what are commonly regarded as high, or acceptable, flow rates, 2·3 litres/min./m.^{2} (Kirklin *et al.*, 1958), or 75–100 ml./kg./min. (Senning, 1958; Varco *et al.*, 1958), with the fact that a value of 2·0 litres/min./m.^{2} or below is the cardiac index usually found in states of shock after certain cases of heart attack, and the fact that the latter value corresponds to 3·3–4·4 litres/min./m.^{2} (cf. the normal cardiac index of 3·5–4·0 litres/min./m.^{2}). Excessive temperature gradients (more than 10°) have been found to be unfavourable during rapid, extracorporeal cooling (Björk and Hultquist, 1962), and it is possible therefore that the heat exchangers may be too efficient. The deliberate increase of the inspiratory carbon dioxide concentration to 10% during hypothermia diminishes these temperature gradients (Broom and Sellick, 1965).

The use of low molecular weight (40,000) dextran is beneficial in lowering the otherwise considerably increased blood viscosity at low temperatures, and perfusion flows are more easily maintained when blood viscosity has been suitably lowered.

Oxygenation of the blood can be considered as adequate if arteriovenous oxygen differences are within normal limits. But whereas an increased arteriovenous oxygen difference may signify a decreased flow rate and an increased oxygen uptake, a decreased arteriovenous oxygen difference may mean decreased oxygen utilization, which is only synonymous with "requirements" in the light of subsequent survival. The differentiation between these two conditions can be made either by assessment of the overall oxygen uptake or by measurement of the blood pH value. It has already been stated that excess acidity is synonymous with inadequate perfusion (p. 522). However, what constitutes a "normal" pH value at temperatures below 26° is a question with which few academic physiologists and biochemists have yet concerned themselves. An increasing metabolic acidosis is a feature of hypothermia. This may be caused by prolonged anaesthesia, although increasing lactacidosis is the most likely cause. While the solubility of carbon dioxide in the blood increases with decreasing temperature, the ionization of haemoglobin and plasma proteins decreases, and so an increased carriage of carbon dioxide results in the virtual maintenance of pH value, *in vitro*, as determined by the similar linear relationship of the plot of log pCO_2 against pH value with decreasing temperature (Brewin *et al.*, 1955). The respiratory regulation of H^+ concentration is basically dependent upon the ratio of the concentrations of bicarbonate to carbonic acid and hence the blood carbon dioxide tension, which is a reciprocal function of ventilation.

$$CO_2 + H_2O \rightleftharpoons H_2CO_3 \rightleftharpoons H^+ + HCO_3'$$

$$[H^+] = K \frac{[H_2CO_3]}{[HCO_3']}$$

$$pH = pK + \log \frac{[HCO_3']}{[H_2CO_3]}$$

However, the normal reduction of oxyhaemoglobin to haemoglobin, as blood traverses the tissues, is diminished by decreasing temperatures, and may be further lowered by artificial hyperventilation during anaesthesia. A relative increase (lack of increase of dissociation) of oxyhaemoglobin concentration will tend to diminish the blood buffering capacity, as oxyhaemoglobin is a stronger acid than haemoglobin and thus is less able to accept H^+ ions. An increase in the concentration of dissolved oxygen at low temperatures has the same effect. In other words, during hypothermia there is a progressive tendency towards a reversal of the normothermic situation in which increasing reduction of oxyhaemoglobin is associated with increasing hydrogen ion acceptance and maintenance of pH value.

The situation is further complicated by the fact that respiratory depression, which results from the combined effects of anaesthesia and decreased temperature, may increase the blood pCO_2, and hence decrease the blood pH value thereby causing respiratory acidosis. A combination of both forms of acidosis is inimical at normal temperatures, where it usually results from severe respiratory or circulatory impairment. Within limits, an increasing pCO_2 will increase oxygen utilization considerably more efficiently than increasing oxygen content. But most clinical efforts have been exclusively expended either in increasing oxygen availability or in attempting to neutralize the acidosis, by hyperventilation or bicarbonate infusion, and sufficient endeavour has not yet been applied to the problem of oxygen utilization, as the whole emphasis of hypothermia has been to diminish oxygen uptake and hence, ultimately, oxygen requirements (some would prefer to say *vice versa*). While the aim of the clinical experiment is the lowering of oxygen consumption to minimum levels, an aim which may be readily achieved, sufficient attention has not yet been paid to the establishment of the optimum conditions of inducing and maintaining hypothermia.

a. Cardiac arrhythmias. Simple surface cooling of the anaesthetized human to temperatures much below 30° has not been found practicable. The tolerance to cardiorespiratory arrest at 30° is about 10 min., long enough for simple heart operations to be carried out but not for the repair of multiple heart defects with which surgeons are becoming increasingly concerned. At this level of conventional moderate hypothermia, the apparently inevitable occurrence of disorders of cardiac rhythm, with consequent premature failure of cardiac output, hastened the development of the alternative artificial aids to oxygenation and circulation that have been mentioned. A search for the actual cause, or causes, of this arrhythmia has incriminated every known variable, as have the various measures designed to prevent its occurrence. It is not now such a serious problem owing to the availability of satisfactory electrical cardiac pace-making techniques which have been developed over the past 15 years.

It is perhaps somewhat surprising that this problem of cardiac arrhythmia has been such a major one, in view of the earlier experimental work on surface cooling. The following account of some of the changes that occur during natural hibernation and accidental hypothermia, together with certain recent experimental work done on surface cooling, suggests possible ways in which this difficulty may be overcome.

The changes preceding and accompanying natural hibernation are complex and not completely investigated, but fine control of local and general circulation down to a body temperature of 5–6°, with the preservation of cardio-respiratory activity, is the dominant feature. During hibernation, the total carbon dioxide content of the blood is raised (Lyman and Chatfield, 1956), though recent determinations of this content are scant. Cold exposure of the unanaesthetized hibernator in the laboratory may be followed by what appears to resemble natural hibernation if carbon dioxide-enriched gas mixtures are breathed (Dubois, 1895a,b,c).

In 1949 it was shown by Giaja and Andjus that the rat could withstand depression of its body temperature to 1·0° and recover, after utilizing progressive, partial asphyxiation during the initial stages of cooling, a technique known as autonarcosis. Further development enabled the realization, by 1956, of subzero temperatures for several hours both in the Norwegian hooded rat, an animal habitually exposed to cold, and the golden hamster, a facultative hibernator, with survival after rewarming in most cases (Andjus *et al.*, 1956). Subjection to these temperatures (0° to −5°) was sometimes associated with supercooling and the absence of ice formation, but more commonly ice formation did occur and calorimetric experiments showed that as much as 50% of the total body water had been converted to ice. Carbon dioxide accumulation during asphyxia was found to be necessary for the successful prosecution of these experiments, and simple hypoxia was not followed by survival. Cardiac arrhythmias were not noted during these cooling experiments, though they did occur sometimes during rewarming. In 1873, Bert first showed that carbon dioxide inhalation, resulting from rebreathing in a closed circuit, depressed the body temperature of the rabbit.

The exciting clinical possibilities of this work were inhibited by its lack of success in larger animals owing to the problems of rewarming larger tissue masses at an appropriate rate. However, the only successful case of human surface cooling to the point of cardiac arrest (9°), without intervening arrhythmia, involved the use of 5% carbon dioxide in oxygen with conventional anaesthesia (Niazi and Lewis, 1958). Experimental work utilizing surface cooling to the point of cardiac arrest in animals has only been successful using carbon dioxide enrichment, while the administration of pure oxygen has not proved a satisfactory alternative gas mixture. Further development of this aspect of the physiology of hypothermia seems to have been suspended because of its lack of immediate success and because of the availability of alternative artificial aids to solving the problem.

Prolonged, accidental human cold exposure is not commonly associated with cardiac arrhythmia. The cooling of body temperatures below 25° has been reported to be followed by survival (Talbott, 1941); and there is a case on record of survival, following about 11 hours cold exposure, at a body temperature of 18° (Laufman, 1951). Cases of prolonged cold exposure who have survived have usually been subjected to gradual, or spontaneous, rewarming, and most attempts at rapid rewarming have been unsuccessful (Duguid et al., 1961). Acute cold water immersion of the unanaesthetized human causes changes similar to those in the anaesthetized patient, both with regard to cooling rate (about 5°/hr.) and the temperature range in which cardiac arrhythmias occur. In these latter examples of acute hypothermia, rapid rewarming at an ambient temperature of about 40° is the most efficient method of revival (Alexander, 1946). However, this does not apply after prolonged hypothermia of several days at around 30° (Bloch, 1965), nor does it appear to be the case after cooling in profound hypothermia, where unduly rapid rates of cooling and rewarming may produce temperature gradients in the body in excess of 10°, with resultant cerebral damage (Björk and Hultquist, 1962). It was noted in 1862 by Walther, and subsequently confirmed in 1943 by Ariel et al., that gradual cooling and rewarming rates were conducive to survival, after surface cooling to 20°, although the use of bloodstream, extracorporeal, cooling usually lowers the body temperature of the core of the patient to 15° within 30–45 min., a situation that the most robust hibernator seldom has to face!

The questions of the depth, and type, of anaesthesia and the optimum rates of cooling and rewarming are critical and not yet sufficiently investigated in the clinical situation. Both hypoxia and deep anaesthesia will diminish the initial metabolic response to cold (increased oxygen uptake) that occurs on cold exposure of the mammal, and the decrement of oxygen uptake with prolongation of cold exposure will then be virtually linear. Experimentally, during surface cooling, the avoidance of deep anaesthesia and hypoxia is not associated with this initial decrease of the metabolic response to cold (B. Broom, unpublished observations), but it is found to influence favourably survival during cold exposure, since it is then possible to preserve cardiovascular and respiratory reflexes down to about 20°, and also to prevent cardiac arrhythmia (Brendel et al., 1958). This more favourable state of affairs may also be obtained by the respiration of a carbon dioxide-enriched gas mixture (Broom, 1963; and unpublished observations). It is interesting to note that the doubling of survival time after cardiorespiratory arrest at 30° is compatible with the explanation that narcotic protection is almost wholly responsible (i.e. the depressant effects of anaesthesia on oxygen uptake), and that this short-term gain currently militates against more favourable survival times at lower temperatures after a longer period of time.

This discussion of some of the physiological problems involved in cardiac surgery under hypothermia has been lengthy because of its complexity and because, in the field of the medical applications of low temperatures, it is only in cardiac surgery that sufficiently extensive use of hypothermia has been made to allow an adequate, though perhaps interim, assessment. The prolongation of ischaemic tolerance by hypothermia has enjoyed considerable application in vascular, renal, hepatic and central nervous system surgery, where elective hypothermia prior to "physiological trespass" is a relatively simple and definitely useful procedure.

b. Other applications. When one considers other uses to which hypothermia has been put, the picture is altogether different. Surface cooling down to around 30° has been employed, advocated and rejected in patients with schizophrenia, head injuries, acute cerebrovascular disease, cerebral damage after cardiac arrest, carbon monoxide and barbiturate intoxication, and in cases of severe fever, burns, haemorrhage, shock and infection. Other occasions in which it has been used are in poor-risk cases before, during or after surgery, as an adjunct to the treatment of cancer, with and without radiotherapy, and in certain cases of neonatal asphyxia immediately after birth. There is experimental evidence that hypothermia may be beneficial in cerebral damage, neonatal asphyxia and states of shock if it is instituted suitably promptly after the insult. The variable clinical pictures and multiplicity of associated treatments makes assessment at the present time impossible. In the two controlled trials of clinical hypothermia so far reported, hypothermia was not found to be of clinical benefit either in the radiotherapy of cerebral tumours (Bloch *et al.*, 1961) or the treatment of certain forms of schizophrenia (Hays *et al.*, 1960).

3. *Future Prospects for Hypothermia*

Subzero tissue refrigeration and storage is already proving of considerable clinical use, and the future needs for whole organ storage are likely to be met, for the technical problems do not appear insuperable. The use of moderate (30°) and profound (15°) hypothermia has an established place as an elective procedure in vascular and cardiac surgery for limited periods of time. The twin developments of pump-assisted oxygenation and circulation, and hyperbaric oxygenation, may supplant hypothermia for short-term surgical purposes. None of these three techniques, alone or in combination, has been designed, or is available at the present time, for operations lasting more than an hour or two. Only hypothermia, with or without mechanical supplementation, is likely to be able to meet future requirements for whole organ transplantation, and to treat otherwise irremediable acute and chronic disease processes, the basic features of which include localized or generalized hypoxia.

Fundamental to these questions are the problems of increasing tissue oxygen utilization, as opposed to tissue oxygen availability, and the validity of equating oxygen availability, uptake and requirements in the 37–0° range. The role of carbon dioxide in this context is in need of adequate assessment, as is the detailed delineation of concomitant circulatory changes.

There is considerable future scope for the local and general applications of low temperatures in medicine and surgery, when the development and application of the appropriate technology takes place. The uses of low temperatures in medicine provide an excellent opportunity for the further integration of the physical sciences into what is becoming the biological science of medicine.

References

Alexander, L. (1946). "Treatment of Shock from Prolonged Exposure to Cold, Especially in Water", C.I.O.S., No. 24, Washington, D.C.

Allen, J. G. Ed. (1958). "Extracorporeal Circulation", Blackwell Scientific Publications, Oxford.

Andjus, R. K., Lovelock. J. E. and Smith, A. U. (1956). *In* "The Physiology of Induced Hypothermia", (Dripps, R. D. Ed.), pp. 125–142. Publ. no. 451, Nat. Acad. Sci. Nat. Res. Council, Washington, D.C.

Ariel, I., Bishop, F. W. and Warren, S. L. (1943). *Cancer Research* **3**, 448.

Åstrand, P-O. and Christensen, E. H. (1964). *In* "Oxygen in the Animal Organism", (F. Dickens and E. Neil, Eds.), pp. 295–303. Pergamon Press, London.

Bernhard, W. F., Carroll, S. E., Schwarz, H. F. and Gross, R. E. (1961). *J. thorac. cardiovasc. Surg.* **42**, 793.

Bert, P. (1873). *Compt. rend. soc. biol. Paris* **5**, 156.

Bigelow, W. G., Callaghan, J. C. and Hopps, J. A. (1950a). *Ann. Surg.* **132**, 531.

Bigelow, W. G., Lindsay, W. K. and Greenwood W. F. (1950b). *Ann. Surg.* **132**, 849.

Björk, V. O. and Hultquist, G. (1962). *J. thorac. cardiovasc. Surg.* **44**, 1.

Blair, E. (1964). "Clinical Hypothermia", McGraw–Hill, New York.

Bloch, M. (1963). *Lancet* ii, 1255.

Bloch, M. (1965). M.D. Thesis: London University.

Bloch, M., Bloom, H. J. G., Penman, J. and Walsh, L. S. (1961). *Lancet* ii, 906.

Blumenstock, D. A., Lampert, N. and Morgado, F. (1965). *J. thorac. cardiovasc. Surg.* **50**, 769.

Boba, A. (1960). "Hypothermia for the Neurosurgical Patient", Blackwell Scientific Publications, Oxford.

Boerema, I., Kroll, J. A., Meyne, N. G., Lokin, E., Kroon, B. and Huiskes, J. W. (1956). *Arch. chir. Neerl.* **8**, 193.

Brendel, W., Albers, C. and Usinger, W. (1958). *Arch. f. d. ges. Physiol.* **266**, 357.

Brewin, E. G., Gould, R. P., Nashat, F. S. and Neil, E. (1955). *Guy's Hosp. Rep.* (London). **104**, 117.

Brierley, J. B. (1963). *Thorax* **18**, 291.

Brock, R. and Ross, D. N. (1955). *Guy's Hosp. Rep.* (London) **104**, 99.

Broom, B. (1963). *Nature, Lond.* **199**, 1155.

Broom, B. and Sellick, B. A. (1965). *Lancet* ii, 452.

Burton, A. C. and Edholm, O. G. (1955). "Man in a Cold Environment", Edward Arnold, London.

Churchill-Davidson, I., Sanger, C. and Thomlinson, R. H. (1955). *Lancet* i, 1091.

Cooper, K. E. (1961). *In* "Hypothermia and the Effects of Cold", (A. S. Parkes, Ed.), pp. 48–51. *Brit. med. Bull.* **17**, 48.

Cooper, K. E. and Ross, D. N. Eds. (1960). "Hypothermia in Surgical Practice", Cassell, London.

Currie, J. (1798). "Medical Reports, on the Effects of Water, Cold and Warm, as a Remedy in Fever and Febrile Diseases", Cadell and Davies, London. *Cited by* Cooper K. E. (1961). *Brit. med. Bull.* **17**, 48.

Dodrill, F. D. (1958). *In* "Extracorporeal Circulation", (J. G. Allen, Ed.), pp. 327–335. Blackwell Scientific Publications, Oxford.

Drew, C. E. and Anderson, I. M. (1959). *Lancet* i, 748.

Dripps, R. D. Ed. (1956). "The Physiology of Induced Hypothermia", Publ. No. 451. Nat. Acad. Sci. Nat. Res. Council, Washington, D.C.

Dubois, R. (1895a). *Compt. rend. soc. biol. Paris* **10**, 149.

Dubois, R. (1895b). *Compt. rend. soc. biol. Paris* **12**, 814.

Dubois, R. (1895c). *Compt. rend. soc. biol. Paris* **12**, 830.

Duguid, H., Simpson, R. G. and Stowers, J. M. (1961). *Lancet*, ii, 1213.

Ehrenhaft, J. L., Claman, M. A., Layton, J. M. and Zimmerman, G. R. (1961). *J. thorac. cardiovasc. Surg.* **42**, 514.

Fay, T. (1940). *New York Sta. J. Med.* **40**, 1351.

Giaja, J. and Andjus, R. (1949). *Compt. rend. Acad. Sci., Paris* **229**, 1170.

Gibbon, J. H. (1937). *Arch. Surg.* **34**, 1105.

Gollan, F. (1959). "The Physiology of Cardiac Surgery: Hypothermia, Extra-corporeal Circulation and Extracorporeal Cooling", Blackwell Scientific Publications, Oxford.

Gollan, F., Grace, J. T., Schell, M. W., Tysinger, D. S. and Feaster, L. B. (1955). *Surgery* **38**, 363.

Hays, P., Wolfson, G., Kirkler, B. and Day, B. (1960). *J. ment. Sci.* **106**, 344.

Horvath, S. M. Ed. (1960). "Cold Injury", (Six Conference, 1958). Josiah Macy Jr. Foundation, New York.

Kappas, A., Palmer, R. H. and Glickman, P. B. (1961). *Amer. J. Med.* **31**, 167.

Kirklin, J. W., McGoon, D. C., Patrick, R. T. and Theye, R. A. (1958). *In* "Extracorporeal Circulation", (J. G. Allen, Ed.), pp. 125–138. Blackwell Scientific Publications, Oxford.

Laufman, H. (1951). *J. Amer. med. Ass.* **147**, 1201.

Leithead, C. S. and Lind, A. R. (1964). "Heat Stress and Heat Disorders", Cassell, London.

Lewis, F. J. (1961). *Int. Abstr. Surg.* **113**, 307.

Lewis, F. J. and Taufic, M. (1953). *Surgery* **33**, 52.

Lyman, C. P. and Chatfield, P. O. (1956). *In* "The Physiology of Induced Hypothermia", (R. D. Dripps, Ed.), pp. 80–122. Publ. No. 451. Nat. Acad. Sci. Nat. Res. Council. Washington, D.C.

Malamud, N., Haymaker, W. and Custer, R. P. (1946). *Milit. Surg.* **99**, 397.

McQuiston, W. O. (1950). *Arch. Surg.* **61**, 892.

Muller, W. H., Littlefield, J. B. and Dammann, J. F. Jr. (1958). *In* "Extracorporeal Circulation", (J. G. Allen, Ed.), pp. 336–341. Blackwell Scientific Publications, Oxford.

Niazi, S. A. and Lewis, F. J. (1958). *Ann. Surg.* **147**, 264.

Parkes, A. S. Ed. (1961). *Brit. Med. Bull.* **17**.

Parkes, A. S. and Smith, A. U. Eds. (1960). "Recent Researches in Freezing and Drying", Blackwell Scientific Publications, Oxford.

Patrick, R. T., Kirklin, J. W. and Theye, R. A. (1958). *In* "Extracorporeal Circulation", (J. G. Allen, Ed.), pp. 272–278. Blackwell Scientific Publications, Oxford.

Pflüger, E. (1878). *Arch. f. d. ges. Physiol.* **18**, 247.

Potts, W. J. (1949). *Ann. Surg.* **130**, 342.

Sealy, W. C., Brown, I. W. Jr., Young, W. G., Smith, W. W. and Lesage, A. M. (1959). *Ann. Surg.* **150**, 627.

Senning, A. (1958). *In* "Extracorporeal Circulation", (J. G. Allen, Ed.), pp. 224–228. Blackwell Scientific Publications, Oxford.

Shafar, J. (1965). *Lancet* **ii**, 431.

Smith, A. U. (1961). "Biological Effects of Freezing and Supercooling", Edward Arnold, London.

Smith, V. M., Sandstrom, R. H., Cruze, K. and Lancaster, R. G. (1964). *Gastroenterology*, **46**, 761.

Starkov, P. M. Ed. (1960). "The Problem of Acute Hypothermia", Pergamon Press, London.

Talbott, J. H. (1941). *New Engl. J. Med.* **224**, 281.

Taylor, A. C. (1959). *Ann. N.Y. Acad. Sci.* **80**, 285.

Varco, R. L., Barnard, C., Dewall, R. A. and Lillehei, R. C. (1958). *In* "Extracorporeal Circulation", (J. G. Allen, Ed.), pp. 164–178. Blackwell Scientific Publications, Oxford.

Vermeulen-Cranch, D. M. E. (1965). *Proc. Roy. Soc. Med.* **58**, 319.

Virtue, R. W. (1955). "Hypothermic Anesthesia", Blackwell Scientific Publications, Oxford.

Wade, O. L. and Bishop, J. M. (1962). "Cardiac Output and Regional Blood Flow", Blackwell Scientific Publications, Oxford.

Walther, A. (1862). *Arch. f. path. u. Physiol.* **25**, 414.

Wangensteen, S. L., Smith, R. B. III., Barker, H. G., Magill, T., Raber, R. and Flood, C. A. (1964). *Gastroenterology*, **46**, 766.

Weiss, L. (1961). *Brit. Med. Bull.* **17**, 70.

Williams, L. K. (1964a). *Physics in Medicine and Biology* **9**, 433.

Williams, L. K. (1964b). *Ann. N.Y. Acad. Sci.* **121**, 99.

Willman, V. L., Zafiracopoulos, P. and Hanlon, C. R. (1958). *In* "Extracorporeal Circulation", (J. G. Allen, Ed.), pp. 295–302. Blackwell Scientific Publications, Oxford.

Yeh, T. J., Ellinson, R. T. and Ellinson, R. G. (1961). *J. thorac. cardiovasc. Surg.* **42**, 782.

Chapter 15

Thermal Energy as a Factor in the Biology of Soils

AMYAN MACFADYEN

*Department of Zoology, University College of Swansea,
Wales*

I. Introduction: Life in the Soil

The distribution of living organisms is neither uniform nor random. Although it is often difficult to decide precisely why an individual occurs in a particular place, there are certain conspicuous regions in space where organisms tend to aggregate. One type of aggregation centre is the interfaces between matter in different states, the boundaries between land and water, water and air and between air and land. Organisms become much less abundant as the observer leaves the interfaces and penetrates the uniform land, water and air masses. Perhaps the most biologically active regions are the shore lines where all three media meet, but next to these must come the upper surface of soil where the ground provides physical support and access to protection from enemies, whilst the air conveys respiratory gases and water vapour, the main raw materials of biological activity.

The extreme localization of life at the ground surface (Fig. 1) is not always appreciated. Almost all soil invertebrates in temperate soils are most abundant within 1 cm. of the surface between the undecomposed litter and the layers beneath. Numbers decline roughly according to an exponential law so that many groups are not found at a depth of 1 dm. from the surface, and only a few cave-dwelling forms attain a metre's depth. The centre of gravity of the great majority of plants is close to the soil surface, and most above-ground animals spend much of their lives supported by the soil surface where they dispose of their excreta and ultimately their corpses. Many insects, whose more conspicuous stages of development take place above ground, spend long periods as soil-dwelling larvae, pupae or eggs.

Whilst the soil surface is the centre of activity of many plants and animals, the actual surface layer is, in many respects, the most extreme from the point of view of its physical properties. At the ground surface

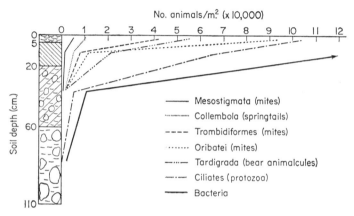

Fig. 1. The vertical distribution of animals in soil. Note that, in all groups, the highest numbers occur in the top 5 cm. After Stöckli (1946).

(unless it is protected by emergent vegetation) the full impact of solar radiation is felt by day, and the greatest loss of long-wave radiation occurs at night. The climatic variability at this surface is thus the most extreme in the whole vertical profile (see Section IV, p. 542). This surface, too, is subject to the most rapid changes of water regime, from flooding to desiccation.

Under normal temperate conditions, soil develops at the ground surface, and consists of the mineral products of weathering together with organic materials from organisms living above and within the soil. The intensity of life in this medium is not widely appreciated. For example, a biologist asked to describe the food chains based on a meadow that is subject to cattle grazing would mention the grass, the cattle in their role as herbivores, man as a carnivore, and perhaps the small mammals and insects which compete with the cattle as consumers of grass. It has recently become apparent that, even in a man-managed system of this kind, only about one-third of the 7,500 kcal. of energy made available by each square metre of herbage annually is consumed by herbirores; perhaps one-sixth is consumed by cattle and one-sixth by other herbivores. The remaining 5,000 kcal., together with the energy from the faeces of the herbivores, are liberated in the decomposition of organic matter by the soil organisms which, in so doing, liberate the nutrients that are otherwise not available for use by the plants (Macfadyen, 1964). Most, perhaps 90%, of the metabolic activity associated with soil decomposition processes is carried out by bacteria, fungi and actinomycetes. These organisms, however, are most intolerant of climatic extremes and, since they are incapable of effective locomotion, spend much time in resting stages or operating below maximum efficiency. Since they also rapidly exhaust localized nutrient supplies, they are highly dependent on the soil fauna (Macfadyen, 1966). These small animals modify the physical structure of soil by their movements and also transport micro-organisms throughout the soil. These effects have been dramatically demonstrated by Witkamp (1960).

Most people consider the soil fauna as being made up of small mammals, earthworms and perhaps a few insect larvae. In fact, some 15 major invertebrate groups are important in soil and occur in great numbers. Average populations beneath a square metre of meadow soil are in the region of:

Protozoa	10^8
Free-living nematodes	10^7
Enchytraeid (white) worms	5×10^5
Oribatid (beetle) mites	5×10^5
Collembola (springtails)	5×10^4
Mesostigmatid (parasitid) mites	2×10^4

In certain soils, different groups of animals become important including millipedes, woodlice, beetle larvae, fly larvae, ants, termites, crickets and small mammals. These animals are mobile throughout most of their lives, and maintain a characteristic vertical distribution. But even the smallest of them probably responds to some extent to climatic change either by vertical movement, demonstrated for mites by Strenzke (1952), or by forming resistant resting stages. Temperature must be one of the most potent factors which dominate the lives of these organisms; hence the importance of thermobiology in soils.

II. The Thermal Energy Budget of a Temperate Soil

Soil is an exceptional substance from the point of view of its thermal properties and different soils vary greatly, for they are complex mixtures of solid, liquid and gaseous materials. The specific heat of a soil usually lies in the range 0·27–0·8 (Sutton, 1953); it is high for dense clays and when much water is present, and low in a sand. The thermal conductivity of a soil also varies with the water content within the range 10^{-2}–10^{-3} cm.^{2}/sec.; maximum values occur at about 12% (w/w) water content. The absorption of solar radiation by a soil varies greatly according to the colour, moisture and texture. Quantitative generalizations about these physical properties are not possible, but in general it is true that soil approaches a perfect black body in its radiation-absorbing properties, although it has a high thermal capacity and is a poor heat conductor. This combination of properties results in very slow penetration of heat through soil, and a consequently rapid attenuation of diurnal and seasonal temperature changes. A wave of temperature change initiated at the soil surface usually travels at 2–3 cm./hr.

The heat balance of temperate soils, especially in relation to solar radiation, is very clearly discussed by Gates (1962), and the theory of soil heat balance by Geiger (1951). Detailed studies on heat transfer through soil have been made by Kristensen (1959) and Coutts (1955), and the physics of meteorology close to the ground surface, including briefly the soil, by Sutton (1953). These works should be consulted for further information.

On average, a 1 cm.^{2} area outside the earth's atmosphere and parallel to the earth's surface receives 2 cal./cm.^{2}/min. of energy in the form of solar radiation; of this, about 43% is within the visible region. On an annual basis, this is equal to 255 kcal./cm.^{2} of energy or, in terms of power, it represents a continuous mean supply of 340 W./m^2. (see Fig. 2.)

Of the 255 kcal./cm.^{2}/year outside the atmosphere, some 24% (61 kcal.) reaches the ground directly by radiation, 17% (43 kcal.) is relayed by diffuse radiation from clouds to the ground, and 6% (15 kcal.) reaches the ground after scattering by the atmosphere and its particles. Thus, 53% fails to reach the ground. The quantity that reaches the ground, namely 119 kcal./cm.^{2}, is equal to 1·2 million kcal./m.^{2}, which is rather more than the average yearly energy intake of a man; it represents a continuous power supply of 160 W./m.^{2} It will be noticed that this is some 600 times the metabolic heat output derived from the decomposition of organic matter, and that the latter can therefore be neglected as a source of heat. It is also some 2,500 times the rate of heat transfer from the centre of the earth, which is about 32 g./cal./cm.^{2}/year. Since the energy reaching the earth's surface is balanced with that lost over the course of a year, all of this heat (120 kcal./cm.^{2}/year) must be lost again from the surface. Depending mainly on the water vapour and cloud contents of the atmosphere, a variable proportion is lost from the soil (or indirectly from covering vegetation) in the form of long-wave radiation. The remainder is dissipated through conduction and convection in the air and through supplying latent heat of vaporization to water.

If the air contains much water vapour, outward going infrared radiation from the soil is intercepted and absorbed in certain distinct wavebands, of which that with a wavelength between 5·4 and 7·9 m. is the

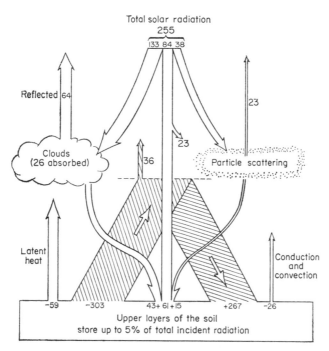

Total solar radiation
255

Reflected 64

Clouds
(26 absorbed)

Particle scattering

36

23

23

Latent heat

Conduction and convection

−59   −303   43+ 61 +15   +267   −26

Upper layers of the soil
store up to 5% of total incident radiation

Fig. 2. A diagram showing the total annual energy balance for a northern temperate soil. The figures indicate the energy in kcal./cm.^{2}/year. Shaded energy streams represent long-wave radiation mainly around 10 μ wavelength. Note that most of this is reflected and contributes a major item in the whole budget. Data from Gates (1962) and other sources; see text.

most important. Because a good absorber is also a good radiator, much of this energy is reradiated to the earth again, a fact familiar to anyone who compares the sensations felt on a cloudy and a clear night under similar conditions of air temperature. A similar blanketing effect occurs due to the carbon dioxide content of the air but, since this is much more uniform and less dense and also mainly concerns wavelengths in the 13·3–17 m. band, the effect is less conspicuous. Nevertheless it is true to say that, in the absence of atmospheric water and carbon dioxide, the surface of the earth would be quite uninhabitable to life as we know it.

18+T.

Under average conditions the loss of long wavelength radiation (i.e. heat) amounts to some 413 W./m.^{2}, of which 375 are reflected and only 56 W. escapes outward. It is evident why regions of clear skies, such as the Sahara, have a far less equable climate than temperate latitudes.

If the water supply to the soil were sufficient, any tendency towards a temperature change would be countered by evaporation or condensation of water. Since the latent heat of vaporization is so great (560 cal./g.), the average excess energy balance after radiant loss of 104 W./m.^{2} would in fact be fully taken up by evaporating 4·2 mm. (0·17 in.) per day of precipitation. Mercifully, however, we are usually spared a steady rainfall of this magnitude (equivalent to 62 in. per year) and, when the soil moisture becomes depleted, its temperature starts to rise. Local regions of high temperature produce convection currents in the air and eventually turbulent mixing; in this way, excess heat is spread through the atmosphere and ultimately dissipated in frictional losses. The rate of heat loss in this way averages 34 W./m.^{2} In drier climates and especially under desert conditions, the shortage of soil water results in much higher surface temperatures and consequent winds during the day.

The thermal properties and consequent avenues of heat exchange are of the greatest importance to soil organisms and, since the penetration of heat into the ground depends on the soil properties, it will be appreciated that simple measurements of air temperature give only a partial indication of the relevant thermal environment. The very steep thermal gradients, and their precise coincidence or change of height relative to the soil surface, can be exploited by animals in particular, so that regions of extreme climate are avoided and preferred regimes are selected. Examples of some of these biological adaptations are discussed in Section V (p. 548).

III. Microclimatic Influences on Heat Exchange at the Soil Surface

As already explained, some of the most potent factors determining heat exchange at the soil surface are components of the regional climate; of these, the water and carbon dioxide contents of the air are conspicuously important. In addition, the general level of air movement and humidity, which are largely determined by the geographical location, control the evaporative and conductive cooling of the soil and are balanced by incident solar radiation.

On a more local scale, important topographical factors affecting the soil heat regime include aspect and ground contours (Geiger, 1951). The combination of a clear dry night and a "frost hollow", into which dense cold air drains from higher ground, can readily produce local frost conditions, in Britain even in summer. The shelter provided by hills and larger trees can radically modify local climate and ameliorate soil temperatures (see Aslyng, 1958; Geiger, 1951; Macfadyen, 1963), and is exploited in the planting of shelter belts.

From the point of view of organisms which live at, or near, the soil surface, however, the most potent influences are the truly microclimatic ones, involving the steep gradients of temperature and air movement that occur very close to the surfaces of soil and plants. Naturally, the growth of a dense tree layer, as in a forest, can completely change the

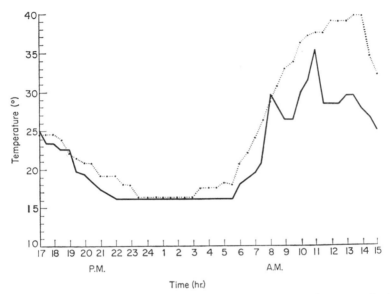

FIG. 3. Diurnal soil temperature regimes in a forest and an adjacent sandy field. The dotted line denotes the temperatures in the sandy field; continuous line, the temperatures in the forest soil. Note that the forest soil temperatures extend over a smaller range, are more erratic (partly due to sun flecks) and are generally cooler. Redrawn from Nørgaard (1945).

climate by intercepting both incident and outgoing radiation and impeding air movement. The region of radiation interception is spread through the depth of the canopy, and this results in smaller temperature gradients. The diurnal temperature range is diminished and the humidity raised (Nørgaard, 1945). Tree shelter also modifies the depth of frost penetration and this, together with transpiration by the trees, changes the whole moisture regime (Coutts, 1958). The mean temperature over the year is often little changed but, climatic extremes are invariably smaller (Fig. 3).

Far shorter vegetation such as grass, even without fully shading the soil, can greatly modify the microclimate, partly by broadening the band

of surfaces at which solar radiation is intercepted but also by diminishing wind movement close to the soil. Whitehead (1951) studied this
problem in a very exposed mountainous region in Italy. He obtained
reasonable confirmation of theoretical considerations which predicted
that the wind was always turbulent at speeds greater than 1 m./sec. and
that the speed then became proportional to the logarithm of the height
above ground. For any uniform surface there is an "extinction height"
below which no air movement due to wind occurs. This height is a
function only of the size of the objects, such as stones or plants, which
are attached to the soil surface and, where these are uniform in size, the
extinction height is about one-thirtieth of their diameter. In practice,
values between 1 cm. and 3 cm. were found even in these very exposed
localities.

Even in the absence of any vegetation, several factors can greatly
modify the soil surface climate. Ludwig and Harper (1958) have shown
that experimental alteration of the soil colour, by the use of soot, lime
and other substances, can so modify the absorption of solar energy as to
produce considerable variations in the surface temperature and,
correspondingly, in the time taken for seeds to germinate (Table I).

TABLE I. *The Effect of Soil Colour on the Surface*
Temperature and the Time Taken for Maize Seeds to
Germinate (Modified from Ludwig and Harper, 1958)

Soil Colour	Max. Temp. (°)	Min. Temp. (°)	Days
White	14·1	6·0	32
Yellow-brown	14·6	6·8	26
Red-brown	17·9	7·2	22
Brown	19·0	7·4	21·5
Dark Grey	19·4	6·9	21
Black	19·5	7·3	20

The temperature columns are the means of the daily maximum and minimum
temperatures respectively during the three weeks period after sowing. The days column
gives the number of days for 50% emergence of seedlings. The colour of the soil was
modified experimentally.

IV. Movement of Heat within Soil

The heat gained by the soil during daytime and in summer is mainly
dissipated to the atmosphere by reradiation, conduction and convection
or by vaporization of water (see Section II, p. 539). Owing to the thermal
properties of soil, relatively little heat penetrates below the surface, but
that which does penetrate is stored in the soil and, at night and in
winter when the thermal gradient is reversed, it is lost again. The
cyclical reversals of temperature gradient result in corresponding
reversals in the direction of heat flow, and these are an important

element in the environment of soil organisms. The higher the thermal capacity and the lower the conductivity of the surface layers, the more effectively will energy be contained in and restricted in the soil. Since the rate of flow of heat through the soil depends on its thermal capacity and on the temperature gradient to which it is subjected, the temperature regime at a given depth can be predicted from these data. The solid material of a hypothetical, dry, non-porous soil has a thermal capacity (number of calories required to heat 1 g. through 1°) which is inversely related to the density, so that:

$$C_v = \frac{C_w}{D} \cong 0\cdot58$$

where C_v = thermal capacity/unit volume
$\quad\quad C_w$ = thermal capacity/unit weight
$\quad\quad D$ = density

With a natural soil, containing air spaces and water, the porosity, P (as a fraction of air volume) and the water content, W (in g. water/g. soil) can be allowed for in the equation:

$$C_v = \frac{0\cdot58(100 - P) + W}{100}$$

Kristensen (1959) calculated the amount of heat which would accumulate during the daytime, and also during the summer months, on the basis of this formula. He estimated the temperature difference from the diurnal (and seasonal) mean for each, arbitrarily limited, soil layer and multiplied this by the thermal capacity. In this way, he showed that, in clear weather in mid-July, the soil in his experiments stored up to 45 cal./cm.^{2} with a peak at about 1900 hours and a minimum at 0700 hours. This is less than 5% of the diurnal input of some 1,000 cal./cm.^{2} During the months May, June and July, the soil was steadily gaining heat at the rate of about 200 cal./cm.^{2}/week, and throughout the whole summer (April through August) it stored some 3,000 cal./cm.^{2}, again about 5% of the total solar energy received at the ground surface. Comparable diurnal values are quoted by Sutton (1953) and summarized in Table II.

The effect of the heat transfer properties of soil on its temperature can be expressed theoretically, either in terms of the heat capacity and temperature gradient as above or by calculating a thermometric conductivity (synonym for thermal diffusivity) constant. Examples of the latter have been given by Sutton (1953), Coutts (1955) and by other authors quoted in these papers. Coutts (1955) presented a simple theoretical treatment in which it is assumed that the diurnal (or seasonal) energy supply is a sinusoidal function of time, and that it can be described by a simple harmonic equation. If this is correct, the ratio

TABLE II. *Daily Heat Storage in Soil under Various Types of Vegetation* (*From Sutton*, 1953)

Type of Soil Cover	Heat Content during Daytime (cal./cm.^{2})
Woods on sandy or "mor" soil	15–24
Moorland	33–43
Bare sandy soil	95–105
Grass on sandy soil	56–67
Bare granite	128

of the amplitudes, θ_1/θ_2, at two depths x_1 and x_2 will be given by the formula:

$$\frac{\theta_1}{\theta_2} = (x_2 - x_1) \left(\frac{\pi}{kT}\right)^{1/2}$$

where T is the period and k a thermal conductivity or diffusivity constant. Transposing this equation gives:

$$k = \frac{\pi}{T} \left[\frac{x_2 - x_1}{\log_e (\theta_1/\theta_2)}\right]^2$$

The phase lag (τ) of the temperature wave at the lower depth relative to the upper is given by:

$$\tau = \tfrac{1}{2}(x_2 - x_1) \left(\frac{T}{\pi k}\right)^{1/2}$$

Coutts (1955) applied this formula to field data obtained from a forest locality in Aberdeenshire (Scotland), and obtained values for k at a depth of between 1 in. and 6 in. (a difference of 12·5 cm.) of 0·0027 –0·0057, which implies a phase lag of 4–5 hours per inch. This was very close to the value observed independently.

Kristensen (1959) also used the relation between annual temperature range and depth to predict the seasonal temperature profile, again using his estimates of soil thermal capacity. When he compared the predictions with observations he found good agreement below a depth of 4 metres.

Under normal conditions, it is clear that the rate of penetration of heat is so slow that an animal has only to burrow some 5 cm. or less to reach a depth at which the diurnal temperature rhythm is reversed, providing a midnight maximum and a midday minimum. This is clearly a factor of importance in the survival of animals inhabiting extreme conditions (see Section V, p. 548). In general, the rapid rate of diminution of diurnal temperature range results in the daily temperature span or "excursion" falling to about half the surface value at 1 cm. depth, one-tenth at 20 cm. and at somewhere between 30 and 70 cm. it is undetectable. Typical results are given by Kristensen (1959), (summarized in Table III) for short grass and bare sand in Denmark, and by Sinclair (quoted in Sutton, 1953) for desert conditions in Arizona (Table IV). In each of these soils, the temperature maxima and minima lag by 2–3 hours for each cm. of depth.

TABLE III. *Maximum and Minimum Temperatures and the Daily Temperature Span of a Temperate Soil as Affected by Depth and Soil Cover (After Kristensen, 1959)*

Position	Height or Depth	Maximum Temperature	Minimum Temperature	Daily Temperature Span
	(cm.)		(°)	
Air	20·0	25·0	15·0	10·0
Under	2·5	36·6	16·3	20·3
Bare	12·5	25·4	20·1	5·3
Soil	25·0	23·3	20·6	2·7
	50·0	19·5	18·6	0·9
Under	2·5	31·9	18·6	13·3
Short	12·5	24·3	20·9	3·4
Grass	25·0	22·2	20·9	1·3
	50·0	19·7	19·1	0·6

TABLE IV. *Effect of Depth on Soil Temperatures in Arizona, U.S.A. Recorded by Sinclair (Quoted in Sutton, 1953)*

Vertical Depth (cm.)	Temperatures (°)			Time Lag (hr.)
	Maximum	Minimum	Range	
0·4	71·5	15·0	56·5	
2·0	62·1	22·0	40·1	1·0
4·0	48·1	23·5	24·6	1·5
7·0	44·1	25·2	18·9	2·0

The magnitudes of the annual temperature cycles also decline with depth but, due to the much longer period, they can be detected at a much greater depth. Theoretically the depth of penetration is proportional to the square root of the duration of the period (Sutton, 1953). Annual variations should therefore penetrate about $\sqrt{365} = 19 \cdot 1$ times as far as diurnal fluctuations of equal amplitude, and Kristensen's (1959) figure of 12 m. for a 0·5° fluctuation is about 20 times the depth at which diurnal fluctuations fell to 0·5°; at 15 m. the annual fluctuation fell to 0·2°.

One important practical consequence of these properties of soil concerns the depth of penetration of frost. Coutts (1955) found in an Aberdeenshire forest that the air temperature fell below 0° on 99 days in 1952. At a depth of only 2·5 cm., there were 87 frosty days; at 15 cm., 9 days; and at 30 cm. there was no frost at all. Potter (1956), investigating the much more continental climate of North Dakota, obtained the results given in Table V, which also illustrate the ameliorating influence of snow cover. It should be remembered, of course, that a great deal of latent heat is absorbed when ice melts to water, and that the conductivity of wet soil also rises somewhat when it is frozen; the first effect predominates and materially delays the rate of change of temperature as the soil cools in autumn and warms again in spring.

TABLE V. *Effect of Snow Cover on the Relation between Depth and Duration of Frost in a North Dakota Soil (From Potter, 1956)*

Depth (cm.)	Weeks of Frost	
	Open Field	Deep Snow
Air	23	23
2·5	21	12
15	13	11
30	10	7
60	5	0
90	1	0
120	0	0

V. Effects of Temperature on the Biological Processes Occurring in Soils

The effects of the thermal environment on soil organisms can be broadly discussed under two headings.

A. EFFECTS OF MEAN TEMPERATURE ON METABOLISM

It is only very broadly true that the metabolic processes of organisms, other than homeotherms, are predictably related to the temperature of the environment. Two laws are commonly quoted in this context (see Wigglesworth, 1965; Kleiber, 1961; Chapter 6, p. 150). Van't Hoff's law, which was originally applied to chemical rections, states that the logarithm of the rate of a metabolic reaction is proportional to the temperature on the Centrigrade scale, while Arrhenius' rule states that the logarithm of the rate is proportional to the reciprocal of the absolute temperature. Since, however, the reciprocal of the absolute temperature is practically a linear function of the temperature on the Centrigade scale in the narrow range within which life occurs (Bělehrádek, 1935), it is not possible on empirical grounds to compare the predictive powers of the two formulae. Further, since the temperature dependence of enzyme-catalysed reactions does not conform strictly to either law (see Chapter 3, p. 62), it can hardly be expected that the behaviour of whole organisms will do so. In fact the Q_{10} value for the total respiration of organisms varies with the temperature range over which it is measured. This has also been shown with the few measurements that have been made on soil invertebrates. For instance in Berthet's (1964b) recent investigation of oribatid mites, Q_{10} values were mainly around 4·0. Microbial respiration tends to approach a $Q_{10} = 2$ rather more closely and, when the carbon dioxide output of intact soil cores was related to temperature, the author found rather consistent values around $Q_{10} = 2·0$ between 10° and 25°.

The unpredictability of laboratory-determined relationships between metabolic rate and temperature is, at first sight, disconcerting. But this is perhaps the least serious difficulty faced by the animal biologist who attempts to generalize from laboratory respirometry to field conditions with the aid of microclimatic measurements. Even under artificial conditions, marked acclimatization to a particular temperature change is usual (Bullock, 1955), and many species have diurnal metabolic rhythms which are innate or easily triggered by other factors such as light. Further, when the steepness of the soil temperature gradients (Section IV, p. 542) is considered in the light of the considerable loco-motory powers even of sluggish soil animals such as the oribatid mites (Berthet, 1964a), the problem of computing the total metabolism in thermally stratified soils appears hopeless. The only studies so far which have attempted such a task have been performed in well-shaded vegetation, and the authors have been forced to assume that the animal's temperature has not departed greatly from that measured at an arbitary depth or, more crudely, that the air temperature can be used as a first approximation (Berthet, 1964b; Healey, 1965; Nielsen, 1949, 1961).

Less direct evidence of the effect of the temperature regime on metabolism can be found in its effect on the length of life of soil organisms. It seems clear that some of the larger soil and litter-dwelling insects, such as beetles, have rather labile life-histories, and the number of generations in the year varies with latitude and presumably temperature (e.g. Larsson, 1939). Among smaller invertebrates, some species of mites and

18*

spiders have fewer annual generations in colder climates and may even require more than one year to complete the life cycle (Bristowe, 1933).

It was shown in Section IV (p. 545) that, although temperature excursion (both diurnal and annual) decreases rapidly with depth, the mean temperature remains nearly constant. Also, since there is a delay in the penetration of a temperature wave to successive depths, a mobile animal should be able to select regions in the soil in such a way as to maintain either higher or lower temperatures than the mean. We are almost entirely ignorant of the extent to which this occurs diurnally, but Strenzke (1952) demonstrated a distinct seasonal downward migration in winter for soil mites in Germany, Macfadyen (1952) for soil arthropods near Oxford, and Nielsen (1956) for enchytraeids in summer in Denmark. However, in Nielsen's (1956) study, temperature and drought were not clearly differentiated, and there was heavy mortality at the time, indicating that the animals probably did not move fast enough.

B. EFFECTS OF EXTREME TEMPERATURES ON THE PHYSIOLOGY, BEHAVIOUR AND RESPONSES OF SOIL ORGANISMS

A major distinction among the higher plants of the world lies between those which are frost-hardy, even if their above-ground parts are cut back, and those which are not. The qualification is, of course, all important as Raunkiaer (1954) realized because, as was shown with the Scottish and North Dakota data (Table V), frost penetrates soil to a surprisingly small extent. But, if sessile plants can avoid the consequences of climatic extremes at the soil surface, animals can do so even more, and many simply avoid altogether the challenge which they offer. They may do this by going elsewhere in the summer or the winter. Many insects and molluscs live as adults in vegetation in the summer, and as eggs or other resting stages in the winter, although their immature stages exploit the resources of the soil in the more equable seasons. Heighton (1964) for instance showed that several British harvestmen (Arachida) spend the winter as eggs and migrate into trees at the height of summer.

On a much shorter time scale, some animals migrate upward from the soil surface to colder strata in the air. A conspicuous example is *Lithyphantes albomaculatus*, a spider which inhabits overhanging lips formed where a sandy road cuts into heathy vegetation. Nørgaard (1948) noticed that the spiders climbed out into their webs in sunshine; they appeared to be sunning themselves, but measurements of the microclimatic profile showed that the spider suspended well above the ground experienced much lower temperatures than one in its retreat near the soil surface.

Nørgaard and other Scandinavian authors have made many studies of the relations between biological behaviour and microclimate in Europe. Conditions are, of course, far more extreme under desert conditions, and Schmidt-Nielsen (1964) gave many detailed examples of the way in which the smaller mammals, which do not have the water-carrying capacity for evaporative cooling or the insulating powers of a thick coat, avoid overheating partly by the possession of long legs (thus keeping above the extreme soil surface) but mainly by burrowing into the sand and exploiting the phase lag of diurnal temperature only a foot or two under the surface. Examples of microclimatic studies on desert invertebrates are few, but it is notable that most desert arachnids have long legs (Cloudsley-Thompson, 1956), and Tervis and Newell (1962) have described how the enormous trombid mites (*Dinothrombium pandorae*) of the Californian deserts remain in deep burrows for several years at a time, and eventually surface when the drought is broken to mate and feast themselves on termites. Conversely, the absorption of heat by rocks in the polar regions provides the short periods of above-zero temperatures which allow completion of the life cycle by those small mites and springtails which live nearest to the South Pole (Dalenus and Wilson, 1958).

If we consider the physiological results of the thermal environment on animals, it is necessary to measure not only the air temperature but also the other factors in the heat balance, including the absorption or reflection of radiant energy, the use of insulating layers of various kinds, and any behavioural peculiarities. This has been done to some extent for man (Schmidt-Nielsen, 1964, Bedford, 1946) and for domestic animals (Kleiber, 1961; Findlay, 1950), but, of those animals which are exposed to the most extreme climatic conditions of all, namely the inhabitants of the soil surface, we are almost entirely ignorant.

In a classical study, Parry (1951) demonstrated that temperatures, measured with thermocouples inside locusts, could be closely simulated with metal and clay models. He was able to measure the effects of colour, size, shape and orientation on temperature, the insulating effect of pubescence, such as is carried by many caterpillars, and the value, as long as the water supply lasts, of evaporative cooling. The survival value of the last factor has been compared in different species of woodlice by Edney (1951). Evidently, the effects of such factors are even more important for minute animals living at the soil surface than they are for larger creatures with greater thermal and water capacities and superior locomotory powers. But these pioneer experiments have not yet been followed up.

There is a type of behaviour experiment which is still widely performed, although consistent and biologically meaningful results are rarely forthcoming. It involves placing animals in a temperature gradient and observing the position between the extremes which they take up. In addition to the various snares common to all such experiments (Macfadyen, 1963), those aimed to discover temperature preferenda of soil invertebrates have been particularly unreliable. Clearly, a small, probably blind animal living in the labyrinthine spaces near the soil surface has a particular need for a means of avoiding being overwhelmed by extreme temperatures and especially by heat. The animal's food, in the form of decaying plant matter or the feeders thereon, is mainly concentrated precisely at the soil surface. An ability to detect and to react kinetically to variations in the temperature of the soil air spaces might ensure their survival. But, in such a complex environment, a far more useful sense organ would be one capable of detecting the direction of origin of infrared radiation. Such organs have been demonstrated in some trombid mites in which a parasitic larva is rendered active by the approach of a potential mammalian host and also in ticks (Homp, 1938; see Carthy, 1958). Why should such organs not be far more widespread among the soil fauna? There is no lack of enigmatic sense organs among such forms, such as the "Rhagidia organs" and "Sig Thor organs" among the mostigmata, the many peculiar solenidia and other hairs in many other mite groups, and the postantennal and antennal organs of collembola. Many of these are paired and potentially capable of use in a directional manner, and it is not impossible that the primary significance of the light-sensitive first legs of many Parasitidae (Bhattacharyya, 1960; Camin, 1953) is as infrared rather than visible light detectors, for most of these forms live almost entirely in the dark and the experimental procedures used would not have distinguished visible from infrared radiation.

VI. A Note on Techniques Especially Relevant in Soil Thermobiology

Methods for temperature measurement in soil can follow normal microclimatic practice provided there is full allowance for the steepness of thermal gradients and the low conductivity of the soil. This means that any temperature detector must be very small, and no thermal leakage must occur along wires which cross steep gradients. Frequently, the biologist wishes to compare the phase lag between maxima and minima at different depths, although these can often be adequately predicted from theory (Section IV, p. 543) backed by preliminary empirical measurements. There is then no alternative to a multichannel recorder using either thermocouples or thermistors. For a discussion of the relative advantages of these detectors, see Macfadyen (1963). The expense and considerable labour involved in deriving mean values from an irregular trace can, however, be avoided if only mean temperatures or maxima and minima are recorded.

A variety of physical and chemical processes are temperature-dependant, and have been used to measure mean temperatures. Brian (1964) used the rate of diffusion of acetic acid through a fine pore, and Berthet (1960) the rate of hydrolysis of sucrose, which can be followed with the aid of a polarimeter. Such methods suffer two disadvantages: firstly, that the apparatus is rather large and therefore unable to discriminate steep gradients; and the second that the Q_{10} value for the reaction is fixed and may not be relevant to the desired measurements. Both of these objections are overcome by the use of temperature-sensitive resistors (thermistors) connected in series with a mercury-alkali (Malory) cell and a simple current integrator (Macfadyen, 1956). Thermistors have sensitive elements less than 1 mm. in diameter, and the integrator can be a silver voltameter with a weighed cathode. A recent improvement (unpublished) substitutes a "Mercron" integrator (Kiryluk, 1962) which can be read in the field with a Vernier caliper. The Q_{10} value of thermistors can also be adjusted to any desired value by the use of a suitable circuit (Macfadyen, 1949).

The measurement of extreme temperatures is not yet well catered for. A simple device due to Dahl (1949a,b) records a frequency distribution curve of temperatures and has been used under snow for periods of six months. A gamma-ray source situated above a slit is moved by a bimetalic strip over a sensitive emulsion, and the density of fogging produced is proportional (within limits) to the time during which a particular temperature occurred. This apparatus is rather large, but the same principle could be employed to record the movement of a moving coil meter connected to a thermistor.

In recent years, the periodical recording of many points on tape, using a battery-operated waterproof "logger", has become possible. This logger can be buried under ground, and the readings collected as infrequently as once a year. Such an apparatus is the d-Mac Limpett Logger (manufactured by d-Mac, Ltd., Glasgow, Scotland).

The recording and measurement of incident radiation, although of major importance in soil biology, lies outside the scope of this chapter since no methods have been developed apart from those normally used for this purpose above ground. The characteristics of different devices are discussed by Gates (1962) and by papers in Bainbridge *et al.* (1966).

VII. Conclusions

We have seen that the soil near the surface in temperate countries is one of the most densely inhabited of all habitats. It contains a very wide range of organisms, and is the site of intense metabolic activity. At the same time, it is the main region of energy exchange from solar radiation by day, and of other forms of energy by day and by night. The physical properties of soil are such that extreme temperature changes, often much greater than those occurring at widely separated geographical localities, are largely confined to a narrow region near the soil surface, but this is precisely the site at which most biological activity takes place. This situation certainly has important effects on the metabolic processes occurring near the soil surface. It demands many special adaptations in the organisms concerned, and it is therefore the more astonishing that very little is yet known about their biology and their behaviour.

References

Aslyng, H. C. (1958). *Oikos* **9**, 282.

Bainbridge, R., Evans, G. C. and Rackham, O., Eds. (1966). "Light as an Ecological Factor", Symp. Brit. Ecol. Soc. Blackwell, Oxford.

Bedford, T. (1946). M. R. C. War. Memo, 17, 2nd. edn. 40 pp. H.M.S.O. London.

Bělehrádek, J. (1935). "Temperature and Living Matter", Gebrüder Borntraeger, Berlin.

Berthet, P. (1960). *Vegetatio* **9**, 3.

Berthet, P. (1964a). *J. anim. Ecol.* **33**, 443.

Berthet, P. (1964b). *Mem. Inst. Roy. Sci. Belg.* No. 152, 152 pp.

Bhattacharyya, S. K. (1960). M.Sc. Thesis: University of Wales (Swansea).

Brian, M. V. (1964). *J. anim. Ecol.* **33**, 451.

Bristowe, W. S. (1933). *Norsk ent. Tidsskrift* **3**, 149.

Bullock, T. H. (1955). *Biol. Rev.* **30**, 311.

Camin, J. H. (1953). Chicago Acad. Sci., Special Publ. No. 10.

Carthy, J. D. (1958). "An Introduction to the Behaviour of Invertebrates", 380 pp. Allen and Unwin, London.

Cloudsley-Thompson, J. L. (1956). *Ann. Mag. nat. Hist. Scr.* 12, **9**, 305.

Coutts, J. R. H. (1955). *Quart. J. Roy. met. Soc.* **81**, 72.

Coutts, J. R. H. (1958). *Forestry* **31**, 167.

Dahl, E. (1949a). *Science* **110**, 506.

Dahl, E. (1949b). *Physiol. Plant.* **2**, 272.

Dalenus, P. and Wilson, O. (1958). *Arkiv. Zool. Ser.* 2, **11**, 23.

Edney, E. B. (1951). *J. exp. Biol.* **28**, 91.

Findlay, J. D. (1950). Hannah Dairy Research Institute Bull. No. 9, 178 pp. Kirkhill, Scotland.

Gates, D. M. (1962). "Energy Exchange in the Biosphere", 152 pp. Harper and Row, New York.

Geiger, R. (1951). "The Climate near the Ground", translated by the author. University Press, Harvard.

Heighton, B. N. (1964). Ph.D. Thesis: University of Durham.

Healey, I. N. (1965). Ph.D. Thesis: University of Wales (Swansea).

Homp, R. (1938). *Z. vergl. Physiol.* **26**, 1.

Kiryluk, W. (1962). Trade literature on Mercron II. Industrial Instruments Ltd., Bromley, Kent, England.

Kleiber, M. (1961). "The Fire of Life: an Introduction to Animal Energetics", 454 pp. John Wiley, New York.

Kristensen, K. J. (1959). *Oikos* **10**, 101.

Larsson, S. G. (1939). *Ent. Medd.* **20**, 277.

Ludwig, J. W. and Harper, J. L. (1958). *J. Ecol.* **46**, 381.

Macfadyen, A. (1949). *Nature, Lond.* **164**, 965.

Macfadyen, A. (1952). *J. anim. Ecol.* **21**, 87.

Macfadyen, A. (1956). *Oikos* **7**, 56.

Macfadyen, A. (1963). "Animal Ecology: Aims and Methods", 2nd edn., 344 pp. Pitman, London.

Macfadyen, A. (1964). *In* "Grazing in Terrestrial and Marine Environments", (D. J. Crisp, Ed.). Blackwell, Oxford.

Macfadyen, A. (1966). *In* "The Ecology of Soil Bacteria", (J. Gray and D. G. Parkinson, Eds.). University Press, Liverpool.

Nielsen, C. O. (1949). *Natura Jutlandica* **2**, 1.

Nielsen, C. O. (1955). *Oikos* **6**, 153.

Nielsen, C. O. (1961). *Oikos* **12**, 17.

Nørgaard, E. (1945). *Flora og Fauna* **51**, 1.

Nørgaard, E. (1948). *Flora og Fauna* **54**, 1.

Parry, D. A. (1951). *J. exp. Biol.* **28**, 445.

Potter, L. D. (1956). *Ecology* **37**, 62.

Raunkiaer, C. (1954). "The Life Forms of Plants and Statistical Plant Geography", 600 pp. University Press, Oxford.

Schmidt-Nielsen, K. (1964). "Desert Animals: Physiological Problems of Heat and Water", 278 pp. University Press, Oxford.

Stöckli, A. (1946). *Schweiz. Zeits. f. Forstwesen.* **8/9**, 23.

Strenzke, K. (1952). *Zoologica* **104**, 173 pp.

Sutton, C. G. (1953). "Micrometeorology", 500 pp. McGraw-Hill, London.

Tervis, L. and Newell, I. M. (1962). *Ecology* **43**, 479.

Whitehead, F. H. (1951). *Ecology* **39**, 330.

Wigglesworth, V. B. (1965). "The Principles of Insect Physiology", 741 pp. 6th edn. Methuen, London.

Witkamp, M. (1960). ITBON (Arnhem) Mededeling No. 46.

Chapter 16

Thermal Energy as a Factor in the Biology of the Polar Regions

J. S. BUNT

Institute of Marine Science, University of Miami,
Florida, U.S.A.

I. Introduction

Life is a delicate phenomenon poised within relatively narrow environmental limits. Nevertheless, individual organisms, species, populations and whole communities always exhibit some degree of resilience to environmental stress. The tolerances displayed under boundary conditions are sometimes remarkable and deserve careful study, for an appreciation of the mechanisms involved can make significant contributions to an understanding of life processes in general. There can be no doubt that thermal stress is a dramatic and outstanding factor influencing polar biology. With increasing facilities and support for arctic and antarctic biological research, our knowledge in this field, although still limited and often descriptive, is steadily becoming more complete and its potential value more apparent.

The present account of the thermobiology of the polar regions has not been written as a detailed review. Rather, it has been designed to provide a wide perspective and, it is hoped, an integrated view. Particular attention has been given to the citation of reviews and of recent, rather than early, papers as these provide most ready access to the literature in particular fields, a literature notoriously scattered and difficult to trace.

II. Physical Environments of the Polar Regions and the Thermal Regime

The tropical, temperate and polar zones of the earth's surface are not sharply delimited. Although discontinuities in climatic and thermal gradients between the equator and the poles are well recognized, their position in time and space is variable so that boundaries are difficult to fix except in arbitrary terms. Because of the relative disposition of land and ocean masses, however, it is true to say that the overall thermal regime increases in severity more rapidly with latitude south of the equator than to the north. For biologists, the arrival at a generally acceptable definition of the polar regions is particularly difficult. Normally, geographic, climatic and biological criteria have been invoked in deciding boundaries. A good deal of compromise is often necessary to reach some form of agreement, although biologists are unanimous that routine meteorological data are inadequate for their purposes. Fortunately, this account does not depend on limits, but is concerned rather with the effects of unmistakably polar thermal regimes on the nature of organisms and their ecology.

In this context, the inclusion of the entire continent of Antarctica in the southern hemisphere, and the treeless tundra and permanently ice-covered regions north of the arctic circle, as the terrestrial component of the polar regions is unlikely to find much disfavour. Of the oceanic areas, we may include as widely representative, those in which water temperatures never or rarely rise more than a few degrees above 0° and which are frozen at the surface during the greater part of the year. It should be emphasized that these criteria will not be allowed to exclude studies undertaken in marginal areas where the results are relevant to the discussion.

Screen temperatures in Antarctica rarely rise above 0° and have been observed to fall as low as $-88 \cdot 3°$ (Anon., 1961). In local situations, which act as radiation traps, conditions may be quite temperate. Thus, Angino et al. (1962) have recorded a temperature of $23 \cdot 9°$ a little over 1 m. above the ice of Lake Bonney in Victoria Land, near McMurdo Sound; rock temperatures as high as $27 \cdot 8°$ have been noted in the Horlick Mountains near the South Pole (Llano, 1962). Fukushima (1959) found pond temperatures up to $10 \cdot 1°$ on Ongul Island (lat. 69°S, long. 39° 35′E), and Goldman (1964) recorded similar values in some lakes of the Taylor Dry Valley in Victoria Land. In general, however, such conditions are of short duration and limited to the summer period.

Mean annual temperatures close to the coast on the relatively mild Antarctic Peninsula are approximately $-11°$. Inland, data available indicate annual means between $-30°$ and $-60°$.

On the Greenland Icecap, mean annual temperatures may be as low as $-30°$. Mean winter air temperatures throughout the arctic range from approximately $-20°$ to $-40°$. Extremes lower than $-50°$ are experienced only rarely. A mean temperature of $10°$ for the warmest month, unheard of in the antarctic, is regarded as a realistic upper limit for the arctic. Extremes may reach $25–30°$. Microclimates are often appreciably warmer than screen data reveal. Bliss (1962) has recorded $38°$ at the soil surface. During 1951, Cook (1955) found mean monthly soil temperatures $1·6$ cm. below the surface at Resolute (lat. $74° 43'$N, long. $95° 59'$W) to rise above $0°$ for only two months. In the same area, Cook and Raiche (1962) found temperatures on the ground surface to rise above $0°$ thirteen times in one day and 170 times during a single summer. This type of information, which reveals thermal patterns within the biosphere, is of much greater value to biologists than screen temperatures but is not widely available. Data such as wind chill factor values, however empirical, are often of greater value than temperature measurements alone.

In contrast with the land, the ocean masses offer a relatively stable thermal regime, sometimes deviating by no more than $0·1°$ from the annual mean as in the bottom waters of McMurdo Sound. Some authors include within the polar marine region areas such as the Bering Sea, where summer surface temperatures may reach $10°$. The thermal range is usually considered to be much narrower, however, and an upper limit of $3–5°$ seems more acceptable.

The thermal regime has a profound influence on the physical environment. The area of Antarctica is $5·5$ million square miles, yet only 3,000 square miles are unencumbered by the vast ice sheet which mantles the continent (Llano, 1962). Greenland is largely covered with ice and much of the arctic barrens are blanketed by snow during the long winter. Permafrost is continuous and the active layer shallow. Plant colonization is impossible where ice hides the land surface, and soil frost phenomena materially affect the nature of plant communities and the distribution of many animals. Snow cover impedes the movement of most animals, aids that of some, and may shorten the growing season for plants. It may also act as an insulating layer and provide shelter. With its reflective properties, snow greatly retards the absorption of radiant heat by soil. Poor drainage due to permafrost leads to the accumulation of water and retards warming.

Massive ice sheets, moving out beyond the coastline, especially in Antarctica, affect the sea bed and its fauna (Tressler and Ommundsen,

1962). The marine habitats provided by extensive floating ice shelves remain almost totally unexplored (Littlepage and Pearse, 1962). The melting of ice in summer introduces large volumes of fresh water to the sea over short periods, and sometimes causes marked local diminutions in salinity (Bunt, 1960, 1964).

The formation of sea ice has great biological significance. The layer, which is commonly 1–3 m. thick, minimizes gas and heat exchange between the hydrosphere and the atmosphere, and considerably modifies the intensity and spectral quality of submarine light. The abrasive action of ice makes effective colonization of the intertidal zone impossible. Annual freezing and thawing of the ice layer, where this occurs, affects the salinity characteristics of the water column, especially near the surface. Sea ice also controls, beneficially and adversely, the activities of marine mammals and birds, predator–prey relationships, and the diversity of species, and it probably has significant influences on the zooplankton. It affords anchorage for a slow growing but rich flora and fauna of micro-organisms. In antarctic waters, ice formation and dispersal are largely annual events, although fast ice may be more or less permanent. Large belts of pack ice persist during the summer. Permanent and heavy pack ice is characteristic of the north polar basin.

Some of the more important physicochemical properties of sea water that are intimately affected by temperature and are of biological significance include: viscosity, the capacity to carry gases and other substances in solution, the concentration of carbon dioxide gas, possibly the degree of polymerization of water molecules (Baird, 1964), and isotopic composition (see Dietrich, 1963, and the results of Crespi et al., 1959). The physicochemical properties of water at different temperatures also affect weathering processes (Jenny, 1941). Under polar conditions, the weathering of rock is mainly physical (see, for example, Blakemore and Swindale, 1958, and Bliss, 1962).

Representative of the many excellent accounts devoted specifically to the terrestrial and marine polar environments are those of Nordenskjöld and Mecking (1928), Dunbar (1951), Kort (1962), Robin (1962), Baird (1964), Deacon (1964) and Phillpot (1964).

III. Thermal Energy and the Biological Characteristics of the Polar Flora and Fauna

For organisms exposed to the severe thermal regimes of the polar regions, it is generally true that biological modifications of some description are essential to survival. The ability to attain degrees of success comparable with those achieved by species under less demanding circumstances must require an additional biological outlay, ultimately measurable in terms of energy expenditure, and reflected in compensatory characteristics of one kind or another at the molecular, cellular or higher levels of organization. The level of efficiency possible will depend upon the nature and genetic potential of the biological material, and the ultimate limits to compensation will be determined by the nature and severity of the thermal regimes.

While some of the possible means of survival or compensation may be shared to some degree by homeotherms and poikilotherms, plants and micro-organisms alike, others may be restricted to specific groups or individual species according to their unique capacities and particular limitations. Characteristics which would ensure success in marine or aquatic environments may not be appropriate on land, and vice versa.

In some instances, temperature, or a pattern of temperatures, may elicit a direct and useful response. However, an innate capacity to respond successfully, but only after a suitable period of exposure, may be equally valuable as may also be characteristics which do not respond to the thermal regime but which happen to be useful against low temperatures or against the unfavourable effects of temperature on some significant factor of the environment.

Even in species which are reasonably well suited to life at high latitudes, certain processes may lack the capacity to overcome the depressive influence of low temperatures. Further, among these forms, there exist some in which abnormalities arise in consequence of this incapacity. Low temperatures may act also by prolonging development and delaying maturity in such a way that, within the latitudinal range of a single species, individuals attain a larger size with increasing latitude. Large individuals may function with relatively greater efficiency under cold conditions than small individuals of the same species.

In discussions concerning the responses and characteristics of organisms exposed to stress, one frequently encounters the terms acclimation, acclimatization and adaptation. Although usage varies, acclimation usually refers to biological responses to changes in temperature, while acclimatization is reserved for responses to climate. The capacity to acclimate or acclimatize is, basically, genetically determined. Adaptation normally implies a more or less permanent change in the genetic constitution appropriate to a particular climate or thermal regime. In principle, however, each of these processes may confer similar characteristics so that distinctions of this type are not always possible.

One or more characteristics may contribute to the variable capacity of polar plants, animals and micro-organisms, terrestrial and aquatic, to resist cold and to maintain efficiency under harsh thermal conditions. These factors are discussed below.

A. BEHAVIOUR

The display of behaviour, which embraces a diverse complex of activities, is found normally only within the Animal Kingdom. While mobility is not essential to behaviour, it greatly extends the advantages inherent in this capacity. Thus, animals which are sessile, or whose movements are restricted either by inherent or external factors, may be subject to temperature stresses, especially on land and in the intertidal zone, which may be avoided or minimized in species in which greater freedom of movement is assured. The fundamental necessity to "weather the storm" probably constitutes one of the most serious biological stumbling blocks presented to the establishment of plant life in the polar regions.

The severity of temperature stresses at high latitudes, as elsewhere, varies with the location and with time. Where the capacity of animals to compensate for unfavourable temperatures in other ways is lacking or limited, behavioural responses or patterns can be most useful when it comes to the selection of habitat.

1. *Migration*

Many species of birds and mammals which breed in the arctic or antarctic are migratory. Their seasonal movements, although not triggered by temperature, ensure that the rigours of the polar winter are avoided. Some of the factors concerned in the general phenomenon of migration have been considered by Fontaine (1954), Marshall (1961), and Allee *et al.* (1961). It should not be assumed that the migrant species are necessarily ill equipped to endure cold. Scholander *et al.* (1950a,b,c) kept arctic gulls in cages over winter at Point Barrow, Alaska, and found them capable of withstanding temperatures as low as −50° without apparent difficulty. However, snow buntings, which are also migratory and are able to endure −40°, lost body temperature rapidly at −50°. For other species, also, migration is probably obligatory as suggested by the data of Irving *et al.* (1955). Kramer (1961) has noted that the homing ability of pigeons is impaired in winter. To my knowledge, the specific effect of temperature on this type of function has not been studied in polar species, although J. Emlen and R. Penney (personal communication) have made field observations of orientation in antarctic penguins. In Arctic Lapland, Snow (1952) observed that many species of birds are able to over-winter in places where human habitation has assured a continuing supply of food. For migrating caribou, winter temperatures in the southern parts of their range are probably no less severe than those prevailing at the same time further north. Certainly, the absence or inaccessibility of food during the long winter, brought about in large part by the direct or indirect effects of extreme temperatures, is a factor of practical if not fundamental significance underlying the migratory habits of many species.

Information on the factors governing the movements of migratory polar fish is limited. Woodhead (1959) discounted the possible significance of temperature in movements of arctic cod. For the Bear Island cod, light is important (Trout, 1957). Wohlschlag (1957) did not find any obvious difference in the environmental temperatures to which migratory and resident forms of the arctic white fish, *Coregonus sardinella*, were exposed.

Vertical and horizontal migrations are well known in zooplankton. Certain aspects of the movements of antarctic zooplankton have been discussed recently by Foxton (1964). For the commoner species, migration is seasonal, and the bulk of the adult animals remain near the surface in summer but descend into deeper waters during the winter. This behaviour has the advantage of keeping the populations close to food supplies and at the same time, as a result of the differences in water flow at the two levels, of maintaining their geographic (thermal) range. It should be added that this pattern also keeps them in relatively warm water, a fact which, though perhaps accidental, could be of some significance in minimizing the need for metabolic compensation. While numerous factors have been implicated in the migratory patterns of planktonic organisms (see, for example, Allee *et al.*, 1961), McLaren (1963), in a re-assessment of this problem, has assigned to temperature a position of principal importance. The movement of many arctic littoral species into deeper water during winter (Brongersma-Sanders, 1957) affords protection against freezing and against the crushing and abrading action of annually formed sea ice.

Whereas metabolic adaptability, rather than behaviour, is perhaps of greater value to aquatic poikilotherms in combating the effects of low but not freezing temperatures, somewhat the reverse is true under the conditions which face terrestrial poikilotherms. Migration, where this occurs, is typically vertical and enables the organisms to avoid severe winter temperatures under some circumstances. The subterranean winter habitat would also ensure greater thermal stability over a period when mobility may have been lost, and may offer additional benefits such as freedom from predation. This type of behavioural pattern, however, does not seem to be common in polar species. The habit is not mentioned in a recent review of adaptations in arctic insects by Downes (1965), who refers, for example, to lepidopteran larvae which hibernate "in exposed areas where little snow accumulates". It is doubtful whether insects which undergo certain stages of their development in the waters of ice-covered lakes should be regarded as migratory, although the pattern of their life cycle automatically affords protection from freezing. Insect forms likely to be migratory are not found in Antarctica (Llano, 1962; Gressitt, 1964). However, Brown (1964) recorded that the larvae of the dipteran, *Calycopteryx moseleyi* sub sp. *minor*, move underground during the Heard Island winter. Behavioural peculiarities, including migration, are obviously ineffectual when temperatures very much below 0° are unavoidable. Under such conditions, a capacity to survive freezing is essential.

2. *Other Types of Habitat Selection*

Habitat selection in direct response to temperature is of common occurrence among terrestrial poikilotherms, particularly arthropods, and is well known in mammals and birds. In the antarctic, Weddell seals haul out on the sea ice in large numbers to bask in the sun on calm, cloudless summer days, but soon return to the water during periods of inclement weather. The striking communal habit of huddle formation adopted by Emperor penguins for added defence against cold has been well described by Prévost (1962). The biotopes of this species have been discussed in some detail by Budd (1961), who took into account the direct and indirect effects of extreme temperatures on behaviour. Many of the smaller arctic mammals and birds, including a number of permanent residents, are unable to endure constant exposure to low temperatures, even temperatures that are likely to be experienced from time to time in the summer. Their ability to provide themselves and their young with a more tolerable thermal regime, either in the form of vegetation shelters (shrews), insulated underground tunnels (lemmings and other rodents), snow burrows (ptarmigan, brown lemming), or nests is basic to survival (Bee and Hall, 1956; Scholander *et al.*, 1950c). For hibernators, such as the arctic ground squirrel (Mayer, 1953), insulated burrows are essential throughout the period of quiescence. In the antarctic, the nesting sites of birds, such as the snow petrel, are characteristically well protected. The fact that the creation or selection of shelter may confer multiple advantages should not be overlooked. In this respect, however, man's responses to the polar environment are unequivocal, for he is basically a tropical species, morphologically and metabolically vulnerable to cold. Classified among the homeotherms, he owes his success at high latitudes almost entirely to behavioural capacities operating through intellect. The phenomenon of creative homeostasis has been discussed by Lewontin (1957).

Downes (1965) has listed a number of instances in which arctic insects are known to rely heavily on an ability to seek out and remain under the influence of temperatures higher than the general environment. As an excellent example of this type of behaviour, Hocking and Sharplin (1965) have described how certain insects locate themselves within arctic flowers which, because of their shape and constant orientation towards the sun, act as efficient radiation traps. Murray (1964) has carried out some interesting studies with the lice of elephant seals in which it was found that a metabolic adjustment to low temperatures would, in fact, be disadvantageous. The parasites multiply only when the host is ashore and then accumulate in the area of the tail flippers where favourable temperatures in the range 27–34° are regularly maintained. In captive animals held under more temperate conditions, the lice spread to other parts of the body.

Wise and Gressitt (1965) have reported recoveries of mites and springtails at a latitude of approximately 85°S in Antarctica, where the temperature of the atmospheric environment is continuously subzero and, even on rock and rubble surfaces receiving direct radiation, rarely above 0°, and then only at the height of summer. Gressitt (1964) has described the way in which these arthropods select microhabitats which are most likely to expose them to favourable temperatures as high as 20° on occasions and how, under adverse conditions, they retreat into rock fissures and under gravel for maximum protection. Movement, for feeding, into more moist and therefore cooler situations, which support mosses and lichens, is possible only under the most favourable circumstances.

In the sea it seems likely that the benthic habit preferred by many species of polar fish is selected not because temperatures are more favourable but because the dangers of freezing from the supercooled state are much greater where there is a likelihood of contact with sea ice (Marshall, 1964).

In addition to the selection of favourable habitats, the attitudes assumed by organisms, particularly homeotherms, can be essential to the maintenance of body temperature. Thus, arctic gulls are found to lower themselves onto, and cover their feet with, the body feathers under extreme conditions (Scholander et al., 1950c; Chatfield et al., 1953). Huskies curl up tightly with their backs to the wind in bad weather to minimize heat loss from poorly insulated parts. Many polar animals have behavioural characteristics which, though not related directly to temperature, equip them more fully against those features of the physical environment which are modelled by temperature. Weddell seals overwintering close to the antarctic coastline maintain breathing holes by chewing at the sea ice. Penguins tend to propel themselves along on ice rather than walking. In animals such as the arctic ground squirrel (Mayer, 1953), the food shortages of the winter are overcome by storage. Some birds are able to overwinter in the arctic (Snow, 1952) either because they are able to search for food beneath the snow or because they possess somewhat catholic feeding habits. Pruitt (1959) has found that barren ground caribou are affected in their movements by the hardness and density of the snow cover.

B. LIFE CYCLES

The nature and pattern of the life cycles of living organisms are composed of physiological, morphological and, in animals, behavioural elements. Together, these characters, and the effect which the thermal regime has upon them, constitute such a distinctive and integrated whole that separate treatment seems both well justified and convenient.

1. *Reproductive Cycle*

Under the thermal stress of low temperatures and other severe conditions, the patterns of life cycles often become modified. The origins of the modifications, which usually involve simplification, are sometimes biological or adaptive, sometimes environmental, and may have survival value. Free living larval stages are curtailed or absent in the life cycles of many arctic and antarctic benthic invertebrates (Gunter, 1957; Holme, 1964), a characteristic which is considered to contribute to the stability of bottom communities (Thorson, 1957). Rust fungi in the arctic exhibit a transitional degeneration with latitude. This ranges from those in which alternate hosts must be in physical proximity to those in which a single host is adequate and, further north, to others in which a sole spore type is characteristic; finally there is a condition in which the parasite exists as a perennial mycelium (Savile, 1963). Transitions similar in principle have been recognized in arctic insects (Downes, 1965). Further, basidiospores are sometimes produced while the fruiting body is still immature. Among the insects, seasonal development is dependent on temperature rather than on light rhythms. Moths and flies often emerge with mature eggs. In *Prosimulium ursinum*, the adults do not even emerge, the eggs being shed on disintegration of the pupae. The existence of apterous forms of normally winged insects, as Downes (1965) and others have indicated, is probably more effective against wind than against temperature although flight is commonly one of the first activities suspended with a fall in temperature.

Genetic phenomena in homeostasis have been discussed by Lewontin (1957), and the probable importance under arctic conditions of polyploidy, heterozygosity and parthenogenesis by Bliss (1962), Downes (1965) and Johnson and Packer (1965). These topics will not be treated further in this account.

Fixed behavioural characteristics closely associated with the reproductive cycle frequently represent a distinct asset and may be prerequisite for survival. Protection of eggs during incubation is almost universal among birds, but the manner in which this is accomplished is at times striking. Emperor penguins do not use nests. Instead, the single egg is placed in the safe keeping of the male bird who carries it on the feet under a special skin fold. A fast is observed throughout the two month incubation period. After hatching, the chicks remain on the feet of the adults until sheer size makes the continuation of this habit impossible. Later, the young birds learn to form crèches which serve, at least in part, to protect them from unfavourable temperatures during this critical stage of development (Prévost, 1962).

The burrowing habits of many of the smaller arctic mammals automatically ensure a degree of warmth for the newly born. Even some of the larger animals, such as the polar bear, retire to snow dens at the time of parturition. Female huskies are capable of remarkable endurance in using their bodies for the protection of the litter under extreme conditions where no other form of shelter is available.

Brood care is not restricted, among poikilotherms, to species of high latitudes, and is not always used to minimize the dangers associated with low temperatures. However, the protection of the young is characteristic of many antarctic marine invertebrates (Holme, 1964) and is sufficiently common in cold waters generally to have led Gunter (1957) to conclude that a relationship between brood care and cold must be assumed. One feels that, in such environments, behaviour of this description is more likely to minimize the possibility of exposure to the indirect rather than to the direct effects of low temperatures.

Other types of behaviour are somewhat comparable in nature to brood care. At Lake Hazen, in the Canadian Arctic, the mosquito, *Aedes nigripes*, oviposits in situations most likely to favour early hatching during the subsequent summer (Downes, 1965). In various species of polar arthropods, dispersal is delayed. This not only tends to maintain the organisms in a suitable microclimate, almost certainly involving factors other than temperature, but also ensures successful mating.

In the polar, as in any other environment, the nature of the component parts of life cycles and their overall pattern may contribute materially to survival and to success. A considerable variety of biological qualities may be involved, and their effects may compensate either for the direct or indirect influences of the thermal regime. As usual, the probable concurrence of influences other than temperature must be recognized.

It will be clear that the advantages inherent in producing large numbers of offspring must be weighed against the difficulties of providing adequate protection during development when a capacity for homeostasis may be latent but not effective (see, for example, Lewontin, 1957; Amadon, 1964). With a few exceptions, the birds and animals of the arctic and antarctic produce few young annually but expend considerable effort in their care. The penguins, among birds, are notable in this respect. However, Watson (1957) found that the mean clutch size of snowy owls on Baffin Island was eight, although it must be added that the hatching period was expanded, and resulted in a spread in the development of the chicks. Rock ptarmigan have been found with six, and willow ptarmigan with nine, eggs in a single clutch (Weeden, 1956). According to Hoyte (1955), small mammals of the genera *Sorex*, *Neomys*, *Clethrionomys* and *Microtus* in arctic Norway tend to produce larger litters than in the south. Moreover, voles born early in the season were sometimes found to breed before the end of summer.

Downes (1965) has remarked upon the fact that egg production in arctic Diptera is particularly low and that, in some species, especially when conditions are severe, a proportion of eggs may be resorbed to favour successful development of the remainder. The large size of individual eggs, also, has been emphasized. A similar phenomenon appears to be common in marine invertebrates (Gunter, 1957) and in fish (Marshall, 1964) where early larval development must be assured.

Egg-laying has often been eliminated altogether from the life cycle, either, one assumes, because of temperature sensitivity in this stage or in order to accelerate development during the short summer season. A number of antarctic benthic invertebrates are known to be viviparous (Holme, 1964) and this trait is of ecological significance for certain arctic insects (Downes, 1965). A form of vivipary is known even in certain species of arctic plants (Bliss, 1962). It should be stressed, however, that, in terrestrial poikilotherms, the egg may be equal or superior in resistance to temperature extremes compared with other stages. Egg-laying is apparently normal for the mite *Maudheimia Wilsoni* (Dalenius and Wilson, 1958).

Viable seeds are produced by many species among the arctic flora (Bliss, 1958); some are capable of germination after remaining frozen throughout the winter, while others lack this capacity e.g. *Salix planifolia* var. *monica*. Under the environmental conditions of the upland tundra, however, reproduction is most successfully achieved by vegetative propagation. At Signy Island, in the maritime antarctic, Holdgate (1964) has found inflorescences produced by *Deschampsia antarctica* and *Colobanthus crassifolius*, although he suspects that mature seeds are rarely formed. In the more northerly sectors of the Canadian Arctic, Savile (1963) has found some fungal parasites limited to perennial mycelium in the crown tissues of the host plants. It would seem from these examples that the thermal regime, and perhaps other factors, have acted to prevent the expression of the normal life habit. There is no indication that the inability to set seed or to produce spores is a permanent characteristic in these organisms.

Murphy (1962) has pointed out that advanced foetal development at birth is characteristic of marine mammals in the polar regions. The pups of the Weddell seal, for example, are delivered directly on to sea ice and first enter the water when only three weeks old. Rapid development in the early stages, and the laying down of insulative tissues, are greatly aided in such creatures by the high fat and protein contents of the milk produced by the mother (White, 1953). On land, infant caribou are subject to exposure from birth. It is not surprising, therefore, that Hart *et al.* (1961) found thermal regulation well established in these animals even at this early stage of development.

An inherent capacity for rapid development, at least during certain stages, appears to be widely used among insects and terrestrial plants as a means of making biological capital of an all too short summer season or even briefer periods of favourable temperatures (Bliss, 1962; Downes, 1965). In describing the biology of *Maudheimia Wilsoni*, Dalenius and Wilson (1958) stressed the fact that, for such organisms, short exposures to relatively high temperatures are of more use than continuous exposure to much lower temperatures with the same overall mean.

The smaller arctic mammals enjoy a capacity for early mating, short gestation and rapid development (Mayer, 1953; Hoyte, 1955; Bee and Hall, 1956) which enable them to complete their main activities before the onset of winter. Similar restrictions apply to most of the arctic and antarctic fauna and especially to those birds which must be in a condition to undertake migration. In this connection, Maher (1964) has emphasized that there is no evidence to support the postulate that arctic passerine birds develop any more rapidly than their close relatives of more temperate regions. Naturally, an adequate food supply is essential for normal rates of development. Food shortages may even prevent onset of the normal breeding cycle in some arctic birds (Marshall, 1952) or at least delay the onset of this activity (Marshall, 1961).

Where rates of development cannot be considered to be unusually rapid, the timing of the reproductive cycle may be all important. The unique winter breeding behaviour of the Emperor penguin is undoubtedly dictated fundamentally by the unequal relationship existing between the time required for the chicks to reach the stage where swimming is possible, and the duration of the summer season. Normally, adult plumage is attained at about the time that the last of the sea ice, including that on which rookeries are located, is broken up and swept out to sea, and when the maturing birds are able to satisfy their increasingly heavy food requirements by their own endeavours. Were the breeding cycle co-incident with that of other antarctic species, the very existence of the Emperor penguin would be placed in jeopardy.

Just as the timing of breeding cycles in the homeotherms is not entirely related to temperature directly, periods of reproductive activity in marine polar invertebrates may be timed to co-incide less with periods of favourable temperature than with the availability of food, the production of which is governed in part by the extent of ice cover and, there-fore, temperature. This fact has been made clear in the review by Gunter (1957). However, the direct effect of temperature should not be dis-counted. Working with amphipods and asteroids in antarctic coastal waters, J. S. Pearse (personal communication) has reached the conclu-sion that, because embryonic development is extremely slow at the prevailing low temperatures, winter spawning is essential to enable the larvae to be ready to take advantage of the summer phytoplankton production. He suggests further, that the slight seasonal change in water temperature of 0·2° in McMurdo Sound (Tressler and Ommund-sen, 1962) could be significant for the synchronization of reproduction.

2. *Growing Period*

The complete cessation of growth during winter is inescapable for terrestrial plants, free-living micro-organisms, and probably for most terrestrial poikilotherms. Some ecto- and endoparasites of homeotherms, notably those of man, may be favoured by the host's microclimate. The growth of extralittoral aquatic plants is hindered more by the absence of light than by the thermal regime. At higher latitudes and altitudes, in the terrestrial arctic and throughout the continent of Antarctica, growth may be restricted to short and irregularly spaced intervals at the peak of summer.

Under these circumstances, it is not surprising to find that many species are equipped to continue growth whenever the opportunity arises. Thus, Savile (1963) recorded that some Pyrenomycetes spend 2–3 years in developing ascospores, and Bliss (1962) quoted several remark-able instances of arctic vascular plants which remain unaffected by freezing during the flowering stage. The inflorescences of one species, *Braya humilis*, are able to continue development through two successive growing seasons. Many lichens and algae are capable of intermittent growth without entering a resistant resting stage. Downes (1965) has described lepidopteran larvae which develop over several seasons with complete cessation of activity at irregular intervals. He suggested that, for many arctic insects, dormancy may be a relatively simple response to cold rather than a diapause under the control of more remote stimuli. The factors controlling dormancy in higher arctic plant life appear to have received little attention, although it would seem likely that at least some species are opportunistic while others probably have definite dormancy patterns and specific requirements for cold exposure. Bliss (1962) found that different cycles of development are followed by the same species in different habitats. Concerning the formation of floral organs, Sørensen's (1941) opinion is quoted that induction may involve low temperature—thermoperiodical adaptation.

Like typical dormancy in plants, the phenomenon of hibernation, which is practised by some homeothermous animals, is not unique to the arctic. The subject has been reviewed by Lyman (1961) and by Matthews (1961). In itself, hibernation does not protect against cold, although the hibernaculum may provide valuable insulation, nor is it induced by lowered temperatures. Rather, it probably serves to carry the organism over a period during which the maintenance of normal activity would be difficult or impossible in the face of seasonal shortages of food. Matthews (1961) recorded that *Citellus citellus* has been observed to enter hibernation at 30°. When the ambient temperature fell below 0° under experimental conditions, most of the hibernating animals died whereas, in their normal, active state, they could withstand environmental temperatures of −15°.

C. MORPHOLOGY

As individual or linked characteristics, the size, form, detailed structure and colour of plants and animals can contribute, often strikingly, to their capacity to withstand thermal stresses. Each of these classes of character may be inherited, although in certain organisms temperature may exert a direct controlling influence. Where this is so, the resultant effect may or may not be of obvious value for survival or homeostasis.

It has frequently been observed that marine poikilotherms tend to increase in size towards the northern, or southern, limits of their thermal range, and that species of the colder seas tend to be larger than closely related forms of more temperate waters (Gunter, 1957; Allee *et al.*, 1961; Kinne, 1963; Brodsky, 1964). Steere (1953) has commented on the comparatively large size of arctic bryophytes. On the other hand, Allee *et al.* (1961) considered that the evidence points towards a general but not unexceptional diminution in size with latitude among terrestrial poikilotherms. A similar condition appears to exist with some fungi (Savile, 1963). Sandon (1924) found that some arctic terrestrial protozoa were larger, and others smaller, than related temperate forms.

Allee *et al.* (1961) have applied Bergmann's rule (see Chapter 12, p. 407) to homeotherms and poikilotherms, and have listed terrestrial poikilotherms among a number of known exceptions. It may be questioned, however, whether Bergmann's rule, and the advantages of heat conservation implicit in it, can be advanced as the sole underlying cause of relative differences in size. Kinne (1963) has noted that, although some large and active freshwater fish may be up to 10° warmer than their surroundings, such differences are not usual. Further, increases in size with range and latitude have been documented within a variety of groups including the marine protozoa. One finds it difficult to accept the proposition that, for such small organisms, a response of this description could contribute in any material degree to heat conservation. Rather, it would appear more probable that, under the cold but relatively constant conditions of the polar seas, large relative size could result simply from long continued development and delayed maturity. It may be added that, at least for many pelagic organisms, density and viscosity would tend to select for a relative diminution in size in warmer waters. Zooplanktonic and phytoplanktonic organisms tend to be more highly ornamented or structurally elaborate in tropical waters, and these morphological embellishments are believed to aid flotation.

Many terrestrial poikilotherms are not metabolically adapted to cold environments. Their smaller size could well result from the need to reach maturity in the course of an all too short and inconstant summer. This argument may be applied equally well to explain the limited size achieved by some of the polar fungi. The contradictory observations with the terrestrial protozoa and the large size of arctic bryophytes suggest that the possible operation of additional factors should not be discounted.

Chamaephytes and hemicryptophytes predominate in the vascular flora of the arctic (Bliss, 1962). Although life form is not selected by thermal conditions alone, temperature is certainly a major influence. The inherent tendency to a prostrate or cushion-like habit is accentuated under thermal stress and becomes increasingly apparent with higher latitude and altitude. Plants of this type benefit not only from the elevated temperatures which prevail close to the surface, but themselves contribute to heat absorption in this stratum (Benninghoff, 1952; Wilson, 1957) and gain further by being insulated to some extent from extreme temperatures when the ground is covered with snow (Bliss, 1962). The shallow rooting habit is a necessary attribute, especially in areas where the active layer is shallow (see, for example, Benninghoff, 1952; Tikhomirov, 1960). The morphological adaptations of antarctic lichens have been described by Dodge (1964) although not with specific reference to temperature. In some species, the thin layers of growth produced on rock surfaces must be of considerable advantage under severe conditions. Llano (1962) reported rock temperatures up to 27·8° at a location only four degrees of latitude from the geographic south pole.

Absorption of long-wave radiation may be favoured, not only by habit but also by the detailed structure of an organism. Vascular plants with abundant epidermal hairs have been reported by several authors to develop earlier than species that are not pubescent (Bliss, 1962). Downes (1965) considered the hairiness of arctic bumble bees, combined with their large size, to be effective in retaining the heat generated by muscular activity. At an ambient temperature of −4°, low enough to impede or arrest the activities of most arctic insects, this species has been observed in normal flight.

Various insects and other arthropods as well as some parts of higher plants, lichens and fungi are dark pigmented. Effective heat absorption, however, is not dependent on true melanism. I have observed small fragments of green algae floating in "self-made" pockets of melt water in otherwise completely frozen antarctic lakes, and incidentally providing a satisfactory milieu for mixed populations of rotifers, tardigrades and other small creatures.

Structural and morphological features with no apparent survival value are often attributable to the thermal regime. The imperfectly formed asci of certain Pyrenomycetes (Savile, 1963) and atypical tests found in arctic and antarctic rhizopods (Sandon, 1924) are perhaps traceable to the influence of temperature. Correlations between temperature and the appearance of certain structures in fish are well known (Gunter, 1957; Kinne, 1963), and the tendency of this group of animals to have greater numbers of vertebrae in colder waters has been formulated as Jordan's rule (Allee et al., 1961).

However useful morphological characters may be in shielding polar poikilotherms against the rigours of their environment, they can scarcely exceed in value or importance the fur, feathers or blubber of the homeotherms. Body insulation is indispensable for warm-blooded animals exposed to cold, especially since basal metabolic rates and body temperatures are inadaptive to climate (Scholander et al., 1950a; Irving and Krog, 1954; Goldsmith and Sladen, 1961). The larger arctic animals and birds, particularly those whose behavioural patterns subject them to constant exposure, are remarkably well equipped in this respect. Thus, the critical temperatures (see Chapter 12, p. 377) of arctic foxes, huskies and arctic gulls probably lie below −40° (Scholander et al., 1950c). The zone of thermoneutrality for larger animals such as the polar bear probably extends at least to −50°. Metabolic heat production increases relatively slowly with increased cold in these species. Scholander et al. (1950b) have shown that a 40% rise in metabolic rate would, in fact, extend the critical gradient from −40° to −70°.

Critical temperatures are not necessarily constant. Irving et al. (1955) recorded values of 8° in summer and −13° in winter for the red fox, and 7° and −12° for porcupines. Species in which the summer and winter values were identical and relatively high either migrate or seek the shelter of burrows. Changes in critical temperature are associated with well known seasonal alterations in pelage which may increase insulation by 10–50% (Fry, 1958). Similar changes have been noted by Hart

19+T.

(1961) in the blubber thickness of the harbour seal. Insulation varies also with the stage of development. Scholander *et al.* (1950a) reported that polar bear cubs and young huskies are able to manage quite well with short fur because their metabolic rates are naturally higher than when fully grown. Infant caribou are very susceptible to adverse conditions (Hart *et al.*, 1961). Lenz and Hart (1960) have shown that the insulating capacity of the fur of these animals may be lost when wind and rain accompany temperatures around 0°. Even fully grown polar animals suffer much greater thermal stress upon wetting of the pelt. Bee and Hall (1956) found that brown lemmings with wet fur died of exposure in only a few minutes. Heat loss through polar bear skin increased 20–25 times when the skins were submerged in still water at 0° (Scholander *et al.*, 1950c). Goldsmith and Sladen (1961) found that Adelie penguin chicks could not prevent a drop in body temperature if immersed before moulting had been completed. According to Bryden (1964) elephant seal pups are probably somewhat poikilothermic at birth, when the blubber thickness is only approximately 0·5 cm. During deposition of the heavy fat layer, a measure of protection is afforded by a temporary coat of fairly thick, black fur.

Heavy insulation is normally associated with a high degree of vasomotor control and a capacity of the unprotected extremities to remain functional at quite low temperatures (Scholander *et al.*, 1950a,b,c; Irving, 1951; Chatfield *et al.*, 1953; Bryden, 1964). This type of control is essential, not only for maintaining internal temperatures against marked winter gradients when at rest, but also for the dissipation of excess heat when in active movement or when exposed to high temperatures in summer. As Scholander *et al.* (1950b) have pointed out, the maintenance of thermoneutrality between − 40° and 30° demands an eleven-fold change in heat dissipation. Although seasonal variations in pelage are undoubtedly of considerable assistance, vasodilation and a rise in skin temperature, particularly in the poorly insulated extremities, must be a major factor in thermoregulation.

Using these facts as his principal argument, Scholander (1955) has made a vigorous attack on the concept of ecological gradients as embodied in Bergmann's and in Allen's rules (Allee *et al.*, 1961; see Chapter 12, p. 407). He has also cited the many exceptions that are known to exist and has expressed the opinion that, to be of adaptive importance, a general convergence towards large, globular species would be expected among the northern homeotherms.

A number of writers have engaged in the controversy over ecological rules. One of the most recent (Schreider, 1964), while leaning towards a "synthetic" view, has presented data based on man, which he considers support the validity of morphological gradients. That there should be a tendency towards an increase in size with latitude, and a reduction in the development of extremities, seems a fundamentally reasonable hypothesis. However, it should be re-iterated that, for many polar species, the provision for efficient heat dissipation, even at quite low temperatures, remains as much a necessity as heat conservation. Further, and equally important, thermal conditions represent but one factor among the many to which organisms are usually exposed. The weighting of individual factors, in turn, will vary from habitat to habitat. Similarly, biological characteristics are likely to be weighted in terms of their adaptive values for each species in its particular environment. Under the circumstances, it would be unrealistic to expect anything approaching complete convergence with respect to any one environmental factor. In this sense, the use of the term "rule" seems unfortunate for it implies immutability.

It may be worth noting here that, whereas Hayward (1965) found large individuals of *Peromyscus* to be more efficient in thermoregulation than small individuals, no evidence was found for a positive correlation between gross climatic conditions and size among the six races studied. Data of this type contradict Bergmann's rule but support the concept on which it is based.

D. PHYSIOLOGY

A number of excellent reviews have been published dealing with the effects of temperature on biological processes and with the physiological aspects of temperature compensation. The accounts of Andrewartha and Birch (1954), Bělehrádek (1957), Allee et al. (1961), Went (1961), Ingraham (1962), McLaren (1963) and Kinne (1963) include discussions of general principles. Concepts of physiological thermal compensation, either in poikilotherms or in homeotherms, have been considered by Bullock (1955), Gunter (1957), Fry (1958), Prosser (1958) and King and Farner (1961). Attitudes and information on some of the probable mechanisms underlying compensation may be found in the accounts of Potter (1958), Depocas (1961), Smith and Hoijer (1962), Rose (1963), Ingraham (1963), Hart (1964) and Benzinger (1964).

A capacity for maintaining metabolic activities under conditions that would be impossibly suboptimum or even lethal for organisms of more temperate origin is the principal requirement for success among species in which tissues are continuously cold. Such are the marine algae and poikilotherms of the arctic and antarctic. On land, where the thermal environment is much less restricted, similar capacities in these groups may be advantageous but not always essential.

The basal metabolic rates of homeotherms are inadaptive to climate.

Of particular importance for polar birds and animals, therefore, are the physiological processes which operate to maintain body temperature and which enable the continuation of function in the exposed extremities. These are ineffective alone and, as mentioned earlier, must be linked intimately with peculiarities of behaviour and morphology. Unfortunately, it will not be possible to treat the subject of thermoregulation further in this account. Reference to the reviews of Hart (1964) and Benzinger (1964) is again recommended.

Little attention has been paid to metabolic temperature compensation among the terrestrial poikilotherms of high latitudes. Scholander *et al.* (1953a) found little or no evidence for a relative elevation in respiratory activity at low temperatures in arctic insects, and Downes (1965) recorded the general observation that most members of this group are dependent on exposure to relatively high temperatures for development and activity. There is no doubt, however, that some are well equipped for activity in cold environments. The stonefly, *Nemoura columbiana*, is able to perform normally and mate at a body temperature of 0°. Many lake insects are apparently cold stenothermal. Dalenus and Wilson (1958) have observed the nymphs of *Maudheimia Wilsoni* developing below 0°. Similar characteristics would be expected in at least some representatives of other invertebrate groups. For example, Dehnel (1955) found the growth of subarctic populations of gastropods in the embryo and larval stages to be 2–9 times faster at a given temperature than in southern populations. However, the difference may have been accentuated by factors other than metabolic compensation. It would be interesting to know something of the metabolic character of arctic helminth parasites (Cameron and Choquette, 1963) the life cycles of which are divided between poikilothermous and homeothermous hosts.

From the available evidence, it is clear that many members of the polar land flora retain their ecological status without the benefit of metabolic compensation. Llano (1962) maintains that some antarctic lichens must be 500–1,000 years old. Growth presumably is restricted to brief periods when moisture is available and absorbed radiant energy creates a favourable microclimate. Scholander *et al.* (1952) found evidence of respiratory adaptation only in the arctic members of the Peltigeraceae and Stictaceae in which oxygen consumption was faster at all temperatures than in their tropical relatives. Scholander and Kanwisher (1959) ascribed minor importance to respiratory compensation among the arctic vascular flora. Such generalizations, especially when based on a single rate process or on particular tissues or organs, are likely to be misleading. The root systems of many arctic vascular plants develop successfully close to 0°, and shoot development is initiated in certain species under a snow cover 50–100 cm. thick (Bliss, 1962). However, lack of adaptation in separate processes may at times exert an important controlling influence. For instance, Bliss (1962) has pointed out that protein synthesis and cell elongation have been considered by some authors to be ill adapted to low temperatures. The possibility should not be overlooked, in examining field data, that a capacity for compensation may be opposed or obscured by other limiting factors such as unfavourable pH values or nutrient deficiencies.

Wager (1941) found the highest values for net carbon assimilation in several East Greenland plants at 20°. However, Q_{10} values in the range 0–20° were apparently lower than for temperate species. The distribution of *Oxyria digyna* appears to be limited mainly by high summer temperatures, when photosynthetic economy is diminished (Mooney and Billings, 1961). Nevertheless, the observation of Bliss (1962), that temperature is the most important limiting factor with regard to plant growth and development in the tundra, suggests that the effectiveness of metabolic compensation, where it occurs, is generally quite limited.

Our knowledge of metabolic adjustments to temperature in the terrestrial free-living micro-organisms is most inadequate. Fortunately there is evidence of a current increase in interest in this area. Among the more specific groups, nitrifying, symbiotic and free-living nitrogen-fixing, cellulose-decomposing and sulphate-reducing bacteria have been isolated from arctic and/or antarctic soils (Rountree, 1938; Jensen, 1951; Krasil'nikov, 1958). Very little is known of their temperature characteristics, although slow nitrification has been reported below 10° (Jensen, 1951). Tedrow and Douglas (1959) found rates of decomposition of organic matter to be very low at 3°, which is the mid-June *in situ* temperature in some arctic soils. Bacteria, algae and protozoa isolated from terrestrial habitats commonly grow optimally in the range 20–30° and very slowly near 0° (Straka and Stokes, 1960; Flint and Stout, 1960).

Micro-organisms which give visible growth in one week in culture media at 0° are generally considered to be psychrophilic (Stokes, 1963). Although this term may be inappropriate (Eddy, 1960), organisms to which it is applicable may be considered to exhibit a degree of metabolic temperature compensation. Since psychrophils are ubiquitous (Stokes, 1963), it is not surprising that they have been isolated in polar habitats. The fact that a capacity for active growth at low temperatures does not seem to be general in the polar microflora and fauna may be explained at least in part from Ingraham's (1962) suggestion that adaptation to a new temperature range may require a large number of mutations, although certain mesophilic spore formers seem to be exceptional in this respect. Krasil'nikov (1958) reported that the temperature optimum for

Bacillus mycoides decreased with latitude. Relatively high microhabitat temperatures, which are quite common in summer notwithstanding low air temperatures, would also favour mesophils with a capacity for survival. Quite recently, Sinclair and Stokes (1965) have isolated obligately psychrophilic yeasts from antarctic materials. They suggest that previous failures to find this type of organism may have resulted from the exposure of samples to lethal conditions prior to isolation. Bunt and Rovira (1955), using refrigerated soils from Macquarie Island (lat. 54° 30′S, long. 158° 57′E), found many bacterial isolates to grow better at 10° than at 25°. Because consistently low but not extreme temperatures are characteristic of subantarctic islands, it would be interesting to know whether metabolic compensation is a more general phenomenon in these areas than in higher latitudes, not only among micro-organisms but also among the plants and invertebrate animals.

While an assumption of metabolic adjustment for low temperatures seems essential for the algae and poikilotherms of the polar seas, there can be no doubt that the degree of compensation varies considerably from species to species. J. S. Pearse (personal communication) has found the rates of development of several benthic invertebrates in McMurdo Sound at the southern end of the Ross Sea to be extremely slow. Thorson (1957) described invertebrates from the East Greenland fiords with up to 12 to 14 year classes. In general, it appears to be accepted that the organisms of colder seas grow more slowly, mature later and live longer than more temperate species (Gunter, 1957), and that metabolic adaptation, although sometimes considerable, is not normally complete (Scholander *et al.*, 1953a). On the other hand, Bandy and Echols (1964) have found isobathyl species of Foraminifera to be independent of temperature control. The amphipod *Themisto libellula* in Hudson Bay, Hudson Strait and South East Baffin Island waters has a life span of two years, which is normal for the species (Dunbar, 1957). Wohlschlag (1961) has discovered that the growth of some antarctic fish is comparable with that of many temperate species.

In the arctic, Scholander *et al.* (1953a) have examined the metabolic temperature characteristics of a range of fish and crustaceans including typically arctic and more wide-ranging forms. It was found that metabolism-temperature curves were displaced relative to those for temperate or tropical species, and showed the type II pattern of acclimation of Precht (Prosser, 1958). Locomotory activity was not affected by low temperatures. However, Fry (1958) has drawn attention to the fact that constancy of activity in poikilotherms may not require temperature compensation. In fish, for example, energy requirements for movement increase in proportion to the square of the swimming speed. No examples of a decreased Q_{10} value for resting metabolism were recorded by Scholander's group. Peiss and Field (1950), working with excized tissues of polar cod, found Q_{10} values for steady state respiration to remain virtually unchanged between 0° and 25°.

A series of interesting studies were carried out by Wohlschlag (1964) with fish from McMurdo Sound where water temperatures average $-1.9°$ and usually deviate no more than $0.1°$. As regards swimming movements, these antarctic fish were all found to be relatively inactive. The fact that the amounts of energy required for swimming were at least twice those of more temperate species appears to be related to the high viscosity of the polar waters. Metabolic levels, determined for four species of the fish *Trematomus* were high, this being evidence for considerable cold adaptation. At the upper temperature range (one or two degrees above 0°; the species are markedly cold stenothermal) basal metabolic levels were little different from those typical of tropical species at 30°. An upward variability in basal metabolism was recorded at temperatures below 0°. Metabolic activity at rest exhibited a variation with season, which may be associated in part with very slight temperature differences between summer and winter.

Dunbar (1954, 1957) has deplored the lack of information on the temperature responses of members of the polar zooplankton. Recently, an investigation was undertaken by McWhinnie (1964) using the antarctic krill, *Euphausia superba*, as experimental material. This species is cold stenothermal and dies within 24 hours at 4°. Measuring oxygen consumption acutely, it was found that, like the crustaceans studied by Scholander *et al.* (1953a), metabolism-temperature curves indicated relatively high activity between 0° and 5°, and no increase in activity above 5°. Q_{10} values were low within the range 0–15°. The pronounced metabolic adjustments displayed by the krill and the antarctic fish reflect the extreme conditions to which these organisms are exposed in nature. Wohlschlag (1964), it should be noted, has discovered that a zoarcid fish, with phylogenetic affinities beyond the antarctic zone, appeared to be less adjusted to cold than the species of *Trematomus*.

Unfortunately, very little is known of the temperature characteristics of the polar marine algae. A capacity for acclimation in *Fucus* was demonstrated some years ago by Harder (Prosser, 1958). Although field studies of photosynthetic carbon dioxide fixation have been undertaken by various investigators, it is difficult to assess the results critically because of a number of complicating factors which could obscure the influence of temperature. Current studies with axenic cultures of diatoms from antarctic sea ice indicate clearly the psychrophilic character of these organisms. Unlike the antarctic fish, however, their net metabolic activity, measured in terms of oxygen production under conditions of adequate illumination, is considerably diminished at temperatures equivalent to those of the habitat of origin. Cell division rates of *Fragilaria sublinearis* have been found to be greatest at around 6°. Nevertheless, light intensities are normally so low beneath the ice that temperature is probably of little importance.

As temperatures fall below 0°, a capacity to survive rather than a capacity to compensate becomes more and more important. A margin of safety is afforded organisms that are able to effect a lowering of the freezing point of their cell contents or to supercool. With increasingly severe conditions, however, a capacity to withstand freezing during one or more stages of the life cycle becomes essential. Chill injury among organisms other than homeotherms is probably rare in the polar regions, although the reported mass mortality of *Pleurogramma antarcticum* (Brongersma-Sanders, 1957) may well have resulted from this cause.

With few exceptions, marine cold-blooded animals and plants cannot survive freezing. Arctic fish are supercooled (Scholander *et al.*, 1957; Smith, 1958; Gordon *et al.*, 1962), and benthic forms can be induced to freeze spontaneously on contact with ice crystals. Species living in shallower water combine supercooling with an increase in the osmotic pressure of their body fluids and avoid this danger under normal circumstances. Although antarctic fish might be expected to have similar characteristics to those from arctic waters, there is apparently a lack of information on this topic (Marshall, 1964). Salt (1961) considers $-30°$ to be a practical limit for supercooling. In many terrestrial habitats, therefore, a capacity to supercool would be unlikely to protect against the dangers of ice formation unless its range were extended by a significant lowering of the freezing point. The inability to tolerate high solute concentrations limits the number of species which might use dehydration to this end.

The ability of many arctic insects to avoid freezing or to survive its effects has been associated with a comparatively high content of glycerol in their body fluids (Downes, 1965). However, there appear to be exceptions. Sømme (1964) has reported eight species containing over 15% glycerol which did not survive freezing. Factors which may delay or suppress freezing have been discussed by Smith (1958, 1961), Salt (1961) and Kinne (1963).

Tolerance of freezing is apparently widespread among polar organisms, although it is not always possible to ascertain from the data available whether organisms exposed to subzero temperatures were themselves in a frozen state. Scholander *et al.* (1953b) found that blackfish survive but are irreversibly damaged by partial freezing. Some littoral organisms successfully tolerate freezing. Kanwisher (1955) found *Mytilus* and *Littorina* fully viable after 6–8 months at or below $-20°$ in Hebron Fiord, Labrador, and later (Kanwisher, 1957) discovered *Fucus*

capable of photosynthesis after long exposure to temperatures as low as
$-40°$. Whether this may be taken as a measure of full viability is
questionable. Apparently the cold hardiness of *Fucus* varies considerably with the season, which indicates a conditioning comparable with
higher plants (Parker, 1960). I have found that most species of micro-
algae isolated from antarctic sea ice are sensitive to freezing under
laboratory conditions although some remain viable after one week at
$-20°$. However, current results indicate that this temperature is probably slowly lethal. In the active state in nature, these organisms are
associated with, but not frozen into, the ice layer (Bunt, 1963).

Resistance to freezing is characteristic of the polar terrestrial flora.
Factors contributing to successful laboratory lyophilization of some
species of antarctic algae have been studied by Holm-Hansen (1963,
1964). Scholander *et al.* (1953b) exposed naturally frozen twigs of arctic
vascular plants and also lichen thalli to $-186°$. Respiration resumed
after the material was thawed but the twigs were unable to develop or
produce leaves. Sakai (1965) considers that development following
exposure to temperature extremes is largely dependent on conditions
that obtained during prefreezing. Although arctic vascular plants do not
suffer from normal winter exposure, resistance may vary during the
reproductive cycle, and in unexpected ways. While some seeds, for
example, are unable to overwinter (Bliss, 1958), the flowers of certain
species withstand short periods of freezing without apparent harm
(Bliss, 1962).

Among the insects, some caterpillars and chironomid larvae (Scholander *et al.*, 1953b; Downes, 1965) survive repeated freezing and thawing
successfully. The latter prepare for winter by slight dehydration but do
not supercool. Dalenus and Wilson (1958) found that *Maudheimia
Wilsoni* can tolerate $-30°$, but not $-70°$, for several days. Temperatures 50–60 degrees below freezing are lethal for the springtail,
Isotoma (Gressitt, 1964). It is believed that both of these species over-
winter in the antarctic mainly in the form of eggs. The survival of some
helminth parasites is undoubtedly favoured by the resistance of the egg
stage (Schiller, 1955; Bauer, 1959).

Free-living protozoa, rotifers, tardigrades and nematodes are sometimes the only invertebrates found over large parts of the arctic and
antarctic land masses. Dixon (1939) has recovered large protozoan
populations from soils frozen over nine months of the year, and Gunter
(1957) reported that representatives of the other groups, when desiccated, survived several hours at $-272°$. Cysts of *Entamoeba histolytica*
in 5% glycerol have remained infective over a period of weeks at $-79°$
(Babbott *et al.*, 1956).

The processes involved in, and the factors affecting, ice formation, as

19*

well as the mechanisms of cell injury and its prevention will not be considered here. Among reviews or papers dealing with one or more of these topics may be listed those of Bělehrádek (1957), Asahino (1959), Salt (1961), Smith (1961), Ingraham (1962), Daubenmire (1962), Kinne (1963) and Farrant (1965).

IV. Thermal Energy and Polar Ecology

The thermal regimes of the polar regions impose powerful restrictions and require pronounced adjustments, not only in individual organisms, but in populations, communities and higher levels of biological organization. To discuss the significance of thermal patterns and those other characteristics of the physical environment affected by temperature in relation to populations, species diversity, food webs, ecosystem structure and productivity would be a mammoth task, even with the relatively limited but wide diversity of information available from studies in high latitudes.

There can be no doubt that these difficulties exist, at least in part, because of the need for unifying principles in ecology. This fact is very well recognized. Among the contributions made towards this goal are the stimulating views expressed by Margalef (1963). Margalef's concept hinges on the recognition that increasing structural complexity is associated with ecosystem evolution and advancement, and that mature ecosystems, rich in information, require less energy for their maintenance than simpler, less organized systems. While this may be true, the concept disturbs me in its present form because it appears to imply that this type of biological maturity represents a thermodynamically ideal state rather than an inevitably imperfect approach to such a state. Because I feel it pertinent to the present topic, I shall digress briefly to explain my views.

I am assuming that the most fundamental characteristic of living systems is a capacity to tend to increase and finally to maintain maximum order, in a steady state, among the matter on which life is based, using an external source of energy. The information content of these component materials would then tend always to be minimum within the limits possible for that steady state. This interpretation appears to accord with current physical concepts of life, though not stated with mathematical rigour (see, for example, Casey, 1962; Setlow and Pollard, 1962). Such a capacity might be most closely realized if all the living and non-living organic materials on earth were in the form of a continuous system of self-sufficient, fully functioning protoplasm. Fortunately for man, such a system seems highly improbable. No organism known is self-sufficient. Even small living organisms require mechanical support.

Ageing appears to be inevitable. The synthesis and maintenance of protoplasm, therefore, requires a division of metabolic labour among several types of organism, each of which must divert matter for the production of micro- and macro-supportive and other metabolically inactive structures. Reproduction is universally essential. To increase the production of protoplasm under favourable conditions, or to tend to maintain its production under stress, further "structure" becomes necessary. According to this argument, it follows that compromise is inevitable and traceable to virtually all levels of biological organization.

Several distinct types of compromise or adjustment, demanded partly by the nature of life and partly by the environment, may be recognized, viz.: biochemical, physiological, structural or morphological, and behavioural. Reproduction is a complex form of adjustment required in part to counteract the effect of ageing. Structural adjustments operate at the cellular, organism and higher levels of biological organization. Behavioural adjustments may be taken to include all forms of activity involving the movements of animals. Probably all forms of adjustment are represented in taxonomic diversity.

This concept, it seems to me, offers a unified and fundamental approach to ecology which could find broad application, either for descriptive or analytical purposes, at any level of organization. It appears to be compatible with Slobodkin's (1962) treatment of production ecology and should enable an objective and perhaps quantitative assessment of ecosystem maturity. For example, if suitable structural criteria could be agreed upon, it might be possible to express this quality in terms of information per unit area or per unit volume. Although more practical units and methods are possible for the measurement of standing crops and productivity, it is difficult to see how information theory concepts could be avoided in analysing the structure of communities and ecosystems in which food web, species diversity, spatial relationships and other similar characteristics must be considered. The difficulties likely to be encountered in such an approach have been discussed by Slobodkin (1962). Whether feedback theory is likely to gain strength in application to ecological problems as it is doing in other fields of biology (see, for example, the Symposium of the Society for Experimental Biology, 1964, no. 18) remains an open question. However, the essentially homeostatic view of ecology as presented here seems to lend itself to this type of treatment. It should be added that, in complex, multispecies biological systems tending to produce maximum protoplasm per unit of usable energy, classic feedback devices seem to be lacking. Instead, chance genetic changes provide a continual supply of potentially but not necessarily useful material. The process, however, is "blind" and cannot be expected always to function with great efficiency. This is especially true under conditions which exhibit marked and erratic fluctuations and which are, in any case, marginal for life.

I should like now to apply this concept of ecology briefly to several aspects of biological organization in the polar regions.

Slobodkin (1962) has shown that it is possible to describe community efficiency by means of the following equation:

$$I = c_i P_i$$

in which I is the energy income and c_i is the maintenance cost for the standing crop, P_i; P_i is usually considered as the total biomass. If, however, P_i were equated with actively metabolizing protoplasm, the c_i term in the equation would include all of the information associated with the organization of the community. Essentially, the standing crop should refer to the negative entropy of the total biological system. In this discussion, however, protoplasm is considered a much more convenient and realistic measure. A breakdown of the c_i term, even in qualitative fashion, should provide a useful means of understanding the types of compromise or adjustment displayed, in the present instance, by polar communities under the thermal stress to which they are exposed.

The first point to be stressed is that, in these terms, Margalef's (1963) ecosystem maturity must be considered only as one possible form of maintenance cost. Polar ecosystems are immature because environmental stresses, among which the thermal regime is but one, limit the extent to which characteristics such as species diversity and the complexity of structure associated with it may be used in maintenance. This is much less so in the stable benthic marine environment than on land. It is often stated that diversity is related to relatively high temperatures (Fischer 1960). However, Margalef's (1963) view that thermal stability is of greater significance in this respect than temperature alone seems reasonable provided time is not limiting. In this context, limited diversity tends to minimize maintenance costs even though it may be counterbalanced in other directions. Ultimately, primary productivity sets the limit to the standing crop of protoplasm, although the proportion of plant biomass existing as actively metabolizing protoplasm may be small. In tundra plants, protein synthesis is apparently slow at low temperatures (Bliss, 1962). A good deal of energy, however, is diverted into carbohydrate reserve materials of high calorific value. Related alpine tundra plants have a high lipid content. While such products permit early summer growth, they are also capable of efficient conversion into animal material when ingested by herbivores. It seems likely that lipid storage is especially active also in the micro-algae of sea ice. My own finding that cultures of these organisms were viable after almost two years' storage in the dark supports this conclusion. It would be interesting to know whether the diversion of photosynthetic products into storage compounds rather than to cell substance in certain species may lead, nevertheless, to an overall increase in the standing crop of protoplasm in the total community.

The largely cellulosic structural components of the vascular plants are capable of ready conversion by herbivores. In the arctic, homeo-therms are prominent in this category so that cellulolytic micro-organisms are able to function in the stable thermal environment of the digestive tract.

The fact that diatoms figure so largely in the polar phytoplankton may be related to the fact that these organisms use silica rather than organic materials as cell wall components. Provided the incorporation of silica was accomplished with an economy of energy expenditure, the character would be expected to lower maintenance costs. Further, the existence of nitrogen-fixing blue-green algae as colonizers in extreme polar habitats is significant. Not only are these organisms among the most self-sufficient forms of life, but structural complexity, even at the subcellular level, is low. Within the strictures of the environment, their efficiency must be high. Viewed in this fashion, the success of blue-green algae under the thermal stresses imposed by hot springs may not be co-incidental. It is interesting to note also the prevalence of lichens at high latitudes and to speculate upon the possible significance of symbiosis under these conditions.

The subdivision of non-photosynthetic organisms into categories such as herbivores, predators and decomposers, is of great practical value but tends to be misleading. In so far as they tend to maximize the standing crop of protoplasm, their functions are identical. Micro-organisms, free-living as well as parasitic, require the co-operation of the herbivore–predator link in order that they may function in the food chain.

In the polar land areas, the activities of the free-living poikilotherms and micro-organisms are severely restricted. The importance of poikilo-therms as herbivores and predators is therefore greatly subordinate to that of the homeotherms. Note, however, the remarkable prevalence of invertebrate intestinal parasites in polar animals. It is interesting that the abundant small mammal herbivores are not as well insulated as the larger forms which predate them. On the arctic barrens, the former are active, not only during the summer, but often throughout the winter when primary production is suspended. Over this period, these species feed on reserve-rich roots and other plant material, and are relatively unaffected by predation. Shelter and warmth is provided to an appreci-able extent by underground tunnels and insulated nests which probably serve a number of generations. This type of behaviour may result not only in a diminution in maintenance costs for the total community but also enable a more efficient conversion into predator material. Even so, the energy expenditure in the maintenance of relatively inconvertible pelage must be considerable. Bee and Hall (1956) have found that brown lemmings change coat no less than six times in their first twelve months of life. Species such as the brown lemming are also rather unstable elements in the community (Pitelka, 1957). The larger arctic animals as a group probably maintain their fur or hair insulation with greater total economy, although it is thicker.

Concerning the limiting influence of the environment on the free-living microflora, it would be of great interest to know whether microbial activity is favoured in the insulated layers of burrows receiving heat from the animal inhabitants and whether keratolytic fungi are active in such situations. Certainly, migratory activity, which is common among polar predators, and perhaps a general lack of annual plants, must remove a considerable load from the thermally stressed and often frozen soil microflora. Although annual losses of biomass limit the standing crop of protoplasm within the polar regions, it must result in a general increase for the world ecosystem provided that energy losses involved in migration are not excessive.

Exploitative processes are especially characteristic of the marine-based ecosystem. Again, primary production is limited to the summer season. The zooplankton, which are forced to build up food reserves, tend to be rich in lipids (Littlepage, 1964). Dunbar (1954) has drawn attention to the fact that the direct dependence of mammals (and the large population of migratory birds) in the arctic zone, on the invertebrate macroplankton rather than on fish has never been explained. An investigation of this problem, in the arctic and antarctic zones, on the postulate that thermoregulators might contribute to the maintenance of protoplasm more efficiently than many poikilotherms, seems worthy of consideration. An assessment of the extent of predation on eggs and immature, imperfectly insulated, individuals both marine and terrestrial should also prove worthwhile.

At this point, one is reminded of the high degree of metabolic cold adaptation of some antarctic fish (Wohlschlag, 1964). Some authors have suggested that the maintenance of cellular activity in the cold might be caused by high concentrations of cellular enzymes. Ingraham (1962) has thrown serious doubt on this proposition on spatial grounds. Intact cells are necessary for the demonstration of adapted activity at low temperature. Could it be that such organisms have achieved a quite fundamental type of adjustment to stress and that the cell contents have a greater degree of order than is found in more temperate organisms? The biophysics of compensation at the cellular level deserves close attention.

In summary, the relative importance of the many possible categories of maintenance cost may be expected to vary from ecosystem to ecosystem and, in total, to tend to be minimum within the limitations imposed by environment. It should be possible to characterize entities of biological organization on this basis, either in general terms or, preferably, by adapting information theory for the purpose. As the standing crop of protoplasm increases with increasing utilization of available energy, the larger and more complex its maintenance is likely to be and the more difficult its analysis. With energy input constant, however, and as evolution tends to maximize the standing crop of protoplasm, and minimize the information content of the system, maintenance costs also must tend to a minimum. Sometimes, perhaps always in one form or another, certain maintenance characteristics of one ecosystem may lend themselves to exploitation by another, removed in space or time.

Finally, a comment on subantarctic Macquarie Island seems appropriate. This extremely isolated small mass of land supports a quite luxuriant vegetation of tussock grass and herbs on the lower slopes and coastal terraces growing atop thick layers of peat. Prior to man's interference, processes of decomposition were unable to keep pace with plant growth. Only a small proportion of the total biomass, including peat, must have been in the form of protoplasm. The efficiency of the communities was low. Then, some years ago, rabbits were introduced. In the perfectly reasonable view of the conservationist, these animals are a menace for they are increasing, consuming the vegetation and creating instability. Large areas of peat from time to time are washed into the sea where decomposition is likely to be accelerated. There can be little doubt that overall efficiency has increased, although, without further interference, it could suffer a dramatic decline. In this situation, geographic isolation rather than temperature has exerted a controlling influence in the past. The question remains, can the arrival of sealers, explorers, and rabbits, be considered a clumsy form of feedback mechanism brought into operation by chance? Further, could this event, or something like it in effect, be reliably predicted?

References

Allee, W. C., Emerson, A. E., Park, O., Park, T. and Schmidt, K. P. (1961). "Principles of Animal Ecology", 837 pp. W. B. Saunders Co., Philadelphia.
Amadon, D. (1964). *Evolution* **18**, 105.
Andrewartha, H. G. and Birch, L. C. (1954). "The Distribution and Abundance of Animals", 782 pp. University Press, Chicago.

Angino, E. E., Armitage, K. B. and Tash, J. C. (1962). *Polar Record* 11, 283.

Anon. (1961). *Polar Record* 10, 409.

Asahino, E. (1959). *Nature, Lond.* 184, 1003.

Babbott, J. G., Babbott, F. L. and Gordon, J. E. (1956). *Amer. J. med. Sciences* 231, 338.

Baird, P. D. (1964). "The Polar World", 328 pp. Longmans, London.

Bandy, O. L. and Echols, R. J. (1964). *Antarctic Res. Ser.* I, 73.

Bauer, O. N. (1959). *Bull. State Scient. Res. Inst. Lake and River Fisheries* 49, 1. (Israel Programme for Scient. Trans., Jerusalem, 1962.)

Bee, J. W. and Hall, E. R. (1956). "Mammals of Northern Alaska", 309 pp. Univ. of Kansas Mus. Nat. Hist., Misc. Pub. 8.

Bělehrádek, J. (1957). *Annu. Rev. Physiol.* 19, 59.

Benninghoff, W. S. (1952). *Arctic* 5, 34.

Benzinger, T. H. (1964). *In* "Homeostasis and Feedback Mechanisms", pp. 49–80. Symposia of the Society for Experimental Biology, no. 18. University Press, Cambridge.

Blakemore, L. C., and Swindale, L. D. (1958). *Nature, Lond.* 182, 47.

Bliss, L. C. (1958). *Arctic* 11, 180.

Bliss, L. C. (1962). *Arctic* 15, 117.

Brodsky, K. (1964). *In* "Antarctic Biology", (R. Carrick, M. Holdgate, and J. Prévost, Eds.), pp. 257–258. Hermann, Paris.

Brongersma-Sanders, M. (1957). *In* "Treatise on Marine Ecology and Paleoecology", (J. W. Hedgpeth, Ed.), pp. 941–1010. Memoir 67, Geological Soc. of America.

Brown, K. G. (1964). *ANARE Reps.* (B)1, 1.

Bryden, M. M. (1964). *Nature, Lond.* 203, 1299.

Budd, G. M. (1961). *The Emu* 61, 171.

Bullock, T. H. (1955). *Biol. Rev.* 30, 311.

Bunt, J. S. (1960). *ANARE Reps.* (B)3, 1.

Bunt, J. S. (1963). *Nature, Lond.* 199, 1254.

Bunt, J. S. (1964). *Antarctic Res. Ser.* 1, 27.

Bunt, J. S. and Rovira, A. D. (1955). *J. soil Sci.* 6, 119.

Cameron, T. W. M. and Choquette, L. P. E. (1963). *Polar Record* 11, 567.

Casey, E. J. (1962). "Biophysics", 335 pp. Chapman and Hall, London.

Chatfield, P. O., Lyman, C. P. and Irving, L. (1953). *Amer. J. Physiol.* 172, 639.

Cook, F. A. (1955). *Arctic* 8, 237.

Cook, F. A. and Raiche, V. G. (1962). *Geogr. Bull.* no. 18, 64.

Crespi, H. L., Archer, S. M. and Katz, J. J. (1959). *Nature, Lond.* 184, 729.

Dalenus, P. and Wilson, O. (1958). *Arkiv för Zoologi* 11, 393.

Daubenmire, R. F. (1962). "Plants and Environment", 422 pp. John Wiley and Sons, Inc., New York.

Deacon, G. E. R. (1964). *In* "Antarctic Biology", (R. Carrick, M. Holdgate, and J. Prévost, Eds.), pp. 81–86. Hermann, Paris.

Dehnel, P. A. (1955). *Physiol. Zool.* 28, 115.

Depocas, F. (1961). *Brit. Med. Bull.* 17, 25.

Dietrich, G. (1963). "General Oceanography", 588 pp. Interscience Publishers, New York.

Dixon, A. (1939). *J. anim. Ecol.* 8, 162.

Dodge, C. W. (1964). *In* "Antarctic Biology", (R. Carrick, M. Holdgate, and J. Prévost, Eds.), pp. 165–172. Hermann, Paris.

Downes, J. A. (1965). *Annu. Rev. Entomol.* 10, 257.

Dunbar, M. J. (1951). Fisheries Res. Bd. of Canada, Bull. 88.

Dunbar, M. J. (1954). *Arctic* **7**, 213.

Dunbar, M. J. (1957). *Canad. J. Zool.* **35**, 797.

Eddy, B. P. (1960). *J. appl. Bact.* **23**, 189.

Farrant, J. (1965). *Nature, Lond.* **205**, 1284.

Fischer, A. G. (1960). *Evolution* **14**, 64.

Flint, E. A. and Stout, J D. (1960). *Nature, Lond.* **188**, 767.

Fontaine, M. (1954). *Biol. Rev.* **29**, 391.

Foxton, P. (1964). *In* "Antarctic Biology", (R. Carrick, M. Holdgate, and J. Prévost, Eds.), pp. 311–318. Hermann, Paris.

Fry, F. E. J. (1958). *Annu. Rev. Physiol.* **20**, 207.

Fukushima, H. (1959). *J. Yokohama Municipal Univ. Ser. C***31**, no. 112.

Goldman, C. R. (1964). *In* "Antarctic Biology", (R. Carrick, M. Holdgate, and J. Prévost, Eds.), pp. 291–300. Hermann, Paris.

Goldsmith, R. and Sladen, W. J. L. (1961). *J. Physiol.* **157**, 251.

Gordon, M. S., Amdur, B H and Scholander, P. F. (1962). *Biol. Bull.* **122**, 52.

Gressitt, J. L. (1964). *In* "Antarctic Biology", (R. Carrick, M. Holdgate, and J. Prévost, Eds.), pp. 211–222. Hermann, Paris.

Gunter, G. (1957). *In* "Treatise on Marine Ecology and Paleoecology", (J. W. Hedgpeth, Ed.), pp. 159–184, Memoir 67, Geological Soc. of America.

Hart, J. S. (1961). *Brit. Med. Bull.* **17**, 19.

Hart, J. S. (1964). *In* "Homeostasis and Feedback Mechanisms", pp. 31–48. Symposium of the Society for Experimental Biology, no. 18. University Press, Cambridge.

Hart, J. S., Heroux, O., Cottle, W. H. and Mills, C. A. (1961). *Canad. J. Zool.* **39**, 845.

Hayward, J. S. (1965). *Canad. J. Zool.* **43**, 309.

Hocking, B. and Sharplin, C. D. (1965). *Nature, Lond.* **206**, 215.

Holdgate, M. (1964). *In* "Antarctic Biology", (R. Carrick, M. Holdgate, and J. Prévost, Eds.), pp. 181–194. Hermann, Paris.

Holm-Hansen, O. (1963). *Physiol. Plant.* **16**, 530.

Holm-Hansen, O. (1964). *Canad. J. Bot.* **42**, 127.

Holme, N. A. (1964). *In* "Antarctic Biology", (R. Carrick, M. Holdgate, and J. Prévost, Eds.), pp. 319–322. Hermann, Paris.

Hoyte, H. M. D. (1955). *J. anim. Ecol.* **24**, 412.

Ingraham, J. L. (1962). *In* "The Bacteria", (I. C. Gunsalus and R. Y. Stanier, Eds.), Vol. 4, pp. 265–296. Academic Press, New York.

Ingraham, J. L. (1963). *In* "Recent Progress in Microbiology", (N. E. Gibbons, Ed.), pp. 201–212. Symposium, 8th. Int. Congr. for Microbiol., 1962. University Press, Toronto.

Irving, L. (1951). *Fed. Proc.* **10**, 543.

Irving, L. and Krog, J. (1954). *J. appl. Physiol.* **6**, 667.

Irving, L., Krog, J. and Monson, M. (1955). *Physiol. Zool.* **28**, 173.

Jenny, J. (1941). "Factors of Soil Formation", 281 pp. McGraw–Hill, New York.

Jensen, H. L. (1951). *Medd. om Grønland* **142**, 23.

Johnson, A. W. and Packer, J. G. (1965). *Science* **148**, 237.

Kanwisher, J. W. (1955). *Biol. Bull.* **109**, 56.

Kanwisher, J. W. (1957). *Biol. Bull.* **113**, 275.

King, J. R. and Farner, D. S. (1961). *In* "The Biology and Comparative Physiology of Birds", (A. J. Marshall, Ed.), Vol. 2, pp. 215–288. Academic Press, New York.

Kinne, O. (1963). *In* "Oceanography and Marine Biology", (H. Barnes, Ed.), Vol. 1, pp. 301–340. Allen and Unwin, London.

Kort, V. G. (1962). *Scient. American* **207**, 113.

Kramer, G. (1961). *In* "The Biology and Comparative Physiology of Birds", (A. J. Marshall, Ed.), Vol. 2, pp. 341–372. Academic Press, New York.

Krasil'nikov, N. A. (1958). "Soil Microorganisms and Higher Plants", Institute of Microbiol., Academy of Sciences of the U.S.S.R., Moscow. Israel Programme for Scientific Translations, 1961.

Lenz, C. P. and Hart, J. S. (1960). *Canad. J. Zool.* **38**, 679.

Lewontin, R. C. (1957). *Cold Spr. Harb. Symp. quant. Biol.* **22**, 395.

Littlepage, J. L. (1964). *In* "Antarctic Biology", (R. Carrick, M. Holdgate, and J. Prévost, Eds.), pp. 463–470. Hermann, Paris.

Littlepage, J. L. and Pearse, J. S. (1962). *Science* **137**, 679.

Llano, G. A. (1962). *Scient. American* **207**, 212.

Lyman, C. P. (1961). Arctic Aeromed. Lab. (Fort Wainwright, Alaska), Tech. Rep. 61–5.

Maher, W. J. (1964). *Ecology* **45**, 520.

Margalef, R. (1963). *Am. Naturalist* **97**, 357.

Marshall, A. J. (1952). *Ibis* **94**, 310.

Marshall, A. J. (1961). *In* "The Biology and Comparative Physiology of Birds", (A. J. Marshall, Ed.), Vol. 2, pp. 307–339. Academic Press, New York.

Marshall, N. B. (1964). *In* "Antarctic Biology", (R. Carrick, M. Holdgate, and J. Prévost, Eds.), pp. 273–278. Hermann, Paris.

Matthews, L. H. (1961). *Brit. Med. Bull.* **17**, 9.

Mayer, W. V. (1953). *In* "Current Biological Research in the Alaskan Arctic", (I. L. Wiggins, Ed.), pp. 48–55. Stanford University Press.

McLaren, I. A. (1963). *J. Fish. Res. Bd Canada* **20**, 685.

McWhinnie, M. A. (1964). *Ant. Res. Ser.* **1**, 63.

Mooney, H. A. and Billings, W. D. (1961). *Ecol. Monogr.* **31**, 1.

Murphy, R. C. (1962). *Scient. American* **207**, 186.

Murray, M. D. (1964). *In* "Antarctic Biology", (R. Carrick, M. Holdgate, and J. Prévost, Eds.), pp. 241–245. Hermann, Paris.

Nordenskjöld, O. and Mecking, L. (1928). "The Geography of the Polar Regions", 359 pp. Amer. Geogr. Soc., Special Pub. no. 8.

Parker, J. (1960). *Biol. Bull.* **119**, 474.

Peiss, C. N. and Field, J. (1950). *Biol. Bull.* **99**, 213.

Phillpot, H. R. (1964). *In* "Antarctic Biology", (R. Carrick, M. Holdgate, and J. Prévost, Eds.), pp. 73–80. Hermann, Paris.

Pitelka, F. A. (1957). *Cold Spr. Harb. Symp. quant. Biol.* **22**, 237.

Potter, V. R. (1958). *Fed. Proc.* **17**, 1060.

Prévost, J. (1962). *New Scientist* **16**, 444.

Prosser, C. L. (1958). *In* "Physiological Adaptation", (C. L. Prosser, Ed.), pp. 167–180. American Physiological Society, Washington.

Pruitt, W. O. (1959). *Arctic* **12**, 158.

Robin, G. de Q. (1962). *Scient. American* **207**, 132.

Rose, A. H. (1963). *In* "Recent Progress in Microbiology", (N. E. Gibbons, Ed.), pp. 193–200. Symposium, 8th. Int. Congr. for Microbiol., 1962. University of Toronto Press.

Rountree, P. M. (1938). *BANZARE Rep.*, Ser. A. Vol. **2**, *part* 7.

Sakai, A. (1965). *Nature, Lond.* **206**, 1064.

Salt, R. W. (1961). *Brit. Med. Bull.* **17**, 5.

Sandon, H. (1924). *Linn. Soc. J. Zool.* **35**, 449.

Savile, D. B. O. (1963). *Arctic* **16**, 17.

Schiller, E. L. (1955). *J. Parasitol.* **41**, 578.

Scholander, P. F. (1955). *Evolution* **9**, 15.

Scholander, P. F., van Dam, L., Kanwisher, J. W., Hammel, H. T. and Gordon, M. S. (1957). *J. cell. comp. Physiol.* **49**, 5.

Scholander, P. F., Flagg, W., Walters, V. and Irving, L. (1952). *Amer. J. Bot.* **39**, 707.

Scholander, P. F., Flagg, W., Walters, V. and Irving, L. (1953a). *Physiol. Zool.* **26**, 67.

Scholander, P. F., Flagg, W., Walters, V. and Irving, L. (1953b). *J. cell. comp. Physiol.* **42**, supplt. 1.

Scholander, P. F., Hock, R., Walters, V. and Irving, L. (1950a). *Biol. Bull.* **99**, 259.

Scholander, P. F., Hock, R., Walters, V., Johnson, F. and Irving, L. (1950b). *Biol. Bull.* **99**, 237.

Scholander, P. F., Walters, V., Hock, R. and Irving, L. (1950c). *Biol. Bull.* **99**, 225.

Scholander, S. I. and Kanwisher, J. T. (1959). *Plant Physiol.* **34**, 574.

Schreider, E. (1964). *Evolution* **18**, 1.

Setlow, R. B. and Pollard, E. C. (1962). "Molecular Biophysics", 545 pp. Pergamon Press, Oxford.

Sinclair, N. A. and Stokes, J. L. (1965). *Canad. J. Microbiol.* **11**, 259.

Slobodkin, L. B. (1962). *Advanc. ecol. Res.* **1**, 69.

Smith, A. U. (1958). *Nature, Lond.* **182**, 911.

Smith, A. U. (1961). "Biological Effects of Freezing and Super-Cooling", Edward Arnold, London.

Smith, R. E. and Hoijer, D. J. (1962). *Physiol. Rev.* **42**, 60.

Snow, D. W. (1952). *Ibis* **94**, 133.

Sømme, L. (1964). *Canad. J. Zool.* **42**, 87.

Sørensen, T. (1941). *Medd. om Grønl.* **125**, 1.

Straka, R. P. and Stokes, J. L. (1960). *J. Bact.* **80**, 622.

Steere, W. C. (1953). *In* "Current Biological Research in the Alaskan Arctic", (I. L. Wiggins, Ed.), pp. 30–47. Stanford University Press.

Stokes, J. L. (1963). *In* "Recent Progress in Microbiology", (N. E. Gibbons, Ed.), pp. 187–192. Symposium, 8th. Int. Congr. for Microbiol., 1962. University of Toronto Press.

Tedrow, J. C. F. and Douglas, L. A. (1959). *Soil Sci.* **88**, 305.

Thorson, G. (1957). *In* "Treatise on Marine Ecology and Paleoecology", (J. W. Hedgpeth, Ed.), pp. 461–534. Memoir 67, Geol. Soc. of America.

Tikhomirov, B. A. (1960). *Canad. J. Bot.* **38**, 815.

Tressler, W. L. and Ommundsen, A. M. (1962). "Seasonal Oceanographical Studies in McMurdo Sound, Antarctica", 143 pp. U.S.N. Hydrographic Office, Tech. Rep. 125. Washington 25, D.C.

Trout, G. C. (1957). *Min. agr. Fish. Food, Fishery Invest.*, Ser. 2, Vol. **21**, no. 6.

Wager, H. G. (1941). *New Phytol.* **40**, 1.

Watson, A. (1957). *Ibis* **99**, 419.

Weeden, R. B. (1956). *Arctic* **9**, 212.

Went, F. W. (1961). *Encycl. plant Physiol.* **16**, 1.

White, J. C. D. (1953). *Nature, Lond.* **171**, 612.

Wilson, J. W. (1957). *J. Ecol.* **45**, 499.

Wise, K. A. J. and Gressitt, J. L. (1965). *Nature, Lond.* **207**, 101.

Wohlschlag, D. E. (1957). *Ecology* **38**, 502.
Wohlschlag, D. E. (1961). *Copeia* no. **1**, 11.
Wohlschlag, D. E. (1964). *Ant. Res. Ser.* **1**, 33.
Woodhead, A. D. (1959). *New Scientist* **6**, 1208.

Author Index

Italic numbers indicate pages on which a reference is listed

A

Aach, H. G., 280, *284*
Abegg, F. A., 264, *284*
Abel, P., 220, *229*
Abercrombie, M., 451, *471*
Abram, D., 172, *210*
Ackerman, L., 316, *346*
Acree, E. G., 222, *230*
Adam, N. K., 142, *145*
Adamiec, A. 105, *113*
Adams, A., 97, *118*
Adams, D. H., 46, *70*
Adams, M. H., 167, *210*, 279, *288*
Adamsons, K., 417, 463, *471*
Adant, M., 166, *210*
Adensamer, E., 387, *406*
Adler, D. J., 110, *113*
Adolph, E. F., 354, *371*, 464, 465, *471*, 486, 496, *508*
Adye, J., 172, *214*
Agate, F. J., Jr. 417, *476*
Aherne, W., 448, *471*
Akagi, J. M., 170, 171, *210*
Akinrimisi, E. O., 95, *113*
Akita, Y., 318, *346*
Aksenova, N. N., 82, *113*
Alabaster, J. S., 386, *406*
Albers, C., 530, *532*
Alberts, B. M., 97, 100, *113, 115*
Albertsson, P. A., 82, *113*
Albury, M. N., 209, *215*
Albus, W. R., 190, *216*
Alderice, D. F., 389, 391, *406, 407*
Aldrich, D. V., 362, *373*
Aldridge, W. G., 82, *113*
Aleinikova, T. L., 91, *113*
Alexander, G., 418, 462, *471*
Alexander, H. E., 83, *122*
Alexander, L., 515, 529, *531*

Alexander, R. A., 223, *229*
Alexandrov, V. Ya., 253, 279, 281, *284*, *285*
Allanson, B. R., 384, 386, 389, *406*
Allee, W. C., 560, 561, 569, 571, 572, 573, *585*
Allen, J. G., 512, *531*
Allen, J. R., 448, *472*
Allen, M. B., 153, 156, 160, 170, *210*, 279, 283, *285*
Allen, T. H., 321, *347*
Allison, J. L., 90, *113*
Almeida, A. M., 359, *372*
Amadon, D., 565, *585*
Amdur, B. H., 386, *401*, 578, *587*
Ander, A., 309, 321, *346*
Anders, F., 309, 321, *346*
Andersen, K. L., 425, *476*
Anderson, B., 427, *471*
Anderson, D. B., 281, *289*
Anderson, E. B., 184, *210*
Anderson, H. M., 125, *146*
Anderson, I. M., 524, *532*
Anderson, J. D., 400, 401, *409*
Anderson, J. F., 317, *349*
Anderson, P. J., 141, *145*
Anderson, W. F., 99, 100, *118*
Andik, I., 431, *471*
Andjus, R., 528, *532*
Andjus, R. K., 528, *532*
Andrewartha, H. G., 340, 341, *346*, 573 *585*
Andronikov (Svinkin), V. B., 361, *370*
Anfinsen, C. B., 25, *71*
Angervall, L., 443, *471*
Angino, E. E., 556, *586*
Angus, D. E., 244, *285*
Anon, 556, *586*
Ansare, A. Q., 242, *285*
Appel, K., 81, *118*

Subject Index

A

Absidia ramosa, 156

Absorption of radiant energy by invertebrates, 365

Absorption of solar radiation by soils, 538

Accidental hypothermia, 515

Acclimation history of invertebrates, 355

Acclimation of invertebrates to temperature, effect of past history on, 356

Acclimation temperature, relation to temperature preferendum in vertebrate poikilotherms, 400

Acclimation to temperature in vertebrates, 376

Acclimatization of vertebrates to temperature, 376

Acclimatization to heat by man, 497

Acclimatization to the polar thermal regimes, 559

Acetylcholine, effect of temperature on accumulation of in insect brains, 326

Achromobacter spp., psychrophilic, 158

Acridines, effect of on melting temperature of DNA, 90

Actinomyces thermophilus, 156

Actinomycetes, thermophilic, 156

Actinomycins, effect of on melting temperature of DNA, 90

Activity in vertebrate poikilotherms, relation to temperature, 390

Activity of enzymes in microorganisms, effect of temperature on, 198

Activity of mammals in relation to cold exposure, 437

Adaptation of invertebrates to temperature, 354

Adaptation of vertebrates to temperature, 376

Adaptation to cold in mammals, 415

Adaptations, morphological, of polar organisms, 571

Adaptive flexibility in plants, 237

Adaptive growth of mammals in relation to cold exposure, 449

Ademsia, temperature in subelytral air spaces in, 297

Adenosine triphosphatase, effect of temperature on insect, 313

thermostability of thermophil, 170

Adipose tissue in rats, loss of during cold exposure, 430

Adrenal cortex, activity of during cold exposure of mammals, 428

Adsorption techniques in studying DNA renaturation, 110

Aerobacter aerogenes, cold shock of, 190

effect of superoptimum temperatures on, 175

effect of temperature on carbohydrate metabolism of, 201

effect of temperature on growth of, 160

effect of temperature on polysaccharide synthesis by, 201

effect of temperature on RNA content of, 198

metabolic injury in, 194

Affinity of β-galactosidase for substrate, effect of temperature on, 276

Age of organism, effect on microbial viability, 185

Age, role of in heat stress in man, 499

Ageratum sp., relationship between optimum day and night temperatures in, 249

Aggregation of proteins, 26

C

F

K

Kidney stones, relation in man to heat exposure, 515

Kidneys of mammals, effect of cold exposure on growth of, 450

Kinetin, effect of on heat resistance of *Nicotiana rustica*, 279

Klebsiella pneumoniae, effect of temperature on virulence of, 203

L

Labial palps of insects, temperature reception by, 323

Lactate dehydrogenase, activity of during cold exposure in mammals, 426

Lactic acid bacteria, effect of temperature on carbohydrate metabolism in, 200

Lactose operon in *E. coli*, effect of temperature on expression of, 276

Lag phase of growth, effect of temperature on, 161

Lambda point, nature of, 8

Lambs, metabolic rates of, 418

Lamellidens marginalis, effect of temperature on protein content of, 361

Lampito mauritii, effect of ions on acclimation to temperature of, 361

Largemouth bass, effect of temperature on cruising speed of, 391

Larvae, effect of chilling insect, 328

Larval development in invertebrates, effect of temperature on, 361

Lassitude, association with living in the tropics in man, 502

Latitudinal differences in acclimation history of invertebrates, 355

Leaf petioles, effect of temperature on movement of materials through, 261

Leaf primordia, effect of temperature on initiation of in plants, 251

Leaf size, effect of temperature on, 251

Leaf temperatures, effect of on leaf temperatures, 255

Leaves, effect of temperature on translocation of materials from, 260

internal temperatures of, 242

Lecithin contents of membranes, 125

Lemmings, activity of in the cold, 437

Lethal effects, of temperature of vertebrate poikilotherms, 381

of temperature on vertebrates, 375

Leuconostoc spp., effect of temperature on dextran production by, 201

Life cycles of organisms in polar regions, 564

Limits of temperature for growth, influence of lipid composition on, 131

Linum usitatissimum, growth of at low temperatures,

Lipase, effect of temperature on activity of, 46

Lipid composition of insects, effect of temperature on, 315

Lipid content of membranes, 125

Lipids, effects of temperature on iodine numbers of, 130

Lipoid liberation theory, 130

Lipopolysaccharide from *Proteus vulgaris*, 514

β-Lipoprotein, effect of freezing on, 130

Lipovitellin, effect of freezing on, 129

Liquid-crystalline structure of phospholipids, 139

Lithyphantes albomaculatus, effect of temperature on behaviour of, 548

Litter size in mammals, effect of cold exposure on, 456

Liver enzymes, activities of during cold exposure of rats, 426

Livers of mammals, effect of cold exposure on growth of, 450

Lizards, critical thermal maxima of, 387

effect of temperature change on respiratory movements in, 402

Local applications of heat in man, 513

Local cooling of humans, 516

Locust, desert, heat exchange in, 296

Locusta migratoria, behaviour of in a temperature gradient, 340

differences between air temperature and thoracic temperature of, 337

P